VITAMINS AND HORMONES

VOLUME 39

VITAMINS AND HORMONES

ADVANCES IN RESEARCH AND APPLICATIONS

Edited by

PAUL L. MUNSON
University of North Carolina
Chapel Hill, North Carolina

EGON DICZFALUSY
Karolinska Sjukhuset
Stockholm, Sweden

JOHN GLOVER
University of Liverpool
Liverpool, England

ROBERT E. OLSON
St. Louis University
St. Louis, Missouri

Consulting Editors

ROBERT S. HARRIS
32 Dwhinda Road
Newton, Massachusetts

KENNETH V. THIMANN
University of California, Santa Cruz
Santa Cruz, California

JOHN A. LORAINE
University of Edinburgh
Edinburgh, Scotland

IRA G. WOOL
University of Chicago
Chicago, Illinois

Volume 39
1982

ACADEMIC PRESS   A Subsidiary of Harcourt Brace Jovanovich, Publishers

New York   London
Paris   San Diego   San Francisco   São Paulo   Sydney   Tokyo   Toronto

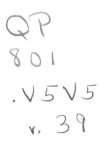

ACADEMIC PRESS, INC.
111 Fifth Avenue, New York, New York 10003

United Kingdom Edition published by
ACADEMIC PRESS, INC. (LONDON) LTD.
24/28 Oval Road, London NW1 7DX

LIBRARY OF CONGRESS CATALOG CARD NUMBER: 43–10535

ISBN 0–12–709839–9

PRINTED IN THE UNITED STATES OF AMERICA

82 83 84 85   9 8 7 6 5 4 3 2 1

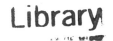

Contents

Leukotrienes: A Novel Group of Biologically Active Compounds

B. SAMUELSSON AND S. HAMMARSTRÖM

Newer Approaches to the Isolation, Identification, and Quantitation of Steroids in Biological Materials

JAN SJÖVALL AND MAGNUS AXELSON

Insulin: The Effects and Mode of Action of the Hormone

RACHMIEL LEVINE

Formation of Thyroid Hormones

J. NUNEZ AND J. POMMIER

Chemistry of the Gastrointestinal Hormones and Hormone-like Peptides and a Sketch of Their Physiology and Pharmacology

VIKTOR MUTT

Contributors to Volume 39

Numbers in parentheses indicate the pages on which the authors' contributions begin.

MAGNUS AXELSON, *Department of Physiological Chemistry, Karolinska Institutet, S-104 01 Stockholm, Sweden* (31)

S. HAMMARSTRÖM, *Department of Physiological Chemistry, Karolinska Institutet, S-104 01 Stockholm, Sweden* (1)

RACHMIEL LEVINE, *Department of Metabolism and Endocrinology, City of Hope Medical Center and Research Institute, Duarte, California 91010* (145)

VIKTOR MUTT, *Department of Biochemistry II, Karolinska Institutet, S-104 01 Stockholm, Sweden* (231)

J. NUNEZ, *Unité de Recherche sur la Glande Thyroide et la Régulation Hormonale, I.N.S.E.R.M., 94270 Bicetre, Paris, France* (175)

J. POMMIER, *Unité de Recherche sur la Glande Thyroide et la Régulation Hormonale, I.N.S.E.R.M., 94270 Bicetre, Paris, France* (175)

B. SAMUELSSON, *Department of Physiological Chemistry, Karolinska Institutet, S-104 01 Stockholm, Sweden* (1)

JAN SJÖVALL, *Department of Physiological Chemistry, Karolinska Institutet, S-104 01 Stockholm, Sweden* (31)

Preface

This volume of *Vitamins and Hormones* is the thirty-ninth in this serial publication of distinguished contributions to biomedical scholarship inaugurated in 1943 by Robert S. Harris and Kenneth V. Thimann, both of whom still participate in the enterprise as Consulting Editors. Volume 39 continues the traditions of its predecessors and, in addition, has some special features.

The international character of the publication is again emphasized by the fact that the authors of the articles in this volume live and work in three different countries; what is unusual is that three of the five articles come from a single outstanding research institution, the Karolinska Institutet. It is unlikely that this record will ever be duplicated.

This is the first volume in which the authors were given the option of including the titles of papers in their lists of references. Four of the five articles include this feature, which, in our opinion, will enhance the usefulness of the references.

Volume 39 also is unusual in not including at least one article that is specifically in the vitamin field. However, the articles on hormones have many implications for nutritional science, including vitamins. Followers of this publication may be assured that the vitamins will continue to be emphasized in future volumes.

It is appropriate to announce that this volume is the last to be supervised by the four undersigned coeditors who have been associated with the enterprise for 14, 13, 12, and 8 years, respectively. We, the publisher, the publication, and its readers are fortunate indeed that our successors will be the eminent scientists and experienced editors Dr. Gerald D. Aurbach, Editor-in-Chief, and Dr. Donald B. McCormick, Associate Editor, and that there will be an outstanding Editorial Board to assist them.

The Editors of *Vitamins and Hormones* have reason to take great satisfaction in the quality of this, their last volume in the series. The first article, by B. Samuelsson and S. Hammarström, is a review of the leukotrienes, major metabolites of arachidonic acid and a novel, newly recognized group of biologically active compounds implicated in immediate hypersensitivity reactions and more generally in the inflammatory process.

Jan Sjövall and Magnus Axelson review newer approaches to the isolation, identification, and quantitation of steroids in biological materials that have contributed to the remarkable progress in steroid analysis in the last fifteen years. The focus is on liquid chromatographic, gas chromatographic, and mass spectrometric methods, with the important subjects of radioimmunoassay and other competitive protein-binding methods left to other authors. Advanced methods of extraction and purification of samples are included.

The third article, on the effects and mode of action of insulin, was appropriately written by Rachmiel Levine, both a pioneer and veteran in insulin research. Dr. Levine has concentrated on the physiological aspects of the integrative role of insulin, both in historical perspective and in the light of recent data obtained by biochemical approaches.

Controversial articles have not been absent from *Vitamins and Hormones* in the past. In the present volume, this role is occupied by the article on formation of thyroid hormones by J. Nunez and J. Pommier. These authors concentrate on the interpretation of results obtained *in vitro* in their own and other laboratories on the thyroid peroxidase system, the iodination reaction, the coupling reaction, and the regulatory effects of iodide and of diiodotyrosine as they relate to the formation of thyroid hormones.

The volume closes with a comprehensive review of the chemistry and biochemistry of the gastrointestinal hormones and hormone-like peptides by Viktor Mutt, director of the laboratory in which many major discoveries and advances in this field have been made. The title implies that the article includes only a "sketch" of the physiology and pharmacology of these peptides, and it is true that only a relatively few of the thousands of scientific papers under these headings could be cited. Nevertheless, the reader will find this article to be an invaluable introduction to the physiology–pharmacology of the subject as well as an authoritative summary of biochemical knowledge about the gastrointestinal peptides.

In closing this Preface, something of a swan song, we would like to express our special appreciation to our colleagues at Academic Press. Their encouragement, stimulation, cooperativeness, and, most of all, their dedication to quality have made our long association memorable and gratifying.

All good wishes for the continued high status of *Vitamins and Hormones* in the scientific community.

PAUL L. MUNSON
EGON DICZFALUSY
JOHN GLOVER
ROBERT E. OLSON

Leukotrienes: A Novel Group of Biologically Active Compounds

B. SAMUELSSON AND S. HAMMARSTRÖM

Department of Physiological Chemistry, Karolinska Institutet, Stockholm, Sweden

I. Transformation of Arachidonic Acid in Polymorphonuclear Leukocytes

The major metabolites of arachidonic acid and 8,11,14-eicosatrienoic acid in rabbit polymorphonuclear leukocytes (PMNL) were originally identified as 5(S)-hydroxy-6,8,11,14-eicosatetraenoic acid and 8(S)-hydroxy-9,11,14-eicosatrienoic acid, respectively (Borgeat *et al.*, 1976). Subsequently, several additional metabolites were detected (Borgeat and Samuelsson, 1979a,b).

Rabbit peritoneal PMNL were incubated with arachidonic acid. Products were isolated and purified by silicic acid chromatography and reverse-phase high-performance liquid chromatography (HPLC). Metabolites were analyzed by infrared (IR) and ultraviolet (UV) spectroscopy and by gas chromatography–mass spectrometry. Figure 1 shows a chromatogram of five products from a typical experiment. The mass spectra of several derivatives of compounds I, II, and III were identical, suggesting that the three compounds were isomers. The spectra demonstrated the presence of hydroxyl groups at C-5 and C-12. Ultraviolet spectra of compounds I–V showed characteristic absorption bands of three conjugated double bonds (Borgeat and Samuelsson, 1979b; Crombie and Jacklin, 1957). Infrared spectrometric analyses

1

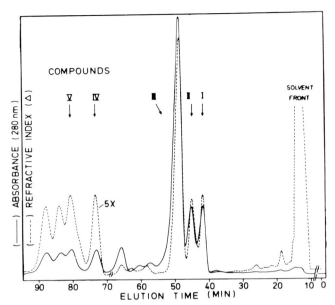

COMPOUNDS

Fig. 1. Chromatogram of dihydroxylated metabolites of arachidonic acid formed by rabbit polymorphonuclear leukocytes. An ether extract was purified by silicic acid column chromatography, and the ethyl acetate fraction was subjected to reverse-phase high-performance liquid chromatography. The traces show ultraviolet absorbance at 280 nm (——) and the change in refractive index (----). Column: μC_{18} Bondapak; solvent: methanol–water, 70 : 30, v/v plus 0.01% acetic acid at 0.3 ml/minute. From Borgeat and Samuelsson (1979b).

demonstrated that the conjugated triene in compounds I and II had all-trans geometry whereas similar analyses indicated the presence of two trans and one cis ethylenic bonds in the conjugated triene of compound III. Steric analyses of the alcohol groups showed that compounds I–III had (S) configuration at C-5 and (R) (compounds I and III) or (S) (compound II) configuration at C-12. The positions of the double bonds were determined by oxidative ozonolyses. The results demonstrated that compounds I–III are stereoisomeric 5,12-dihydroxy-6,8,10,14-eicosatetraenoic acids (Fig. 2). The trivial name leukotriene B_4 has been assigned to compound III (cf. below).

Mass spectrometric analyses of compounds IV and V indicated the presence of hydroxyl groups at C-5 and C-6. The ultraviolet spectra of compounds IV and V were identical (Fig. 2) and showed the presence of conjugated trienes in these molecules too. Owing to the limited amounts of material available, infrared spectrometry and steric analyses of the alcohols were not done. The mass spectrometric and ul-

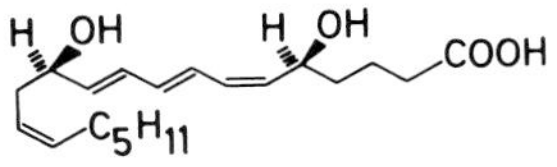

5S, 12R-DHETE
III

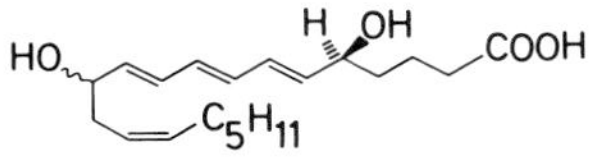

5S, 12R-DHETE (E,E,E,Z) I
5S, 12S-DHETE (E,E,E,Z) II

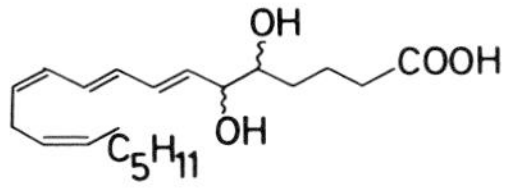

5,6-DHETE
(TWO ISOMERS) IV, V

FIG. 2. Structures of dihydroxylated metabolites of arachidonic acid in rabbit polymorphonuclear leukocytes. DHETE, dihydroxyeicosatetraenoic acid.

traviolet spectrometric data suggested that compounds IV and V were diastereoisomeric 5,6-dihydroxy-7,9,11,14-eicosatetraenoic acids. Based on the proposed mechanism of formation (see below), compounds IV and V have (*S*) configuration at C-5 and are epimeric at C-6 (Fig. 2; Borgeat and Samuelsson, 1979b).

II. Evidence for an Epoxide Intermediate in the Formation of Dihydroxyeicosatetraenoic Acids

The structures and stereochemistry of the products mentioned above indicated that they might be formed from a hydrolyzable intermediate. The following experiments demonstrated that this was the case (Borgeat and Samuelsson, 1979c). Rabbit PMNL were incubated with arachidonic acid under an atmosphere of $^{18}O_2$. The products, purified by HPLC, were esterified with diazomethane and subjected to catalytic hydrogenation. The presence and position of ^{18}O in the molecules were determined by mass spectrometry. Compounds I–V each contained a single atom of ^{18}O located at C-5. The 5*S*-hydroxyeicosatetraenoic acid was also labeled at C-5. These data showed that the hydroxyl groups at C-5 in the metabolites of arachidonic acid in Fig. 2 are derived from molecular oxygen. Incubation of rabbit peritoneal PMNL in $H_2{}^{18}O$-enriched buffer confirmed that the hydroxyl groups at C-12 in compounds I–III originated in water (Fig. 3). Based on these observations it seemed conceivable that arachidonic acid was transformed into an unstable intermediate that would undergo nucleophilic attack by water, alcohols, and other nucleophiles.

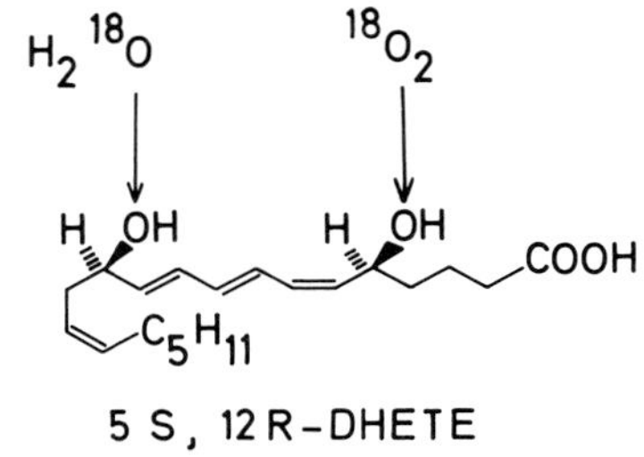

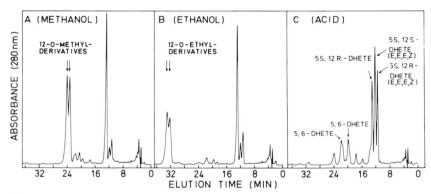

5 S, 12 R – DHETE

FIG. 3. Origin of oxygen in hydroxyl groups of 5(S),12(R)-dihydroxy-6,14-*cis*-8, 10-*trans*-eicosatetraenoic acid.

To test this hypothesis, rabbit peritoneal PMNL were incubated for 30 seconds with arachidonic acid prior to addition of excess methanol (A), excess ethanol (B), or 1 N HCl (C). After extraction and silicic acid column chromatography, the products were analyzed by reverse-phase HPLC. The chromatograms in Fig. 4 show the patterns of products obtained (ethyl acetate eluates from silicic acid chromatograms). The chromatograms after trapping with methanol (or ethanol) indicated the presence of two incompletely separated components of equal size. Their ultraviolet spectra were identical to those of compounds I and II. Infrared spectrometry suggested that the conjugated triene had all-trans geometry. Gas chromatographic–mass spectrometric analyses of multiple derivatives showed that the components of each pair were

FIG. 4. Reverse-phase high-performance liquid chromatography (RP-HPLC) chromatograms of the products obtained upon addition of (A) 10 volumes of methanol; (B) 10 volumes of ethanol; and (C) 0.2 volume 1 N HCl to suspensions of polymorphonuclear leukocytes incubated for 30 seconds with arachidonic acid. The samples were fractionated by silicic acid column chromatography, and the ethyl acetate fractions were analyzed by RP-HPLC (Nucleosil C$_{18}$): solvent, methanol–H$_2$O, 75 : 25, v/v, + 0.01% acetic acid at 1 ml/minute. From Borgeat and Samuelsson (1979c).

isomeric and carried hydroxyl groups at C-5 and alkoxy groups at C-12. Steric analyses showed that the C-5 alcohol groups had (S) configuration. Although configurations at C-12 were not determined, it seems clear that the new components were the C-12 alkoxy derivatives of compounds I and II (Fig. 2). The data indicate the formation of a metabolite of arachidonic acid in leukocytes that can react easily with alcohols. Interestingly, there was always an inverse relationship between the amounts of compounds I and II and the 12-O-alkyl derivatives.

The stability of the intermediate was determined in the following way. Rabbit PMNL were incubated with arachidonic acid for 45 seconds before addition of acetone to stop enzymatic activity. At different time intervals, aliquots of the mixture were transferred to flasks containing methanol. The relative amounts of metabolites were estimated by HPLC. Figure 5 shows the decay of the intermediate, measured as the 12-O-methyl derivative, at pH 7.4 and 37°C ($t_{1/2} = 3-4$ minutes). Simultaneously, the concentrations of compounds I, II, IV, and V increased with time. The concentrations of compound III and 5-hydroxy-6,8,11,14-eicosatetraenoic acid remained constant (not shown). This suggests that compounds I, II, IV, and V are formed nonenzymatically by hydrolysis of a common unstable intermediate, whereas compound III arises by enzymatic hydrolysis of the same

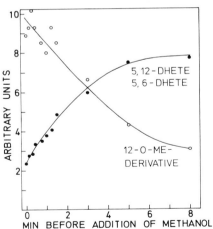

FIG. 5. Time course of the formation of compounds I, II, IV, or V (●——●) and of the disappearance of the unstable intermediate measured as 12-O-methyl compounds I and II (○——○) in a mixture of water–acetone, 1:1, v/v, at pH 7.4 and 37°C. Prostaglandin B$_2$ was added as an internal standard for quantitation by reverse-phase high-performance liquid chromatography. From Borgeat and Samuelsson (1979c).

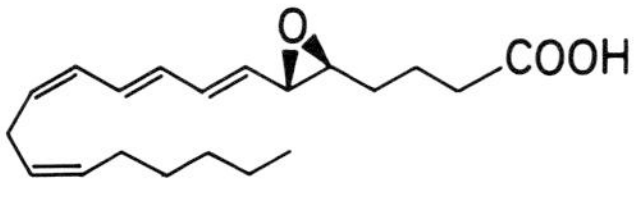

Leukotriene A_4

FIG. 6. Structure of the intermediate in dihydroxy acid formation.

intermediate. Similar experiments performed at acid and alkaline pH indicated that the intermediate was acid-labile and somewhat stabilized at alkaline pH.

Based on these data, it was proposed that the intermediate was 5,6-oxido-7,9,11,14-eicosatetraenoic acid (Fig. 6) (Borgeat and Samuelsson, 1979c). Hydrolsis of epoxides is acid-catalyzed, and opening of allylic epoxides is favored at allylic positions (C-6 in this case). This agreed with the retention of ^{18}O at C-5 observed in compounds IV and V. A mechanism for the formation of compounds I–V from the epoxide intermediate has been proposed (Borgeat and Samuelsson, 1979c). Except for compound III, these are formed by chemical hydrolysis of the epoxide through a mechanism involving a carbonium ion. The latter adds hydroxyl anion preferentially at C-6 and C-12 to yield four isomeric products that contain the stable conjugated triene structure. Compound III is formed by enzymatic hydrolysis of the epoxide, since it is optically active at C-12 and is formed only in the presence of nondenatured leukocyte proteins. This unstable epoxide has been given the trivial name leukotriene A_4 (Samuelsson *et al.*, 1979; Samuelsson and Hammarström, 1980).

III. STRUCTURE OF SLOW-REACTING SUBSTANCE OF ANAPHYLAXIS (SRS-A)

The term SRS (slow-reacting substance) was introduced by Kellaway and Trethewie (1940) for a smooth-muscle contracting factor appearing in the perfusate of sensitized guinea pig lungs after treatment with specific antigen. Subsequently, it was suggested that SRS is an important mediator in asthma and other immediate hypersensitivity reactions (Orange and Austen, 1969; Austen, 1978). Immunologically released SRS, usually referred to as SRS-A, is considered to be released together with other mediators (e.g., histamine and chemotactic factors) after interaction of IgE molecules, bound to membrane receptors, with antigens such as pollen (Fig. 7). Quantitative determinations of 5-hydroxyeicosatetraeonic acid (5-HETE) and leukotriene B_4 in human

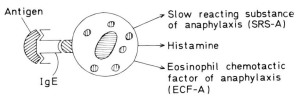

FIG. 7. Classical theory of mediator release in allergic asthma.

PMNL showed that the formation of these compounds was stimulated by the ionophore A23187 (Borgeat and Samuelsson, 1979d). This was of interest, since previous studies had shown that this ionophore stimulated release of SRS from various cells. The UV absorption spectrum of leukotriene B_4 (λ_{max} around 270 nm) was also similar to that reported for SRS-A (Orange *et al.*, 1973; Morris *et al.*, 1978).

After having surveyed published procedures (see Orange and Moore, 1976) for generation of SRS, a new system (murine mastocytoma cells) that gave a better yield of SRS was found. The mouse mast cell tumor was propagated in the peritoneal cavity of syngeneic mice (Murphy *et al.*, 1979). The SRS was generated after preincubation with [$^3H_8$]arachidonic acid or labeled cysteine and challenging with ionophore A23187 in the presence or the absence of unlabeled cysteine. Incubation mixtures were centrifuged; supernatants were mixed with ethanol to 80%, filtered, and evaporated to dryness. Pure SRS was obtained by treating the residue with base and chromatographing it on columns of Amberlite XAD-8 and silicic acid followed by two steps of reverse-phase HPLC (Fig. 8). Purifications were monitored by bioassay on isolated guinea pig ileum in the presence of atropine and pyrilamine maleate. Reversal of contractions by the antagonist FPL 55712 (Augstein *et al.*, 1973) was used as a criterion of SRS activity. A preparation of SRS from ionophore-challenged human leukocytes was used to standardize the contractile response. Purified mast cell tumor SRS gave a characteristic ultraviolet spectrum with λ_{max} at 280 nm (Fig. 9). This absorption and the biological effect were highly correlated during HPLC purification (Fig. 9), suggesting that the UV absorbance was a property of the SRS. The spectrum resembled that of leukotriene B_4 but was shifted 10 nm bathochromically, indicating that SRS contained an auxochrome α to a conjugated triene. Incubations with [$^3H_8$]arachidonic acid and [^{35}S]cysteine yielded purified SRS that contained ^3H and ^{35}S (Fig. 8). Dual isotope experiments with [3-^3H, ^{35}S]cysteine and [U-^{14}C, 3-^3H]cysteine indicated that the carbon atoms and hydrogen at C-3 of cysteine were incorporated in the SRS. Purified material from incubations with [$^3H_8$]arachidonic acid was treated with

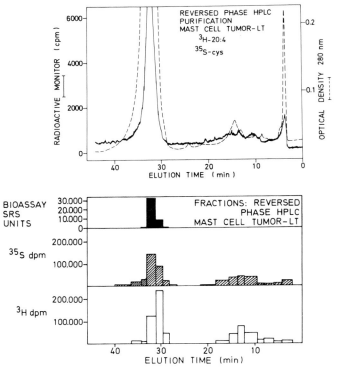

FIG. 8. *Upper panel:* Reverse-phase high-performance liquid chromatography (RP-HPLC) (Nucleosil C_{18}, methanol–water, 65:35, v/v, + 0.01% acetic acid) of mast cell tumor leukotriene C, purified by silicic acid chromatography and Polygosil C_{18} RP-HPLC. The tumor cells were prelabeled with [$^3H_8$]arachidonic acid and [^{35}S]cysteine. A radioactivity monitor and an ultraviolet detector (280 nm) were connected in series after the HPLC column. *Lower panel:* Biological activity of ^3H and ^{35}S contents of fractions collected during the RP-HPLC. From Murphy *et al.* (1979).

Raney nickel. The desulfurized product was esterified, purified by silicic acid chromatography, and analyzed by gas–liquid radio-chromatography after trimethylsilylation. The mass spectrum of the major radioactive component was identical to that of similarly de-rivatized 5-hydroxyarachidic acid (Fig. 10). This suggested that the entire carbon skeleton of arachidonic acid had been converted to SRS and that the molecule had a hydroxyl group at C-5. The material was further degraded by reductive ozonolysis. [1-^3H]-1-Hexanol was iden-tified by cochromatography with unlabeled reference material on reverse-phase HPLC and gas–liquid radiochromatography (Fig. 11).

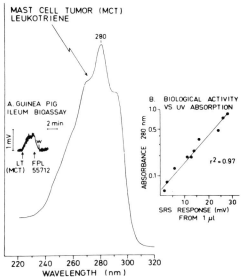

FIG. 9. Ultraviolet spectrum of a slow-reacting substance, SRS (leukoctriene C), from mast cell tumor. *Inset A:* Contraction of guinea pig ileum after addition of UV-absorbing material. Note the addition of FPL 55712 at the second arrow. *Inset B:* Correlation between the log absorbance at 280 nm from a purification of the mast cell tumor-leukotriene C and the biological response on isolated guinea pig ileum (least-square linear regression). LT, leukotriene. From Murphy *et al.* (1979).

This demonstrated that the SRS molecule had retained the Δ^{14} double bond of arachidonic acid. Because of this, an experiment with soybean lipoxygenase, which proved to be essential for the determination of the locations of the remaining double bonds and of the auxochrome, was performed. This lipoxygenase, which is specific for methylene-interrupted *cis,cis*-1,4-pentadienes, introduces a molecule of oxygen at the W6 carbon atom of the pentadiene (Hamberg and Samuelsson, 1967). Incubation of purified SRS with lipoxygenase gave a 28 nm bathochromic shift, showing that the conjugated triene was extended to a tetraene. The experiment demonstrated that the SRS molecule had double bonds at $\Delta^{7,9,11}$ and was thus a cysteine-containing derivative of 5-hydroxy-7, 9, 11, 14-eicosatetraenoic acid. The sulfur-containing substituent was attached at C-6 for the following reasons.

1. The products obtained after oxidative and reductive ozonolysis (1,5-pentanedioic acid and 1-hexanol, respectively) excluded substitution at C-1 through C-5 and at C-15 through C-20.

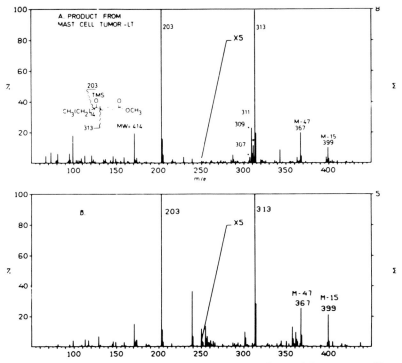

FIG. 10. (A) Mass spectrum of a radioactive product obtained from mast cell tumor leukotriene after Raney nickel desulfurization and conversion to methyl ester, trimethylsilyl-ether derivative. (B) Mass spectrum of the methyl ester, trimethylsilyl (TMS) derivative of 5-hydroxyarachidic acid. From Murphy *et al.* (1979).

2. A sulfur substituent at C-7 through C-12 would give a greater bathochromic shift of the ultraviolet spectrum than that observed (10 nm, cf. above).

3. Substitution at C-13 or C-14 would prohibit conversion of the SRS by soybean lipoxygenase.

4. A thioether bond α to a conjugated triene (i.e., at C-6 or C-13) gives a 10-nm bathochromic shift (Koch, 1949).

Failure to isolate alanine after Raney nickel desulfurization suggested that other amino acids were present. Amino acid analyses of acid-hydrolyzed SRS showed that the molecule contained equimolar amounts of glycine and glutamic acid (1 mol of each per mole of SRS). The yield of ½-cystine was about 0.4 mol per mole of SRS. End group (dansyl method and hydrazinolysis) and sequence analyses (dansyl–Edman

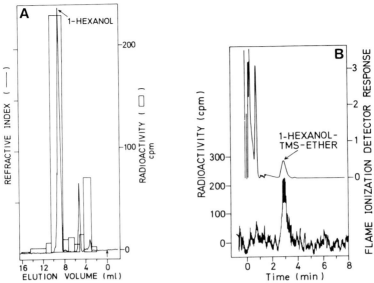

FIG. 11. Reductive ozonolysis of mast cell tumor leukotriene C from [^{3}H$_8$]arachidonic acid: *Left:* High-performance liquid chromatography (HPLC) of ether-extractable products. 1-Hexanol was added as internal reference (μC$_{18}$ Bondapak; methanol–water, 1:1, + 0.01% acetic acid at 1 ml/minute). Radioactivity was determined after addition of Instagel to HPLC fractions. *Right:* Gas–liquid radio chromatogram of ether-extractable products (trimethylsilyl derivative). 1-Hexanol was added prior to derivative formation (1.6% OV-1 at 52°C). From Murphy *et al.* (1979).

procedure) demonstrated that the peptide substituent was γ-glutamylcysteinylglycine (glutathione). The structure of the SRS was therefore 5-hydroxy-6-S-glutathionyl-7,9,11,14-eicosatetraenoic acid (Murphy *et al.*, 1979; Hammarström *et al.*, 1979). The structural work is summarized in Fig. 12. It has been confirmed by a total organic synthesis of leukotrienes developed by E. J. Corey and his associates (1980).

The synthetic routes that are stereospecific (Fig. 13) provided several isomers. One of these, 5(S)-hydroxy-6(R)-S-glutathionyl-7,9-*trans*-11,14-*cis*-eicosatetraenoic acid (**1**, Fig. 13; Hammarström *et al.*, 1980) was identical with SRS of biological origin. This work represents the first structure determination of a slow-reacting substance of anaphylaxis. The compound has been designated leukotriene C$_4$ (Samuelsson *et al.*, 1979; Samuelsson and Hammarström, 1980). Additional stereochemical studies have shown that another component of SRS from murine mastocytoma cells (provisionally referred to as

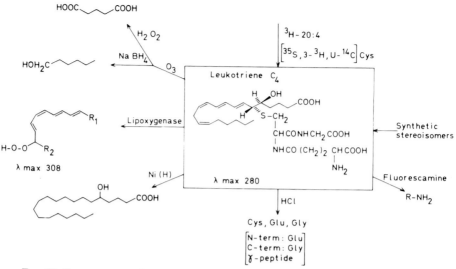

F<small>IG</small>. 12. Precursor experiments and chemical and enzymatic transformations of mouse mast cell tumor leukotriene (slow-reacting substance).

LTC-2) is 5(S)-hydroxy,6(R)-S-glutathionyl-7,9,11-*trans*-14-*cis*-eicosatetraenoic acid (Fig. 2) (11-*trans*-LTC₄) (Clark *et al.*, 1980).

Rat basophilic leukemia (RBL) cells, stimulated with ionophore A23187, produced an SRS that was less polar than LTC₄ (Örning *et al.*, 1980). Its UV spectrum was indistinguishable from that of LTC₄, and a similar spectral change was observed when LTC₄ and RBL SRS were treated with soybean lipoxygenase. Desulfurization with Raney nickel yielded 5-hydroxyarachidic acid. This suggested that the fatty acid part of the molecule was identical to that of leukotriene C₄. The amino acid composition of RBL SRS differed from that of LTC₄ by the absence of glutamic acid. Cysteine and glycine were obtained in the same yields as from LTC₄, and the sequence of the dipeptide substituent was cysteinylglycine as determined by Edman degradation. LTC₄ from mastocytoma cells was treated with γ-glutamyltranspeptidase (GGTP). This yielded a product that was identical to RBL SRS by several criteria: UV spectroscopy, amino acid and sequence analyses, conversion by lipoxygenase, HPLC, and biological activity on guinea pig ileum. The identity suggested that the stereochemistry of LTC₄ and RBL SRS is the same, since the methods used for the comparisons are known to distinguish stereoisomers of LTC₄. The structure is therefore 5(S)-hydroxy-6(R)-S-L-cysteinylglycyl-7,9-*trans*-11,14-*cis*-eicosatetraenoic acid (designated leukotriene D₄ (Samuelsson and Hammarström, 1980)). Leukotriene D₄ is 3–10 times more potent than LTD₄ in

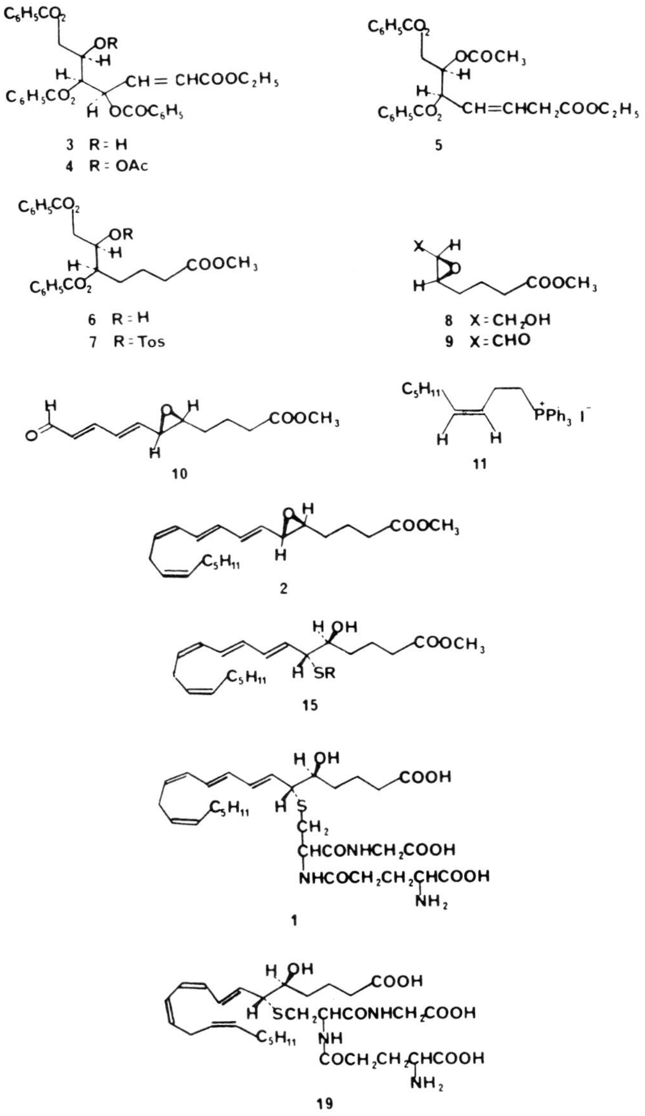

FIG. 13. Chemical synthesis of leukotriene C_4 (1) and 9-*cis*-leukotriene C_4 (19). 2,3,5-Tribenzoyl-D-ribose was converted to 3 by reaction with ethoxycarbonylmethylene triphenyl phosphorane. The monoacetate 4 gave rise to 5 by treatment with zinc amalgam and HCl and to 6 after catalytic hydrogenation and transesterification in methanol. The monotosylate (7) was converted to the epoxide (8) in the presence of K_2CO_3, and the epoxyaldehyde (9) was obtained from 8 using Collins reagent. Condensation with 1-lithio-4-ethoxybutadiene and methanesulfonyl chloride gave 10, which reacted with 11 to yield leukotriene A_4 methyl ester (2). Treatment of 2 with glutathione and triethylamine and alkaline hydrolysis afforded leukotriene C_4 (1). 9-*cis*-Leukotriene C_4 (19) was similarly obtained from 9-*cis*-leukotriene A_4 methyl ester. Modified from Corey *et al.* (1980).

the guinea pig ileum bioassay, and the onset of the contraction is shorter for LTD$_4$.

IV. Biosynthesis of Leukotrienes

A. Leukotrienes A$_4$ and B$_4$

The chemical synthesis of leukotriene C$_4$, described above, also provided leukotriene A$_4$ (Corey *et al.*, 1980). A method based on methylation at alkaline pH and rapid extraction, after addition of synthetic methyl leukotriene A$_4$ methyl ester, permitted the isolation of natural [1-^{14}C]leukotriene A$_4$ (Rådmark *et al.*, 1980a). Chromatographic and chemical comparisons revealed identity, thus establishing beyond doubt the structure of the epoxide intermediate in the formation of dihydroxyeicosatetraenoic acids described above. Other experiments with PMNL pretreated with an inhibitor of leukotriene biosynthesis (BW 755C), showed that synthetic leukotriene A$_4$ was transformed into the same products as was arachidonic acid in the absence of inhibitor (Fig. 14) (Rådmark *et al.*, 1980b). One of the products (compound III, leukotriene B$_4$) was formed enzymatically, whereas compounds I, II, IV, and V were derived nonenzymatically from the epoxide as originally suggested (Borgeat and Samuelsson, 1979c). Additional experiments (Samuelsson, 1982) have demonstrated the formation of leuko-

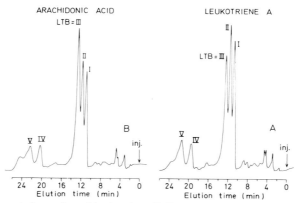

Fig. 14. Enzymic formation of leukotriene B. Reverse-phase high-performance liquid-chromatography chromatograms of products isolated from incubation of polymorphonuclear leukocytes with 5(S)-*trans*-5,6-oxido-7,9-*trans*-11,14-*cis*-eicosatetraenoic acid (A), or with arachidonic acid and ionophore A23187 (B). The solvent system was methanol–water–acetic acid, 75:25:0.01 v/v/v. From Rådmark *et al.* (1980b).

triene B_4 from 5(S)-hydroperoxy-6-*trans*-8,11,14-*cis*-eicosatrienoic acid (5-HPETE). The results prove the originally suggested pathway for the biosynthesis of leukotriene B_4 (Borgeat and Samuelsson, 1979c). This pathway involves initially a lipoxygenase-catalyzed formation of 5-HPETE from arachidonic acid followed by isomerization of two double bonds (6-*trans* to 7-*trans* and 8-*cis* to 9-*trans*) and elimination of hydroxyl anion from the hydroperoxy group to give leukotriene A_4 (cf. Fig. 17 below).

B. LEUKOTRIENES C_4 AND D_4

Leukotriene C_4 is a C-6 glutathione derivative of 5-hydroxy-7,9,11,14-eicosatetraenoic acid (see above). Because of the structural similarity with leukotriene A_4, it seemed likely that leukotriene C_4 was formed from the epoxide by glutathione conjugation (Murphy *et al.*, 1979; Hammarström *et al.*, 1979). The following experiments were therefore performed. Short incubations of mastocytoma or basophilic leukemia cells in the presence of arachidonic acid and ionophore A23187 were terminated by addition of acidic methanol (Hammarström and Samuelsson, 1980). Products were purified by chromatography on Amberlite XAD-8 and silicic acid, and the material eluted from silicic acid with ethyl acetate was analyzed by reverse-phase HPLC. Two compounds with the same chromatographic behavior as diastereoisomeric 5-hydroxy-12-methoxy-6,8,10-*trans*-14-*cis*-eicosatetraenoates were formed. The structures were confirmed by ultraviolet spectroscopy and gas-liquid chromatography–mass spectrometry. The formation of these stable derivatives of leukotriene A_4 demonstrated that the proposed epoxide intermediate is formed during biosynthesis of leukotriene C_4 by mastocytoma cells as well as during the biosynthesis of leukotriene D_4 by basophilic leukemia cells.

Time-course analyses revealed an early, transient accumulation of leukotriene A_4 (maximum after about 30 seconds of incubation) that preceded the formation of leukotrienes D_4 and 11-*trans*-D_4 in the leukemia cells (Fig. 15) and the synthesis of leukotrienes C_4 and 11-*trans* C_4 by mastocytoma cells (Hammarström and Samuelsson, 1980). Other experiments with synthetic leukotriene A_4 showed that this compound was converted enzymatically to leukotrienes C_4 and 11-*trans* C_4 by mastocytoma cells and human leukocytes, pretreated with the inhibitor of arachidonic acid metabolism, BW 755C (Fig. 16) (Rådmark *et al.*, 1980c). The experiments described above confirm the originally proposed (Murphy *et al.*, 1979; Hammarström *et al.*, 1979) pathway for the biosynthesis of slow-reacting substance of anaphylaxis: It involves

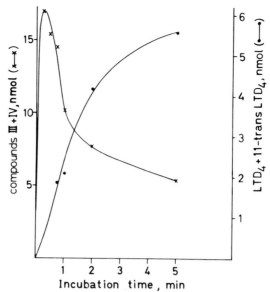

FIG. 15. Temporal relationship between the formation of 5-hydroxy-12-methoxyeicosatetraenoic acids (compounds III, and IV) and the biosynthesis of leukotriene D_4 (LTD$_4$), plus 11-*trans*-leukotriene D_4 (●——●) in basophilic leukemia cells. From Hammarström and Samuelsson (1980).

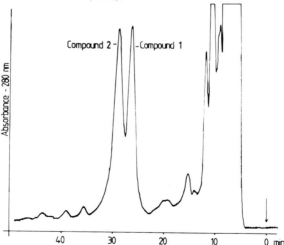

FIG. 16. Reverse-phase high-performance liquid chromatography (HPLC) chromatogram of products obtained from leukotriene A_4 incubation of human polymorphonuclear leukocytes. The incubation was stopped with ethanol after 10 minutes, saponified, and extracted with XAD-8 resin. The extract was purified by silicic acid chromatography. The fraction active on the guinea pig ileum bioassay was evaporated and injected onto the HPLC column (Whatman, Partisil). This was eluted with methanol–water–acetic acid, 70:30:0.1, pH 5.1, at 4 ml/minute; UV detection, 280 nm. From Rådmark *et al.* (1980c).

formation of leukotriene A_4 from arachidonic acid via 5-HPETE, as described above, followed by glutathione conjugation of leukotriene A_4 with scission of the epoxide at C-6 (Fig. 17).

Leukotriene C_4 is a precursor of leukotriene D_4, as suggested by the observations that (a) enzymatic conversion of leukotriene C_4 to leukotriene D_4 occurs in basophilic leukemia cells (Orning et $al.$, 1981) and (b) inhibitors of the enzyme involved prevent the formation of leukotriene D_4 by basophilic leukemia cells and lead to accumulation of

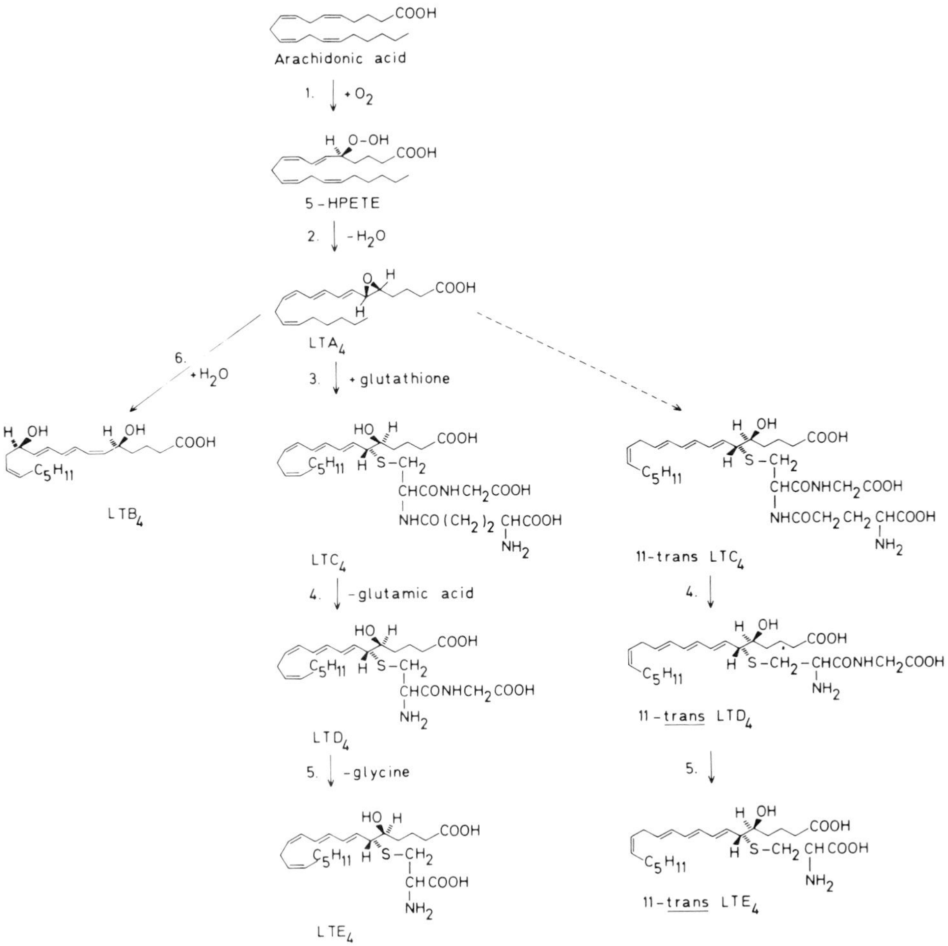

FIG. 17. Transformation of arachidonic acid to leukotrienes. Reactions: 1. Lipoxygenase; 2. leukotriene A synthetase; 3. glutathione S-transferase; 4. γ-glutamyltranspeptidase; 5. leukotriene D dipeptidase; 6. leukotriene A hydrolase.

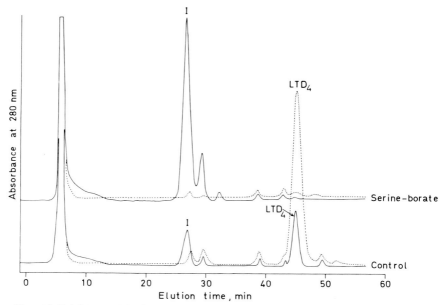

FIG. 18. Inhibition of leukotriene D_4 (LTD$_4$) biosynthesis in RBL-1 cells by L-serine borate complex. The figure shows high-performance liquid chromatograms of methanol–ethyl acetate, 1:1, v/v (----) and methanol eluates (——) from silicic acid chromatographies. The upper curves show chromatograms of material from RBL-1 cells treated with ionophore A23187 plus arachidonic acid and L-cysteine after addition of serine·borate (20 mM). The lower curves show chromatograms from the corresponding experiment without serine·borate. From Örning and Hammarström (1980).

leukotriene C_4 (Fig. 18) (Örning and Hammarström, 1980; Örning *et al.*, 1981).

C. LEUKOTRIENES FORMED FROM OTHER POLYUNSATURATED FATTY ACIDS

Addition of 5,8,11-eicosatrienoic acid to mastocytoma cells stimulated with ionophore A23187 resulted in the formation of two additional products (I and II) besides leukotrienes C_4 and 11-*trans*-C_4 (Hammarström, 1981a). The UV spectrum of compound I had an absorbance maximum at 279 nm and shoulders at 291 and 269 nm, indicating that the molecule contained a conjugated triene with an allylic thioether substituent. The shift of the spectrum of approximately 1 nm compared to the spectrum of leukotriene C_4 (λ_{max} 280 nm) is due to the absence of a Δ^{14} double bond (see below). Treatment of compound I with

Raney nickel yielded 5-hydroxyeicosanoic acid as judged by gas-liquid chromatography – mass spectrometry. Amino acid analyses gave similar results as for LTC$_4$, i.e., approximately 1 mol of glutamic acid, 1 mol of glycine, and approximately 0.3 mol of cysteine per mole of compound I. Incubations with γ-glutamyltranspeptidase transformed compound I to a less polar derivative (compound III), which lacked glutamic acid. This suggested that compound I contained an N-terminal glutamic acid attached by its γ-carboxyl group. Glycine was C terminal, as judged by hydrazinolysis showing that the peptide part of compound I was glutathione. Oxidative ozonolysis of compound I gave two products as determined by gas-liquid chromatography – mass spectrometry analyses of methyl ester derivatives, i.e., nonanoic acid and 1,5-pentanedioic acid. These results demonstrated that compound I lacked a Δ^{14} double bond and provided direct evidence for the location of the conjugated triene chromophore at $\Delta^{7,9,11}$. The formation of nonanoic acid also excluded attachment of glutathione at C-13. No spectral change was observed when compound I was incubated with soybean lipoxygenase. This is in agreement with the absence of a Δ^{14} double bond. The structure of compound I is therefore 5-hydroxy- 6-S-glutathonyl-7,9,11-eicosatrienoic acid (leukotriene C$_3$; Fig. 19) (Hammarström, 1981a). It is likely that the stereochemistry is analogous to that of LTC$_4$ [5(S), 6(R)-7,9-*trans*-11-*cis*].

The UV spectrum of compound II was shifted 2 nm hyposochromatically (λ_{max} at 277 nm) compared to the spectrum of leukotriene C$_3$. This suggests that the conjugated triene had all-trans configuration (cf. Clark *et al.*, 1980). The amino acid composition and the conversion of compound II by γ-glutamyl transpeptidase to a less polar derivative (compound IV) suggested that the peptide parts of compounds I and II were identical. The relative HPLC elution time of compound II compared to leukotriene C$_3$ was similar to the relative elution time of 11-*trans* leukotriene C$_4$ compared to leukotriene C$_4$. Based on these data, compound II was tentatively identified as 11-*trans* leukotriene LTC$_3$. Compound III was obtained by treatment of compound I with γ-glutamyl transpeptidase. The UV spectrum was not affected by this reaction, and amino acid analyses showed that compound III lacked glutamic acid. Compound III is therefore 5-hydroxy-6-S-cysteinylglycyl-7,9,11-eicosatrienoic acid, leukotriene D$_3$ (Fig. 19). Similarly, compound IV is the cysteinylglycine analog of 11-*trans*-leukotriene C$_3$, 11-*trans*-leukotriene D$_3$ (Hammarström, 1981a).

Addition of 5,8,11,14,17-eicosapentaenoic acid to mastocytoma cells stimulated with ionophore A23187 induced the formation of a new product in addition to leukotriene C$_4$ (compound V) (Hammarström,

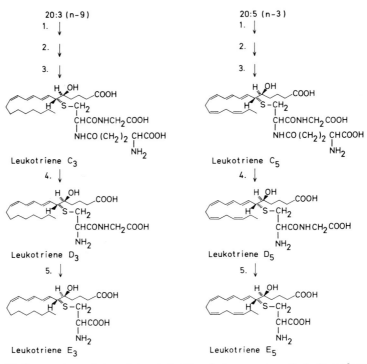

FIG. 19. Conversions of eicosatrienoic (n-9) and eicosapentaenoic (n-3) acids to leukotrienes.

1980). Compound V was eluted earlier than leukotriene C_4 during HPLC, as would be expected if it contained additional double bonds. The UV spectrum was identical to that of leukotriene C_4, and treatment with soybean lipoxygenase produced the same spectral shift as was earlier reported for leukotriene C_4 (λ_{max}, $280 \rightarrow 308$ nm; shoulders, $270 \rightarrow 295$ and $291 \rightarrow 232$ nm). Compound V, therefore, contains double bonds at the same positions as leukotriene C_4 ($\Delta^{7,9,11,14}$) and has an allylic thioether substituent at C-6 (the double bonds at Δ^{11} and Δ^{14} have cis geometry; cf. Murphy *et al.*, 1979). Treatment of V with Raney nickel yielded 5-hydroxyeicosanoic acid and corresponding mono-, di-, tri-, and tetra-unsaturated species were more abundant than in spectra of desulfurized leukotriene C_4. This suggested that compound V differs from leukotriene C_4 by the presence of an additional double bond. It was assumed that the position and geometry of this double bond is the same as in the precursor eicosapentaenoic acid (Δ^{17}-*cis*). Compound V was converted by γ-glutamyltranspeptidase to a less polar derivative (compound VI). The amino acid composition and carboxy-terminal analyses (showing glycine as the only residue) indicated that the peptide substituent of V was glutathione. The structure of compound V was therefore 5-hydroxy-6-S-glutathionyl-7,9,11,14,17-eicosapentaenoic acid (leukotriene C_5; Fig. 19) (Hammarström, 1980). It was assumed that the stereochemistry at C-5 and C-6 as well as the geometry of the Δ^7 and Δ^9 double bonds were the same as in leukotriene C_4. Based on its mode of formation and relative elution behavior on HPLC, compound VI is the cysteinylglycine analog of leukotriene C_5 (5-hydroxy-6-S-cysteinylglycyl-7,9,11,14-17-eicosapentaenoic acid, leukotriene D_5; Fig. 19).

The conversions of [$^3H_6$]5,8,11-eicosatrienoic acid to leukotriene C_3 and leukotriene D_3 (Hammarström, 1981a), and [U-^{14}C]eicosapentanoic acid (n-3) to leukotriene C_5 and leukotriene D_5 (Hammarström, 1981b) have been demonstrated. The identifications of radioactive products were based on cochromatography on HPLC before and after treatment with γ-glutamyltranspeptidase. The conversion of [$^3H_6$]eicosatrienoic acid (n-9) to leukotriene C_3 proceeded without appreciable change in specific activity. This permitted the preparation of [$^3H_6$]leukotriene C_3 of close to theoretical specific activity for use in metabolic experiments (see below).

D. NOMENCLATURE

The fundamental importance of the biosynthetic pathways described and the cumbersome systematic names of the compounds involved suggested the introduction of a trivial name for these entities. The term

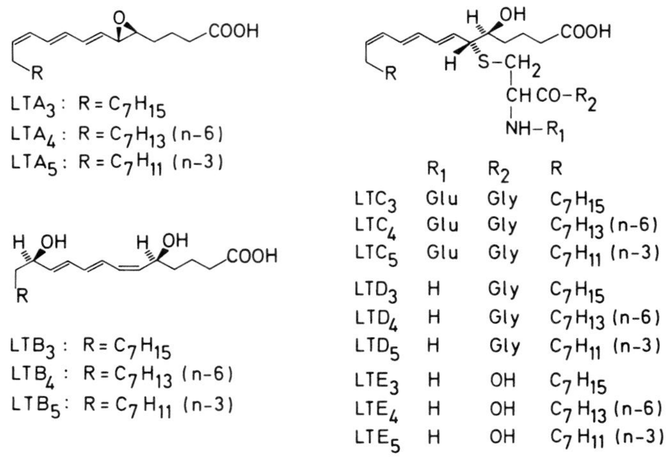

FIG. 20. Nomenclature for leukotrienes. From Samuelsson and Hammarström (1980).

"leukotriene" was chosen (Samuelsson *et al.*, 1979) because these compounds were first detected in leukocytes and the common structural
feature is a conjugated triene. Various members of the group have been
designated alphabetically (Fig. 20): leukotrienes A are 5,6-oxido-7,9-
trans-11-*cis*; leukotrienes B, 5(*S*),12(*R*)-dihydroxy-6-*cis*-8,10-*trans*;
leukotrienes C, 5(*S*)-hydroxy-6(*R*)-*S*-γ- glutamylcysteinylglycyl-7,9-
trans-11-*cis;* leukotrienes D, 5(*S*)-hydroxy-6(*R*)-*S*-cysteinylglycyl-7,9-
trans-11-*cis;* and leukotrienes E,5(*S*)-hydroxy-6(*R*)-*S*-cysteinyl-7,9-
trans-11-*cis*-eicosapolyenoic acids (Samuelsson and Hammarström,
1980). Since various precursor acids can be converted to leukotrienes
containing 3–5 double bonds, a subscript denoting this number is used
(Fig. 20). Leukotriene A_4 is thus the epoxy derivative of arachidonic
acid, which can be further transformed to leukotrienes B_4, C_4, D_4, and
E_4 as detailed in Fig. 17.

V. METABOLISM OF LEUKOTRIENES

The metabolism of leukotriene C_3 has been investigated using
tritium-labeled material of high specific activity, and with the label in
the fatty acid part of the molecule (Hammarström, 1981c). The results
showed that guinea pig lung homogenates rapidly converted leukotriene C_3 to leukotriene D_3. Liver and kidney homogenates did not
catabolize leukotriene C_3 appreciably. This was apparently due to high
tissue concentrations of glutathione, which prevented leukotriene D_3
formation. In contrast, leukotriene D_3 was rapidly metabolized by liver
and kidney homogenates by hydrolysis of the peptide bond to give
5-hydroxy-6-*S*-cysteinyl-7,9,11-eicosatrienoic acid (leukotriene E_3)
(Bernström and Hammarström, 1981; Hammarström, 1981c). An enzyme catalyzing the latter transformation has been partially purified
from kidney (Bernström and Hammarström, 1981). This enzyme preparation also converted leukotrienes D_4, 11-*trans* D_4, and D_5 to corresponding E leukotrienes (Fig. 19). *In vivo* experiments in the guinea
pig (Hammarström, 1981c) and the mouse (Appelgren and Hammarström, 1982) have shown that leukotriene C_3 metabolites are excreted primarily via bile (feces). The metabolism of leukotrienes was
recently reviewed in greater detail (Hammarström, 1982).

VI. OCCURRENCE OF LEUKOTRIENES

Leukotriene B_4 was originally obtained from polymorphonuclear
leukocytes harvested from the peritoneal cavity of rabbits after glyco-

gen injections (Borgeat and Samuelsson, 1979a). The same system was also used to demonstrate the intermediate formation of leukotriene A_4 (Borgeat and Samuelsson, 1979c). Leukotrienes C_4 and D_4 were first isolated from mouse matocytoma (Murphy et al., 1979; Hammarström et al., 1979) and rat basophilic leukemia cells (Örning et al., 1980; Parker et al., 1980; Morris et al., 1980a), respectively. Subsequently, leukotriene formation was demonstrated in other cells and tissues. Leukotriene A_4 is formed as an intermediate in mouse mastocytoma and rat basophilic leukemia cells (Hammarström and Samuelsson, 1980), leukotriene B_4 by human peripheral leukocytes (Borgeat and Samuelsson, 1979d), rat polymorphonuclear leukocytes (Ford-Hutchinson et al., 1981), rat neutrophils (Siegel et al., 1981), and rat macrophages (Doig and Ford-Hutchinson, 1980).

Leukotriene C_4 has been isolated from rat basophilic leukemia cells (Örning and Hammarström, 1980; Örning et al., 1981), rat monocytes (Bach et al., 1980a), human peripheral leukocytes (Hansson and Rådmark, 1980), mouse peritoneal macrophages (Rouzer et al. 1980), and anaphylactic rat peritoneal cavity (Lewis et al., 1980a). Formation of leukotriene D_4 has been observed in rat monocytes (Bach et al., 1980b), human lung (Lewis et al., 1980a), guinea pig lung (Morris et al., 1980b), cat paws (Houglum et al., 1980), and anaphylactic rat peritoneal cavity (Lewis et al., 1980a). The latter two systems also appeared to produce some leukotriene E_4 (Houglum et al., 1980; Lewis et al., 1980b).

VII. Biological Effects of Leukotrienes

The suggested importance of SRS-A in asthma and anaphylactic reactions (Orange and Austen, 1969; Austen, 1978) and the structure elucidation of SRS-A as leukotrienes C_4 and D_4 (Samuelsson et al., 1980) have stimulated interest in the biological effects of these and other leukotrienes. Leukotrienes C_4 and D_4 (0.1–1.0 nM) caused concentration-dependent contractions of guinea pig ileum, but did not contract rabbit duodenal strips in concentrations up to 50 nM (Hedqvist et al., 1980). The guinea pig ileum is the classical preparation for determinations of the biological activity of SRS-A in relation to histamine. It was observed that, on a molar basis, histamine was less than 200 times as active as leukotriene C_4, suggesting that one unit of SRS-A (i.e., 5 ng of histamine hydrochloride) corresponds to approximately 0.2 pmol of leukotriene C_4. Leukotriene C_4 also contracted uterine strips from virgin (0.1–1.0 nM) and adult ovariectomized (1.0–100 nM) guinea pigs in a dose-dependent manner and was approximately 300 times more potent than histamine in these systems. In contrast, uterine horns from rats in artificial estrus did not respond to leukotriene C_4 (100 nM) and histamine (10 μM), but contracted vigorously to 100 nM PGE_2. Another effect of leukotrienes C_4 and D_4 was to increase vascular permeability of guinea pig skin. At a dose of 0.1 pmol injected intradermally, these leukotrienes, after 30 minutes, produced blue spots due to leakage of circulating Evans blue of significantly greater intensity and size than those caused by NaCl (solvent) or histamine (0.1 nmol). Pulmonary effects of leukotrienes were of particular interest in view of the suggested mediator role of SRS-A in anaphylactic reactions. Injections into the jugular vein of leukotriene C_4 or histamine caused dose-related and parallel increases in insufflation pressure in anesthetized and artificially ventilated guinea pigs (Fig. 21). Leukotrienes C_4 and D_4 in doses of 89 and 120 pmol, respectively, caused 100% increase in insufflation pressure. Fourteen nanomoles of histamine were required to produce the same increase in insufflation pressure. The leukotrienes were at least as potent when given as aerosols, indicating that the increase in insufflation pressure was due to bronchoconstriction. The results agree with previous information on biological effects of impure preparations of SRS-A from cat paws (Strandberg and Hedqvist, 1975).

The pulmonary effects of leukotrienes C_4 and D_4 were further investigated on isolated strips from guinea pig, human, and rabbit lung.

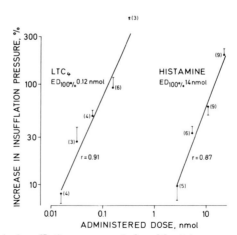

FIG. 21. Increase in insufflation pressure induced by intravenous injections of leukotriene C_4 (LTC_4) and histamine in artificially ventilated guinea pigs. Shown are mean values $\pm$ SE; (n) = number of observations from 12 experiments. Regression lines were calculated according to the method of least squares. From Hedqvist et al. (1980).

Lower absolute doses and lower doses relative to histamine were required to induce parenchymal as compared to tracheal contractions in guinea pigs. This indicates that leukotrienes are particularly active on peripheral airways, as was previously suggested for SRS-A (Drazen *et al.*, 1979). Rabbit bronchial strips did not respond to leukotrienes C_4 and D_4 in concentrations up to 100 nM, whereas human bronchi proved to be remarkably sensitive to these compounds. Thus, leukotrienes C_4 and D_4 caused dose-dependent, long-lasting contractions of human bronchial strips (Dahlén *et al.*, 1980). Contractions induced by histamine readily disappeared after changing of the bath fluid, whereas the responses to both leukotrienes C_4 and D_4 were difficult to reverse even by repeated washings. In fact, a contraction obtained by a high dose of leukotriene C_4 (100 nM), although reversible by isoproterenol (1 μM), reappeared when the added drugs were washed out. The SRS-A antagonist FPL 55712 (Augstein *et al.*, 1973; 1–10 μM) reversed contractions of human bronchi induced by leukotrienes C_4 or D_4 without affecting histamine responses. Blockade of muscarinic and histamine (H-1) receptors by atropine (1 μM) and mepyramine (1 μM), respectively, had no effect on the leukotriene C_4-induced contractions. Repeated administration of leukotrienes caused tachyphylaxis. Therefore, noncumulative administration of drugs was chosen. Dose-response curves obtained for histamine and leukotriene C_4 were parallel and gave similar maximum values, but the leukotriene C_4 curve was markedly to the left of the histamine curve (Fig. 22). According to the calculated regression lines, a 100% increase in resting tension was obtained with 6.3 nM leukotriene C_4 as compared to 10 μM histamine. Thus, on a molar basis, leukotriene C_4 is over 1000 times more potent than histamine in causing contractions of isolated human bronchi. Prostaglandin $F_{2\alpha}$, another effective bronchoconstrictor (Hedqvist and Mathé, 1977), was 500 times less potent than leukotriene C_4.

Leukotriene A_4 was less potent than leukotrienes C_4 or D_4 and as potent as histamine in causing contractions of human bronchial strips. It was not determined whether the effect was due to partial conversion to leukotrienes C_4 and/or D_4 in the bronchial preparations.

Leukotrienes C_3, C_5, E_4, and 11-*trans*-E_4 induced similar types of contractions of trachea and lung parenchyma as leukotriene C_4 (Dahlén *et al.*, 1982). The responses were antagonized by FPL 55712. On guinea pig ileum, dose-response curves indicated that leukotrienes C_3, C_4, and C_5 were approximately equipotent and that 11-*trans*-leukotriene C_3 was 5–10 times less active (Hammarström, 1980, 1981a). Leukotriene D_3 induced similar types of contractions of guinea pig ileum as leukotriene D_4 with regard to time of onset and duration.

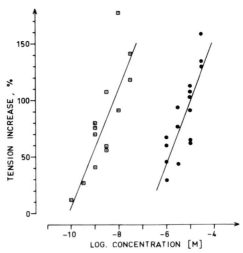

FIG. 22. Contraction responses of isolated human bronchi to histamine and leukotriene C_4 (LTC$_4$) plotted on a semilogarithmic scale. Regression lines were calculated according to the method of least squares. $ED_{100\%}$ is dose of agonist increasing tension 100% above resting level (5 mN). Results are for 13 strips obtained from eight subjects. ●, Histamine, $n = 16$; $ED_{100\%} = 1.0 \times 10^{-5}$ M; $y = 375 + 55$ X; $r = 0.82$. ⊡, LTC$_4$, $n = 13$; $ED_{100\%} = 6.3 + 10^{-9}$ M; $y = 529 + 52$ X; $r = 0.83$. From Dahlén et al. (1980).

Its potency was comparable to that of leukotriene D_4. Leukotrienes E_4 and 11-*trans*-E_4 were 8–12 times less potent than leukotriene C_4 (Bernström and Hammarström, 1981) in this system.

Leukotriene B_4 is a potent chemotactic and chemokinetic agent (Ford-Hutchinson et al., 1980; Goetzl, 1980; Malmsten et al., 1980). 6-*trans*-leukotriene B_4 (compound I) and 6-*trans*-12-epi-leukotriene B_4 (compound II) also induced directed and random motion of human polymorphonuclear leukocytes, but were less potent than leukotriene B_4 (Table I). In the concentration range 10^{-9} to $10^{-5} M$, 5(S)-hydroxy-6-*trans*-8,10,14-*cis*-eicosatetraenoic acid (5-HETE) and leukotriene C_4 did not induce migration different from that of control cells.

At high concentrations (2.5×10^{-5} to $2.5 \times 10^{-3} M$) indomethacin inhibited leukocyte migraion induced by the chemotactic peptide formyl-methionyl-leucyl-phenylalanine (fMLP, $10^{-7} M$), whereas an enhancement was observed at $2.5 \times 10^{-6} M$ indomethacin. No effect was observed at $2.5 \times 10^{-7} M$ or lower. The lipoxygenase–cycloxygenase inhibitor 5,8,11,14-eicosatetraynoic acid (ETYA, 2.5×10^{-5} to $2.5 \times 10^{-4} M$) inhibited both spontaneous and fMLP-stimulated migration of leukocytes. The results with indomethacin and ETYA are compatible with the concept that leukotriene B_4 formation is

TABLE I

THE ABILITY OF LEUKOTRIENE B_4 AND COMPOUNDS I AND II TO INDUCE A STIMULATED
MIGRATION OF NEUTROPHILS[a]

Concentration (M)	Distance to leading front cells (mm)	
	Leukotriene B_4	Compounds I and II
10^{-5}	0.40 ± 0.09[b]	0.35 ± 0.15*
10^{-6}	0.56 ± 0.01**	0.25 ± 0.14
10^{-7}	0.50 ± 0.07**	0.10 ± 0.05
10^{-8}	0.27 ± 0.01*	0.13 ± 0.04
10^{-9}	0.13 ± 0.02	0.11 ± 0.03

** $p < 0.01$, * $p < 0.05$ in comparison with measures for unstimulated cells (Wilcoxon's signed rank test).

[a] The unstimulated migration never exceeded 0.13 mm in any examination. Mean $\pm$ SD values for polymorphonuclear leukocytes from five different subjects (each sample in triplicate).

[b] Polymorphonuclear leukocytes showed a desensitized pattern of stimulated migration.

involved in the chemotactic response. The stereospecificity in the response to leukotriene B_4 isomer further supports this notion.

These results demonstrate that the biological effects are not confined to immediate hypersensitivity reactions but also include inflammation through the increase in permeability of microvasculature induced by leukotrienes C_4 and D_4 and the chemotactic and chemokinetic effects of leukotriene B_4.

ACKNOWLEDGMENTS

This work was supported by grants from the Swedish Medical Research Council (03X-217 and 03X-5914) and the Swedish Cancer Society (1503-02X).

REFERENCES

Applegren, L. E., and Hammarström, S. (1982). Distribution and metabolism of leukotriene C_3 in the mouse. *J. Biol. Chem.* **257**, 531–535.

Augstein, J., Farmer, J. B., Lee, T. B., Sheard, P., and Tatersall, M. L. (1973). Selective inhibitor of slow reacting substance of anaphylaxis. *Nature (London)* **245**, 215–217.

Austen, K. F. (1978). Homeostasis of effector systems which can also be recruited from immunologic reactions. *J. Immunol.* **121**, 793–805.

Bach, M. K., Brashler, J. R., Hammarström, S., and Samuelsson, B. (1980a). Identification of leukotriene C-1 as a major component of slow reacting substance from rat mononuclear cells. *J. Immunol.* **125**, 115–117.

Bach, M. K., Brashler, J. R., Hammarström, S., and Samuelsson, B. (1980b). Identification of a component of rat mononuclear cell SRS as leukotriene D. *Biochem. Biophys. Res. Commun.* **93**, 1121–1126.

Bernström, K., and Hammarström, S. (1981). Metabolism of leukotriene D by porcine kidney. *J. Biol. Chem.* **256**, 9579–9582.

Borgeat, P., and Samuelsson, B. (1979a). Transformation of arachidonic acid by rabbit polymorphonuclear leukocytes. Formation of a novel dihydroxyeicosatetraenoic acid. *J. Biol. Chem.* **254**, 2643–2646.

Borgeat, P., and Samuelsson, B. (1979b). Metabolism of arachidonic acid in polymorphonuclear leukocytes. Structural analysis of novel hydroxylated compounds. *J. Biol. Chem.* **254**, 7865–7869.

Borgeat, P., and Samuelsson, B. (1979c). Arachidonic acid metabolism in polymorphonuclear leukocytes: Unstable intermediate in formation of dihydroxy acids. *Proc. Natl. Acad. Sci. U.S.A.* **76**, 3213–3217.

Borgeat, P., and Samuelsson, B. (1979). Arachidonic acid metabolism in polymorphonuclear leukocytes: Effects of ionophore A23187. *Proc. Natl. Acad. Sci. U.S.A.* **76**, 2148–2152.

Borgeat, P., Hamberg, M., and Samuelsson, B. (1976). *J. Biol. Chem.* **251**, 7816–7820, correction (1977) **252**, 8772.

Clark, D. A., Goto, G., Marfat, A., Corey, E. J., Hammarström, S., and Samuelsson, B. (1980). 11-*trans*-leukotriene C: A naturally occurring slow reacting substance. *Biochem. Biophys. Res. Commun.* **94**, 1133–1139.

Corey, E. J., Clark, D. A., Goto, G., Marfat, A., Mioskowski, C., Samuelsson, B., and Hammarström, S. (1980). Stereospecific total synthesis of a slow reacting substance of anaphylaxis, leukotriene C-1. *J. Am. Chem. Soc.* **102**, 1436–1439.

Crombie, L., and Jacklin, A. G. (1957). *J. Chem. Soc.* 1632–1646.

Dahlén, S. E., Hedqvist, P., Hammarström, S., and Samuelsson, B. (1980). Leukotrienes are potent constrictors of human bronchi. *Nature (London)* **288**, 484–486.

Dahlén, S. E., Hedqvist, P., Hammarström, S., and Samuelsson, B. (1981). Importance of cysteinyl-substituent for leukotriene broncho-constrictor potency. *Proc. Natl. Acad. Sci. U.S.A.* **78**, 3887–3891.

Dahlén, S. E., Hedquist, P., and Hammarström, S. (1982). *Eur. J. Pharmacol.*, in press.

Doig, M. V., and Ford-Hutchinson, A. W. (1980). *Prostaglandins* **20**, 1007–1019.

Drazen, J. M., Lewis, R. A., Wasserman, S. I., Orange, R. P., and Austen, K. F. (1979). Differential effects of a partially purified preparation of slow reacting substance of anaphylaxis on guinea pig tracheal spirals and parenchymal strips. *J. Clin. Invest.* **63**, 1–5.

Drazen, J. M., Austen, K. F., Lewis, R. H., Clark, D. A., Goto, G., Marfat, A., and Corey, E. J. (1980). Comparative airway and vascular activities of leukotrienes C-1 and D *in vivo* and *in vitro*. *Proc. Natl. Acad. Sci. U.S.A.* **77**, 4354–4358.

Ford-Hutchinson, A. W., Bray, M. A., Doig, M. W., Shipley, M. E., and Smith, M. J. H. (1980). Leukotriene B, a potent chemokinetic and aggregating substance released from polymorphonuclear leukocytes. *Nature (London)* **286**, 264–265.

Ford-Hutchinson, A. W., Bray, M. A., Cunningham, F. M., Davidson, E. M., and Smith, M. J. H. (1981). Isomers of leukotriene B_4 possess different biological potencies. *Prostaglandins* **21**, 143–152.

Goetzl, E. J. (1980). The unique roles of mono-hydroxy-eicosatetraenoic acids (HETE's) in the regulation of human eosinophil function. *In* "The Eosinophil in Health and Disease" (A. Mahmoud and K. F. Austen, eds.), pp. 167–184. Grune & Stratton, New York.

Hamberg, M., and Samuelsson, B. (1967). On the specificity of the oxygenation of unsaturated fatty acids catalyzed by soybean lipoxygenase. *J. Biol. Chem.* **242**, 5329–5335.

Hammarström, S. (1980). Leukotriene C_5: a slow reacting substance derived from eicosapentaenoic acid. *J. Biol. Chem.* **255**, 7093–7094.

Hammarström, S. (1981a). Conversion of 5,8,11-eicosatrienoic acid to leukotrienes C_3 and D_3. *J. Biol. Chem.* **256**, 2275–2279.

Hammarström, S. (1981b). Conversion of ^{14}C-labeled eicosapentaenoic acid (n-3) to leukotriene C_5. *Biochim. Biophys. Acta* **663**, 575–577.

Hammarström, S. (1981c). Metabolism of leukotriene C_3 in the guinea pig. Identification of metabolites formed by lung, liver and kidney. *J. Biol. Chem.* **256**, 9573–9578.

Hammarström, S. (1982). *Adv. Prostaglandin, Thromboxane Leukotriene Res.* **9**, 83–101.

Hammarström, S., and Samuelsson, B. (1980). Detection of leukotriene A_4 as an intermediate in the biosynthesis of leukotriene C_4 and D_4. *FEBS Lett.* **122**, 83–86.

Hammarström, S., Murphy, R. C., Samuelsson, B., Clark, D. H., Mioskowski, C., and Corey, E. J. (1979). Structure of leukotriene C: Identification of the amino acid part. *Biochem. Biophys. Res. Commun.* **91**, 1266–1272.

Hammarström, S., Samuelsson, B., Clark, D. A., Goto, G., Marfat, A., Mioskowski, C., and Corey, E. J. (1980). Stereochemistry of leukotriene C-1. *Biochem. Biophys. Res. Commun.* **92**, 946–953.

Hansson, G., and Rådmark, O. (1980). Leukotriene C_4: Isolation from human polymorphonuclear leukocytes. *FEBS Lett.* **122**, 87–90.

Hedqvist, P., and Mathé, A. (1977). Lung function and the role of prostaglandins. *In* "Asthma Physiology, Immunopharmacology and Treatment" (L. M. Lichtenstein and K. F. Austen, eds.), pp. 131–146. Academic Press, New York.

Hedqvist, P., Dahlén, S. E., Gustafsson, L., Hammarström, S., and Samuelsson, B. (1980). Biological profile of leukotrienes C_4 and D_4. *Acta Physiol. Scand.* **110**, 331–333.

Houglum, J., Pai, J.-K., Atrache, V., Sok, D.-E., and Sih, C. J. (1980). *Proc. Natl. Acad. Sci. U.S.A.* **77**, 5688–5692.

Kellaway, C. H., and Trethewie, E. R. (1940). The liberation of a slow-reacting smooth muscle stimulating substance in anaphylaxis. *Q. J. Exp. Physiol. Cogn. Med. Sci.* **30**, 121–145.

Koch, H. P. (1949). Absorption spectra and structure of organic sulphur compounds. Part I. Unsaturated sulphides. *J. Chem. Soc.* 387–394.

Lewis, R. A., Austen, K. F., Drazen, J. M., Clark, D. A., Marfat, A., and Corey, E. J. (1980a). Slow reacting substances of anaphylaxis: Identification of leukotrienes C-1 and D from human and rat sources. *Proc. Natl. Acad. Sci. U.S.A.* **77**, 3710–3714.

Lewis, R. A., Drazen, J. M., Austen, K. F., Clark, D. A., and Corey, E. J. (1980b). Identification of the C(6)-S-conjugate of leukotriene A with cysteine as a naturally occurring slow reacting substance of anaphylaxis (SRS-A). Importance of the 11-*cis* geometry for biological activity. *Biochem. Biophys. Res. Commun.* **96**, 271–277.

Malmsten, C. L., Palmblad, J., Udén, A.-M., Rådmark, O., Engstedt, L., and Samuelsson, B. (1980). Leukotriene B_4: A highly potent and stereospecific factor stimulating migration of polymorphonuclear leukocytes. *Acta Physiol. Scand.* **110**, 449–451.

Morris, H. R., Taylor, G. W., Piper, P. J., Sirois, P., and Tippins, J. R. (1978). Slow-reacting substance of anaphylaxis. Purification and characterization. *FEBS Lett.* **87**, 203–206.

Morris, H. R., Taylor, G. W., Piper, P. J., Samhoun, M. N., and Tippins, J. R. (1980a). Slow reacting substances (SRSS): The structure identification of SRSS from rat basophilic leukemia (RBL-1) cells. *Prostaglandins* **19**, 185–201.

Morris, H. R., Taylor, G. W., Piper, P. J., and Tippins, J. R. (1980b). Structure of slow reacting substance of anaphylaxis from guinea pig lung. *Nature (London)* **285**, 104–106.

Murphy, R. C., Hammarström, S., and Samuelsson, B. (1979). Leukotriene C: A slow reacting substance from murine mastocytoma cells. *Proc. Natl. Acad. Sci. U.S.A.* **76**, 4275–4279.

Orange, R. P., and Austen, K. F. (1969). Slow reacting substance of anaphylaxis. *Adv. Immunol.* **10**, 105–144.

Orange, R. P., and Moore, E. G. (1976). The effect of thiols on the immunologic release of slow reacting substance of anaphylaxis: II. Other *in vitro* and *in vivo* models. *J. Immunol.* **116**, 392–397.

Orange, R. P., Murphy, R. C., Karnovsky, M. L., and Austen, K. F. (1973). The physicochemical characteristics and purification of slow reacting substance of anaphylaxis. *J. Immunol.* **110**, 760–770.

Örning, L., and Hammarström, S. (1980). Inhibition of leukotriene C_4 and leukotriene D_4 biosynthesis. *J. Biol. Chem.* **255**, 8023–8026.

Örning, L., Hammarström, S., and Samuelsson, B. (1980). Leukotriene D: A slow reacting substance from rat basophilic leukemia cells. *Proc. Natl. Acad. Sci. U.S.A.* **77**, 2014–2017.

Örning, L., Bernström, K., and Hammarström, S. (1981). Biosynthesis of leukotrienes E in rat basophilic leukemia cells. *Eur. J. Biochem.* **120**, 41–45.

Parker, C. W., Falkenhein, S. F., and Huber, M. M. (1980). Sequential conversion of the glutathionyl side chain of slow reacting substance (SRS) to cysteinyl-glycine and cysteine in rat basophilic leukemia cells stimulated with A-23187. *Prostaglandins* **20**, 863–886.

Rådmark, O., Malmsten, C., Samuelsson, B., Goto, G., Marfat, A., and Corey, E. J. (1980a). Leukotriene A: Isolation from human polymorphonuclear leukocytes. *J. Biol. Chem.* **255**, 11828–11831.

Rådmark, O., Malmsten, C., Samuelsson, B., Clark, D. A., Goto, G., Marfat, A., and Corey, E. J. (1980b). Leukotriene A: Stereochemistry and enzymatic conversion to leukotriene B. *Biochem. Biophys. Res. Commun.* **92**, 954–961.

Rådmark, O., Malmsten, C., and Samuelsson, B. (1980c). Leukotriene A_4: Enzymatic conversion to leukotriene C_4. *Biochem. Biophys. Res. Commun.* **96**, 1679–1687.

Rouzer, C. A., Scott, W. H., Cohn, Z. A., Blackburn, P., and Manning, J. M. (1980). Mouse peritoneal macrophages release leukotriene C in response to a phagocytotic stimulus. *Proc. Natl. Acad. Sci. U.S.A.* **77**, 4928–4932.

Samuelsson, B. (1982). Unpublished observations.

Samuelsson, B., and Hammarström, S. (1980). Nomenclature for leukotrienes. *Prostaglandins* **19**, 645–648.

Samuelsson, B., Borgeat, P., Hammarström, S., and Murphy, R. C. (1979). Introduction of a nomenclature: Leukotrienes. *Prostaglandins* **17**, 785–787.

Samuelsson, B., Hammarström, S., Murphy, R. C., and Borgeat, P. (1980). Leukotrienes and slow reacting substance of anaphylaxis (SRS-A). *Allergy* **35**, 375–381.

Siegel, M. I., McConnell, R. T., Bonser, R. W., and Cuatrecasas, P. (1981). The production of 5-HETE and leukotriene B in rat neutrophils from carrageenan pleural exudates. *Prostaglandins* **21**, 123–132.

Strandberg, K., and Hedqvist, P. (1975). Airway effects of slow reacting substance, prostaglandin $F_{2\alpha}$ and histamine in the guinea pig. *Acta Physiol. Scand.* **94**, 105–111.

VITAMINS AND HORMONES, VOL. 39

Newer Approaches to the Isolation, Identification, and Quantitation of Steroids in Biological Materials

JAN SJÖVALL AND MAGNUS AXELSON

Department of Physiological Chemistry, Karolinska Institutet, Stockholm, Sweden

I. INTRODUCTION

Progress in steroid analysis has been remarkable in the last 15 years. Much of our present knowledge in steroid endocrinology could not have been acquired without the development of radioimmunoassay and other competitive protein-binding methods. These methods have provided the sensitivity and speed required for measurement of physiological concentrations of steroid hormones in large series of samples (see Gray and James, 1979). Parallel with this development, both liquid and gas–liquid chromatographic methods have been markedly improved and mass spectrometers have become available for routine use. The most important advance in this area has been the successful combination of gas chromatography and mass spectrometry (GC–MS)

31

for analysis of molecules as large as steroids (Ryhage, 1964; Stenhagen, 1964; Watson and Biemann, 1964).

Immunoassay and GC–MS are complementary methods. GC–MS is important as a reference method to test and validate the specificity of an immunoassay. The steroid composition of biological samples taken under different physiological and pathological conditions can be characterized by GC–MS, and immunoassays may then be developed for detailed studies of selected steroids in larger numbers of samples. Other analytical techniques are available, e.g., based on enzymatic reactions, fluorescence, or luminescence, but the simplicity, speed, and specificity of immunoassays and other protein-binding methods are usually superior for determination of steroid concentrations in body fluids. Important information about the physiology and pathophysiology of steroid hormones is further derived from determinations of turnover and production rates. Such metabolic studies are usually carried out with radioactive tracer techniques. Recent advances in GC–MS technology have resulted in an increased use of nonradioactive isotopes. Common to analytical methods and metabolic studies is the need for extraction and separation techniques. Similar principles are used, but the requirements for chromatographic purification decrease with increasing specificity of the method of detection and quantitation.

It is not possible to cover all aspects of steroid analysis in one chapter. We have limited this review to methods with which we have some personal experience. Thus, immunoassays and other competitive protein-binding methods are excluded. There are many important lines of development in this field, e.g., nonisotopic immunoassays, monoclonal antibodies, new binding systems, antigens labeled with iodine, automation, combination with high-pressure liquid chromatography. References to work in several of these areas can be found in reviews by Jeffcoate (1977), Pratt and Woldring (1977), Felber (1978), Pratt (1978), Exley (1979), and Landon et al. (1979). Excellent reviews of a variety of methods for analysis of individual steroids and for determination of their production rates are found in the third volume of "Hormones in Blood," edited by Gray and James (1979). Our review is focused on liquid chromatographic, gas chromatographic, and mass spectrometric methods. We have tried to indicate how these methods can be integrated into analytical systems. The discussion of extraction and sample purification is relevant for all types of steroid analysis.

GC–MS has been used to a relatively limited extent in clinical and endocrinological studies in spite of its ability to separate, identify, and specifically quantitate steroids in biological materials. This is because most GC–MS methods lack the speed and simplicity that characterize immunoassays. Furthermore, complete characterization of a steroid profile in tissues and body fluids is often considered of limited endocrinological value compared to analysis of selected steroids with known biological functions. This assumption can be tested only when simpler and more rapid methods for analysis of metabolic profiles of steroids become available. At present, the combination of chromatographic separation with mass spectrometric detection seems to offer the best basis for such methods. We have attempted to review work that may be relevant for development in this area, but the list of references is not intended to be complete. Since future analytical systems should be automated, emphasis has been put on methods that are amenable to automation. Although the discussion has been limited mainly to hormonal steroids, the applicability of a method to other classes of compounds has been considered important, as has the potential for future improvements and simplifications.

A general method for analysis of steroids by GC–MS may be subdivided into four main steps: (a) extraction, group separation, or purification; (b) hydrolysis of conjugates, group separation, or purification; (c) derivatization, purification; (d) GC–MS analysis. Depending on the particular sample to be analyzed and the steroids to be determined, different steps in this procedure may be omitted. Thus, in the simplest case a steroid present in high concentration may only require extraction and GC–MS. Since this is impossible in most cases, it is important to choose methods for group separation and purification that can be used for a wide range of steroids. In this way analytical systems may be constructed that require only minor modifications or additions of selective steps to be applied to a wide variety of analytical problems. These considerations have determined the order in which different methods are discussed.

II. EXTRACTION OF STEROIDS

Although elimination of separate extraction steps must be the ultimate goal in the development of methods for steroid analysis, this has not yet been achieved. The commonly used extraction procedures may be divided into two groups: those employing solvents and those utilizing solids.

A. EXTRACTION WITH SOLVENTS

Solvent extraction has long been the most common first step in steroid analysis. However, it is often time-consuming and emulsions may form, which result in poor recoveries. Solvents are often selected in order to give partial purification of the steroids to be studied, and this can lead to difficulties in recovery and reproducibility between samples. Even when the most highly purified commercially available solvents (e.g., nanograde) are used, solvent impurities will contaminate the sample. Obviously, this is always a problem, but it is most pronounced with the large solvent volumes frequently used in extraction steps. Finally, with the increasing awareness of the long-term toxicity of many solvents, it is desirable to reduce the amount and number of solvents used.

1. *Unconjugated Steroids*

A variety of solvents has been used for extraction of unconjugated steroids from biological fluids. A new procedure based on the well-known salting-out effect was described by Stillwell et al. (1973). A large amount of powdered anhydrous potassium carbonate was added to urine or diluted plasma, which was then extracted with ethyl acetate. Yields of steroids with polarities ranging from that of cholesterol to those of cortisol and estriol were nearly quantitative, and solvent volumes could be kept small. Obviously a large amount of extraneous material will be extracted, and further purification will be necessary in most cases. However, both cortisol and estriol in plasma from pregnant women could be determined directly by GC–MS after derivatization.

A modification of liquid–liquid extraction for isolation of drugs from blood and urine has been described by Breiter et al. (1976). The aqueous fluid to be extracted is absorbed in a column bed of dry diatomaceous earth, which is then eluted with a suitable solvent. The method has been used for extraction of steroids in plasma (Wehner and Handke, 1979; Schöneshöfer et al., 1981) and urine (Ende et al., 1980; Fotsis et al., 1980). Column beds ready for use are available (Extrelut), but it is necessary to wash the bed material exhaustively to remove a variety of contaminants (Ende et al., 1980). The main advantage of the technique is that time-consuming use of separatory funnels is avoided and that solvent volumes can be reduced. The pH and concentration of the sample can also be conveniently adjusted before absorption in the column. The method is not new; it can be compared with the method of absorbing a sample in the stationary phase in dry support prior to application on a chromatography column. A method of this type, combined with salting-out, was employed by Siiteri (1970) for extraction of conjugated steroids in urine. The steroids may be subfractionated by a suitable choice of solvents for the elution. It is possible that further development of this technology can lead to simplified methods, particularly for extraction of tissue steroids. However, liquid–solid methods as described below can be considerably improved and are potentially more useful for extraction of aqueous samples.

Analysis of steroids in tissues is likely to assume an increasing importance in studies of pathological processes where steroid hormones or their precursors and metabolites may play an etiological or modifying role. Quantitative extraction of steroids from tissues without formation of artifacts is difficult, and few studies have been carried out in this area. One problem is that conventional recovery experiments with addition of radioactively labeled steroids are not valid; it is a minimum requirement that added steroids are quantitatively recovered. The only way in which yields can be determined accurately is to use tissues from animals that have been given labeled steroids and are in isotopic equilibrium. Since such experiments are not possible in most instances, it is necessary to evaluate recoveries indirectly. It is of particular importance to use solvents that penetrate both hydrophilic and hydrophobic structures in the tissues. Methods that are based on extractions either with nonpolar (e.g., diethyl ether) or polar (e.g., methanol) solvents are unlikely to be satisfactory.

There are many reports of analyses of steroids in tissues where final quantitation has been performed by GC–MS (see Sections V,D and E) or radioimmunoassay. In most cases conventional solvent extraction has been employed, and it is often impossible to evaluate the efficiency of the extraction process. A combination of liquid and solid extraction has also been described (Albert *et al.*, 1978). In this case the extract, obtained with dimethoxymethane–methanol, 4:1 (v/v), is evaporated with silicic acid, which is then eluted with suitable solvents. Considering the lability of many steroids on adsorbent surfaces and the reactivity of dimethoxymethane, this type of extraction technique cannot be recommended.

Since chloroform–methanol is known to extract lipids of a wide polarity range (see Radin, 1969), we have used a 1:1 (v/v) mixture to extract steroids from corpus luteum and other tissues (Axelson *et al.*, 1974b, 1975, 1981b). It is possible that hexane–isopropanol, 3:2 (v/v), will prove to be useful in many cases (Hara and Radin, 1978). Another method to establish good contact between solvent and tissue has been described by Batra and Bengtsson (1976). They digested uterine tissue in aqueous sodium hydroxide with sodium dodecyl sulfate for 2–3 hours and were then able to extract progesterone quantitatively with ethyl acetate. This procedure could probably be converted to a filter-bed method employing absorption of the aqueous mixture in diatomaceous earth. However, alkali-labile steroids cannot be extracted in this way. An alternative method would be to digest the tissue with a mixture of enzymes and then to extract the aqueous solution with a solid. Since protein binding is a major factor in preventing extraction of steroids, conditions have to be selected that minimize this binding.

2. *Conjugated Steroids*

Methods for extraction of conjugated steroids in urine and blood have been excellently reviewed by Pasqualini (1967) and Siiteri (1970). Most of the old methods have now been replaced by the solid extraction methods discussed in Section II,B. However, there has been an important development in the field of ion-pair extraction. The major conjugated steroids are charged and may be extracted into organic solvents as ion pairs with a nonpolar cation. This principle was used in the steroid field for the first time by McKenna and Norymberski, who extracted sulfates of less polar steroids as salts with methylene blue and pyridine (see Siiteri, 1970). A further development was described by Kushinsky and Tang (see Siiteri, 1970), who used an organic solution of a liquid ion exchanger for extraction of steroid conjugates. Hofmann (1967) showed that conjugated bile acids could be extracted as tetraheptylammonium salts, and this work led to a series of studies by Mattox *et al.* (1972a,b) on the extraction of conjugated steroids by solutions of different nonpolar amines in organic solvents. Further detailed studies of the extraction of polar taurine, glycine, glucuronic, and sulfuric acid conjugates were performed in Schill's laboratory (Fransson and Schill, 1975a,b), where much of the basic work on ion-pair extraction has been carried out (see Schill, 1974, 1981; Schill *et al.*, 1977). The extraction methods described by these groups have rarely been used in steroid analysis, possibly because they require removal of the quaternary ammonium ions and appear to be technically tedious. However, the principle is simple and the method could be considerably simplified, particularly by transformation into a column extraction technique (see Section II,B) and by combining it with a reversed-phase partition purification step (see Section III,B).

An important aspect of ion-pair formation is that biological materials may contain organic cations giving ion pairs with conjugated steroids. These ion pairs may be partly extracted with organic solvents used for supposedly selective extraction of unconjugated steroids. They can also behave as neutral compounds in subsequent purification steps.

B. Extraction with Solids

A variety of adsorbents and liquid-coated supports have been used for extraction of steroids from aqueous solutions. The early development has been reviewed by Pasqualini (1967) and Siiteri (1970). There are obvious technical advantages over liquid–liquid extractions in having column beds that retain steroids from solutions. Development of solid extraction methods has accelerated in the last few years and has involved three main types of adsorbents: polystyrene resins, substituted crosslinked dextrans, and substituted porous silica.

1. *Polystyrene Resins*

The description by Bradlow (1968) of a method for extraction of steroids by the neutral polystyrene resin Amberlite XAD-2 represents a major advance in steroid analysis. The matrix structure of the resin is similar to that of ion exchangers previously tried for extraction of steroids from aqueous solutions (see Pasqualini, 1967; Siiteri, 1970). However, owing to a combination of adsorption, ion exchange, and restricted diffusion in the resin matrix, the latter attempts were not very successful. Since Amberlite XAD-2 has a rigid porous matrix and should not contain charged groups, several of these problems are avoided. Neutral Amberlite resins (XAD-2, XAD-4, XAD-7) have now been widely used for many years for extraction of steroids from aqueous solutions. However, problems have been noted in several laboratories. Polar steroid conjugates are either incompletely adsorbed and partly eluted when the column is washed with water (e.g., Matsui *et al.*, 1975; Derks and Drayer, 1978c) or they are bound in such a way that they are not eluted with methanol (Bradlow, 1977; Yapo *et al.*, 1978).

Evidently the properties of Amberlite XAD-2 have changed during the past 10 years, although changes in the manufacture have not been reported (Bradlow, 1977). Various methods have been used to overcome the difficulties. Losses in the water wash have been reduced by decreasing the volume of water used (Matsui *et al.*, 1975; Derks and Drayer, 1978), which has the obvious drawback that inorganic ions are eluted with the steroids. The firm binding of polar conjugates, particularly pronounced with steroid disulfates, can be overcome by a wash with triethylamine sulfate and water before elution with methanol (Bradlow, 1977). This has the negative effect that triethylamine will contaminate the steroids and influence further treatment of the sample (e.g., hydrolysis, ion exchange). The effect of triethylamine sulfate was originally thought to be due to formation of triethylammonium salts of the steroid sulfates. However, the mechanism is probably much more complex, as seen from the study of Rotsch and Pietrzyk (1980). Formation of electrical double layers, ion exchange, and ion-pair formation may all be involved. More recent studies indicate that Amberlite XAD-2 has ionic sites with high affinity for sulfate anions (Axelson and

Sahlberg, 1981). Thus, nearly quantitative recoveries of steroid disulfates are obtained if the resin is washed with sodium sulfate and water before elution with methanol. In this way, the use of organic cations can be avoided and subsequent steps in the analytical sequence are simplified.

When steroids are to be extracted from aqueous solutions containing proteins, conditions must be chosen that minimize specific and nonspecific protein binding. This can be achieved by elevating the temperature (see Westphal, 1971). Plasma steroids can be extracted by Amberlite XAD-2 at 45°C if 4 volumes of 10% ammonium sulfate are first added to the plasma sample (Spiegelhalder, 1971, cited by Schindler and Sparke, 1975). All unconjugated steroids studied can be extracted by passing plasma diluted with one volume of saline through a bed of Amberlite XAD-2 at 64°C (Axelson and Sjövall, 1974). Steroid monosulfates and glucuronides are also extracted by this method, whereas disulfates are only partially retained by the polymer. Addition of triethylamine sulfate to the diluted plasma results in quantitative extraction also of this group of conjugates (Axelson and Sahlberg, 1981). It is not known whether this is due to ion-pair formation or to a decrease of the ionic interaction between the disulfates and plasma proteins.

Various solvents have been used to elute steroids from Amberlite XAD-2. Methanol was used in the original procedure. Depending on the nature of the steroids and other components in the sample, an additional, less polar, solvent may be required. Stepwise elution can also be used to achieve some purification. Hexane has been used to displace water in the void volume and to remove nonpolar lipids (Makino and Sjövall, 1972), and selective elution with a suitable solvent may be used. However, for quantitative elution of all steroids in the presence of lipids it is advisable to use the sequence methanol, methanol–chloroform, 1:1 (v/v) (Axelson and Sahlberg, 1981).

Numerous modifications of Bradlow's original procedure (1968) have been published. Some authors prefer Amberlite XAD containing phenyl substituents (XAD-4 or XAD-7), and others use batch rather than column techniques. Knowledge of the factors influencing sorption and elution as discussed above should make it possible for the individual scientist to select appropriate conditions. A technically important development is to perform the extraction with small particles of porous polymer packed in a micro precolumn that, after appropriate washing, can be directly attached to the beginning of the chromatographic system to be used for purification or analysis of the sample (Ishii et al., 1978). Another interesting possibility is to perform microchemical reactions when the steroid is adsorbed to the polymer (Roginsky *et al.*, 1975). The validity of such procedures must be documented by careful studies of possible side reactions.

2. *Substituted Dextran Gels*

Sephadex gels substituted with alkyl chains form good stationary phases in alcohol–water mixtures (Ellingboe *et al.*, 1970a). Gels with an appropriate degree of substitution to be just wetted by water, e.g., Lipidex 1000 (containing 10%, w/w, of C_{12}–C_{14} alkyl chains), function as nonpolar adsorbents. If water containing lipid-soluble compounds is passed through a small bed of Lipidex 1000, these compounds are extracted and can then be eluted with methanol or chloroform–methanol (Dyfverman and Sjövall, 1978). High flow rates can be used, e.g., 5–10 ml/minute. Less polar steroids, e.g., testosterone and progesterone, are quantitatively retained whereas cortisol moves more rapidly through the column bed. Such polar steroids can be retarded if 5% *n*-pentylamine is added to the aqueous solution. The amine will also inhibit protein binding and disrupt lipoproteins (Dyfverman and Sjövall, 1978; unpublished results). In the presence of pentylamine, unconjugated plasma steroids of low and medium polarity are extracted (together with lipids) at room temperature. In the absence of amine, steroids of lower polarity can be extracted at an elevated temperature (see above; Dahlberg *et al.*, 1980). Lipidex 1000 can be used to extract unconjugated steroids released by enzyme hydrolysis. If only steroids of low polarity (containing three oxygen substituents or less) have to be extracted, no pentylamine has to be added and a highly purified extract is obtained (Tetsuo *et al.*, 1980).

Phenolic steroids are extracted only at an acidic pH, i.e., not as phenolate anions. Also, in other respects, extraction with Lipidex 1000 shows analogies with a solvent extraction. Thus, it differs from the adsorption on hydrophilic Sephadex G-10 observed with some steroids (Muller *et al.*, 1974). Conjugated steroids, because of their water solubility, are poorly extracted by Lipidex 1000. Studies of the extraction of conjugated bile acids have shown that addition of decyltrimethylammonium bromide to the aqueous solution results in formation of ion pairs that are extracted by Lipidex 1000 (Dyfverman and Sjövall, 1979). It is possible that this principle could be used for charged steroid conjugates (see also Section II,A,2).

A different and selective extraction procedure has been described by Nilsson *et al.* (1979). Nilsson *et al.* coupled immunoglobulin against transcortin to Sepharose 4B and used a bed of this material to adsorb the cortisol–transcortin complex from plasma. After elution of the complex with buffer, cortisol could be extracted and analyzed by high-pressure liquid chromatography (HPLC). The immunosorbent principle could probably be used in different forms for extraction and purification of a variety of steroids. This is illustrated by a paper by Glencross *et al.* (1981) describing the use of estradiol antiserum coupled to Sepharose to extract estradiol from biological fluids. Elution with aqueous acetone yielded a highly purified extract for analysis with radioimmunoassay.

3. Substituted Porous Silica

The rapid development of HPLC has led to synthesis of various types of so-called bonded phases, i.e., silica particles to which organic substituents have been attached. Materials of this type can be used for extraction of substances from aqueous solutions. In an important paper, Shackleton and Whitney (1980) described the use of Sep-Pak C_{18} cartridges for extraction of steroids from urine and enzyme hydrolyzates. These cartridges, about 1×1 cm, contain octadecylsilane bonded-phase packing that will adsorb conjugated as well as unconjugated steroids from an aqueous solution. Thus, while the alkyl substitution is similar to that of Lipidex 1000, the mechanism of steroid sorption is different. Sep-Pak C_{18} behaves more as a polar adsorbent and does not quantitatively extract cholesterol and other nonpolar lipids. In this way it resembles Amberlite XAD-2, but it has a much higher capacity. Thus, steroids in 100 ml of urine may be extracted on one cartridge, and the flow rate can be kept very much higher than with the polystyrene polymer, e.g., 30 ml/minute.

The use of Sep-Pak C_{18} cartridges for extraction of steroids from plasma and milk has been studied by Axelson and Sahlberg (1981). Extraction is performed at 64°C to minimize protein binding, and triethylamine sulfate has to be added to give quantitative yields of steroid disulfates (cf. Amberlite XAD-2 above). Triethylamine sulfate also seems to affect the interaction between steroids and chylomicrons so that quantitative yields of steroids from milk can be obtained even when the lipids are not quantitatively extracted.

When the different solid extraction systems are compared, the method utilizing Sep-Pak C_{18} cartridges appears to be superior for analysis of total steroid profiles. It will largely replace methods based on Amberlite XAD-2 because it is much more rapid, gives better yields of polar corticosteroid metabolites (Shackleton and Whitney, 1980), does not give problems due to ion exchange, and has a much higher capacity. Lipidex 1000 may be used when only unconjugated steroids of low and medium polarity are to be analyzed. In this case it is particularly useful for rapid extraction of enzyme hydrolyzates. It is also the method of choice for extraction of cholesterol and other nonpolar lipids. When both lipids and total steroids are to be recovered, a combination of Lipidex 1000 and Sep-Pak C_{18} may be used, the aqueous effluent from the Lipidex bed being directly passed through the Sep-Pak cartridge.

Further improvements of the solid extraction procedures can be expected. In particular, there is a need for such methods in analyses of steroids in tissues. Protein binding is the main problem and new methods for displacement of steroids from binding sites are needed. One may consider the use of nonselective displacers, e.g., sulfhydryl group reagents (cf. Coty, 1980) or synthetic steroids to displace specific endogenous steroid hormones from their sites (cf. McGinley and Casey, 1979). Such methods combined with the use of Lipidex 1000 and Sep-Pak C_{18} may provide new ways for analysis of steroids in target organs.

III. Purification and Isolation Procedures

The need for purification of steroids prior to the final analysis varies greatly. In all analytical procedures there has to be a balance between the different steps. If the extraction is selective and the detection specific, e.g., selected ion monitoring with a high-resolution GC–MS system, the intermediate purification can be minimal. The same is true when the steroid concentration is high. The choice of purification procedure also depends on the nature of the analysis; it is obvious that analyses of metabolic profiles of total steroids or classes of conjugates require methods that differ from those needed for analysis of a single steroid. The methods may also differ depending on whether the steroids have to be isolated for structure determination or for quantitative analysis. In order to structure the following discussion, methods have been subdivided according to their potential resolving power, i.e., whether they are useful for isolation of individual steroids or better suited for isolation of groups of compounds. For more comprehensive information regarding separation of steroids, the reader is referred to the book by Heftmann (1976).

Important characteristics of all good isolation and purification procedures are that they should be nondestructive, give high yields, and be simple and rapid. A potential for automation is also important to permit use in clinical laboratories and other situations where the number of samples is large. Several methods that are presently used do not fulfill these criteria. This is particularly true of adsorption chromatographic methods, especially when the adsorbent is used in thin layers and the steroids become exposed to oxygen and heat. Since it is very difficult to achieve 100% recoveries in a purification scheme, radioactively labeled steroids are often added to the extracts and correction for low recoveries are based on the yield of radioactivity. However, it is rarely shown that the radioactivity in the final sample represents the steroid added, not the transformation products. Thus, correction for low yields with the aid of radioactive tracers may give grossly misleading results. An example was given by Morreal and Dao (1975). Estrogens were lost after thin-layer chromatography (TLC) and extraction of the silica gel, whereas recovery of added radioactive tracers were good. In this case the chemical transformation occurred in connection with the extraction of the gel and evaporation of the extract. Incorporation of ascorbic acid into the layer improved the results.

Similar additions of antioxidants have been used for a long time to prevent decomposition of steroids in TLC (for references see Lisboa, 1969; Doerr, 1971; Morreal and Dao, 1975). However, addition of reagents may give rise to other artifacts, and the most satisfactory method would be to eliminate reactive materials and solvents from the analytical scheme. This may not be easy since a simple evaporation step may lead to large losses, possibly due to adsorption and decomposition on the glass surface and to reactions between the steroid and other compounds in the extract. The nature of the glass and the solvent may determine the extent of the loss, as described by Burstein (1976) for some 11-oxygenated steroids. There are many similar reports of losses, not only of labile steroids such as α-ketolic steroids, catechol estrogens, 18-oxygenated C_{21} steroids, but also of seemingly stable steroids. We have noted large irreversible losses of bile acid methyl esters when stored as trimethylsilyl (TMS) ethers in hexane in borosilicate glass tubes; these losses are prevented if the samples are stored in methanol and rederivatized before analysis. Probably the TMS ethers react with the glass surface. Most problems with losses become more severe as the amount of steroid decreases and the purity of the biological extracts increases. It is therefore important to select solvents that are as inert as possible and to try to use siliconized glass and Teflon as the only materials with which the extract come into contact.

A. SEPARATION INTO INDIVIDUAL COMPONENTS

The analytical need for separation into individual components has decreased as the specificity of the detection and quantitation methods have increased. With presently available methods for quantitation (see

Section V), isolation of groups of compounds is usually sufficient for quantitation of individual components. The most important recent advance is the use of high-pressure liquid chromatography (HPLC) for separation (and quantitation) of individual steroids. However, some important applications of the older methods should also be mentioned.

1. *Paper and Ion-Exchange Chromatography*

A comprehensive review of paper chromatography appeared in 1967 (Dominguez, 1967). The most interesting development in this field was published subsequently by Mattox and co-workers. In a series of papers they described the use of "liquid ion exchangers" as components of solvent systems for separation of steroid glucosiduronic acids (Mattox et al., 1972c, 1975a,b). Addition of tetraheptylammonium chloride to the mobile phase and KCl to the stationary phase of Zaffaroni- or Bush-type systems (see Bush, 1961) results in a marked increase of the mobility of the glucuronides, which otherwise remain at the starting line. The authors suggested that the partition between the two phases occurred predominantly by an ion-exchange process. In retrospect, the systems are examples of ion-pair chromatography, which is now widely used for separation of charged compounds in partition chromatographic systems (see Section III,A,2). Mattox et al. (1976) also used reversed-phase systems where the nonpolar tetraheptylammonium ions served as stationary phase in the paper, and aqueous solutions of KCl as the mobile phase. Both ion-pair formation and hydrogen bonding seemed to play a role in the chromatographic behavior of steroid glucuronides. The interesting observation was also made that tetraalkylammonium salts influenced the mobility of unconjugated steroids (cf. Section II,B,2). The papers by Mattox et al. (1975b, 1976) contain an abundance of information about the influence of various functional groups on the mobility in different systems. As an aid in the selection of solvents, equations were formulated to characterize resolving properties of chromatographic systems. A procedure was described that was tested on 163 unconjugated steroids in seven TLC systems (from Lisboa, 1969), and on 61 C_{21} steroids of moderate polarity in nine paper chromatographic systems (Mattox and Litwiller, 1979; Mattox et al., 1979). It is difficult to evaluate the practical importance of the method. Perhaps it will be useful in the selection of HPLC systems that could be designed from the paper chromatographic systems.

The separation of individual molecular species of steroid conjugates has also been studied by Kornel and co-workers (Kornel and Saito 1975; Kornel et al., 1975). The systems were of the Bush type, containing neither acids nor bases, to avoid formation of steroid artifacts. The low mobility of the conjugates was compensated for by letting the mobile phase overrun, resulting in very long times of development (up to 90 hours). Some systems included boric acid to improve separation of cortisol metabolites with a glycerol side-chain structure. The separations of individual conjugated steroids were impressive, and the systems have been used in detailed studies of conjugated cortisol metabolites in human urine and blood. In the study cited, 22 monoglucuronides and 7 diglucuronides were identified, both with respect to steroid structure and site of conjugation. The studies also indicated the importance of subfractionation of conjugated steroids prior to analysis of metabolic profiles as discussed in Section VI,A.

Ion-exchange chromatography is playing an increasingly important role in the separation of steroid conjugates. Early results using polystyrene resins were not encouraging (see Bush, 1961; Pasqualini, 1967). After Hähnels separation of estrogen conjugates on DEAE-Sephadex (see Pasqualini, 1967), this method has been improved and become increasingly used, particularly in studies of the metabolism of natural and synthetic estrogens. Hobkirk and Nilsen (1970) used a linear gradient of aqueous sodium chloride to separate individual estrogen conjugates and also achieved some resolution of conjugated neutral steroids (Hobkirk and Davidson, 1971). The separations are only partly due to ion exchange. Estrogen conjugates are eluted later than corresponding conjugates of neutral steroids, and separations of individual sulfated neutral steroids are also most likely due to interactions with the polysaccharide matrix. This is supported by the effect of methanol on the mobilities (Fotsis et al., 1981). When lipophilic ion exchangers are used in aqueous ethanol or methanol (see Section III,B,1), individual mobility differences disappear, and separations depend on the acid strength of the conjugate. Various modifications of the methods of Hähnel and of Hobkirk and Nilsen (1970) have been made. Isocratic elution with aqueous sodium chloride may be advantageous depending on the mixtures to be separated (Musey et al., 1977). The drawback with all the methods is that the separations are slow and the compounds are obtained in large volumes of aqueous sodium chloride.

2. High-Pressure Liquid Chromatography

The HPLC of steroids has been reviewed by Heftmann and Hunter (1979). The literature is growing very rapidly, and it is often difficult to find innovative studies among the routine separations obtained by use of commercially available instruments, columns, and packing materials.

Published separations are still often trivial compared to the separations obtained with TLC (see Lisboa, 1969) and paper chromatography (see Bush, 1961; Dominguez, 1967), except for the speed with which they are obtained. However, the potential of HPLC for efficient, rapid, and quantitative separations both on an analytical and a preparative scale is much greater than that of the older methods, and the possibilities of automation are obvious.

Early separations of steroids by HPLC were achieved with adsorption chromatography or reversed-phase partition chromatography with two immiscible solvent phases. In one of the first applications, a nonpolar amine coated on a trifluoroethylene polymer was used as stationary phase, and interesting effects of different functional groups were observed (Siggia and Dishman, 1970). After preparation of silica supports with covalently bound functional groups (e.g., long alkyl, phenyl, cyanoalkyl, nitro, or pyrrolidone groups), reversed-phase systems can be obtained with water containing a suitable percentage of methanol, isopropanol, acetonitrile, tetrahydrofuran, or dioxane as mobile phase. Thus, stability problems associated with the use of two immiscible solvent phases are avoided. The systems are analogous to those previously developed based on alkylated Sephadex (see Section III,B,2). In straight-phase systems, hydrophilic silica particles are stationary phases together with polar components of the mobile phase, which may consist of mixtures of hydrocarbons, chlorinated hydrocarbons, alcohols, and water. Nonaqueous systems of the conventional adsorption chromatography type are also used.

Since detailed information can be obtained in the review by Heftmann and Hunter (1979), only a few examples will be given where comparisons of different systems have been made in the separation of a larger number of steroids from biological extracts. O'Hare et al. (1976) used three solvent gradients (methanol–water, acetonitrile–water, and dioxane–water) in a reversed-phase system with an octadecylsilane bonded phase to separate 43 steroids in studies of steroid secretion by human adrenal and testis cell cultures. Later, they compared the properties of different types of octadecylsilane bonded phases and found each to exhibit different selectivity toward certain functional groups (Nice and O'Hare, 1978). Studies of this type will undoubtedly result in the manufacture of improved stationary phases. A more superficial comparison of systems for separation of synthetic steroid drugs has been made (Tymes, 1977).

In a study of testicular steroids, Cochran and Ewing (1979) separated 14 steroids by reversed-phase chromatography. Celite columns had to be used for preliminary group separation. Considering the efficiency of the latter separations, it should be possible to improve the HPLC system considerably. Combinations of reversed-phase and adsorption systems have been used to fractionate C_{18} and C_{19} steroids in studies of ovarian and testicular steroid metabolism (Satyaswaroop *et al.*, 1977; Kautsky and Hagerman, 1979). The paper by Kautsky and Hagerman exemplifies the value of HPLC in metabolic studies with radioactively labeled steroids, and it also illustrates the need for preliminary purification as discussed in Section III,B.

Lin *et al.* (1980) compared reversed-phase and adsorption chromatography for separation of 25 isomeric $C_{21}O_2$ steroids. It was concluded that a combination of reversed-phase and adsorption chromatography is needed to resolve complex mixtures. Other comparisons, aiming at the selection of systems suitable for separation of clinically important steroid hormones prior to immunoassays, have been made (Schöneshöfer and Dulce, 1979). With the steroids studied, and the need for evaporation of solvents prior to assays, an adsorption system using hydroxyl-substituted silica and nonaqueous solvents was superior to other systems. Schöneshöfer *et al.* (1981) have published a detailed evaluation of automated HPLC as a means of purifying a large number of steroids before radioimmunoassay. A DIOL column was used in a hexane–isopropanol gradient. A similar type of system has been used by Williams and Goldzieher (1979) for separation of ethynyl estrogens and their metabolites. These studies clearly illustrate the value of the hydroxyl-substituted phases, both for purification of individual steroids and for separation of mixtures of radioactively labeled metabolites.

Since one of the advantages of HPLC over GLC is that the compounds do not have to be volatilized, HPLC should be particularly useful for isolation and analysis of conjugated steroids. Van der Wal and Huber (1974, 1977, 1978) have made extensive studies of the separation of estrogen conjugates and have obtained impressive results. The early systems were based on cellulose ion exchangers. While ion exchange is a major factor in the separations (e.g., glucuronides elute before sulfates, a free phenolic hydroxyl group increases retention), other mechanisms also operate to give separations according to steroid structure. In later studies, the same authors (1978) compared a variety of bonded phases with and without ion exchanging groups with conventional ion exchangers and ion-pair chromatography. It is not possible to summarize the results in a limited space, and the original paper should be consulted for a choice of systems. Very rapid separations of estrogen conjugates (2 minutes) were achieved on octadecyl silica with phosphate buffer containing cetyltrimethylammonium bromide as the mobile phase. The latter was assumed to adsorb to the surface of the substituted silica and act as an ion-pairing agent to retard the steroid conjugates. However, it is not clear whether ion-pair formation occurs in the aqueous phase as is the case in the ion-pair extraction method using Lipidex 1000 (see Section II,B,2).

Musey *et al.* (1978) studied the separation of estrogen conjugates with a strong anion exchanger bonded on silica. Their results were more promising than those of van der Wal and Huber (1978) with similar materials from other manufacturers. While the Dutch group had problems with long-term stability of the packing material, Musey *et al.* did not report such problems. The two groups also used different mobile phases; Musey *et al.* used aqueous NaCl, similar to the system with DEAE-Sephadex (see Section III,A,1).

Ion-pair chromatography, pioneered by Schill and co-workers (1977, 1981), has also been applied to the separation of steroid conjugates. Fransson *et al.* (1976) used a straight-phase system, and since this makes the direct injection of biological fluids impossible, Hermansson (1978) studied reversed-phase systems in which a stationary phase of pentanol was coated on octadecyl silica. Phosphate buffer containing a quaternary ammonium ion was used as mobile phase. Reversed-phase adsorption systems in which a low percentage of pentanol was added to the mobile phase in the absence of the hydrophobic counterion were also studied (Hermansson, 1980).

The detection of steroids in HPLC is a problem when the compounds have no specific UV-absorption. Derivatization with UV-absorbing or fluorescent reagents has been used to increase sensitivity and specificity in quantitative work (see Section V,A). HPLC-separations of the cortoic acids as p-bromophenacyl esters have been reported (Farhi and Monder, 1978). These and similar derivatives have been used in analyses of fatty acids and bile acids. High-sensitivity detection of estrogens has been obtained by allowing the phenolic hydroxyl to react with dansyl chloride to yield a fluorescent derivative (Schmidt *et al.*, 1978). The 3-keto group of neutral steroids can be converted into a dansyl hydrazone (Kawasaki *et al.*, 1979). An interesting possibility is to use an enzyme reactor containing an immobilized enzyme at the end of the column. Cholesterol oxidase was used in this way to convert steroids with the cholesterol A,B-ring structure into UV-absorbing 3-keto-4-ene steroids (Ögren *et al.*, 1980). Estrogens, in particular catechol estrogens, are suitable for electrochemical detection, and this method is likely to become of considerable importance, e.g., in studies of catechol estrogens in brain (Shimada *et al.*, 1979; Smyth and Frischkorn, 1980).

In connection with their work on this method, Shimada *et al.* (1979) also achieved a reversed-phase separation of the 1- and 4-glutathione conjugates of 2-hydroxyestrone.

The development of HPLC techniques is only in its beginning. Besides the technical improvements that can be made, exemplified by the micro-liquid chromatography of Ischii and co-workers (1978), one may expect development of new packing materials giving better resolution and higher efficiencies. An example is the use of bonded pyrrolidone for separation of estrogens (Mourey and Siggia, 1980). Liquid crystals are being tested as stationary phases, and bonded phases with properties of liquid crystals may be developed (Taylor and Sherman, 1979, 1980). There are already automated systems for purification of compounds before immunoassay, GC–MS, or mass spectrometry (de Ridder and van Hal, 1978), and these could be coupled to automated precolumns extracting the steroids from the biological fluid before the separation (see e.g., Ischii *et al.,* 1978). At the present stage of development it should be possible to construct automated systems of the reversed-phase type combining, e.g., Sep-Pak C_{18} extraction (see Section II,B,3), lipophilic ion exchange filtration (see Section III,B,1), and HPLC.

B. SEPARATION INTO GROUPS

Group separations can be made simple, inexpensive, and rapid. Unless there is a particular need for isolation of individual steroids, a suitable group separation step is usually the most convenient way to purify biological extracts. Groups can be defined as steroids that have the same substituents (e.g., glucuronides, sulfates, phenolic steroids, 3-keto-4-ene steroids) or are within a certain polarity range. High-resolution methods discussed in Section III,A may be used for group separations. However, the low-resolution methods discussed in this section are usually simpler and cheaper and have the higher capacity needed of methods to be used as the first step in the sample purification.

1. *Based on Mode of Conjugation*

Steroid metabolites are excreted largely in a conjugated form. Conjugation is a substrate-selective process and may determine the metabolic fate of the steroid. Thus, analysis of steroids of a defined conjugate class is more informative than analysis after initial hydrolysis of the total mixture.

Since the conjugate classes differ in acidity, they may be separated by anion-exchange chromatography. When hydrophilic ion exchangers are used in water, nonionic interactions result in separation of individual steroids (see Section III,A,1), and such systems are less suitable for group separations. The synthesis of lipophilic ion exchangers from Sephadex LH-20 (Ellingboe *et al.*, 1970b; Almé and Nyström, 1971) provided materials that permitted rapid ion exchange with high capacity in organic solvents. Small columns of diethylaminohydroxypropyl Sephadex LH-20 (DEAP-LH-20, Lipidex-DEAP) were used by Setchell *et al.* (1976a) to obtain group separation of unconjugated steroids, monoglucuronides, monosulfates, and disulfates. Aqueous ethanol was used as solvent, and acetate buffers were chosen to be compatible with enzymatic hydrolysis after removal of the ethanol. A modified elution sequence also permitted separation of A-ring from D-ring glucuronides of estrogens (Setchell *et al.*, 1979). Before application on DEAP-LH-20, the biological extract had to be passed through a strong cation exchanger in H^+ form. If this step was omitted, steroid conjugates were sometimes eluted in the neutral fraction, possibly due to formation of ion pairs with organic cations. The lipophilic cation exchanger originally used had a low capacity, and subsequent work has shown that commercially available SP-Sephadex can be used in 70% methanol and is preferable because of its higher capacity (Tetsuo *et al.*, 1980). A lipophilic cation exchanger, sulfohydroxypropyl Sephadex LH-20 (SP-LH-20), has been synthesized (Axelson and Sjövall, 1979); it has the additional advantage that it can be alkylated to reduce its polarity further.

Problems with the use of DEAP-LH-20 have been encountered in some laboratories. These are probably related to the fact that it is a weak ion exchanger. For example, if the amount of organic acids is high in a pathological sample, the effluent from the cation exchanger must be neutralized before passage into DEAP-LH-20 to permit adequate sorption of the steroid conjugates. These problems are largely avoided by use of the stronger triethylamino derivative, TEAP-LH-20 (Axelson *et al.*, 1981c). This ion exchanger has been used in OH^- form in a simplified method for separation of conjugated steroids in urine (Axelson *et al.*, 1981c) and plasma (Axelson and Sahlberg, 1981). An alternative method using commercially available DEAE-Sephadex in methanol has also been developed (Fotsis *et al.*, 1981). This gives a separation of conjugated estrogens from corresponding conjugates of neutral steroids, which is an advantage in analysis of estrogens, since separations of unconjugated estrogens from neutral steroids on an ion exchanger results in partial destruction of alkali-labile estrogens (see Section III,B,3,a). The major disadvantage is that the chromatography is more time-consuming than that using TEAP-LH-20.

Methods other than ion exchange have also been used for separation and isolation of groups of steroid conjugates. Thus, mono- and disulfates of neutral steroids in urine and plasma have been analyzed in great detail (see Section VI,A) after group separation on Sephadex LH-20 with 0.01 M NaCl in methanol–chloroform as eluent (Sjövall and Vihko, 1966b; Jänne et al., 1969). The sodium salts of the sulfates have different mobilities and separate from unconjugated steroids and glucuronides that elute early together with lipids. The solvents have also been modified for separation of estrogen conjugates (Tikkanen and Adlercreutz, 1970). The columns and solvent volumes have to be larger than with ion exchangers, and the method is not suitable for isolation of glucuronides.

High-voltage electrophoresis has been used by Kornel and co-workers (Miyabo and Kornel, 1974; Kornel and Saito, 1975). In their extensive studies of cortisol metabolites in plasma, several electrophoretic runs were required for complete separation of conjugate classes. This may be due to a low capacity, and ion exchange chromatography therefore seems more suitable for the preliminary group separation.

Although chromatography on lipophilic ion exchangers in organic solvents seems to be the simplest and most rapid method for group separation of steroid conjugates, it should be emphasized that only common types of conjugates have been studied. However, the method is flexible, and systems could probably be developed for isolation of mixed and unusual conjugates. If present, positively charged conjugates could probably be separated on the lipophilic cation exchanger.

Since mass spectrometric, GC–MS, and LC–MS methods have not yet reached the stage that permits analysis of complex mixtures of conjugated steroids (see Section IV), it is necessary to hydrolyze the conjugates. This is usually the most uncontrolled and time-consuming step in sample preparation procedures. Enzymatic hydrolysis may be incomplete due to enzyme specificity, e.g., poor hydrolysis of sulfate esters at C-17, C-20, and C-3α(5α) by most sulfatase preparations (see Bradlow, 1970). Solvolysis of sulfates may result in undesired side reactions. A recent evaluation of different hydrolytic procedures for urinary steroids has been made by Vestergaard (1978). Problems due to the presence of enzyme inhibitors of low (e.g., sugar acids and lactones) and high molecular weight can be eliminated by Amberlite XAD-2 (or Sep-Pak) extraction (Graef et al., 1977; Albrecht et al., 1975). Addition of sodium sulfate decreases the effect of a high molecular inhibitor (Graef et al., 1977; Nishikaze and Kobayashi, 1977), but this will obviously inhibit sulfate hydrolysis. Enzyme preparations often contain compounds that interfere in GC–MS analyses or radioimmunoassays. Filtration of the enzyme–buffer solution through Amberlite XAD-2 (Carlström and Sköldefors, 1977) or Lipidex 1000 (Tetsuo *et al.*, 1980) is a suitable way to remove such contaminants immediately before use.

Elevated temperatures have long been used to increase rates of hydrolysis. When preparations of *Helix pomatia* were employed, the yield of steroids was the same after a few hours at 50–55°C as with conventional prolonged incubations at lower temperatures (Albrecht *et al.*, 1975; Nishikaze and Kobayashi, 1977). High concentrations of enzyme have to be used at these temperatures. Another possibility to increase the rate of hydrolysis is to add a low percentage of solvent to the incubation mixture. Pesheck and Lovrien (1977) obtained a ninefold increase of glucuronidase activity upon addition of 5% *t*-butanol, and showed that this was due to a cosolvent effect on V_{max} as well as to a decrease of the substrate inhibition. It is possible that improved hydrolytic methods can be developed by use of such solvent effects.

2. *Based on Polarity*

The most common way to purify unconjugated steroids is to try to remove contaminants more and less polar than the steroid to be determined. Column adsorption chromatography has long been used for this purpose. Group fractionation on small silicic acid columns (see Jänne *et al.*, 1969) is still being used in many laboratories. However, there is an obvious risk for chemical transformation and loss of polar steroids on these columns. Magnesium oxide, described as a superior adsorbent (Kawahara *et al.*, 1980), appears to have similar drawbacks judging from the recoveries of simple steroids, which were 62–83%. Scandrett and Ross (1976) separated corticosteroids on polyamide layers and found this method superior to the use of Sephadex LH-20 in the same solvent system. Recoveries were the same for the two methods.

Because of their inertness and relative simplicity in use, coated Celite and lipophilic Sephadex derivatives have been the most frequently used column materials. Celite columns carrying ethylene or propylene glycol as stationary phase (Siiteri, 1963) have a high loading capacity. Volatile solvents, e.g., isooctane containing ethyl acetate and in some cases an alcohol, have been used as mobile phase in separations of less polar steroids, such as estrogens, androgens, and progestins, before radioimmunoassay (Abraham *et al.*, 1970, 1972). The method is less suitable for compounds with high polarity (e.g., corticosteroids) particularly before GLC, since an increase of the polarity of the mobile phase results in elution of nonvolatile stationary phase.

In liquid–gel chromatography with lipophilic Sephadex derivatives, the stationary phase is created by the gel and solvent components (Sjövall *et al.* 1968b; Ellingboe *et al.*, 1970a). Depending on the polarity of the derivative and the solvents used, the stationary phase becomes more (straight-phase system) or less (reversed-phase system) polar than the mobile phase.

The early derivatives, methyl and hydroxypropyl Sephadex, do not swell in nonpolar solvents, and the latter, Sephadex LH-20, has been widely used for separation of steroids in straigh-phase systems prior to GC–MS or immunoassay. Solvents are often based on mixtures of a hydrocarbon (hexane, cyclohexane, benzene, heptane, or isooctane), a chlorinated hydrocarbon (chloroform or methylene chloride), and an alcohol (methanol, ethanol, or *t*-butanol), in some cases with addition of water (Nyström and Sjövall, 1968; Eneroth and Nyström, 1967; Murphy, 1971; Carr *et al.*, 1971). The polarity of the solvent may be controlled by the amount of alcohol added. The alcohol content is usually less than 10% in separations of less polar estrogens (Lisboa and Strassner, 1975), androgens and progestins (Murphy, 1971; Murphy and d'Aux, 1975; Golder and Sippel, 1976; Ganjam, 1976; Bègue *et al.*, 1976), and alcohol was omitted in separations of vitamin D_3 metabolites (Holick and de Luca, 1971). When more polar steroids are to be purified, e.g., corticosteroids or estrogens, the hydrocarbon may be omitted. Methylene chloride containing a low percentage of methanol has been frequently used (Murphy, 1971; Sippel *et al.* 1975; Scandrett and Ross, 1976; Thomas *et al.* 1977). Alternatively, the chlorinated hydrocarbon is omitted with a simultaneous increase of the alcohol content (Seki, 1967; Setchell and Shackleton, 1973; Lebel *et al.* 1975). Rao *et al.* (1979) used such a system (benzene–methanol, 85 : 15) in a study of estrogen metabolites in bovine liver, and separated unconjugated steroids as well as a glucoside and a glucosiduronic acid conjugate. Seki and Sugase (1969) have used butanol with 1% water for separation of corticosteroids. Although Sephadex derivatives are less compatible with solvents containing carbonyl groups, ethyl acetate or acetone have been used in a few systems (Sippel *et al.*, 1978; Gips *et al.*, 1980). Reversed-phase chromatography on Sephadex LH-20 in water has been used for purification of aldosterone and other corticosteroids (Kachel and Mendelsohn, 1979).

The synthesis of Sephadex derivatives containing long alkyl (Ellingboe *et al.*, 1968, 1970a), hydroxycholanyl (Anderson *et al.*, 1973a), or hydroxycyclohexyl residues (Anderson *et al.*, 1973b) has provided stable hydrophobic materials, which swell in a wide range of solvents and can be used both for straight-phase and reversed-phase chromatography. Straight-phase systems with Lipidex 5000 (hydroxyalkyl Sephadex LH-20) are usually more suitable for separation of less polar steroids than systems using Sephadex LH-20. Solvents usually consist of a hydrocarbon (petroleum ether, hexane, cyclohexane, benzene, or toluene) and a low percentage of a chlorinated hydrocarbon (chloroform or methylene chloride) (Ellingboe et al., 1970a). Such systems have been widely employed for separation of androgens and progestins prior to GC–MS or radioimmunoassay (Holmdahl and Sjövall, 1971; Ruokonen and Vihko, 1974; Jänne et al., 1974; Apter et al., 1975, 1976; Hammond et al., 1977; Fairclough et al., 1977). Nonpolar 16-androstenes have been separated by use of n-pentane with 0.5% cyclohexane (Bicknell and Gower, 1975). Solvents for separation of polar steroids often contain an alcohol (ethanol, isopropanol, t-butanol) (Anderson et al., 1974a,b; Boreham et al., 1978; Goldzieher et al., 1978), but benzene (Anderson et al., 1974a,b; Berthou et al., 1976) or light petroleum–chloroform, 1:1 (Apter et al., 1975) have also been used. As a guide in the choice of solvent polarity, the mobilities of a number of steroids on Lipidex 5000 in hexane–chloroform mixtures and hexane–t-butanol are listed in Tables I and II.

Reversed-phase chromatography has been employed for purification of nonpolar compounds such as 16-androstenes with 75% aqueous methanol (Ruokonen and Vihko, 1974) and vitamin D_3 in methanol (De Leenheer and Cruyl, 1978). Such systems provide simple means for removal of nonpolar lipids from extracts of tissues or plasma. A mixture of methanol–water–chloroform, 9:1:2, or 72% aqueous methanol, gives rapid elution of steroid hormones, while cholesterol and other neutral lipids are retained on the column (Axelson et al., 1974b; Axelson and Sjövall, 1974; Tetsuo et al., 1980). These systems are also formed with hydroxylalkylated ion exchangers (Axelson and Sjövall 1977, 1979; Tetsuo et al., 1980).

When selecting a gel–solvent system for separation of steroids according to polarity, it is usually most convenient to use a straight-phase system in which solvents are volatile and readily removed. Systems with Lipidex 5000 are more suitable for less polar steroids (see Anderson et al., 1974a). In contrast to Sephadex LH-20, this gel swells in the nonpolar solvents, e.g., hexane–chloroform, that have to be used in such separations. Systems based on Sephadex LH-20 are usually better for polar steroids, since more-polar solvents can be used with this gel, e.g., cyclohexane–ethanol (Setchell and Shackelton, 1973) or hexane–chloroform–ethanol–water (Nyström and Sjövall, 1968). Reversed-phase systems are best suited for preliminary fractionation of the crude biological extract.

TABLE I

RELATIVE ELUTION VOLUMES[a] OF C_{19} STEROIDS ON LIPIDEX 5000 IN SOLVENTS OF DIFFERENT POLARITY

Steroid[b]	Solvent system[c]			
	H–C 9:1	H–C 8:2	H–C 7:3	H–t-BuOH 9:1
$A^{4,16}$-3-one	0.19	0.43	0.35	—
A^4-3,17-one	0.24	0.34	0.55	0.49
19-nor-A^4-3,17-one	0.46	0.42	—	0.57
A^4-15α-ol-3,17-one	—	3.05	2.24	1.50
A^4-17α-ol-3-one	0.70	0.81	—	0.67
A^4-17β-ol-3-one	0.79	0.88	1.00	0.67
19-nor-A^4-17β-ol-3-one	0.84	1.00	—	0.74
17α-Me-A^4-17β-ol-3-one	0.43	0.61	0.77	0.60
5αA-17β-ol-3-one	—	—	—	0.57
A^4-1β,17β-ol-3-one	—	—	5.58	—
A^4-2α,17β-ol-3-one	1.59	1.48	1.35	—
A^4-4,17β-ol-3-one	0.92	1.10	1.11	—
A^4-11α,17β-ol-3-one	—	—	6.00	—
A^4-14α,17β-ol-3-one	—	3.91	3.01	—
A^4-15β,17β-ol-3-one	—	—	3.86	—
A^4-16α,17β-ol-3-one	—	—	7.42	—
A^4-16β,17β-ol-3-one	—	3.37	2.70	—
A^4-19,17β-ol-3-one	—	—	5.46	—
A^5-3β-ol-17-one	0.79	0.97	1.04	0.54
$A^{5,15}$-3β-ol-17-one	0.92	1.06	1.19	0.65
A^5-3β,16α-ol-17-one	—	—	2.55	1.04
5βA-3α,11β-ol-17-one	—	3.55	2.82	1.20
5αA-3β,12β-ol-17-one	1.16	1.16	1.24	0.80

[a] Relative to that of P^4-17α-ol-3,20-one, which had the following elution volumes expressed as total column volumes: 6.0 in H–C, 9:1; 2.6 in H–C, 8:2; 1.5 in H–C, 7:3; and 3.5 in H–t-BuOH, 9:1.

[b] A = androstane; superscript indicates position of double bond; Greek letters, configuration of hydroxyl groups.

[c] H = light petroleum; C = chloroform; t-BuOH = tertiary butanol.

The major disadvantage with liquid–gel chromatographic systems is that the flow rates must be low because of restricted diffusion in the gel phase. This problem may be solved by use of smaller gel particles that can give very high column efficiencies (Nyström and Sjövall, 1968; Sjövall et al., 1968b). Advantages with lipophilic gels are inertness and low bleed, giving high yields and little contamination, high sample capacity, ease of column preparation, and possibility of repeated use. Several of the papers cited have described automated or semiauto-

TABLE II

RELATIVE ELUTION VOLUMES[a] OF C_{21} STEROIDS ON LIPIDEX 5000 IN SOLVENTS OF DIFFERENT POLARITY

Steroid[b]	Solvent system[c]			
	H–C 9:1	H–C 8:2	H–C 7:3	H–t-BuOH 9:1
P^4-3,20-one	0.21	0.33	0.49	0.45
P^4-20α-ol-3-one	0.51	—	—	—
P^4-20β-ol-3-one	0.44	—	0.66	—
P^5-3β-ol-20-one	0.67	0.90	0.99	0.48
$P^{5,16}$-3β-ol-20-one	0.56	0.89	1.00	0.50
P^4-3,11,20-one	0.32	0.42	0.50	—
6α-Me-P^4-3,11,20-one	0.27	0.42	0.47	—
P^4-6β-ol-3,20-one	1.32	1.12	—	0.70
5βP-3α,6α-ol-20-one	—	—	4.64	—
5αP-3β-ol-7,20-one	—	1.20	1.22	0.88
P^4-11α-ol-3,20-one	1.78	1.42	1.26	1.22
5βP-3α,11α-ol-20-one	—	—	2.28	1.48
P^4-11β-ol-3,20-one	1.38	1.12	1.07	1.23
6α-Me-11β-ol-3,20-one	1.17	1.00	—	1.08
5βP-3α,11β,20β-ol	—	—	4.69	—
P^4-15α-ol-3,20-one	—	—	1.53	—
P^4-15β-ol-3,20-one	—	—	1.27	—
P^4-16α-ol-3,20-one	—	1.59	1.30	0.93
P^5-3β,16α-ol-20-one	—	—	3.76	1.04
5βP-3α,16α-ol-20-one	—	3.16	—	—
P^4-17α-ol-3,20-one	1.00	1.00	1.00	1.00
P^5-3β,17α-ol-20-one	—	2.80	2.10	1.16
P^4-21-ol-3,20-one	0.43	0.55	0.68	0.75
5βP-20β,21-ol-3-one	—	3.45	2.79	1.21
P^4-15α-ol-3,11,20-one	—	3.77	2.47	2.54
P^4-17α-ol-3,11,20-one	—	1.91	1.57	1.63
P^4-21-ol-3,11,20-one	—	—	0.83	1.76
5βP-3α,21-ol-11,20-one	—	2.81	2.15	1.80
P^4-11β,21-ol-3,20-one	—	3.25	2.25	2.07
P^4-6β,11α-ol-3,20-one	—	>5	6.2	2.28
P^4-15α,21-ol-3,20-one	—	4.32	3.16	3.30
P^4-15β,21-ol-3,20-one	—	3.76	2.58	3.12
P^4-17α,21-ol-3,20-one	—	4.47	3.03	1.70
P^4-11β,17α,21-ol-3,20-one	—	—	>10	—

[a] Relative to that of P^4-17α-ol-3,20-one, which had the following elution volumes expressed as total column volumes: 6.0 in H–C, 9:1, 2.6 in H–C, 8:2, 1.5 in H–C, 7:3, and 3.5 in H–t-BuOH, 9:1.

[b] P = pregnane; superscript indicates position of double bond; greek letters, configuration of hydroxyl groups.

[c] H = light petroleum; C = chloroform; t-BuOH = tertiary butanol.

mated multicolumn systems for purification of steroids prior to radioimmunoassays, and these are equally useful for GC–MS analysis of selected groups of steroids.

3. Based on Specific Substituents

A few selective isolation procedures for unconjugated steroids have been described that are based on the presence of a specific substituent. These procedures may be used when only one group of steroids is of interest and will increase the specificity and usually simplify the analysis.

a. *Phenolic Steroids.* Conventional separations of estrogens from neutral steroids are based on partition between an organic solvent and aqueous alkali. This is a crude method, and polar neutral steroids as well as stronger acids will appear in the phenolic fraction. A more selective method was described by Eberlein (1969), who used the strong anion exchanger Amberlite AG1-X2 in carbonate form to sorb phenolic estrogens from a solution in methanol. They could then be eluted with aqueous methanol. This or similar procedures have been used in several laboratories (see Adessi *et al.,* 1975; Pierrat *et al.,* 1976; Cohen *et al.,* 1978). Obviously other phenolic compounds will appear in the eluate. Since losses of steroids may occur on polystyrene resins (see Siiteri, 1970), it is better to use lipophilic ion exchangers without adsorptive properties. Triethylaminohydroxypropyl Sephadex LH-20 in OH^- form takes up phenolic steroids from a variety of solvents. The estrogens can then be quantitatively eluted by saturation of the solvent with CO_2 (Axelson and Sjövall, 1977). This method has been used for analysis of estrogens in plasma (Axelson and Sjövall, 1977), urine, and tissues (Axelson *et al.,* 1981b,c). A disadvantage is the destruction of catechol estrogens by the strongly basic ion exchanger. This group could be recovered in better yields with DEAE-Sephadex in base form in methanol containing ascorbic acid (Järvenpää *et al.,* 1979; Fotsis *et al.,* 1980). Since estrogens are less firmly sorbed by the weaker ion exchanger, there is a risk of losses if the columns are washed with large volumes of solvent. Catechol estrogens have also been isolated by partition between an organic solvent and aqueous borate buffers containing ascorbic acid (Gelbke *et al.,* 1976). A quantitative evaluation of the method by GC–MS is still lacking. However, studies of borate complex–anion exchange chromatography, as used in carbohydrate separations, might yield a useful method.

b. *3-Ketosteroids.* Most of the biologically active neutral steroids possess a 3-keto group. A method for selective isolation of these compounds for GC–MS analysis is based on the observation that oximes of ketosteroids are positively charged in methanol and are retained by a lipophilic strong cation exchanger (Axelson and Sjövall, 1976). Oximes of 17- and 20-ketosteroids are eluted much faster than those of 3-ketosteroids. Originally, sulfoethyl Sephadex LH-20 was used as the ion exchanger, but it has been replaced by the sulfohydroxypropyl derivative (SP-LH-20), which can be synthesized with 10 times higher capacity (Axelson and Sjövall, 1979). This permits use of smaller columns and selective isolation also of 17- or 20-ketosteroids. The mobilities depend on position and number of oxime groups and on the presence of neighboring groups. The method is selective, relatively rapid, and gives high recoveries. Since trimethylsilyl ethers of oximes are not always favorable for GC–MS, the unsubstituted oximes may be converted into methyloximes prior to analysis (Axelson, 1978).

c. *Ethynyl Steroids*. Synthetic steroids that possess an ethynyl group are widely used for contraception. Selective isolation of this group is important, since the steroids and their metabolites are usually present in low concentrations in tissues and body fluids. The ability of silver ions to form complexes with the triple bond has been utilized. Early methods used silica gel or Florisil impregnated with silver nitrate (Ercoli *et al.*, 1964; Kulkarni and Goldzieher, 1969) and were less suitable for analysis of trace amounts of ethynyl steroids. Pellizari *et al.* (1973) showed that the silver form of sulfoethyl cellulose retained ethynyl steroids and developed a method for isolation of these compounds. This method was simplified, and the capacity was increased by use of the silver form of SP-Sephadex (or SP-LH-20) in aqueous methanol. Hexyne was added as displacing agent to elute the ethynyl steroids (Tetsuo *et al.*, 1980). The purity and recoveries of the steroids were high. The main problem, specific for ion exchangers in silver form, was leakage of silver ions that interfered with subsequent extraction and derivatization. This was overcome by use of a short bed of ion exchanger in acid form as a trap. The column preparation has been simplified, and elution of ethynyl steroids can be conveniently achieved with acetylene in methanol (Andersson *et al.*, 1981).

4. General Purification Scheme

Neutral and ion-exchanging derivatives of Sephadex and Lipidex can be used in the design of generally applicable methods for isolation of steroids from biological materials. The synthetic procedures are simple and can be used to prepare derivatives with desired properties both with respect to ion-exchanging groups and polarity (see Ellingboe *et al.*, 1970a,b; Almé and Nyström, 1971; Setchell *et al.*, 1976a; Axelson and Sjövall, 1974, 1977, 1979; Testsuo *et al.*, 1980). As new derivatives have been synthesized, the purification schemes have been improved and simplified. The principle has been to use a series of small gel bed filters that retain either the steroids or the unwanted material.

At present, the following sequence may be suggested. The desalted biological extract (see Section II), dissolved in 72% methanol, is filtered through hydroxyalkylated SP-LH-20 in H^+ form. This nonpolar bed retains organic bases and lipids such as cholesterol. Neutral and acidic steroids appear in the effluent, which is directly passed through a bed of TEAP-LH-20. This filter retains phenolic steroids, acidic conjugates, and acidic contaminants. Neutral steroids can be collected in the effluent for further purification according to polarity or presence of a 3-keto group. In many cases they are sufficiently purified for derivatization, provided that the reaction mixture is filtered through Lipidex 5000 prior to GC–MS analysis (see Section IV,B,2,a). If present, neutral conjugates can also be isolated from this fraction.

The cation exchanger contains basic compounds that may be of interest for analysis. These may be recovered, e.g., by elution with dilute ammonia or buffers. A GC–MS analysis of tamoxifen and one of its metabolites has been based on this principle (Daniel et al., 1979). Basic steroid drugs and possibly existing basic conjugates could be isolated in the same way. In addition to positively charged steroids, fatty acid esters of less polar C_{19} and C_{21} steroids are likely to be retained by the cation exchanger in the reversed-phase system. Such compounds have been found in steroidogenic tissue (Albert et al., 1980). If present in a biological extract, they could be isolated by elution of the cation exchanger with methanol–chloroform.

The anion exchanger contains the phenolic steroids and acidic conjugates that can be separately eluted as described above. This is more conveniently done if the lipids have been removed in the preceding filter rather than on a nonpolar anion exchanger as originally described (Axelson and Sjövall, 1977).

When conjugated steroids are analyzed, the hydrolyzed fractions should be passed through the anion exchanger a second time. Compounds that remain acidic after the hydrolysis are retained, and neutral steroids are eluted in purified form. This is also important for the derivatization, since acidic compounds can influence the reactions and decrease the stability of the derivatives. Partition between a solvent and alkaline water has been used for the same purpose in many methods. This is not recommended, since polar steroids can be lost in the water phase. The anion exchanger is also useful for purification of acidic unconjugated steroids, as exemplified in bile acid analysis (Almé et al., 1977). An ion-exchange procedure was also used by Boreham et *al.* (1978) for purification of steroidal spirolactones, which could be isolated as acids and purified as lactones using a combination of DEAE-Sephadex and Lipidex 5000 columns. Cortoic acids could also be conveniently isolated on an ion exchanger. In all cases, derivatization reaction mixtures are best purified by rapid filtration through Lipidex 5000.

IV. IDENTIFICATION OF STEROIDS

There are two main types of identification problems in biomedical research: (*a*) identification of previously known steroids, e.g., in analyses of metabolic profiles; and (*b*) identification of new steroids. In the former case, GC–MS is usually sufficient, with or without comparison with authentic compounds, and with or without use of microchemical reactions. The same may be true in the latter case when the number of substituents is small [e.g., $C_{21}O_3$ steroids (Sjövall and Sjövall, 1968)]. However, mistakes in assignment of stereochemistry of polyhydroxylated steroids can be made when only GC–MS is used to analyze products of derivatization and microchemical reactions [e.g., $C_{21}O_5$ steroids (Gustafsson and Sjövall, 1968); $C_{21}O_6$ steroids (Setchell *et al.*, 1976c)]. The mistakes mentioned were corrected by further comparisons with authentic steroids (Eriksson, 1976) or by nuclear magnetic resonance (NMR) analysis (Setchell *et al.*, 1978). The latter example illustrates that GC–MS, NMR, and microchemical reactions is the most powerful combination for identification of steroids. In many cases, NMR requires more material than is available, and identifications by GC–MS may have to be tentative. Proton NMR spectra can be obtained with several micrograms, whereas a few milligrams are needed for ^{13}C NMR. Since the authors have no personal experience with NMR techniques, and since most biomedical studies are made with HPLC, GLC, or GC–MS, this review is limited to identification by mass spectrometric methods. For information about NMR spectrometry of steroids, the reader is referred to reviews by Caspi and Wittstruck (1967) on proton NMR and by Blunt and Stothers (1977) on ^{13}C NMR.

A. MASS SPECTROMETRY BY DIRECT INLET SYSTEMS

The fragmentation of underivatized steroids with a direct inlet system and electron impact ionization has been studied for a long time, and the major fragmentation reactions are known for most common steroids. Four groups in particular have performed systematic studies of mechanisms of fragmentation and formation of diagnostically significant ions: the groups of Djerassi, Budzikiewicz, and Spiteller and the Russian group. Several reviews of this work have been published (Budzikiewicz *et al.*, 1964; Budzikiewicz, 1972, 1980; Spiteller-Friedman and Spiteller, 1969; Zaretskii, 1976). The extensive studies by Djerassi and co-workers have aimed at the elucidation of fragmentation mechanisms with high-resolution mass spectrometry and isotope labeling, exemplified by studies of substituted progesterones (Hammerum and Djerassi, 1975) and α,β-unsaturated 3-ketosteroids (Brown and Djerassi, 1980). In the course of this work a large number of selectively deuterated steroids have been synthesized (see Tökés and Throop, 1972; Brown and Djerassi, 1980). This work is particularly important in view of the increasing use of stable isotopes in metabolic studies (see Section VI,B).

Spiteller and co-workers have made systematic studies to define key ions and key differences (fragment losses) as an aid in localizing substituents on the steroid skeleton. They have reported on the fragmentation of $C_{19}O_3$ steroids substituted with hydroxyl or keto groups at C-3, C-11, and C-17 (Obermann *et al.*, 1971a,b), C-3, C-6, and C-17 (Hammerschmidt and Spiteller, 1973a,b), C-3, C-12, and C-17 (Zietz and Spiteller, 1974), C-3, C-16-, and C-17 (Grote and Spiteller, 1976), of $C_{19}O_4$ steroids substituted at C-3, C-11, C-16, and C-17 (Richter and Spiteller, 1976), of $C_{19}O_3$ steroids substituted at C-3, C-6, and C-20 (Grupe and Spiteller, 1978) and at C-3, C-11, and C-20 (Ende and Spiteller, 1971, 1973). The differences in fragmentation reactions of steroids with A/B cis or trans configuration have been studied by all four groups (see Ende and Spiteller, 1975; Zaretskii, 1976). The studies of underivatized steroids are mentioned because general information on fragmentation is given that is helpful in identification of hormonal steroids also in the form of derivatives more suitable for GC–MS analysis.

The interpretation of mass spectra can be made manually or by computer. Simple and helpful tabulations of key ions and key differences have been published by von Unruh and Spiteller (1970a,b,c). The key ions and differences in 1730 spectra of steroids were used in a computer-aided system for determination of partial structures of unknown steroids (Spiteller *et al.*, 1978). This is the simplest type of computer interpretation and can be very helpful in analyses of metabolic profiles, provided that a sufficiently comprehensive library of spectra of the appropriate derivatives has been collected. An important primary assumption [as in the system of Reimendal and Sjövall (1973a); see Section IV,B,3) is that the spectrum is due to a steroid.

There are several advanced and generally applicable computer techniques for mass spectral identification. A recent summary of available methods was published by McLafferty and Venkataraghavan (1979) and the reader is referred to this paper for references. One method involves comparison of the unknown spectrum with library spectra. Several systems have been described since the first report by Biemann (1962). A new program (Damen *et al.*, 1978) was applied to the identification of underivatized steroids. The library contained 524 spectra of mainly underivatized steroids and the same library was used by Varmuza (1976), who compared different search methods. A factor of major importance is the mode of selection of peaks to be compared. The best results are obtained when a probability weighting of masses and abundances is used (McLafferty and Venkataraghavan, 1979). This permits calculation of the probability that a match occurs by chance. Another important method is the reverse search where the program finds out whether the peaks of the reference spectrum are present in the unknown spectrum. This method is particularly useful when spectra represent mixtures of compounds, e.g., in analyses of metabolic profiles. The 524 spectra mentioned above have also been used by Rotter and Varmuza (1978) in a study of pattern recognition (learning machine) systems for interpretation of steroid spectra. Seventeen structural features could be predicted with a high probability (71–100%). However, these methods are less likely to become generally useful in biomedical analyses.

Lederberg, Djerassi, and co-workers have applied "artificial intelligence" methods to the interpretation of mass spectra. The methods have been extensively tested on mass spectra of estrogens (Smith *et al.*, 1973a,b), alkyl-substituted progesterones (Hammerum and Djerassi, 1975), and keto-androstanes (Buchanan *et al.*, 1976). The program uses high-resolution mass spectral data, including molecular ions and metastable peaks. While such data may still be difficult to obtain in most biomedical studies, the results of the interpretation of spectra of mixed estrogen are impressive (Smith *et al.*, 1973b). With an increasing availability and use of high-resolution mass spectrometry, the systems may become of great practical importance. The present limitations of these heuristic search methods are discussed by Buchanan *et al.* (1976).

The group at Cornell has described a third type of search and interpretation system called STIRS (self-training interpretive and retrieval system) (see McLafferty and Venkataraghavan, 1979). This system has not yet been specifically tested on a group of steroids.

The reasons for using direct inlet mass spectrometry rather than GC–MS in biomedical studies may be difficulties in obtaining molecular ions of the derivatives most suitable for GLC, thermal lability or absence of a volatile derivative, or a need to analyze other derivatives or the underivatized steroid. In spite of the use of low temperatures and low energy of the bombarding electrons it may not be possible to obtain well-defined molecular ions. This makes interpretation of spectra, both manually and by computers, more difficult. Furthermore, the mass spectrometric conditions influence the fragmentation processes, making library comparisons more difficult. Although there are many examples of instrumental differences, these are not as serious as originally believed in identification work. However, the condition of the ion source may affect the fragmentation patterns markedly. The ion source may be contaminated with previous biological samples, or active sites may be present inside the source. This was shown to be the reason for changes in the fragmentation of sterols in an electropolished source (Wegmann, 1978). As in the case of GC–MS, the method of transfer of the sample into the ion source is of great importance both for the sensitivity and the fragmentation pattern. The group at Baylor has shown that labile steroids should be evaporated from glass probe tips that are first siliconized and then coated with SE-30 prior to application of the sample (Thenot *et al.*, 1979).

Electron impact ionization at the energies commonly used results in extensive fragmentation. While this is important in identification work, it decreases sensitivity in quantitative analyses, and information about the molecular weight of the steroid may not be obtained. Various other ionization methods have therefore been used. Relatively few fragment ions are produced with chemical ionization, where ionization occurs by an ion-molecule reaction and quasi-molecular ions are formed. After the early applications in the steroid field (Fales *et al.*, 1969; Michnovicz and Munson, 1974), it has been used in numerous biomedical applications involving direct mass spectrometry, GC–MS, and LC–MS. Various reagent gases, such as methane, isobutane, and ammonia, have been used. References to these applications can be found in the reviews mentioned in Section IV,B. A development in this area is the study of negative ions produced by chemical ionization. Roy *et al.* (1979) investigated the hydroxyl ion negative chemical ionization mass spectra of 35 steroids of the cholestane series. Intense $(M-1)^-$ ions were obtained in almost all cases. The total yield of ions was somewhat higher than the yield of positive ions in chemical ionization with methane, but the authors did not consider this to be a definitive analytical advantage. However, the negative ion spectra can become very useful in the analysis of steroids with free hydroxyl groups.

Desorption chemical ionization is another method that may become of particular importance for LC–MS combinations. The sample is placed on a gold tip (coated with SE-30) in the source, and the same reagent gases are used as in conventional chemical ionization (Carroll *et al.*, 1981). Nowlin *et al.* (1979) used isobutane in a study of plasma desorption mass spectra of underivatized steroids, including $C_{21}O_5$ corticosteroids. MH^+ ions were obtained with steroids containing a keto group, but steroids having only hydroxyl groups gave $(MH-n18)^+$ ions showing the successive losses of water from the quasi-molecular ion. Loss of side chain from 17-hydroxycorticosteroids was also observed. The advantage with plasma desorption ionization is that the sample is ionized directly, without a separate vaporization step that will decompose thermally labile steroids.

The group at Baylor has developed atmospheric pressure ionization mass spectrometry (Carroll *et al.*, 1974) that can be used for direct injection of biological extracts and is compatible with capillary column GLC and HPLC. Ions are produced by reaction with ions of the carrier liquid or gas, the primary source of electrons being a ^{63}Ni foil or a corona discharge. The ions (positive or negative) enter the low-pressure region of the mass spectrometer through a small aperture in one of the reaction chamber walls. Horning *et al.* (1978) have reviewed their work in this area. Few steroids have been studied (see Section IV,C), but the spectra are expected to resemble those obtained with conventional chemical ionization. Sensitivity in the femtogram range has been obtained with some compounds.

Some special techniques for mass spectral identification of steroids have been described. Kruger *et al.* (1979) applied mass-analyzed ion kinetic energy spectroscopy (MIKES) to the analysis of steroids. The method involves chemical ionization in a high-resolution mass spectrometer. The ions are separated in the magnetic sector, and selected metastable or stable ions are excited and fragmented by collision with a target gas. The fragment ion kinetic energies are then scanned with the electrostatic analyzer. It is difficult to evaluate the future of this method; the analyses of dehydroepiandrosterone and testosterone in urine used as examples could have been more easily done by conventional GC–MS.

The combined mass spectrometry–mass spectrometry systems developed by McLafferty and his co-workers (see McLafferty, 1980) are yet outside the analytical reality of biomedical laboratories. In these systems, the first mass spectrometer acts as a separating system that provides selected ions for further fragmentation and analysis in the second mass spectrometer. It is obvious that such systems can be very powerful in analyses of complex biological mixtures. Applications in the steroid area have not yet been published.

Conjugated steroids constitute a special problem in mass spectrometric analysis. They are thermally labile and have high molecular weights. Three different approaches have been used: (a) ionization by special methods; (b) derivatization to produce volatile compounds; and (c) a combination of (a) and (b). The field desorption technique, reviewed by Beckey and Schulten (1975), has been used to obtain mass spectra of glycosides including the sodium salts of testosterone glucuronide (Schulten and Games, 1974) and estriol-16α-glucuronide from pregnancy urine (Adlercreutz et al., 1974b). Peaks were observed at M^+ of the undissociated acids and at $(M+1)^+$ of the sodium salt. Ions corresponding to the aglycons were also seen. A more common use of this method has probably been prevented by practical difficulties both in sample preparation and in the field desorption technique. The plasma desorption ionization method mentioned above has also been reported to yield mass spectra of steroid sulfates and glucuronides as well as of bile acids (Nowlin et al., 1979). Further development in this area can be expected, especially in combination with HPLC.

Mass spectra of derivatized steroid glucuronides have been studied by several groups. Horning and co-workers showed that steroid glucuronides could be analyzed by GLC and mass spectrometry as methyl ester trimethylsilyl ether derivatives (see Horning, 1968).

Similar studies of steroid N-acetylglucosaminides were made by Nambara et al. (1971). However, the mass spectra of the derivatives of neutral steroid glucuronides are not very informative, and molecular ion peaks are small or absent (see Spiegelhalder et al., 1976). The main value of the mass spectrum is that it defines the compound as a glucuronide and indicates the general type of steroid. Similar information is given by mass spectra of permethylated steroid glucuronides (Thompson and Desiderio, 1972). Molecular ion peaks are small also when chemical ionization is used. However, when pyridine was added to ammonia or isobutane, prominent ions were observed at $(M+80)^+$ of the pertrimethylsilylated glucuronide of testosterone (Johnson et al., 1978). However, the spectra give little information about the steroid structure.

The situation is different for glucuronides of estrogens. These have been studied as trimethylsilyl (TMS) ether ester derivatives (Spiegelhalder et al., 1976), but Miyazaki et al. (1976) found the n-propyl ester TMS ether derivatives more suitable. Thompson (1976) analyzed permethylated derivatives. In all cases important ions due to fragmentation of the steroid moiety were observed, and the site of conjugation (aliphatic or aromatic) could be determined. An interesting transfer of one TMS ether group from the glucuronyl moiety to the steroid occurs in the fragmentation of TMS ethers of estrogen 3-glucuronides.

B. GAS CHROMATOGRAPHY–MASS SPECTROMETRY

Several books have described the development and applications of GC–MS. A review that contains references to most of these books has been published (Milberg and Cook, 1978). A series of reviews on GC–MS by Gudzinowicz (1977) have also appeared. Information about the development of GC–MS up to the late 1970s and its applications in the steroid area can be found in the excellent reviews by Brooks and Middleditch (1973a,b, 1975, 1977, 1979) and by Burlingame and co-workers (Burlingame and Johanson, 1972; Burlingame et al., 1974, 1976, 1978, 1980).

The early applications of GC–MS to the analysis of steroids were mainly qualitative and led to the identification of a large number of steroids in blood, urine, bile, and feces. References to this literature are found in reviews, e.g., by Engel and Orr (1972), Milne (1971), and Brooks and Gaskell (1980). Lately, applications of GC–MS have been more concerned with analyses of metabolic profiles, quantitative analyses, and metabolic studies. Some reviews have appeared (e.g., Setchell, 1979; Adlercreutz, 1980). The vast literature makes it impossible to cover all applications, and we will only attempt to discuss some points of practical importance in the use of GC–MS.

1. *Gas Chromatographic System*

Packed columns have been used for a long time in analysis of steroids. However, the efficiency of such columns is often too low even when a mass spectrometer is used as detector. Development of open tubular glass capillary columns has greatly improved specificity of the analyses. The high resolving power and the reduction of peak width, column bleed, and adsorption result in enhanced sensitivity. However, the lack of stability at high temperature was an early problem due to the tendency of the liquid film to break up into droplets. There were also problems with the injection system and the connection to the ion source, leading to losses of labile steroids. Several solutions to these problems have been published. An excellent review on the use of glass capillary columns in steroid analysis has been written by Shackleton (1981).

a. Glass Capillary Columns. Coating with common nonpolar stationary phases is readily obtained by static or dynamic procedures after deactivation of the glass wall. Silylation is widely used for deactivation of glass and has been performed at elevated temperature using mixtures of hexamethyldisilazane–trimethylchlorosilane (Novotny and Zlatkis, 1970), dimethyldichlorosilane (German and Horning, 1973), and mixtures of hexamethyldisilazane and diphenyltetramethyldisilazane (Grob *et al.*, 1979a,b). At present, the latter method appears to give the most inert glass surface. Before silylation, the columns were leached with acid to remove metal oxides and to open the silica structure.

Surface-active agents forming monomolecular layers on the glass wall, e.g., benzyltriphenylphosphonium chloride, have also been used prior to coating with nonpolar phases (Rutten and Luyten, 1972). In our experience, such columns are easy to prepare, have satisfactory chromatographic properties, and cause little adsorption of common steroid derivatives.

A different approach to making thermally stable nonpolar columns was used by German and Horning (1973). The silanized glass wall was coated with silanized silica powder (Silanox), which served to retain the stationary phase. The procedure resembles techniques for preparation of support-coated open tubular (SCOT) columns. Silanox, however, is probably not attached to the wall. The rough surface of columns of this type increases the volume of stationary phase and the loading capacity, which is a major advantage.

Nonpolar stationary phases have also been chemically attached to the glass wall. A polymeric product obtained from dimethyldichlorosilane was made to react *in situ* under base-catalyzed conditions, forming a stable coating (Madani *et al.*, 1976; Rigaud *et al.*, 1976). Columns coated with more polar phases could also be prepared with methyl-phenyl polysiloxane polymers (Madani and Chambaz, 1978). Both types of columns yielded excellent separations of steroid *O*-methyloxime-trimethylsilyl derivatives. The columns were stated to be highly stable, but actual studies of column bleed with GC–MS were not made.

Although columns coated with nonpolar phases are most suitable for general applications, polar stationary phases may be required for specific separations (Sandra *et al.*, 1979). Such columns are more difficult to prepare. Deactivation of the glass wall is less important than for nonpolar columns, whereas wetting of the glass wall presents problems. Soft (soda lime) glass capillaries etched with dry HCl gave a layer of sodium chloride crystals on the surface that could be coated with polar phases (Alexander and Rutten, 1973). A disadvantage is that the method is limited to soft glass. Grob described a method in which a layer of barium carbonate crystals was produced on the glass surface by treatment with barium hydroxide and CO_2 (Grob and Grob, 1976; Grob et al., 1977). This method can be used for most types of glass, producing almost neutral thermostable columns. The treated surface may then be coated with polar phases.

The efficiency of SCOT columns prepared with various materials has been evaluated for use in steroid analysis (Deelder et al., 1976; Thomas, 1980). An advantage with these columns is their higher capacity. A high temperature nematic liquid crystal has been used as stationary phase for selective separation of epimeric 3-hydroxysteroids (Zielinski et al., 1976).

Capillary columns made of quartz have become commercially available. The major advantages, compared to conventional glass capillaries, are that they are flexible and almost unbreakable. One may expect rapid development in coating procedures for these columns.

b. *Injection Systems.* Several injection systems for glass capillary columns have been used in steroid analysis. Splitters were originally employed, but results were unsatisfactory in quantitative work. An improved splitter with a short packed precolumn was then described, which ensured gas-phase rather than aerosol splitting (German and Horning, 1972, 1973). With this method, MO-TMS derivatives (Section IV,B,2,a) could be injected together with the derivatizing reagents without decomposition (Thenot and Horning, 1972b). As with other splitters, however, the loss of sample is a disadvantage.

The entire sample is analyzed when liquid on-column or solid injection techniques are used. The former has been described by Grob and Grob (1978). Since the sample is not concentrated to dryness on a surface, volatile samples can be injected, and degradation of labile compounds is avoided. The major disadvantages are that only small volumes can be conveniently injected and that the solvent may damage the column.

Solid injection after evaporation of the solvent can be performed with a "falling needle" (van den Berg and Cox, 1972) or "falling capillary tube" (Bailey et al., 1974; Lawrence et al., 1974) system. With these systems, the solvent will not interfere with the analysis, but labile compounds may decompose during evaporation of the solvent. High precision can be obtained with both systems, and the vials can be used for automatic sampling (Shackleton and Honour, 1976; Fantl and Gray, 1977).

Gastight connections are made by hard or elastic fittings. The former are made of graphite, organic polymers, or mixtures of these and are used for glass capillary–metal connections. An elastic fitting, Kalrez, appears not to have the disadvantages of other elastic fittings, such as bleeding, loss of elasticity, and sticking to glass and metal (Grob, 1978). A simple device for thermostable coupling of two glass capillaries consists of a Teflon tube compressed in a metal capsule (Axelson and Sjövall, 1977). Thermoshrinkable Teflon tubing is simple to use, but does not give leak-free connections in GC–MS work.

c. *Interfaces to Ion Source.* The use of conventional molecule separators with addition of extra carrier gas at the end of the capillary column is convenient since the separator does not have to be reconstructed. The flow through the column is easy to control, and a simple valve may be used (Maume and Luyten, 1973). However, losses of labile steroids are known to occur owing to presence of metal surfaces in the separator. A single-stage adjustable jet separator has been used to diminish this problem (Axelson and Sjövall, 1977). No extra gas was added and metal surfaces were deactivated by coating with a thin layer of water glass coated with benzyltriphenylphosphonium chloride (Axelson, 1977).

When the pumping capacity is sufficiently large, the capillary column may be directly connected to the ion source (Thome and Young, 1976). A form of direct coupling is the widely used open-split connection (Henneberg *et al.,* 1975a,b). Columns are easy to change, and valves are not required. Depending on the split ratio, part of the sample is lost. A number of all-glass connections have been developed (Dürbeck *et al.,* 1978a,b; Henneberg *et al.,* 1978; Stan and Abraham, 1978; Schmid *et al.,* 1979). The all-glass interfaces, after appropriate deactivation, have been shown to give much better yields of labile compounds than the platinum–iridium capillaries originally used. Obviously, adsorptive losses occurring in the ion source will not be avoided.

2. *Derivatization*

Since most steroids cannot be directly subjected to gas chromatography, it is necessary to protect hydroxyl and usually also keto groups. An excellent book on derivatization in chromatography has been published by Blau and King (1977). The choice of derivative depends on the type of analysis, and three major needs may be distinguished: analysis of metabolic profiles, quantitation, and identification of selected steroids.

a. *Trimethylsilyl Ethers and O-Methyloximes.* When mixtures that contain a variety of steroid structures are to be analyzed, reactions with a wide range of applicability, yielding single derivatives with good GLC and GC–MS properties, should be chosen. At present the fully reacted *O*-methyloxime (MO)-trimethylsilyl (TMS) ether derivative appears to be most versatile for analysis of endogenous steroids (Thenot and Horning, 1972a). Methyloximes are prepared prior to acid-catalyzed silylation in order to prevent enol-TMS ether formation. The 11-keto group does not react under the usual reaction conditions. Hindered keto groups that require longer reaction times for complete conversion include the 20-keto group in dexamethasone (having a 16α-methyl group) and medroxyprogesterone acetate (having a 17α-acetoxy group) (Thenot and Horning, 1972c). Some steroids are partly destroyed by the reaction conditions. This is the case with aldosterone, its metabolites, and 18-hydroxylated precursors and their metabolites. Reaction at room temperature overnight has been used for these steroids (Honour and Shackleton, 1977; Shackleton and Honour, 1977). The different reaction rates of keto or hydroxyl groups, largely dependent on sterical hindrance, may be utilized in structure elucidation (Vouros and Harvey, 1973a; Axelson, 1978). A disadvantage with MO derivatives is the formation of *syn/anti* isomers that may separate also on nonpolar phases. More important in quantitative analysis is their acid lability (Thenot and Horning, 1972b), resulting in losses particularly upon contact with metal surfaces (Axelson, 1977). Such surfaces must be well deactivated, particularly in analysis of MO derivatives of small amounts of 3-keto-4-ene steroids.

Keto groups may also be converted into TMS ethers (enols) in the presence of a nucleophilic agent, usually potassium acetate (Chambaz *et al.*, 1972, 1973). Different reagents and reaction conditions for this base-catalyzed reaction have been studied by Gleispach (1974). Although the derivatives show excellent GC–MS properties in analysis of urinary steroids (e.g., Nicosia *et al.*, 1973; Egger *et al.*, 1978), quantitative conversion of all steroids into single derivatives appears to be difficult to achieve. This is also the case when trimethylbromosilane is used as the catalyst (Aringer *et al.*, 1971). Thus, TMS-enol-TMS ethers are less versatile than MO-TMS derivatives for studies of metabolic profiles, but they can be very useful in analyses of specific steroids. The molecular ions are often abundant and can be used for selected ion monitoring. Estrogens and neutral steroids with few, and stable substituents can usually be analyzed after conversion of hydroxyl groups into TMS ethers, leaving keto groups intact.

Nonvolatile reagents are conveniently removed by filtration of the reaction mixtures through a short bed of Lipidex 5000 (Axelson and Sjövall, 1974, 1977). This method can be used for purification of most derivatives when a polar group is converted into a nonpolar derivative. All compounds in the sample that do not change their polarity in the derivatization reaction are thereby removed. Sephadex LH-20 has also been used for this purpose (Engel *et al.*, 1970) but gave partial hydrolysis of TMS ethers.

   b. *Other Silyl Ethers and Oximes.* A variety of substituted silyl derivatives have been used in analyses of organic compounds, including steroids (see Poole and Zlatkis, 1979). These derivatives are generally less susceptible to hydrolysis and often give only a few prominent ions of high mass, which makes them suitable for quantitation by selected ion monitoring (see Section V). These advantages were first demonstrated by Kelly in 1974 for the *t*-butyldimethylsilyl (t-BDMS) derivative of steroids (see Kelly and Taylor, 1976a,b). Keto groups were derivatized as *t*-BDMS oximes. The derivatives have been prepared under various conditions using *t*-butyldimethylchlorosilane (Kelly and Taylor, 1976b; Gaskell and Brooks, 1976) or *t*-butyldimethylsilylimidazole (Quilliam and Westmore, 1977). The latter reagent was also used for a base-catalyzed formation of enol ethers of keto groups (Blair and Phillipou, 1978). The rates of reaction with hydroxyl groups in common positions were studied by Phillipou *et al.* (1975). The sterically hindered hydroxyl groups at C-11 and C-17 (tertiary) could not react under the conditions used, and a 20β-hydroxy group reacted more slowly than one at 20α. The stability of the derivatives in acid was also investigated (Hosoda *et al.*, 1975), and *t*-BDMS derivatives were much more stable than TMS ethers.

   The GC–MS properties have been studied in detail by several groups. A *t*-BDMS group increases the retention time of a steroid considerably compared to a TMS group (Harvey, 1977a). Thus, *t*-BDMS ethers are less suitable derivatives for polyhydroxy compounds. Mass spectrometric fragmentation is usually limited owing to the steric crowding of the large alkyl group providing abundant (M-alkyl)$^+$ ions. Thus, the derivatives are less suitable for structural studies but are very useful for quantitative analysis by selected ion monitoring (see Section V). *t*-BDMS derivatives are also useful in NMR analysis (Hosoda *et al.*, 1977) and in synthetic work (Hosoda *et al.*, 1975).

   The useful properties of TMS and *t*-BDMS derivatives encouraged investigations of other alkyldimethylsilyl ethers: ethyl-DMS , propyl-DMS (Miyazaki *et al.*, 1975, 1977a,b, 1979), allyl-DMS (Phillipou, 1976; Blair and Phillipou, 1977; Harvey, 1977a), and various halogenated derivatives, e.g., chloromethyl-DMS (Brooks and Middleditch, 1972), trifluoropropyl-DMS, heptafluoropentyl-DMS, and pentafluorophenyl-DMS (Morgan and Poole, 1974, 1975; Poole and Morgan, 1975). The latter derivatives are useful for GLC with electron capture detector as well as for GC–MS.

   Cyclotetramethylenealkylsilyl ethers have also been prepared (Quilliam and Westmore, 1977, 1978; Quilliam *et al.*, 1977). The retention times of alkyldimethylsilyl ethers increase with increasing size of the alkyl group, and this property can be used to separate steroids according to number of hydroxyl groups (Miyazaki *et al.*, 1977b). Mass spectrometric fragmentation and acid-lability decrease with increasing size of the alkyl group (Harvey, 1978; Poole and Zlatkis, 1979).

Trialkyl, e.g., triethyl, tripropyl, and tributylsilyl, ethers have GC–MS properties similar to those of alkyldimethylsilyl derivatives. Thus, the spectra usually contain fewer ions than those of TMS ethers. Abundant ions are produced by elimination of one of the alkyl groups, but successive elimination of C_nH_{2n} fragments also occurs (Harvey, 1977b, 1978).

As mentioned above, sterically crowded silyl oxime derivatives of steroids may be prepared (Kelly and Taylor, 1976a,b). In contrast to TMS-oximes (Brooks and Harvey, 1970), these derivatives usually give abundant ions of high mass.

The GC–MS behavior of oximes substituted with ethyl (Brooks and Harvey, 1970), butyl, pentyl (Baillie *et al.*, 1972), and benzyl groups (Devaux *et al.*, 1971a,b) has also been studied. Because of the increased retention times, the larger derivatives may be prepared to separate ketonic from nonketonic steroids (Devaux *et al.*, 1971a,b). However, long retention times and need for higher temperatures are inconvenient. The alkoxy group is readily lost upon electron impact, but preparation of these derivatives may aid in the determination of the position of a keto group.

Halogenated oximes, e.g., 2-chloroethyloximes, may be used to increase the specificity in GC–MS analysis since they permit selected ion monitoring of the two peaks caused by the chlorine isotopes (Brooks and Middleditch, 1971; Nambara *et al.*, 1976). Pentafluorobenzyloximes have been used for GLC with electron capture detection (Nambara *et al.*, 1975; Koshy *et al.*, 1975).

c. Other Derivatives. Heptafluorobutyrates (HFB) of hydroxysteroids or enols of ketosteroids have long been employed for high-sensitivity analysis with electron capture detection (see Clark and Wotiz, 1973; Dehennin and Levisalles, 1976). The HFB esters of saturated steroids usually have less affinity for thermal electrons. Increased sensitivity for these steroids was obtained by preparation of 1-heptafluorobutanoyl-2-propenyl ether derivatives (Dehennin and Scholler, 1975). Since quantitative yields were obtained only for steroids with axial hydroxy groups at C-3 and C-17, the use of this derivative appears to be limited.

The HFB esters of steroids have been extensively used for selected ion monitoring GC–MS. They have short retention times and usually abundant molecular ions, which results in high sensitivity (see Section

V,D). HFB anhydride, as well as other perfluoroacylating agents, has been employed for direct derivatization of sulfate esters of steroids (Touchstone and Dobbins, 1975; Murray and Baillie, 1979). The perfluoro esters of the parent steroids were formed. Only 3-sulfates of estrogens and steroids with a 3β-hydroxy-5-ene structure reacted in this way. An analogous reaction was proposed to occur with some silylating reagents. The reaction may serve to simplify sample preparation or to discriminate between aromatic and nonaromatic sulfate esters.

Methylation of hydroxyl groups with methylsulfinyl carbanion and methyl iodide has been studied by Leclercq (1974). When 17-ketosteroids were allowed to react, both C-16 hydrogen atoms were replaced by methyl groups. The method may find some use in analysis of hydroxysteroids with unhindered hydroxyl groups and in analyses of simple glucuronides (see Section IV,A). The advantages are short retention times, little mass increase upon derivatization, and chemical stability. Steroid acids are usually analyzed as methyl esters. Phenolic hydroxyl groups are readily methylated, and a quantitative method for analysis of catechol estrogens is based on the use of extractive alkylation to yield the diethyl ether derivative (Rosenfeld and Taguchi, 1978).

Substituted boronates form cyclic derivatives selectively with proximal hydroxyl groups. Thus, these esters are particularly useful as a complement to other derivatives for GC–MS characterization of polyhydroxysteroids, such as 1,2- and 1,3-diols and corticosteroids (17,20-diols, 20,21-diols, and 17,20,21-triols) (Brooks and Harvey, 1971). Since boronation shifts the equilibrium between 20-oxosteroids and hemiacetal forms toward the latter, they give single products of steroids like 18-hydroxy-11-deoxycorticosterone (Gaskell et al., 1976) and aldosterone (Gaskell and Brooks, 1978), steroids that may be difficult to characterize by GC–MS.

Dimethylphosphinic esters (Vogt et al., 1974) and dimethylthiophosphinic esters (Jacob and Vogt, 1978) of monohydroxysteroids have been employed for high-sensitivity GLC analysis with an alkali flame ionization detector. Since the reagent for the former derivative takes long to prepare and is unstable, the latter derivative appears to be superior. The yields of steroids tested were 70–100%.

Keto groups of steroids can be converted into ethylenedioxyderivatives (ethylene acetals) by percolating a mixture of the steroid and ethylene glycol in tetrahydrofuran through a cation exchanger in H^+ form. The derivative appears in the eluate (Dann et al., 1979). Derivatization by filtration through a bed of catalyst is a useful procedure also in other reactions, e.g., formation of acetonides (Dann et al., 1979).

3. *Retention Times and Mass Spectra*

The quantitative relationships between structure and mobility have long served as the basis for identification of steroids by chromatographic methods (see Bush, 1961). In the ideal case, each group gives a logarithmic contribution (positive or negative) to the true retention volume, i.e., retention time. For use in identification work, retention times are therefore best expressed as retention indices (RI) or methylene units (MU, retention index $\times$ 10^{-2}), which are based on the linear relationship between the logarithm of the retention time and the number of carbon atoms in a series of n-alkanes (see Horning, 1968). These units have largely replaced relative retention times, which show larger variations with temperature. However, RI and MU values are also temperature-dependent, and Mori and Sato (1973) showed that steroid numbers, introduced by VandenHeuvel and Horning (see Horning, 1968) were less variable in analyses of steroids. Edwards (1978b) measured temperature coefficients of MU values for a number of steroids and proposed a method to correct for the temperature variation.

Because of the often predictable changes caused by introduction, derivatization, transformation, epimerization, or elimination of functional groups, retention times have played an important role in identification and structure determination of steroids by GC–MS. Lists of relative retention times, RI or MU values are found in many papers dealing with analysis of metabolic profiles (Section VI,4), derivatization methods (Section IV,B,2), and identification of steroids (see below). A systematic study of the contribution of keto groups and their oximes to steroid numbers was made by Nambara and Iwata (1973), using a series of androstanones. Extensive studies of group contributions to retention times on a dimethylpolysiloxane column were made by Vandenheuvel (1974, 1975a,b,c, 1977). Androstanes substituted at C-3, C-11, and C-17, and pregnanes substituted at C-3, C-11, C-17, C-20, and C-21 were analyzed as partial TMS ethers. Simple microchemical reactions were used to modify the functional groups, to prepare reference compounds on a small scale, and to identify steroids.

While retention times can provide important information about stereochemistry, particularly when combined with microchemical reactions and with use of polar stationary phases, the mass spectra will aid in establishing a general steroid structure and possible positions of the functional groups. There is a vast literature on mass spectra of steroids in connection with the use of GC–MS for identification purposes. TMS ethers and methyloximes are the predominant derivatives used, and Table III gives the mass increments required for calculation of

TABLE III

MOLECULAR WEIGHTS OF STEROIDS AND CHANGES CAUSED BY SUBSTITUTION OR
DERIVATIZATION

Contributing groups	Mass increment upon substitution
Cholestane	372
Pregnane	288
Androstane	260
Estrane	246
Ketone	14
Methyloxime	43 (29)[a]
Hydroxyl	16
Trimethylsiloxy	88 (72)[a]
Carboxyl	44
Methyl(ene)	14
Double bond	−2

[a] Mass increment upon derivatization of a substituent.

molecular weights of these derivatives and their homologs. It is beyond the scope of this review to discuss the mass spectra. However, as an aid in the preliminary evaluation of spectra, Tables IV–VI list a number of ions encountered in analyses of C_{19} and C_{21} steroids from biological sources. To limit the number of possible fragmentations, all hydroxyl groups are converted into TMS ethers, and only a keto group at C-11 remains unreacted in the preparation of MO-TMS derivatives. It should also be emphasized that the formation of ions from a particular steroid structure is greatly influenced by other structural features of the steroid. Thus, the ions listed are not found in all steroids with the structure indicated, nor are they exclusively formed from these structures. Also, there are diagnostically important fragmentations that lead to ions of low abundance. A difficulty in the interpretation of spectra of TMS ether derivatives is the possibility of migration of the TMS group during fragmentation (see Gaskell *et al.*, 1975; Smith *et al.*, 1976; Brooks and Gaskell, 1980). Table IV gives several examples of such rearrangement ions. Another problem is to decide whether a spectrum represents a pure steroid or a mixture of compounds. This is best resolved by use of repetitive scanning and computer construction of chromatograms of selected ions found in the spectra. However, even this method may fail if the mixtures are too complex or the efficiency of the GLC column is insufficient. Mixtures of isomeric steroids may be very difficult to resolve.

TABLE IV

COMMON FRAGMENT IONS AND LOSSES SEEN IN MASS SPECTRA OF TRIMETHYLSILYL (TMS)
AND METHYLOXIME (MO)-TMS DERIVATIVES OF C_{19} AND C_{21} STEROIDS

Fragment ion or loss[a]	Elemental composition	Possible structures in steroid derivative
−29	C_2H_5	3,6-TMS; 3-TMS-6-one
−30	CH_2O (C-18 or -19)	19-TMS-3-one; 18-TMS-17-one
−47	—	6-TMS-4-ene-3-MO
−56	C_3H_4O (C-1,2,3)	3-TMS-5-ene-17-, 11- or 20-one
−56	—	6-TMS-4-ene-3-one
103, −103	CH_2OTMS	18-, 19- or 21-TMS
−116	C_2H_3OTMS	1- or 2-TMS-4-ene-3-one
124	$C_8H_{12}O$	(4-ene)-3-one
125, 137, 153	—	4-ene-3-MO
129	C_3H_4OTMS	5-ene-3-TMS, 17-TMS(C_{19}), 2,3-TMS
−129	C_3H_4OTMS	5-ene-3-TMS, some 3,6-TMS, 3-TMS-11,17-one
133	—	1-TMS-4-ene-3-MO
138	A-ring, C-19	5β-3,6-MO
142, 143	$C_4H_{5(6)}$ OTMS	4-ene-3-TMS, 3-enol-TMS, 2,3-TMS, (1,3-TMS)
−142	—	4-ene-3-TMS
143	—	3,11-TMS
−143	—	4-ene-3,6-TMS, 6-TMS-3-one
−144	—	3-TMS-11-one
−145	—	3,6(β)-TMS
147	$(CH_3)_2SiOTMS$	Di- and poly-TMS
191	$CH(OTMS)_2$	C_{19}-(11,15,16,17,18)-di(tri)-TMS. C_{21}-poly-TMS
217, (218, 219)	$C_3H_3(OTMS)_2$	1,3-TMS, C_{19}-15,(18),17-TMS
243	$C_5H_5(OTMS)_2$	17,20,21-TMS, 3,7-TMS

[a] Fragment losses, −, from molecular ion or after loss of trimethylsilanol (−90).

Tables IV–VI do not include generally occurring ions due to loss of a methyl group (−15) or trimethylsilanol (−90). Loss of water (−18) usually indicates the presence of a free hydroxyl group, although it is seen to some extent also with free keto groups. A trimethylsiloxy group (−89) is often lost in steroids with vicinal or a large number of TMS groups. Ions due to the ABCD-ring skeleton with one (m/z 257), two, three, and four (m/z 251) double bonds and with or without carbonyl groups (+14) are often given by C_{21} steroids. Corresponding ions from C_{19} steroids are at even-numbered masses.

References to mass spectra of TMS, MO-TMS, and other derivatives of steroids suitable for GC–MS analysis can be found in the reviews by Engel and Orr (1972), Brooks and Middleditch (1973a,b, 1975, 1977, 1979), and Brooks and Gaskell (1980). In most original publications,

TABLE V

SOME TYPICAL FRAGMENT IONS AND LOSSES IN MASS SPECTRA OF TRIMETHYLSILYL (TMS)
AND METHYLOXINE (MO)-TMS DERIVATIVES OF COMMON NATURALLY OCURRING C_{19}
STEROIDS

Fragment ion or loss[a]	Possible sites of substitution			Probable origin
	TMS	MO	Keto	
−47	—	—	C-7,17	—
−56	—	—	C-17	D ring
87	—	C-17	—	D ring
−103	C-16,17	—	—	C-17
116 or 117	C-15 or 16	—	C-17	—
129	C-17	—	C-16	C-16,17
−131[b]	C-7,17 or 18,17	—	—	D ring
−131	C-15,16	—	C-17	C-16,17
133	C-16 or 17	C-17 or 16	—	—
143	C-15 or 17	—	C-17 or 16	D ring
−144	C-15 or 16 or 17	—	C-17 or 16	D ring
156,184,199	C-3,11	—	C-17	—
158	C-18 or 19	—	C-17	—
158	C-17	C-16	—	C-16,17
169,182	C-11,17	—	—	—
169	C-18	—	C-17	—
174,−174	C-16 or 17	C-17 or 16	—	D ring
196	C-16	—	C-17	—
205	C-16,17	—	—	C-16,17
223	C-6(β),17	—	—	C,D rings

[a] Fragment losses, −, from molecular ion or after loss of trimethylsilanol (−90).
[b] Also with 12,17-TMS.

TABLE VI

SOME TYPICAL FRAGMENT IONS AND LOSSES IN MASS SPECTRA OF TRIMETHYLSILYL (TMS)
AND METHYLOXIME (MO)-TMS DERIVATIVES OF
COMMON NATURALLY OCCURRING C_{21} STEROIDS

Fragment ion or loss[a]	Possible sites of substitution			Probable origin
	TMS	MO	Keto	
−43	—	—	C-20	Side chain
−44	C-15 or 20	—	C-11	C-11,12
−85(86)	—	—	C-20	Side chain, D ring
100, 87, 70	—	C-20	—	Side chain, C-16,17
−99, −86	—	C-20	—	Side chain, C-16,17

TABLE VI (*Continued*)

Fragment ion or loss[a]	Possible sites of substitution			Probable origin
	TMS	MO	Keto	
117	C-20	—	—	Side chain
−117	C-17,20	—	—	Side chain
−131	C-21	—	C-20	Side chain
152	C-15,21	C-20[b]	—	—
−152	C-18,21	C-20	—	—
156	C-20[c]	—	—	Side chain, D ring
156, 188	C-17 or 16	C-20	—	Side chain, C-16,17
156, 157, 141	C-16,20	—	—	Side chain, D ring
157, 159, 172, 186	C-16	—	C-20	Side chain, D ring
−159	C-15,16	—	C-20	Side chain, C-16,17
161	C-3,6 or 11,21	—	—	—
170	C-15	C-20	—	Side chain, D ring
−171	C-15	—	C-20	Side chain, D ring
172	C-15 or 16	—	C-20	Side chain, D ring
−174	C-11,21 or 15,21	C-20	—	Side chain, C-17
175, 188	C-21	C-20	—	Side chain, C-16,17
−187	C-21	C-20	—	Side chain, C-16,17
201	C-15 or 20	C-20 or 16	—	Side chain, D ring
−205	C-17,20,21	—	—	Side chain
260	C-15,21 or 16,21	—	C-20	Side chain, D ring
276	C-16,21	C-20	—	Side chain, C-16,17
276, 246, 244	C-17,21	C-20	—	Side chain, C-16,17
289	C-15,21	C-20	—	Side chain, D ring

[a] Fragment losses, −, from molecular ion or after loss of trimethylsilanol (−90).
[b] A 4-ene-3-MO structure was also present.
[c] With a 16,17-double bond.

spectra of a few steroids found in the biological samples are reported. Systematic studies using isotope labeling to support fragmentation mechanisms are less frequent and are exemplified by analyses of steroids with a 3-TMS-5-ene structure (Brooks et al., 1973), androstanes with TMS groups at C-3,7,17 (Stock and Spiteller, 1974), at C-11 or C-16 (Vouros and Harvey, 1972b, 1973b), at C-16,17 (Grote and Spiteller, 1977). Mechanisms of fragmentation of steroids with a 6-TMS group have recently been studied (Harvey and Vouros, 1979), and the results confirm and extend previous results of studies of naturally occurring steroids. A series of 6α-hydroxylated cortisol metabolites were synthesized and their structures were determined by GC–MS analysis, microchemical reactions, and NMR spectroscopy (Derks and Drayer, 1978a). Several of these metabolites were identified as quantitatively important steroids in urine from infants (Derks and Drayer, 1978b) and baboons (Setchell et al., 1978).

TMS and MO-TMS derivatives of 15,17- and 16,17-dioxygenated C_{19} steroids in urine and bile have been analyzed, and previous GC–MS results have been confirmed and extended (Matsui and Hakozaki, 1978; Begue et al., 1979a). Additional data on $C_{19}O_3$ steroids have been provided by Kerebel et al. (1977), and on pregnane derivatives and progesterone metabolites by Padieu and co-workers (Desgres et al., 1976; Begue et al., 1978a,b). Shackleton and Taylor (1975) used GC–MS to characterize some 3,15,16,17- and 3,16,17,18-tetrasubstituted androstanes in urine from infants. Shackleton and coworkers (Shackleton and Honour, 1977; Honour and Shackleton, 1977; Shackleton et al., 1979b; Bokkenheuser et al., 1979) as well as Maume and associates (Prost and Maume, 1974; Bournot et al., 1975) have made detailed studies of TMS and MO-TMS derivatives of 18-hydroxylated corticosteroids and aldosterone metabolites. C_{21}-Carboxylic acid metabolites have also been analyzed (Senciall and Dey, 1976; Shackleton et al., 1980b).

The GC–MS properties of various substituted oximes derived from ketosteroids have been studied in detail by Brooks and co-workers (Allen et al., 1969; Brooks and Harvey, 1970; Baillie et al., 1972; Smith and Brooks, 1976). The value of converting keto groups into methyloximes for GC–MS identification is evident from Tables V and VI. The position of these groups may be determined, and mass spectra of MO derivatives of 3,6-diketosteroids permit differentiation between a 5α- and 5β-configuration (Allen et al., 1969). This was useful both for the differentiation between 6- and 7-substitution and for establishment of the 5β configuration of 6α-hydroxytetrahydrocortisol in urine (Setchell et al., 1978).

Estrogen derivatives have been extensively studied by Adlercreutz and co-workers (see Adlercreutz and Luukkainen, 1970; Adlercreutz and Martin, 1976; Adlercreutz, 1980; and references to work by this group in Section V,D). A systematic GC–MS study of catechol estrogens as TMS and methyl ethers was performed by Hoppen and Siekmann (1974). Estetrols and estriolones in pregnancy urine were analyzed by Taylor and Shackleton (1977) and were compared with the androstanes substituted at C-3, -16, -17, -18, or -15 mentioned above.

Steroid drugs and their metabolites give typical mass spectra due to the alkyl or other substituents not present in naturally occurring steroids (Brooks et al., 1971a; Stillwell et al., 1972; Middleditch et al., 1973; Ward et al., 1975, 1977; Braselton et al., 1977). This can serve as the basis for selected ion monitoring in screening for misuse, e.g., of anabolic steroids (Ward et al., 1975, 1977). Epoxy metabolites can also be analyzed by GC–MS (Siekmann et al., 1980).

While TMS and MO-TMS derivatives are most suitable for preliminary identification purposes, mass spectra of many other derivatives have been studied. References can be found in Section IV,B,2. Some derivatives have received particular attention because of their usefulness in identification work or in quantitative GC–MS. For example, mass spectra of alkyl boronates of steroids with different combinations of oxygen substituents at C-17α,20, and 21 have been studied by Brooks et al. (1971b), who showed the value of these derivatives in determination of the structure of the side chain in corticosteroids. Some formate derivatives were analyzed by Pettit and King (1979). Although loss of formic acid is the predominant reaction leading to few ions of diagnostic importance, formates are formed upon periodate oxidation of glucuronides and may be analyzed to determine the site of conjugation (Almé and Sjövall, 1980).

The usefulness of t-BDMS derivatives for selected ion monitoring is well established. Detailed studies of the mass spectra of these and other sterically crowded trialkylsilyl ethers have been made by Quilliam and Westmore (1977). Gaskell et al. (1979a) used linked field scanning in a double-focusing mass spectrometer to determine the fragmentation pathways for t-BDMS ethers of eight isomeric androstanediols. While the intensities of ions in low-resolution spectra were often similar, differences in the relative importance of fragmentation pathways leading to the same ions permitted differentiation between the isomers.

4. Microchemical Reactions

When retention indices and mass spectra of the derivative are not sufficient to establish identity with an authentic steroid derivative, simple microchemical reactions can be carried out on a submicrogram scale. Also in cases when agreement between retention times and mass spectra are obtained, it may be advisable to analyze several derivatives with different stationary phases and to compare products of microchemical reactions. This is especially true when packed GLC columns are used and many isomeric forms of a steroid are possible. Identical retention times and mass spectra of the biological compound and a reference steroid do not necessarily signify identity in such cases.

The microchemical reactions may be performed with conventional chemicals or by enzymatic reactions with stereospecific enzymes. The commercial availability usually limits the latter to dehydrogenase and oxidase reactions. Examples of the use of steroid dehydrogenases are found in papers by Gustafsson and Sjövall (e.g., 1968) while Brooks and co-workers have performed extensive studies on the use of cholesterol oxidase as an aid in the characterization of 3-hydroxysteroids (see Brooks and Smith, 1975; Smith *et al.*, 1978).

Microchemical reactions and determination of changes in mobility caused by these reactions have been used for a long time (see Bush, 1961; and more recently Vandenheuvel, 1974, 1975a,b,c, 1977). Essentially the same reactions are still used, now in combination with GC–MS. Simple reactions are chromic acid oxidations (selective or complete), reductions with sodium borohydride or lithium aluminum hydride, hydrogenation of double bonds, periodate cleavage of vicinal glycols or α-ketolic structures. These reactions are combined with derivatization reactions specific for the types of functional groups formed. Examples of these procedures from our own work can be found in Gustafsson *et al.* (1968), Gustafsson and Sjövall (1968), Sjövall and Sjövall (1968), and Setchell *et al.* (1976c, 1978). Formation of acetonides from vicinal glycols (of cis but not trans configuration in the rings) is a useful reaction (Adlercreutz and Luukkainen, 1968; Sjövall and Sjövall, 1968; Shackleton *et al.*, 1970; Baillie *et al.*, 1975), as is the formation of alkylboronates from 1,2- and 1,3-diols (Brooks and Harvey, 1971; Gaskell *et al.*, 1976; Gaskell and Brooks, 1978).

The position and configuration of hydroxyl groups influence the rates of derivatization markedly. Conditions and reagents in trialkylsilylation reactions can be varied in order to give information about the localization of hydroxyl groups (see Section IV,B,2). The same is true of reactions of keto groups, both with silylating reagents to form enol ethers and with unsubstituted and substituted hydroxylamine hydrochlorides to form oximes. The oxime exchange reaction rates can also be helpful in determining positions of keto groups (Axelson, 1978).

Whenever microchemical reactions are performed, it is important to ascertain that the product(s) observed are derived from the compound(s) seen in the chromatogram of the unreacted material. This material may be more complex than is evident from the GLC analysis: peaks may be due to mixtures of compounds, and steroids may be present that are not detected until after the microchemical reaction. For these reasons it is important to work in a quantitative or at least semiquantitative way and to compare peak areas given by assumed precursors and products.

Interpretation of mass spectra both of the original steroid and its conversion products can be greatly aided by use of reagents labeled with stable isotopes. Hydrogens α to carbonyl groups can be replaced by deuterium (see Tökés and Throop, 1972), which can then be stabilized against back-exchange on the GLC column by reduction of the keto group. Comparisons of spectra of the steroid reduced with unlabeled and ^{2}H-labeled hydrides are often helpful. Deuterium-labeled trimethylsilylating reagents have been extensively used as an aid in the interpretation of spectra and in studies of fragmentation reactions (Vouros and Harvey, 1973a; Vouros, 1973). Such reagents have also been used to prepare internal standards for quantitation by selected ion detection (see Section V,D,1). Miyazaki et al. (1977c) have prepared trimethylsilylimidazole containing one trideuteromethyl group. Reaction of the steroid with a mixture of this and the unlabeled reagent creates ion clusters where the relationships between the peaks depend on the number of derivatized groups. This can be helpful both for interpretation of spectra and for establishing whether or not a spectrum represents a single compound. Unlabeled homologs of derivatizing reagents can be used for similar purposes when the retention time relationships are known (e.g., Miyazaki et al., 1977b; Harvey, 1978; Halket and Lisboa, 1980).

The oxygen of keto groups is exchangeable in $H_2^{18}O$ under acidic conditions. The rates of exchange differ widely depending on the electronic and steric environment of the carbonyl group (Lawson et al., 1969). This reaction can be used both as an aid in the interpretation of spectra of the original ketosteroid and of spectra obtained following reduction of the keto group (Vouros and Harvey, 1972a). Derivatization of keto groups with $^2H_3$-methoxyamine or ^{14}N-hydroxlamine hydrochlorides may also aid in the identification of ketosteroids.

The site of conjugation of steroids can also be determined using microchemical reactions. Acetylation followed by solvolysis and trimethylsilylation may identify the site of sulfation (Cronholm, 1969; Gustafsson and Sjövall, 1969). Some sulfate esters can be directly derivatized without need for solvolysis or enzyme hydrolysis (Touchstone and Dobbins, 1975; Murray and Baillie, 1979). Periodate cleavage of a glucuronide will result in a formate ester that can be localized after conversion of other hydroxyl groups into TMS ethers or carbonyl groups (exemplified in Almé and Sjövall, 1980).

C. Liquid Chromatography–Mass Spectrometry

This method, LC–MS, is likely to become very important in future steroid analysis. Recent reviews include those of Arpino and Guiochon (1979), Dawkins and McLafferty (1978), McFadden (1980), Games (1980), and Privett and Erdahl (1978). So far there are few applications in the steroid area. This is because capillary column GC–MS yields superior separations, and because good LC–MS systems permitting mass spectrometry of underivatized, conjugated steroids without need for vaporization are still lacking.

There are three principally different modes of transferring the sample into the ion source. Scott et al. (1974), McFadden et al. (1976), and Privett and Erdahl (1978) deposit the effluent on a moving wire or belt, and the solvent is evaporated prior to introduction, vaporization, and ionization of the sample. The problem with this system in steroid analysis is the poor volatility and thermal lability of many steroids. In the method of Privett and Erdahl (1978) the sample is converted to hydrocarbons prior to ionization, and this makes it less useful in steroid analyses. The Finnegan system (McFadden, 1980) has been used by Games (1980) and co-workers in analyses of underivatized glucuronides and bile acid conjugates. The results of these studies are awaited with interest. A system for solvent removal with a silicone membrane separator (Jones and Yang, 1975) is unlikely to be useful in steroid analyses.

Horning and co-workers have used atmospheric pressure ionization (see Section IV,A) of the entire or part of the effluent, followed by analysis of the ions in a quadrupole mass spectrometer (Horning et al., 1974; Carroll et al., 1975). This results in a solvent-mediated ionization with prominent quasi-molecular ions. Examples of LC–MS separations of progesterone and 11-ketoprogesterone were shown. However, further applications in steroid analysis have not appeared.

McLafferty and co-workers (Arpino et al., 1974) first described the method of introducing part of the effluent from a HPLC column into a chemical ionization source. The solvent serves as the ionizing reagent. High pumping capacities, preferably with large cold traps, are required. A solvent flow rate of 10 μl/minute could be maintained. Problems encountered with this method are that the inlet capillary gets plugged with sample residues and that the need for ion source cleaning increases. A few simple steroids were studied.

In attempts to increase the percentage of effluent introduced into the ion source, Takeuchi *et al.* (1978) used a jet separator in combination with the micro liquid chromatography columns of Ishii *et al.* (1978). Thus, the total effluent from the micro columns (8 μl/minute) could be accepted by the mass spectrometer and sensitivities in the nanogram range were obtained. The problem is the vaporization of nonvolatile compounds, and continued work by this group (Tsuge *et al.*, 1979) has resulted in an interface that uses a stream of helium to produce fine droplets that are led into the ion source via the collecting part of the separator.

A direct connection of micro liquid chromatography columns to a mass spectrometer was described by Henion and Maylin (1980). The effluent was led through a narrow capillary probe into the chemical ionization source. The probe tip orifice was 30–35 μm, but problems with plugging were not discussed. About 20 pg of phenothiazine tranquilizers could be analyzed using selected ion monitoring.

A different system to vaporize the entire effluent has been described by Vestal and co-workers. In a recent version (Blakely *et al.*, 1980) an oxyhydrogen flame vaporizes and nebulizes the effluent around a jet similar to that used by Tsuge *et al.* (1979). Nonvolatile compounds such as nucleotides could be analyzed at nanogram sensitivity, and this system appears to be promising for analysis of nonvolatile steroids.

The coupling of reversed-phase ion-pair chromatography with mass spectrometry has been studied by Karger and co-workers (Karger *et al.*, 1979; Kirby *et al.*, 1980). This is an important problem, since ion-pair chromatography is likely to be widely used for separation of steroid conjugates. A segmented-flow extractor was placed between the liquid chromatograph and the mass spectrometer, and the organic extract was then deposited on a moving belt. Solvent was evaporated, and the ion pairs could be ionized. The observed properties of ion pairs in electron impact and chemical ionization mass spectrometry should stimulate corresponding studies of ion pairs of steroid conjugates.

It is clear that LC–MS techniques develop very rapidly. Some instruments and interfaces are already commercially available. However, it will probably take several years before separating efficiencies and sensitivities become comparable to those obtained by capillary column GC-MS. The time when intact unconjugated steroids can be efficiently separated and identified as is presently done with unconjugated steroid derivatives is probably a decade away.

V. QUANTITATION OF STEROIDS

Although precision is also of importance, specificity is the most important quality of a quantitative analytical method. The historical development shows that the specificity of a method is always lower than originally believed. This is repeatedly seen with colorimetric, radioisotopic, enzymatic, and immunological methods of steroid analysis, and it is true also of many mass spectrometric methods. Recovery experiments are often performed to estimate the accuracy of a method. It is obviously a minimum requirement that an added compound can be estimated; the problem is to ascertain that the value obtained for an untreated sample is due to the compound thought to be measured. In spite of some limitations, mass spectrometric, and GC–MS techniques have been extremely important in improving the specificity of steroid analyses.

A quantitative method consists of two parts to be matched: sample preparation and quantitative measurement. With increasing specificity of the measuring method, sample preparation can be simplified. This has often been done in immunoassays and GC–MS analyses, resulting in questionable specificity of many methods, particularly when concentrations of steroids are low. When retention time is the only criterion of specificity, as in HPLC and GLC, the column efficiency is very important, and independent proof of specificity, e.g., by GC–MS analysis, should in most cases be presented. In the examples given below it is often difficult to evaluate specificity. The reader interested in using a method should test the specificity with the particular samples to be studied.

A. HIGH-PRESSURE LIQUID CHROMATOGRAPHY

Vestergaard (1973) has made the most extensive routine use of column liquid chromatography in quantitative analyses of urinary steroids. The systems were developed before the time of HPLC, and similar separations could probably be obtained more rapidly now. However, the detailed descriptions of the methods and their optimization is valuable reading for anyone working with steroid analysis (see Vestergaard et al., 1978).

Since the introduction of commercial HPLC instruments, an increasing number of quantitative HPLC methods have been published. Modifications and improvements are often published at short intervals, possibly reflecting methodological deficiencies when biological problems are studied.

Because of their clinical interest, high concentrations in plasma, and UV absorption, cortisol and related synthetic steroids have been the subject of a large number of studies. Different packing materials and mobile phases have been used, both reversed-phase systems (Scott and Dixon, 1979; Smith, 1979; Reardon *et al.*, 1979; Kabra *et al.*, 1979) and straight-phase adsorption systems (De Vries *et al.*, 1980; Rose and Jusko, 1979; Frey *et al.*, 1979). Among the more elegant and rapid methods is that of van den Berg *et al.* (1977) with a *p*-nitroaniline bonded silica in a straight-phase system. Tests of interference by different compounds were made in most studies, and the particular types of plasma samples to be analyzed determined the choice of system. The specificity and sensitivity of methods for use in studies of adrenal steroid biosynthesis and metabolism (Chan *et al.*, 1977; Gallant *et al.*, 1978) still appear insufficient except in special applications. To improve sensitivity, Kawasaki *et al.* (1979) allowed the 3-keto group to react with dansyl hydrazine to obtain a fluorescent derivative. In this as well as several other studies, a comparison was made with radioimmunoassay. Although the correlations were generally good, it may be noted that the immunoassay gave higher values at low levels of cortisol. Dansyl derivatives were also used by Schmidt *et al.* (1978) for analysis of estrogens, but the specificity of this method in analysis of urine samples was studied only in a preliminary way.

A method for analysis of vitamin D and its metabolites in plasma illustrates the potential of HPLC to measure low concentrations when it is combined with suitable prepurification steps (Lambert *et al.*, 1977). The plasma was extracted, and vitamin D metabolites were collected separately in a straight-phase chromatography on Sephadex LH-20. They were then quantitated by HPLC in a reversed-phase system with a UV detector. The 1,25-dihydroxy metabolite was estimated by adsorption-HPLC and quantitation with a ligand binding assay. The concentration of the latter metabolite was about 35 pg/ml plasma. This is an elegant example showing superiority of HPLC over GC–MS in analysis of labile steroids.

The combination of HPLC with detection by immunoassay has an obvious potential value. Schöneshöfer *et al.* (1981) have evaluated such a system in detail. Eleven steroids were studied, and appropriate steroid bands were collected with an automatic system. Forty samples could be handled in 1.5 days without any manual manipulation. The results indicated marked overestimation (100%) of aldosterone and cortisol in urine by radioiimmunoassay without HPLC separation. Recoveries of added radiolabeled steroids varied between 87 and 100%. Further development of this methlology can be expected.

B. Gas-Liquid Chromatography

Quantitative analysis of metabolic profiles of steroids in urine is mostly performed with GLC and a flame ionization detector (FID) (see Section VI,A). Satisfactory specificity is obtained when a high-resolution glass capillary column is used, and the samples contain high concentrations of steroids. Specificity and sensitivity can be further increased by use of selective purification methods (see Section III,B,3). Thus, the precision for duplicate analysis of estrone after selective isolation of a phenolic fraction was 3.2% when the concentration in urine was more than 10 ng/ml and 8.0% when the concentration was at or below 5 ng/ml (Fels et al., 1979). Quantitation by GLC with glass capillary columns has been discussed in detail by Shackleton (1981), and applications to the analysis of steroid profiles are reviewed in Section VI,A,1–3.

The FID response varies considerably for different steroids. Mass response factors based on peak areas of MO-TMS derivatives of major urinary neutral steroids ranged from 0.40 for androsterone to 1.16 for pregnanetriol, compared with cholesteryl butyl ether (Pfaffenberger and Horning, 1977; Maume et al., 1979). Part of the variations may be due to losses in the GLC system. Thus, for accurate determinations with FID, response factors are required for each compound. Three 6α-hydroxylated cortisol metabolites in human neonatal urine were quantified as their MO-TMS derivatives with reference compounds specifically synthesized for this purpose (Derks and Drayer, 1978b). Since it may not be possible to prepare every reference substance in pure form, approximations of response values have to be made. The molar FID response of underivatized steroids has been shown to be linearly related with both proportional and constant factors to an effective carbon number (Edwards, 1978a). A similar study of derivatized steroids has not been made. In the absence of the appropriate reference steroid, the response may be assumed to be the same as that of a similar steroid.

Electron capture detection has been used for a series of underivatized substituted 17α-acetoxyprogesterones (Koshy, 1976). The response was largely dependent on the structure of the steroids, and highest sensitivity was obtained with melengestrol acetate (6-dehydro-6-methyl-16-methylene-17α-acetoxyprogesterone). Obviously, the specificity of the analysis increases when compounds do not have to be converted into electron capturing derivatives. Endogenous steroids are usually converted into haloalkyl derivatives (see Section IV,B,2,b,c). The precision in analyses of reference mixtures of HFB derivatives of 50 or 500 pg each of seven estrogens was better than 2–7% and 1%

respectively (Kern and Brander, 1979). However, as with all analytical techniques, the specificity and sensitivity are considerably lower when steroids in biological materials are analyzed. This is particularly true when packed columns are used, and analyses such as those of pregnenolone and pregnanolone isomers in human myometrium (Mickan and Zander, 1979) should be carried out with glass capillary columns.

C. High-Resolution Mass Spectrometry

Biological samples, even in a purified form, give ions of every nominal mass if the sensitivity of the mass spectrometer is set reasonably high. There are two ways to decrease this biological noise: (a) use of a GLC column as a fractionating inlet; or (b) use of a high resolution mass spectrometer. In the latter case, resolution may be set so that the interference is reduced to ions having the same elemental composition. Snedden and Parker (1976) have used the method for quantitative determination of estrogens and progesterone in human ovarian tissue. Dried tissue was introduced on the direct inlet probe with and without added standard (Snedden and Parker, 1971). The probe was heated, and currents of the molecular ions of estrone, estradiol, estriol, and progesterone were monitored at a resolution of 10,000. Calibration curves linear down to 1 ng of steroid and recoveries of steroids added to plasma were 81–93%. The general value of this method is difficult to assess; the use of dried tissue makes it rapid. On the other hand, this limits the usefulness to tissues that contain high concentrations of steroids (above 1 ppm based on dry weight). One may assume that contamination of the ion source is a problem.

D. Gas Chromatography–Mass Spectrometry

No doubt GC–MS is one of the most versatile and accurate methods for quantitative determination of steroids. Its use in biomedical research and clinical chemistry has been reviewed by several authors (e.g., Lehmann and Schulten, 1978; Björkhem, 1979). A comprehensive and useful book on quantitative mass spectrometry has been written by Millard (1978), and papers from two symposia on quantitative mass spectrometry in life sciences have been published (de Leenheer and Roncucci, 1977; de Leenheer et al., 1978). Quantitative GC–MS can be performed in four ways: (a) by repetitive scanning of the entire mass range; (b) by repetitive scanning of a limited mass range of interest; (c) by repetitive switching between a few selected m/z values; and (d) by monitoring of a single m/z value. When repetitive scanning methods are used, computer acquisition of data is required for construction of selected ion current chromatograms. The switching methods and single-ion monitoring permit analog recording of the chromatograms.

Single-ion monitoring gives the highest sensitivity, since the current of ions of interest is measured continuously and optimal signal : noise ratio is achieved. Repetitive scanning of the entire mass range is the least sensitive method, since most of the measuring time is spent on m/z values without interest and on valleys between peaks. Comparisons of the sensitivities (Reimendal and Sjövall, 1972; Middleditch and Desiderio, 1973; Axelson et al., 1974a), have shown that repetitive scanning of complete spectra is at least 100 times less sensitive than repetitive scanning of a narrow mass range. The former method is useful for screening and measurements of complex mixtures, while switching between selected ions is used when a few specific steroids are to be accurately determined at low concentrations.

Instrumentation for GC–MS is continuously being improved for quantitative work, especially in connection with analysis of molecules differing in content of heavy isotopes (see Section VI). Atmospheric pressure ionization with counting of ions can yield sensitivities in the low femtogram range (see Reynolds et al., 1977). Development of electrooptical detection systems will permit continuous monitoring of ions within a limited mass range and should give sensitivities similar to that of single-ion monitoring for all ions within this range (Dreyer et al., 1974; Boettger et al., 1977; Hedfjäll and Ryhage, 1979). Major limiting factors will be the stability of the steroids in the column and interface to the ion source, and the background noise due to other compounds.

Quantitative GC–MS is carried out with the aid of internal and external standards. The former can either be the steroid or steroid derivative to be measured labeled with heavy atoms, or an isomer or homolog having a different retention time. The isotopically labeled steroid is added in excess and serves both as a conventional internal standard and as a carrier to decrease losses in the column and interface (Samuelsson et al., 1970). Cases have been described where the isotopically labeled version of the standard does not act as a carrier (see Millard, 1978), but the carrier effect has been obtained in all studies of steroids (see Reiffsteck et al., 1980). It has also been proposed (see Millard, 1978) that two internal standards should be used to increase sensitivity; one labeled with heavy atoms and acting as carrier, and the other having a different retention time but giving ions of the mass to be used for single-ion monitoring.

When external standards are used, i.e., separate injections of known amounts of the steroid to be measured, an internal standard should be added to all sample and standard solutions in amounts sufficient to avoid adsorption. This standard serves to correct for errors in injection volumes (Axelson et al., 1974a,b).

1. Isotopically Labeled Standards

In theory, isotope dilution with selected ion-monitoring GC–MS is one of the most accurate techniques for quantitative analysis of steroids. The isotopically labeled version of the steroid is added to the biological sample prior to purification. The ratio between labeled and endogenous compound is determined with high precision by GC–MS (see Björkhem, 1979; De Leenheer and Cruyl, 1980). The labeled steroid may contain a small amount of unlabeled molecules, and the endogenous compound has molecules that contain stable isotopes in natural abundance. Appropriate equations have to be used to compensate for this mutual interference (Yamamoto and McCloskey, 1977; Colby and McCaman, 1979; Schramm et al., 1979a,b). Schramm et al. (1979b) give an example of a published formula that is valid only when the interference is equal for the labeled and unlabeled steroid. In many studies such errors have been avoided by analysis of known mixtures and construction of calibration curves. The interference is decreased by use of a standard containing many heavy atoms. However, if too many deuterium or tritium atoms are introduced, isotope effects can result in separation of labeled and unlabeled steroid, both during purification and on the GLC column.

Steroids labeled with either radioactive (^{3}H or ^{14}C) or stable (^{2}H or ^{13}C) isotopes have been used as standards. The latter are preferable since radiation hazards are avoided. However, radioactively labeled steroids in high purity are commercially available and have therefore been frequently used. They also permit checks of recovery through the purification procedure, and determination of the amount added by scintillation counting.

Most methods have been developed for measurement of unconjugated steroids of moderate polarity in plasma (see Setchell, 1979). A limited number of studies deal with urine (Romanoff and Brodie, 1976; Björkhem et al., 1975b; Björkhem, 1979; Johnson et al., 1979a) and milk (Bhaskar et al., 1979). The standard is added to plasma, which is then extracted with an organic solvent of suitable polarity. In a few cases (Björkhem et al., 1975c; Siekmann et al., 1978) a period of equilibration at elevated temperature is allowed before extraction.

However, this is frequently omitted and the distribution of added standard between serum proteins may not be the same as that of the endogenous steroid. This is particularly important in analyses of milk, and we have not found the extraction method used by Bhaskar *et al.* (1979) to be quantitative when tested after appropriate equilibration of a labeled steroid with the milk sample.

After extraction, the steroid is usually purified in a single step using TLC (Björkhem *et al.*, 1974a,c; Siekmann *et al.*, 1976; Baba *et al.*, 1979; Moneti *et al.*, 1980) or chromatography on columns of silicic acid (Vestergaard *et al.*, 1975), Sephadex LH-20, or Lipidex (e.g., Zamecnik *et al.*, 1978; Siekmann, 1979; Knuppen *et al.*, 1979). When steroids are present in high concentration, no purification may be required, e.g., cortisol in plasma (Björkhem *et al.*, 1974).

In most cases only one steroid is analyzed at a time. This permits use of the most favorable derivative, giving intense ions of high mass and optimal sensitivity and specificity (see Section IV,B,2). Commonly employed derivatives for simple steroids include HFB esters (e.g., Siekmann *et al.*, 1970, 1976, 1978; Siekmann, 1979; Björkhem *et al.*, 1975c; Knuppen *et al.*, 1979), trifluoroacetate esters (Vestergaard *et al.*, 1975; Baba *et al.*, 1979), and the favorable *t*-BDMS ethers (see Moneti *et al.*, 1980). TMS ethers have been used in analyses of estrogens (Adlercreutz *et al.*, 1974c,d, 1975, 1978; Björkhem *et al.*, 1975a,b), and MO-TMS derivatives for analysis of cortisol (Björkhem *et al.*, 1974) and norethindrone (Bhaskar *et al.*, 1979).

Tritium-labeled steroids have been used as standards in analyses of testosterone using tetra-labeled (Vestergaard *et al.*, 1975) or di-labeled (Siekmann *et al.*, 1970; Breuer and Siekmann, 1975; Moneti *et al.*, 1980) species, and in analyses of dihydrotestosterone (Breuer and Siekmann, 1975), 5α-androstane-3α,17β-diol (Moneti *et al.*, 1980), ethynylestradiol (Siekmann *et al.*, 1978), cortisol and aldosterone (Siekmann *et al.*, 1970; Breuer and Siekmann, 1975) with di-labeled analogs. The high specific radioactivity is a disadvantage. If a glass capillary column is used and the standard contains four tritium atoms, isotope separations on the column may lead to differences in the adsorptive loss of standard and endogenous steroid.

The amount of radioactivity is less, and no isotope separation occurs with ^{14}C-labeled steroids. Methods for analysis of several estrogens (Siekmann, 1979) and 3-ketosteroids (Björkhem *et al.*, 1974, 1975a,c; Siekmann *et al.*, 1976; Siekmann, 1979; Jeannin *et al.*, 1978) have been based on the use of such standards. The small mass difference and the isotopic impurity of the labeled steroid may result in decreased accuracy and precision.

Development of selected ion monitoring techniques has stimulated work on the synthesis of steroids labeled with stable isotopes. Since it is cheaper and simpler to introduce several ^2H than ^{13}C atoms, most work has been done using deuterium-labeled steroids. Methods have been described for analysis of many endogenous steroids: estrone, estradiol, estriol, and 2-hydroxyestrone (Björkhem et al., 1975b; Breuer and Siekmann, 1975; Zamecnik et al., 1978; Knuppen et al., 1979), dehydroepiandrosterone (Johnson et al., 1980), testosterone (Baba et al., 1979), and progesterone (Johnson et al., 1979a). 25-Hydroxy vitamin D_3 was analyzed as the 3-t-BDMS-25-TMS derivative (Björkhem and Holmberg, 1978). The synthetic steroids 16α-cyano-3β-hydroxy-5-pregnen-20-one cyclopentyl ether (Gaskell et al., 1977), norethindrone (norethisterone) (Bhaskar et al., 1979; Fotherby et al., 1979), dianabol (Björkhem et al., 1980), and medroxyprogesterone acetate (Phillipou and Frith, 1980) have also been determined with ^2H-labeled standards.

The precision and accuracy of the methods depend on the concentration of the steroid, the isotopic purity of the internal standard, and the purity of the sample. The precision is often better than 1%, and the methods have been used as reference methods in clinical chemistry (see Björkhem, 1979). Comparisons with radioimmunoassay have been part of several of the studies cited, and the correlations between the methods have differed depending on the methods compared. Particularly in the low concentration range, radioimmunoassays tend to give higher values.

Since relatively few isotopically labeled steroids are available, several methods have been developed that are based on the use of a labeled derivatizing reagent. When many groups in the steroid are derivatized, e.g., as perdeuterio-TMS ethers, the mass differences may become too large, and isotope effects may result in separation of standard and endogenous steroid. The technique has been extensively used in analyses of estrogens in different biological fluids (Adlercreutz, 1974, 1977; Adlercreutz et al., 1974c,d, 1975, 1978) and in analyses of corticosteroids in adrenal cell cultures (Maume et al., 1973, 1976). Rosenfeld and Taguchi (1978) used the di(perdeuterio)ethyl ether as standard to determine 2-hydroxyestradiol, which was isolated by extractive ethylation. Some C_{21} steroids in urine were analyzed as acetates, with deuterioacetates as carriers (Romanoff and Brodie, 1976). Obviously, corrections for losses in the purification of endogenous steroids cannot be made when deuterated TMS ethers are used as standards. However, it is a useful alternative in analyses of metabolic profiles. It is important to establish that exchange of labeled and unlabeled TMS groups does not occur under the conditions used.

2. *Other Standards*

Since labeled steroids are frequently not available, it may be necessary to use a homolog, isomer, or other closely similar steroid as internal standard. Alternatively, the authentic steroid is used as external standard. These methods have been used in many studies, often without detailed evaluation of accuracy and precision. Some examples that illustrate advantages and disadvantages with different procedures will be given.

In order to permit single-ion monitoring, internal standards are often used that give molecular or fragment ions of the same mass as the steroid to be determined. Stillwell *et al.* (1974) analyzed norethisterone with norgestrel as the internal standard. The TMS-enol-TMS derivatives were used, which give intense molecular ions suitable for selected ion monitoring. Brooks and Middleditch (1971) evaluated sensitivity and linearity in quantitations of 17α-alkylated 17β-hydroxysteroids by single ion monitoring. The limit of detection was about 10 pg for several compounds lacking a 3-hydroxy group, and losses due to adsorption were not seen in the 50–100 pg range. This is unusual for an underivatized steroid and indicates the importance of a 3-hydroxyl group for such losses. The authors also employed chloromethyl-dimethylsilyl ethers to be able to use the $^{35}Cl : ^{37}Cl$ ratio in appropriate ions to support the specificity of the analyses.

Urinary estra-1,3,5-triene-3,15α,16α,17β-tetrol, was analyzed by Kelly (1971), with a 4-methyl-1,15α,16α,17β-tetrol analog as internal standard. The intense ion at m/z 191, due to a silyl migration in the D ring (Gustafsson *et al.*, 1969), was monitored. The limit of measurement was as high as 5 ng, which illustrates the background problems at this low mass. However, the precision was 6% for the entire procedure, which was very good compared to other methods at that time.

A thorough study of the analysis of testosterone and progesterone in plasma was performed by Dehennin *et al.* (1974). The 17β-hydroxy group was converted into an acetate and the 3-keto-4-ene structure into an enol heptafluorobutyrate. In this way intense molecular ions of high mass were obtained. Two standards were synthesized, 4-methyl-19-nortestosterone and 4-ethyl-4-androstenedione, which gave molecular ions of the same mass as testosterone and progesterone, respectively. The study described a number of the problems encountered in selected ion detection without use of labeled carrier materials. While adsorptive losses appeared to be below 20 pg, a marked increase in response was caused by contaminating substances arriving to the ion source at the same time as the steroid to be measured. From their experiments, Dehennin *et al.* (1974) concluded that the increased response was due to an effect in the ion source. The same phenomenon was observed in analyses of MO-TMS derivatives of ethynylestradiol, norethisterone, and norgestrel from urine and plasma with single ion monitoring (Tetsuo *et al.* 1980). These authors considered the effect to be due to a carrier action of the contaminating compounds, particularly in the separator and ion source. The phenomenon has been further studied in detail by Reiffsteck *et al.* (1980). The ability of a steroid to act as a carrier for another steroid depended on the structures of the two compounds, deuterated analogs acting as ideal carriers. The increased response was due to effects both in the column and ion source. In their early studies, Dehennin *et al.* (1974) had sufficient amounts of contaminants to maximize and linearize the response for the steroids measured. In the study of Tetsuo *et al.* (1980), glass capillary columns were used, and the purity of the samples was high. This diminished the carrier effect, and quantitations were made with external standards injected between each sample. In a study of the concentration of estradiol in the nuclear fraction of rat uteri, the carrier effect was essentially compensated for by injection of appropriate amounts of the external standard (estradiol) about 2 minutes before and after the injection of the biological sample (Axelson *et al.*, 1981b).

Corticosteroids with a hydroxyl group at C-18 present special analytical problems since they are labile and can exist in different isomeric forms. Maume and co-workers (see Bournot *et al.*, 1975) and Shackleton and Honour (1977) have developed procedures for the analysis of these steroids. MO-TMS derivatives were used, and conditions required for quantitative conversion were studied in detail. Shackleton and Honour (1977) used an epimer of the steroid to be analyzed as internal standard. Urinary tetrahydroaldosterone was analyzed by an analogous procedure (Honour and Shackleton, 1977).

In many methods an internal standard is selected to permit correction for losses during the purification without giving ions of the same mass as the steroid to be analyzed. Adlercreutz *et al.* (1974a) used medroxyprogesterone as standard in analyses of megestrol acetate, which contains an additional double bond. Since the 17-acetoxy-20-keto structure makes the steroid thermally labile, different derivatives were studied. The 3-methyloxime was used that was formed under mild conditions without reaction at the hindered C-20. Seamark *et al.* (1977) measured steroid production by ovarian follicles in culture and perfused human ovaries, with selected ion monitoring of enol-trifluoroacetates of *t*-BDMS derivatives. 19-Norandrostenedione and 19-nortestosterone served as internal standards for steroids of low and medium polarity, respectively. These groups were separated on Lipidex 5000 to avoid problems with interference in the GC–MS analysis.

Complex steroid mixtures have been analyzed by repetitive scanning techniques with external standards. Mono- and disulfate conjugates of several isomers of 16α-hydroxypregnanolones and -pregnanediols in plasma of pregnant women were measured by repetitive accelerating voltage scanning of an appropriate narrow mass range followed by computer calculation of areas in selected ion current chromatograms (Baillie et al., 1976). This study illustrates the complexity of the steroid sulfate mixture in plasma in pregnancy, 24 steroids being identified. The mixture of unconjugated steroid metabolites is equally complex. Only some of these steroids have been estimated in a semiquantitative way from selected ion current chromatograms obtained by repetitive scanning of partial (m/z 250–480) mass spectra (Axelson and Sjövall, 1977).

Steroids in bovine corpora lutea have also been measured with repetitive magnetic scanning and external standards (Axelson et al., 1974b, 1975). Again, the steroid mixture was found to be more complex than was previously realized, and the quantitative composition was different from that obtained in studies with other methods.

In summary, quantitation of steroids by GC–MS without use of standards labeled with heavy atoms is less accurate than when such standards are used. Adsorptive losses modified by various nonspecific carrier effects will decrease the precision of the measurements. The linearity of the response has been impoved by use of packed columns and less sample purification, but it is obvious that this decreases the specificity. In spite of the problems, it is often necessary to use unlabeled internal or external standards, particularly when complex mixtures of partly unknown composition are to be quantitated.

E. GAS CHROMATOGRAPHY–HIGH-RESOLUTION MASS SPECTROMETRY

The problems with interference by contaminating compounds and background peaks in low-resolution GC–MS may be solved by better sample purification and use of glass capillary columns. An alternative is to use a high-resolution mass spectrometer. Millington and Griffiths and co-workers have used this method extensively in studies of tissue concentrations of various steroids (Millington et al., 1974; Millington, 1975, 1977). A packed column was attached via a Watson-Biemann separator to the mass spectrometer operating at a resolution of 10,000. The drop in sensitivity of about 90%, compared to that at resolution

1000, was compensated for by the increased signal : noise ratio. Tissue samples were extracted, lipids were removed by a solvent partition, and aliquots corresponding to 0.5 g of tissue or 2.5 ml of plasma were analyzed as TMS or t-BDMS ethers together with epimeric internal standards, with single-ion monitoring. The main advantage compared to low resolution GC–MS is the reduced need for sample purification. Selection of more suitable derivatives with respect to uniqueness and abundance of ions to be monitored may result in higher sensitivity. Data showing the number of interfering ions of the same integer mass but with different elementary composition clearly indicated that GC–MS with low resolution can be an unspecific method unless samples are properly purified or ions of high mass are monitored (see Millington, 1977).

The method has been used in studies of estrogens and C_{19} steroids in breast tumor tissue (Millington et al., 1974; Maynard et al., 1977) and of C_{19} steroids in hyperplastic prostatic tissue (Millington et al., 1975). In the latter case purification of extracts by TLC was needed to ensure sufficient sensitivity and specificity. For compounds with good GLC properties giving intense ions, concentrations down to 10 pg per gram of tissue could be estimated. In most cases concentrations were much higher. The method has also been used for validation of radioimmunoassays of estradiol (D. W. Wilson et al., 1977).

Development of these methods has been continued by Gaskell and Pike (1978), who used t-BDMS derivatives because of their higher stability and prominent ions at $(M-57)^+$. Sample extracts and derivatives were purified on microcolumns of Lipidex 5000 in reversed-phase systems and Sephadex LH-20 in straight-phase systems. Different $C_{19}O_2$ steroids in plasma and saliva were analyzed at concentrations above 0.5 ng per milliliter of plasma and 25 pg per milliliter of parotid fluid. The need for high resolution was clearly illustrated, showing that low-resolution detection can give erroneously high values. However, it should be noted that ions of relatively low mass were monitored (around m/z 350), and this is known to be nonspecific at low resolution.

Gaskell and Millington (1978) have also described a method in which fragmentations occurring in the first field free region of the high-resolution mass spectrometer (metastable ions) are monitored. This method is very specific and sensitive, provided that a transition gives a metastable ion of high intensity. Dihydrotestosterone in plasma was measured as the t-BDMS derivative without interference, by monitoring the reaction m/z 347 → m/z 271. The detection limit was about 20 pg of injected steroid. A similar method was used for analysis of testosterone in hamster prostate (Gaskell et al., 1979b), and a comparison was made with conventional selected ion monitoring both at high and low resolution. The results demonstrate that low resolution is not sufficiently specific when ions of intermediate mass are monitored. However, the possible elimination of interference by use of a capillary column was not tested.

VI. Analysis of Metabolic Profiles and Studies of Metabolism

A. Metabolic Profiles

The goal in analyses of metabolic profiles is the quantitation of each individual steroid. This includes separate analysis not only of each group of conjugates of a steroid, but also of the positional isomers arising by conjugation at different sites. This is important for the interpretation of analytical results, since different conjugates of a steroid may have different metabolic origins. There are many examples of this situation; an illustrative one is the selective influence of an ethanol-induced change of the hepatic redox state on plasma levels of 3- and 17-sulfates of 5α-androstane-$3\alpha,17\beta$-diol (Cronholm and Sjövall, 1970). It is also obvious that the order in which reduction, hydroxylation, and conjugation takes place in the sequential metabolism of steroids may vary and that the metabolic fate of an unconjugated steroid differs from that of the conjugated one. The differences in hydroxylation of conjugated and unconjugated steroids are typical examples (e.g., Diczfalusy 1969; Einarsson et al., 1976; Gustafsson and Ingelman-Sundberg, 1976; Baillie et al., 1975b).

However, the technical development has not yet reached a stage when such detailed analyses can be carried out within a reasonable time frame. The LC–MS combination may change this situation in the future. At present, analyses of metabolic profiles are simplifications, where information about molecular species of steroids is lost in one way or another. There are three principal means by which analyses are simplified.

1. Conjugated steroids are hydrolyzed, and the resulting mixture of unconjugated steroids is analyzed with or without preceding group fractionation.
2. One or a few groups of steroids is first isolated and the analysis is performed after cleavage of conjugates.
3. Unconjugated steroids and known groups of conjugates are separated, and each group is analyzed after hydrolysis of conjugates.

1. *Analysis after Initial Hydrolysis*

Methods for analysis of steroid profiles by GLC were pioneered by E. C. Horning and co-workers (Gardiner and Horning, 1966; Horning and Horning, 1971). An important factor in the development was the use of combined MO-TMS derivatives. Although the analytical results were remarkable, there were deficiencies in the methodology that were largely eliminated by the same group. Thus, the original method of derivatization gave incomplete conversion of hindered hydroxyl groups into TMS ethers. Thenot and Horning (1972a) established conditions for conversion of all keto groups except at C-11 into MO derivatives and of all hydroxyl groups into TMS derivatives. Incomplete separations on packed columns constituted another problem. Changes of stationary phase, although helpful for separation of certain groups of steroids, resulted only in overlaps between other steroids. Conversion of ketosteroids into O-benzyloximes was used in analyses of steroids in infants, since a separation of ketosteroids from hydroxysteroids was achieved (see Section IV,B,2,b). However, quantitative derivatization of hindered groups in corticosteroids cannot be obtained, and the method is not useful for general purposes. Separation problems were greatly reduced by the use of Silanox-SE-30 glass capillary columns (see Section IV,B,1). An excellent description of a method with these columns to analyze metabolic profiles of steroids in human urine was given by Pfaffenberger and Horning (1975). This method was used in studies of steroids in healthy men and women and in women with breast tumors (Pfaffenberger and Horning 1975; Pfaffenberger *et al.*, 1977, 1978). Sex differences were noted in ratios between certain 5β and 5α reduced $C_{19}O_2$ and $C_{21}O_5$ metabolites, and there were interesting correlations between the $5\beta:5\alpha$ ratios and presence of breast tumors. It is known that 5α steroids are sulfated to a higher degree than 5β steroids (see Pasqualini, 1967) and that the extent of biliary excretion is different for the two types of steroids (see e.g., Laatikainen and Karjalainen, 1972). It is therefore a drawback that the method of Pfaffenberger and Horning starts with hydrolysis.

Glass capillary columns developed by other workers were also used in analyses of metabolic profiles of steroids. The first application was by Völlmin, who combined the partial MO-TMS derivatization procedure of Gardiner and Horning (1966) with analysis on columns prepared according to Grob (for references see Curtius *et al.*, 1975). As discussed above, the derivatization procedure is not satisfactory for many corticosteroid metabolites. Ros and Sommerville (1971) used a similar method and also attempted to use the TMS-enol-TMS derivatization technique of Chambaz *et al.* (1972). Partial and incomplete derivatization of some groups make this reaction less suitable in profile analyses (see Section IV,B,2). Luyten and Rutten (1974) used their type of capillary columns and solid injection system and pointed out the advantage of using persilylated MO-TMS derivatives. Bailey *et al.* (1974) studied the quantitative aspects of capillary GLC with columns of the Novotny type (see Section IV,B,1). They found that automatic solid injection could be used with good reproducibility. However, only TMS ether derivatives were used, so that most corticosteroid metabolites of the C_{21} series were not included in the profiles. A study with particular emphasis on automation and quantitation was carried out by Fantl and Gray (1977). Glucuronidase hydrolysis limited their profiles to glucuronides, and TMS-enol-TMS derivatives were used.

Leunissen and Thijssen (1978) evaluated accuracy and reproducibility of extraction, hydrolysis, solvolysis, and quantitation of urinary steroid profiles by glass capillary GLC. The study was performed with urine containing metabolites of several radioactively labeled steroids given to the subjects to monitor recoveries. MO-TMS derivatives were used, but the method of preparation appears less satisfactory than that of Thenot and Horning (1972a) and takes a longer time. Since direct solid injection was used, the reagents had to be removed prior to injection. This was done by filtration through Lipidex 5000 (see Section IV,B,2,a) or by partition between methylene chloride and dilute sulfuric acid. The possible hydrolysis of labile TMS ethers (e.g., of phenolic steroids) with the latter method was not studied. A similar analytical approach was used by Phillipou *et al.* (1978). However, these authors used SCOT columns, the efficiencies of which were insufficient judging from the chromatograms shown.

Shackleton and co-workers have published the most systematic series of studies with capillary column GLC and GC–MS to analyze metabolic profiles of steroids in urine of neonatal infants and children with abnormal steroid synthesis. This work is discussed in the excellent review by Shackleton (1981), which also describes a number of other applications of glass capillary column GLC to the analysis of steroid profiles in patients with different diseases. After the early studies with packed columns (see Horning *et al.*, 1969; Gustafsson *et al.*, 1970; Shackleton *et al.*, 1971, 1973; Devaux *et al.*, 1971b), Shackleton and Honour (1976) described a method where glass capillary columns (20 m OV-101) were used with an automatic solid injection system. Quantitation was based on the use of two internal standards, one with a short and one with a long retention time. Response factors and precision were studied, as were the conditions for derivatization. In most cases persilylated MO-TMS derivatives were used, purified by filtration through Lipidex 5000. The analysis starts with enzymatic hydrolysis of urine. This results in loss of certain steroid sulfates that are not substrates of the enzymes used. After extraction with Amberlite XAD-2, the hydrolyzed steroids are purified by chromatography on Sephadex LH-20 (see Section III,B,2). When necessary, a group fractionation is made that permits analysis of minor components and overlapping peaks. Since this increases the number of fractions to be analyzed, the automatic injection system is very useful.

The method has been used to study steroid profiles in urine of an infant with a salt-losing syndrome (Shackleton and Snodgrass, 1974) and in urine of infants with defects in aldosterone biosynthesis (Shackleton et al., 1976), 21-hydroxylation (Shackleton, 1976; Taylor et al., 1978), and 17α-hydroxylation (Honour et al., 1978). GC–MS with selected ion monitoring was frequently used in addition to analysis of complete profiles in order to search for early changes in specific metabolites. An interesting study of congenital adrenal hypoplasia (Shackleton et al., 1979a) illustrates the value of steroid profile analysis. Virtual absence of 3β-hydroxy-5-ene steroids in an infant was combined with normal excretion of cortisol metabolites, indicating separate localization of control systems for the formation of these steroids in the fetal adrenal. Another profile analysis indicated that abnormalities in the metabolism of steroids in the liver might be associated with hypertension (Shackleton et al., 1980a). Studies of this type may be even more important than those concerned with inherited defects of steroid synthesis since they may reveal new diseases secondary to disturbed metabolism of steroids (Ulick et al., 1977). Using similar methods, Shackleton and co-workers have also analyzed metabolic profiles of steroids in urine from monkeys. Species differences in steroid metabolism have been defined, and references to this work can be found in the paper by Setchell et al. (1976b).

Independently of the studies of Shackleton and co-workers, Reiner and Spiteller (1975) investigated metabolic profiles of steroids in urine of the newborn with the aid of glass capillary gas chromatography and mass spectrometry. They summarized mass spectrometric results for 42 compounds as TMS derivatives. The limitations of the derivatization method with respect to incomplete reactions and enol ether formation is seen from this and other studies by Spiteller and co-workers (see below).

Several other groups have used methods similar to those of Horning or Shackleton and their co-workers to analyze metabolic profiles of steroids in urine. Anderson et al. (1974a,b, 1977) studied profiles of steroids in urine of the newborn. They used packed columns and circumvented the problem of insufficient resolution in three ways: (a) separate solvolysis and hydrolysis of sulfates and glucuronides, respectively; (b) group separation of steroids by straight-phase or reversed-phase chromatography on hydroxyalkoxypropyl Sephadex (Lipidex 5000); (c) preparation of different substituted oximes of ketosteroids. The method to separate sulfates and glucuronides by solvolysis–hydrolysis is not quantitative, but the major aim was to characterize the steroid composition qualitatively.

Studies of a similar nature were carried out by Bègue et al. (1976) in order to identify further the steroids in urine of pregnant women. Steroids were enzymatically hydrolyzed, extracted with solvent, and group-fractionated on Sephadex LH-20. The steroids in 12 fractions were analyzed as TMS ethers. It follows from the discussion above that this methodology will exclude certain steroid sulfates, highly polar steroids, and most cortisol metabolites from the profiles. The complexity of the steroid mixture is evident from the list of 48 identified steroids, which does not include any $C_{19}O_4$, $C_{21}O_4$, $C_{21}O_5$, or $C_{21}O_6$ steroids. The same method was used to study the steroid profile in a pregnant woman with a virilizing luteoma (Bègue et al., 1977). Thirty-nine steroids were identified and many were quantitated. As expected, androgenic C_{19} steroids were produced in large amounts and were excreted partly in hydroxylated form.

Further studies of pathological pregnancies have been reported by this group (Bègue et al., 1979b; Losty et al., 1979). Unfortunately solvent extraction methods were used, and the profiles lack information on tetra-, penta-, and hexaoxygenated steroids. The same is true of the recent analyses of steroid profiles in amniotic fluid (Peltonen et al., 1979). Glass capillary columns were used to separate TMS ethers of steroids first liberated by β-glucuronidase, then by Helix pomatia enzymes. As discussed above, profiles obtained in this way will lack several sulfated steroids as well as polar steroids. In addition, the latter steroids would be partly removed in the silicic acid chromatography used to purify the steroid fractions (see Section III,B,2).

2. Analysis of Limited Groups

The first GLC and GC–MS analyses of this type were concerned with steroid sulfates in plasma. After qualitative studies (Sjövall and Vihko, 1966a, 1968; Sjövall et al., 1968a), a quantitative method was developed for separation of steroid mono- and disulfates and quantitation of individual steroids as TMS ethers by GLC and GC–MS (Jänne et al., 1969). The methods of purification and derivatization limited the analyses mainly to steroids with two and three oxygen substituents. Steroid sulfate profiles in plasma, urine, bile, and feces of men and of nonpregnant and pregnant women were analyzed (see Sjövall, 1970; Eriksson *et al.*, 1970; Jänne and Vihko, 1970; Jänne, 1971; Laatikainen and Karjalainen, 1972). A large number of studies were published in this area by the Swedish and Finnish groups.

Interesting abnormalities in the concentrations of sulfated steroids of the pregnane series were found in pregnant women with intrahepatic cholestasis of pregnancy (Sjövall and Sjövall, 1970). This disease was further studied with regard to steroid profiles in feces and urine and the influence of antibiotics on the profiles (see Eriksson *et al.*, 1972) Similar methods were used to study profiles of steroid glucuronides in urine, but again the methods of purification and derivatization limited the profiles to steroids with two or three oxygen substituents and excluded most corticosteroid metabolites (see Viinikka and Jänne, 1973). The same gel chromatographic separation of steroid sulfates was used for analysis of partial steroid profiles in urine of infants with 21-hydroxylase deficiency (Viinikka *et al.*, 1973) and 3β-hydroxysteroid dehydrogenase deficiency (Laatikainen *et al.*, 1972). Shackleton (1974) used essentially the same method for studies of urinary steroid profiles in orangutan and rhesus monkey infants and compared the results with those obtained with humans (Gustafsson *et al.*, 1970; Shackleton *et al.*, 1971). A similar conjugate separation was used by Ludwig *et al.* (1977) in qualitative studies of metabolic profiles of mono- and disulfated steroids in plasma from humans.

Improved purification of hydrolyzed steroids was obtained by use of DEAP-LH-20 and Lipidex 5000 (see Section III,B,1,2), and several new steroids were found in these profiles. Using the same procedures, Spiteller and co-workers have investigated steroid profiles in uremia (Ludwig *et al.*, 1978) and psoriasis (Ludwig-Köhn *et al.*, 1979). These studies are largely qualitative, but they provide GLC data for many steroids and indicate marked abnormalities in the profiles. The importance of separating conjugate groups prior to hydrolysis is evident. Such separations were not done in a study of steroid profiles in urine of hirsute women (Egger *et al.*, 1978). The most striking abnormality in 50% of the patients was a 10- to 100-fold increase of dehydroepiandrosterone. Since many androgen precursors and metabolites are sulfated, such studies should have included prior isolation of these conjugates.

Whereas metabolic profiles of glucuronidated and sulfated neutral steroids can usually be analyzed by capillary column GLC with flame ionization detection and identification of peaks by GC–MS, estrogenic steroids are usually present in amounts that require the use of a mass spectrometer as a detector. Profiles of estrogens have been extensively studied by Adlercreutz and co-workers. Their early methods were very complex owing to the need for purification of sufficient amounts of steroids for GLC analysis (see Adlercreutz and Luukkainen, 1968). With the development of selected ion detection methods it has been possible to simplify the analytical procedures. Since the analyses have usually involved selected ion monitoring, this work is discussed in Section V,D,1. A review by Adlercreutz (1980) has been published.

The phenolic group permits selective isolation of estrogens by ion-exchange chromatography (see Section III,B,3,a). This has opened new possibilities for analysis of estrogen profiles. Adessi et al. (1975) isolated urinary estrogens from hydrolyzed pregnancy urine and analyzed them as TMS ethers on packed GLC columns. With their present availability, glass capillary columns should be used to ascertain the specificity (Fels et al., 1979). Unconjugated estrogens in plasma from pregnant women could be analyzed by capillary column GLC after a simple isolation on TEAP-LH-20 (see Section III,B,3,a) (Axelson and Sjövall, 1977). Adlercreutz and co-workers have improved the isolation methods with regard to the alkali-labile estrogens (Fotsis et al., 1980, 1981), and methods for analysis of metabolic profiles of estrogens by GLC or GC/MS will probably soon be available in a greatly simplified form.

There are few examples of metabolic profiles of unconjugated neutral steroids. This is due both to the difficulties in isolating a sufficiently pure neutral steroid fraction and to the low concentrations of these steroids. Repetitive scanning GC–MS with MO-TMS derivatives and a glass capillary column permitted semiquantitative analyses of 13 neutral steroids in plasma from pregnant women (Axelson and Sjövall, 1977). Subfractionation according to polarity was not used in the purification procedure, and mostly progesterone metabolites were detected. However, the method is not sufficiently sensitive for most hormones unless isotopically labeled standards are added and a number of preselected ions are monitored.

Profiles of steroids with polarities between those of progesterone and corticosterone have been analyzed in bovine corpus luteum (Axelson et al., 1975). Maume and co-workers (Delaforge et al., 1974; Maume et al., 1976, 1979) have made extensive studies of steroids produced by cultures of adrenocortical cells. In the early work packed GLC columns were used and the steroid mixture was separated by TLC into three fractions. Capillary columns gave greatly improved separations and specificity (Maume et al., 1979). The results indicate that GC–MS is still required for identification of the steroids while quantitation can be achieved with capillary column GLC of MO-TMS derivatives. Preliminary studies of steroid metabolite profiles in liver have been made with a similar method (Delaforge *et al.*, 1974). Profiles of steroids produced by perfused ovaries have also been analyzed (Seamark *et al.*, 1977).

A method has been developed for analysis of profiles of cortoic acids, acidic metabolites of cortisol (Shackleton *et al.*, 1980b). The isolation procedure is conventional, consisting of solvent extractions, and the acids are analyzed as methyl ester TMS ethers on Carbowax glass capillary columns. This group of compounds should be well suited for isolation by ion-exchange chromatography.

3. *Analysis of Multiple Groups*

With the introduction of simplified methods for group separation of steroid conjugates, it has become practical to analyze profiles of several groups of steroid conjugates in the same sample. Setchell *et al.* (1976a) used glass capillary columns to analyze profiles of MO-TMS derivatives of steroids after group fractionation on DEAP-LH-20 (see Section III,B,1,a). An advantage with this procedure is that different types of conjugates are separated and that the most suitable conditions for hydrolysis can be selected for each fraction. Similar methods have been developed for bile acids (Almé *et al.*, 1977). However, there are groups of conjugates that will not be obtained as isolated fractions (e.g., mixed conjugates, conjugates of acidic steroids), and positional isomers are eluted as mixtures. Furthermore, the method is time-consuming when all fractions have to be analyzed separately. With improved methods that involve Sep-Pak extractions (see Section II,B,3) and TEAP-LH-20 (see Section III,B,1), a profile analysis can be completed in 2 days.

The method of Setchell *et al.* (1976a) has been used in studies of steroid excretion in the baboon (Setchell *et al.*, 1976b) and the squirrel monkey (Setchell *et al.*, 1977). The papers by Setchell *et al.* contain GC–MS data for a large number of steroids in different conjugate fractions. The large proportion of unconjugated steroids in urine from baboons (Setchell *et al.*, 1976b) may be artifactual in spite of the attempts to avoid hydrolysis (see Section III,B,1).

The importance of conjugate separation prior to GLC of the hydrolyzed steroids is well illustrated by a study of placental sulfatase deficiency (Taylor and Shackleton, 1979). Both ion exchange and Sephadex LH-20 separations of conjugate classes were used to analyze steroid profiles in urine and blood. The maternal plasma levels and daily urinary excretion of steroid sulfates were highly elevated. The excretion of 1β- and 6α-hydroxylated metabolites of cortisol (see Taylor *et al.,* 1978; Derks and Drayer 1978b) in the urine of some of the infants also appeared to be increased. The study exemplifies the value of recent analytical methods in defining defects in steroid metabolism.

A study of the acute effects of ethanol on the metabolic profiles of steroids in urine (Axelson *et al.,* 1981a) also exemplifies the importance of separation of conjugated steroids before hydrolysis. The main effects, as on plasma steroids, were on ratios between sulfated 17-keto : 17-hydroxysteroids. These effects would hardly be noticeable in a total metabolic profile of hydrolyzed steroids.

If one compares the different methods for analysis of metabolic profiles of steroids, it appears advisable to use a method that separates conjugates into groups. Direct hydrolysis of urine should be avoided because of the risks of incomplete hydrolysis of some steroids. Solvent extractions should also be avoided, since polar steroids are lost. Derivatization techniques may have to be varied depending on the particular class of steroids under study. Glass capillary columns should be used, since packed columns do not give the separations required.

There are several problems to be solved in the analysis of steroid profiles. Quantitations often have poor accuracy and precision, and the sensitivity is too low for profiles of unconjugated steroids in blood and tissues. Positional isomerism in conjugation is not taken into account in available methods. However, at the present rate of progress in liquid chromatography and GC–MS, these problems are likely to be solved within a few years.

4. *Computer Evaluation of GC–MS Data*

A goal in the development of GC–MS methods for analysis of metabolic profiles of steroids is to have an automated system in which data are evaluated by computer. This is true whether repetitive scanning of complete (or partial) mass spectra or selective monitoring of a few *m/z* values is employed. The computer should locate the steroids in the chromatogram, suggest a structure based on retention times and mass spectra, and estimate the amount based on peak areas in specific fragment or total ion current chromatograms. An automated system of this type has not yet been developed for steroids, but semiautomated procedures have been described. A book on data acquisition and computer evaluation of GC–MS analyses and mass spectra has been published (Chapman, 1978).

The main problems in developing a completely automated system are (*a*) insufficient resolution of steroids on the GLC column; (*b*) background due to column bleed and, more important, sample constituents;

(c) variations in yields of ions due to losses of steroid on the column or in the interface to the mass spectrometer and to variations in the condition of the ion source; (d) lack of reference compounds for preparation of artificial steroid profiles. Obviously, the difficulties in automated evaluation increase as the signal : noise ratio decreases. Simpler computer programs that are functional when tested on synthetic mixtures of steroids may not be useful when applied to analyses of biological mixtures.

The methods to locate steroids in the GC–MS chromatograms obtained by repetitive scanning are based on computer search for peaks in individual ion current chromatograms. This can be done in a selective or nonselective way. In the former case, a limited number of m/z values known to be present in spectra of steroids are selected (Reimendal and Sjövall, 1972, 1973b). The number can be limited so that only specific groups of steroids are detected, and relative retention time limits can be given so that the search is made only within a certain range of retention times (Axelson et al., 1974a). This procedure has been used in a semiautomated way for quantitative analysis of the excretion of about 30 bile acids in urine (Bremmelgaard and Sjövall, 1979). Sweeley and co-workers have made extensive use of this type of search in a more sophisticated form and combined it with reverse library searches for analyses of metabolic profiles of urinary acids (see Sweeley et al., 1974; Gates et al., 1978). Baty and Wade (1974) have described a more specialized method for computer evaluation of steroid analyses. Each spectrum is reduced to the 30 most abundant ions above a certain mass limit, and the retention time of the scan is noted. A reverse library search is then made for the 10 most intense m/z values of the library spectrum. This method will also detect the elution of overlapping compounds.

In the nonselective, unbiased search, all ion current chromatograms are used. Depending on the type of analysis, amount of steroids, noise level, etc., limits have to be set to define a peak in one of these chromatograms and the intensities and numbers of peaks required to indicate elution of a steroid (or other compound). This method will resolve mixed GLC peaks, provided that the mass spectra of the compounds are different and that the m/z values maximize in different scans. It has been used in steroid analyses in our laboratory for a number of years (Reimendal and Sjövall, 1973a). A similar procedure was employed by Biller and Biemann (1974), who used all m/z values maximizing in two neighboring scans to obtain a reconstructed mass spectrum of the compound(s) having a GC peak maximum at this retention time. The summed intensities of these m/z values were also used to obtain a "mass resolved gas chromatogram" that has a greatly improved apparent resolution.

A more sophisticated program to detect compounds and resolve mixtures was described by Dromey et al. (1976). The approach was more statistical, and compounds were located by looking for "clusters" of maximizing peaks. Noise levels and background variations were also considered. Compounds in a mixture giving rise to 4% of the total ion current and separated by 1.5–2 scan times from another component could be detected (provided mass spectra were sufficiently dissimilar). The background subtraction method also provided better spectra for library search and interpretation. Smith et al. (1977) used this CLEANUP program to obtain the total ion current peak area for the resolved components. The relative concentrations of each compound could then be estimated by comparison with the peak area of suitable internal standards. Comparison with historical libraries of GC–MS data provided information about the identity of the compounds or their occurrence in similar samples analyzed previously. Unknown spectra were automatically added to the library as were spectra of known compounds when the quality of the new spectrum was better.

Sweeley and co-workers have continued their work on the development of increasingly refined methods for computer evaluation of GC–MS data obtained in analyses of metabolic profiles (Blaisdell and Sweeley, 1980a,b; Blaisdell et al., 1980). All masses are taken into account and the programs can resolve mixtures of up to 10 overlapping compounds differing in retention times by less than one scan. The method for localizing and resolving compounds is combined with a reverse library search for identification, and two programs, SVIA and LIANAL, accomplish the detection of unknown compounds and compounds whose spectra are in the library, respectively. The total ion current profile of each compound is also obtained and can be used for quantitative estimations although the accuracy of such estimations remains to be determined (c.f. Smith et al., 1977).

Less sophisticated methods for evaluation of GC–MS analyses containing overlapping components have been described. Halket (1979) used matrix rank analysis and principal components analysis to resolve a mixture of steroids. The potential of this method in analysis of metabolic profiles cannot be evaluated since it was tested only on a simple mixture.

The identification of a compound is best accomplished by reverse library search procedures (Sweeley et al., 1974; Gates et al., 1978; Blaisdell and Sweeley, 1980b; Smith et al., 1977; Baty and Wade,

1974). At present, the methods for computer interpretation of spectra (see Section IV,A and Chapman, 1978) are too complex and time-consuming for analyses of metabolic profiles. Furthermore, when the analyses are limited to steroids, simpler methods are sufficient. For routine analyses, when most steroids are known and many isomers are present, it would be sufficient to base tentative identifications on retention indices and characteristic ions and fragment losses. Since the general structure of a steroid is usually given by its molecular weight, Reimendal and Sjövall (1973a) have described a program that will locate potential molecular ions in a spectrum assumed to be due to a steroid. Simple common fragment losses are used in the search, and the permitted number and types of substituents are restricted depending on the derivatization method used in the analysis. The search is an aid in the manual interpretation of spectra, and, although mixtures are detected, the number of molecular ions suggested is usually larger than the number of steroids present.

Quantitation is based on peak areas in chromatograms constructed either using selected ions (Reimendal and Sjövall, 1972; Axelson *et al.,* 1974a; Sweeley *et al.,* 1974; Gates *et al.,* 1978) or total ion current of the individual components after computer resolution of overlapping peaks (Smith *et al.,* 1977; Blaisdell and Sweeley, 1980a,b). In the method of Axelson *et al.* (1974a), the current of the selected ions are converted into total ion current for comparison with the total ion current given by internal and external standards. This conversion can be done when the relative contribution of the selected ions to the total ionization is known from reference spectra or can be calculated by the computer from spectra of pure compounds in the analysis. This presents a problem when reference compounds are not available and when relative intensities can vary with the conditions of the GC–MS system. The methods of Smith *et al.* (1977) and Blaisdell and Sweeley (1980a,b) reduce errors due to these problems, but in the absence of empirically determined mass response factors, quantitative analyses of metabolic profiles will remain relative.

Considerable improvements in the computer evaluation of GC–MS analyses of metabolic profiles have been made during the last few years. Use of glass capillary columns will decrease the problems with overlapping compounds and background noise, but the narrow peaks will create problems of resolution and quantitation when fewer spectra are obtained over each peak. However, computer evaluation of GC–MS profiles is likely to become a routine method within a few years. As has been necessary in the studies cited above, it will probably be done off-line, i.e., after all the GC–MS data have been acquired and stored on a disc or magnetic tape. The time required for evaluation and printing of results is also likely to decrease; at present it is about the same as the actual GC–MS analysis.

B. STUDIES WITH STABLE ISOTOPES

The development of GC–MS methods has led to a rapid increase in the use of stable isotopes for studies of biosynthesis, metabolism, and turnover of steroids (see bibliographies by Klein and Klein, 1978, 1979). Besides the elimination of radiation hazards, there are several advantages with the use of stable isotopes. For example, GC–MS permits determination of the number of heavy atoms in a molecule as well as the relative abundances of each labeled species in one analysis, often requiring only a few nanograms of substance. Multiple labeling at different positions may be used to follow several metabolic processes simultaneously, and the sites of labeling can sometimes be directly determined from the mass spectrum. Isotope effects are smaller with deuterium than with tritium, but the problems with metabolic and chemical lability of the label is the same. There are also several drawbacks with the use of stable isotopes. Most important are the analytical problems, with lack of accuracy at low levels of labeling and frequent need for lengthy purification procedures to eliminate interfering ions produced by other components in the sample.

Abundances of unlabeled and labeled molecules are measured by selected ion monitoring (see Klein *et al.*, 1975) or by repetitive scanning of the entire mass range or part of it (see Axelson *et al.*, 1974a). The former method is best suited for studies of pharmacokinetics and turnover and when only one species of labeled molecules is involved. The scanning methods are needed when many species of labeled molecules are involved and when many fragment ions have to be screened for isotope content. As in other quantitative applications of GC–MS, accuracy and precision increase as the time spent on measuring the ions of interest increases. However, there are many potential sources of error, both instrumental (see Matthews and Hayes, 1976) and in the calculation of isotopic composition from the GC peaks produced by the different species of molecules (see Biemann, 1962). In our experience, the main sources of error (besides instrumental ones) in analyses of the isotopic composition of steroids are: interference by ions from contaminating compounds, isotope separations, and difficulties in finding the correct baseline for mass spectrometric and GLC peaks. Under optimal conditions it should become possible to measure less than 0.1 atom% excess of heavy isotopes as demonstrated in studies of amino acids (Matthews *et al.*, 1979).

Labeling with stable isotopes has been used in many studies of reaction mechanisms in steroid formation and metabolism. It is outside the scope of this review to discuss these studies, but a few references to methodologically interesting papers will be given. Björkhem (1971, 1972) used an elegant combination of labeling with ^{14}C, ^3H, and ^2H to determine isotope effects and rate-limiting steps in steroid hydroxylations. The mechanism of side chain cleavage in the formation of pregnenolone from cholesterol has been studied with mixtures of $^{16}O_2$ and $^{18}O_2$ (Burstein and Middleditch 1974; see also Engel and Orr, 1972) and with ^{18}O-labeled intermediates (Duque et al., 1978). Combinations of ^2H- and ^{18}O-labeling have been used by Shimizu (1978, 1979) in studies of the formation of C_{19} steroids from pregnenolone in boar testis.

The relative contribution of exogenous and endogenous cholesterol to the formation of pregnenolone in adrenal mitochondrial preparations has been determined by combining radioactivity measurements with GC–MS analyses of $^{14}C : {}^{12}C$ ratios in precursor and product (Björkhem and Karlmar, 1975). The principle of this method is generally applicable and useful in studies of biosynthetic reactions that may be compartmentalized and in studies of transformations of water-insoluble compounds in vitro. A preference for endogenous precursors was found by Seamark et al. (1977), who added $[16-{}^2H_1]$ pregnenolone to sheep ovarian follicles in culture and analyzed steroids released into the medium. These authors emphasized the difficulties in measuring monodeuterated steroids, and the precision was lower than reported by Axelson et al. (1974a).

Labeling with deuterium has been used in studies of coupling between redox reactions and compartmentation of coenzymes used in steroid oxidoreductions. Deuterium is introduced at a carbon carrying a hydroxyl group, and the transfer of this deuterium to reducible substrates in vivo is measured. A coupling between the oxidation of ethanol and the reduction of several sulfated 17-ketosteroids has been demonstrated in this way in man (Cronholm and Sjövall, 1970). An analogous coupling with reduction of 20-ketosteroids was not found, and experiments with rats have indicated that different pools of NAD(P)H are used in different steroid oxidoreductions (Cronholm, 1972; Cronholm and Fors, 1976). Similar studies with ^2H-labeled steroids have shown specific coupling between steroid oxidoreductions (Cronholm and Rudqvist, 1979). ^2H- and ^{13}C-labeled ethanols have also been administered as precursors of acetate, cholesterol, bile acids, and steroids (Cronholm et al., 1974).

Such experiments have provided information about the cholesterol pools serving as precursors of bile acids and steroids. These studies also illustrate the possibility of using proton–deuteron decoupled ^{13}C NMR for detailed investigations of deuterium labeling at individual carbon atoms of the steroid, in addition to the estimation of ^{13}C-labeling patterns (Wilson *et al.*, 1974; Cronholm *et al.*, 1979). However, the amount of steroid needed is still too large for most biomedical applications. Another possibility to analyze molecules containing both ^{13}C and ^{2}H is to use ultra-high resolution mass spectrometry. At a resolution of 100,000, ions containing ^{13}C can be separated from the corresponding ions containing ^{2}H, as illustrated in studies of the biosynthesis of cholesterol and bile acids from ethanol (D. M. Wilson *et al.*, 1977).

An alternative to labeling of reduced cofactors with ^{2}H or acetate with ^{2}H or ^{13}C is to label the oxygen substituents of the steroids. This has been done *in vivo* by letting rats inhale [18]O_2 via a tracheal cannula for 30 minutes. Extensive labeling of the hydroxyl groups of bile acids occurred (Björkhem and Lewenhaupt, 1979). This method could probably be used in studies of steroid turnover and metabolism.

When metabolism is studied with stable isotopes, it is much more difficult to find the metabolites than when radioactivity can be monitored. The twin-ion technique (Braselton *et al.*, 1973) is a very useful aid. A 1 : 1 mixture of unlabeled and labeled steroid is administered, and mass spectra of the metabolites will show the typical twin ions of the mixture (provided that the label is metabolically stable). This method has been used only in a few studies of steroid metabolism (Braselton *et al.*, 1973; Morfin *et al.*, 1980; Sahlberg *et al.*, 1981), but its importance can be expected to increase. For example, GC–MS studies of the metabolism of steroid drugs (e.g., Braselton *et al.*, 1977) would be aided by the use of a twin-ion technique.

Turnover and metabolism of naturally occurring steroids can be studied by administration of steroids labeled with stable isotopes. Pinkus *et al.* (1971, 1979) used [2]H-labeled estrogens to measure production rates of estrogens in pregnant and nonpregnant women. They isolated estrogens from urine, determined their ^{2}H content, and calculated production rates with mathematical models as developed for radioactive tracers. However, for analytical reasons the amount of [2]H-labeled estrogen administered has to be much larger than a true tracer dose, and the mathematics may not apply. The extent to which steady states are disturbed is not known, and endogenous production could conceivably be depressed or clearance rates be increased by the exogenous dose of steroid. It is, therefore, interesting to note that values for production rates of estradiol and estrone were similar to those obtained in radioactive tracer experiments. A similar observation was made by Johnson *et al.* (1979b), who measured the production rate of pregnenolone using [7,7-[2]H_2]pregnenolone. Baba *et al.* (1980) found that plasma levels and urinary excretion of endogenous testosterone were not influenced by a 20-mg oral dose of [19,19,19-^{2}H$_3$]testosterone. However, the number of subjects studied by Pinkus *et al.* (1971, 1979), Johnson *et al.* (1979b), and Baba *et al.* (1980) was small, and it is yet too early to evaluate the possible effect of a disturbance of steady state caused by the labeled steroid.

When production and metabolic transformation rates are determined from the labeling of steroids in blood it is necessary to take pool expansions caused by the labeled steroids into consideration. A mathematical model described by Nystedt (1980) was used by Baillie *et al.* (1980) in a study of the metabolism of sulfated pregnanolone and pregnanediol isomers in pregnant women. This study illustrates the use of multiple labeling with deuterium to enable simultaneous calculations of rates of steroid skeleton turnover, oxidoreduction, hydroxylation, and sulfation. Metabolically stable ^{2}H atoms were located at C-11, a ^{2}H atom at C-20 served to indicate oxidation of a 20-hydroxy group, and a ^{2}H atom was introduced at C-3 to monitor possible hydrolysis of the sulfate ester followed by oxidation to a 3-keto steroid. While the latter reaction was not observed in pregnant women, an analogous study showed that it was a major reaction in the male rat, followed by 2α-hydroxylation (Baillie *et al.*, 1975a). Rates of hydroxylation of the intact sulfate could be measured in the pregnant women, 16α-hydroxylation being predominant for isomers with a 3β,5α configuration and 21-hydroxylation for the 3α,5α isomers (Baillie *et al.*, 1975b, 1978). These studies provide examples of the value of stable isotope labeling, and problems of analysis and treatment of kinetic data were discussed.

The use of stable isotopes in metabolic studies will undoubtedly increase. When low abundances of heavy atoms can be measured more accurately, problems with pool expansions can be eliminated. Steroids labeled with multiple ^{13}C atoms may become available so that problems with undesirable isotope effects and the biochemical and chemical lability of the ^{2}H label can be avoided.

VII. CONCLUSIONS

The development of GC–MS methods can be expected to continue. Capillary column technology will be improved, as will the methods for coupling of columns to the ion source. This will lead to decreased losses of labile steroids, and sensitivity can be increased with improved methods of ionization. A more widespread use of GC–MS in routine applications will require simplifications of the instrumentation, both mechanically in the capillary column and GC–MS interface parts and in the systems for computer evaluation of data. Automation of analyses of metabolic profiles will be necessary because of the large amount of information acquired in a short period of time.

Sample preparation and purification procedures are frequently rate-limiting in steroid analyses. Many of the new column extraction and chromatographic techniques can be automated, and it should be possible to construct systems in which the biological fluid is injected at one end and a purified steroid extract is collected at the other.

Development of HPLC methods is only at its beginning. Improved LC–MS systems are required to permit evaluation of the specificity, as is now done with GLC analyses. In the future it should become possible to analyze intact conjugates by such methods.

ACKNOWLEDGMENTS

This review could not have been completed without the unfailing assistance of Ms Agneta Sjövall during the preparation of the manuscript. Work carried out in the authors' laboratory was supported by the Swedish Medical Research Council, Karolinska Institutet, Magn. Bergvalls Stiftelse, and the World Health Organization.

REFERENCES

Abraham, G. E., Tulchinsky, D., and Korenman, S. G. (1970). Chromatographic purification of estradiol-17β for use in radio-ligand assay. *Biochem. Med.* 3, 365–368.

Abraham, G. E., Buster, J. E., Lucas, L. A., Corrales, P. C., and Teller, R. C. (1972). Chromatographic separation of steroid hormones for use in radioimmunoassay. *Anal. Lett.* 5, 509–517.

Adessi, G. L., Eichenberger, D., Nhuan, T. Q., and Jayle, M. F. (1975). Gas chromatography profile of estrogens: Application to pregnancy urine. *Steroids* 25, 553–564.

Adlercreutz, H. (1974). Analysis of natural and synthetic hormonal steroids in biological fluids by mass fragmentography. *In* "Mass Spectrometry in Biochemistry and Medicine" (A. Frigerio and N. Castagnoli, eds.), pp. 165–181. Raven, New York.

Adlercreutz, H. (1977). Quantitative mass spectrometry of endogenous and exogenous steroids in metabolic studies in man. *Int. Symp. Quant. Mass Spectrom. Life Sci. Proc.* pp. 15–28.

Adlercreutz, H. (1980). Biomedical application of the mass spectrometry of steroid hormones. *In* "Advances in Mass Spectrometry" (A. Quayle, ed.), Vol. 8, pp. 1165–1179. Heyden, London.

Adlercreutz, H., and Luukkainen, T. (1968). Gas phase chromatographic methods for estrogens in biological fluids. *In* "Gas Phase Chromatography of Steroids" (K. B. Eik-Nes and E. C. Horning, eds.), pp. 72–149. Springer-Verlag, Berlin and New York.

Adlercreutz, H., and Luukkainen, T. (1970). Identification and determination of oestrogens in various biological materials in pregnancy. *Ann. Clin. Res.* 2, 365–380.

Adlercreutz, H., and Martin, F. (1976). Oestrogen in human pregnancy faeces. *Acta Endocrinol. (Copenhagen)* 83, 410–419.

Adlercreutz, H., Nieminen, U., and Ervast, H.-S. (1974a). A mass fragmentographic method for the determination of megestrol acetate in plasma and its application to studies on the plasma levels after administration of the progestin to patients with carcinoma corporis uteri. *J. Steroid Biochem.* **5,** 619–626.

Adlercreutz, H., Soltmann, B., and Tikkanen, M. J. (1974b). Field desorption mass spectrometry in the analysis of a steroid conjugate, estriol-16α-glucuronide. *J. Steroid Biochem.* **5,** 163–166.

Adlercreutz, H., Tikkanen, M. J., and Hunneman, D. H. (1974c). Mass fragmentographic determination of eleven estrogens in the body fluids of pregnant and nonpregnant subjects. *J. Steroid Biochem.* **5,** 211–217.

Adlercreutz, H., Nylander, P., and Hunneman, D. H. (1974d). Studies on the mass fragmentographic determination of plasma estriol. *Biomed. Mass Spectrom.* **1,** 332–339.

Adlercreutz, H., Martin, F., Wahlroos, Ö., and Soini, E. (1975). Mass spectrometric and mass fragmentographic determination of natural and synthetic steroids in biological fluids. *J. Steroid Biochem.* **6,** 247–259.

Adlercreutz, H., Martin, F., and Lindström, B. (1978). Gas chromatographic and mass spectrometric studies on oestrogens in bile—2. Men and non-pregnant women. *J. Steroid Biochem.* **9,** 1197–1205.

Albert, J., Geller, J., Stoeltzing, W., and Loza, D. (1978). An improved method for extraction and determination of prostate concentrations of endogenous androgens. *J. Steroid Biochem.* **9,** 717–720.

Albert, D. H., Ponticorvo, L., and Lieberman, S. (1980). Identification of fatty acid esters of pregnenolone and allopregnenolone from bovine corpora lutea. *J. Biol. Chem.* **255,** 10618–10623.

Albrecht, B. H., Kusalasai, K., and Hagerman, D. D. (1975). Rapid enzyme hydrolysis of urine extracts for estriol analysis. *Steroids* **25,** 587–590.

Alexander G., and Rutten, G. A. F. M. (1973). Preparation of polar phase coated open tubular columns for steroid analysis. *Chromatographia* **6,** 231–233.

Allen, J. G., Thomas, G. H., Brooks, C. J. W., and Knights, B. A. (1969). The determination of stereochemistry at C-5 of 3,6-dioxygenated steroids. *Steroids* **13,** 133–142.

Almé, B., and Nyström, E. (1971). Preparation of lipophilic anion exchangers from chlorohydroxypropylated Sephadex and cellulose. *J. Chromatogr.* **59,** 45–52.

Almé, B., and Sjövall, J. (1980). Analysis of bile acid glucuronides in urine. Identification of 3α,6α,12α-trihydroxy-5β-cholanoic acid. *J. Steroid Biochem.* **13,** 907–916.

Almé, B., Bremmelgaard, A., Sjövall, J., and Thomassen, P. (1977). Analysis of metabolic profiles of bile acids in urine using a lipophilic anion exchanger and computerized gas-liquid chromatography-mass spectrometry. *J. Lipid Res.* **18,** 339–362.

Anderson, R. A., Brooks, C. J. W., and Knights, B. A. (1973a). Preparation and evaluation of a chiral derivative of Sephadex LH-20. *J. Chromatogr.* **75,** 247–259.

Anderson, R. A., Knights, B. A., and Brooks, C. J. W. (1973b). Preparation and evaluation of a hydroxycyclohexyl derivative of Sephadex H-20. *J. Chromatogr.* **82,** 337–342.

Anderson, R. A., Defaye, G., Madani, C., Chambaz, E. M., and Brooks, C. J. W. (1974a). Lipophilic gel and gas-phase analysis of steroid hormones. Application to the human newborn. *J. Chromatogr.* **99,** 485–494.

Anderson, R. A., Chambaz, E. M., Defaye, G., Madani, C., Baillie, T. A., and Brooks, C. J. W. (1974b). Steroids in the human newborn; lipophilic gel separation and gas phase analysis. *J. Chromatogr. Sci.* **12,** 636–641.

Anderson, R. A., Chambaz, E. M., Defaye, G., Madani, C., Joannou, G., and Brooks, C. J. W. (1977). Identification of urinary androstenetetrol in the newborn and its assay in a patient with a placental enzymatic defect. *In* "Research on Steroids" (A. Vermeulen, A. Klopper, F. Sciarra, P. Jungblut, and L. Lerner, eds.), Vol. 7, pp. 589–594. North-Holland Publ., Amsterdam.

Andersson, S. H. G., Axelson, M., Sahlberg, B.-L., and Sjövall, J. (1981). Simplified method for the isolation and analysis of ethynyl steroids in urine. *Anal. Lett.* **14**, 783–790.

Apter, D., Jänne, O., and Vihko, R. (1975). Lipidex chromatography in this radioimmunoassay of serum and urinary cortisol. *Clin. Chim. Acta* **63**, 139–148.

Apter, D., Jänne, O., Karvonen, P., and Vihko, R. (1976). Simultaneous determination of five sex hormones in human serum by radioimmunoassay after chromatography on Lipidex-5000. *Clin. Chem.* **22**, 32–38.

Aringer, L., Eneroth, P., and Gustafsson, J.-A. (1971). Trimethylbromosilane catalyzed trimethylsilylation of slow reacting hydroxy- and oxosteroids in gas chromatographic-mass spectrometric analysis. *Steroids* **17**, 377–398.

Arpino, P. J., and Guiochon, G. (1979). LC/MS coupling. *Anal. Chem.* **51**, 682A–701A.

Arpino, P., Baldwin, M. A., and McLafferty, F. W. (1974). Liquid chromatography-mass spectrometry II—Continuous monitoring. *Biomed. Mass Spectrom.* **1**, 80–82.

Axelson, M. (1977). Deactivation of gas chromatographic systems for quantitative analysis of MO-TMS derivatives of steroids at the picogram level. *J. Steroid Biochem.* **8**, 693–698.

Axelson, M. (1978). Exchange of oxime functions: A useful reaction in GC-MS analysis of steroids. *Anal. Biochem.* **86**, 133–141.

Axelson, M., and Sahlberg, B.-L. (1981). On solid extraction of steroids and steroid conjugates in biological fluids. *Anal. Lett.*, in press.

Axelson, M., and Sjövall, J. (1974). Separation and computerized gas chromatography–mass spectrometry of unconjugated neutral steroids in plasma. *J. Steroid Biochem.* **5**, 733–738.

Axelson, M., and Sjövall, J. (1976). Selective liquid chromatographic isolation procedure for gas chromatographic–mass spectrometric analysis of 3-ketosteroids in biological materials. *J. Chromatogr.* **126**, 705–716.

Axelson, M., and Sjövall, J. (1977). Analysis of unconjugated steroids in plasma by liquid-gel chromatography and glass capillary gas chromatography–mass spectrometry. *J. Steroid Biochem.* **8**, 683–692.

Axelson, M., and Sjövall, J. (1979). Strong non-polar cation exchangers for the separation of steroids in mixed chromatographic systems. *J. Chromatogr.* **186**, 725–732.

Axelson, M., Cronholm, T., Curstedt, T., Reimendal, R., and Sjövall, J. (1974a). Quantitative analysis of unlabeled and polydeuterated compounds by gas chromatography–mass spectrometry. *Chromatographia* **7**, 502–509.

Axelson, M., Schumacher, G., and Sjövall, J. (1974b). Analysis of tissue steroids by liquid-gel chromatography and computerized gas chromatography–mass spectrometry. *J. Chromatogr. Sci.* **12**, 535–540.

Axelson, M., Schumacher, G., Sjövall, J., Gustafsson, B., and Lindell, J. O. (1975). Identification and quantitative determination of steroids in bovine corpus luteum during oestrous cycle and pregnancy. *Acta Endocrinol.* **80**, 149–164.

Axelson, M., Cronholm, T., Sahlberg, B.-L., and Sjövall, J. (1981a). Changes in the metabolic profile of steroids in urine during ethanol metabolism in man. *J. Steroid Biochem.* **14**, 155–159.

Axelson, M., Clark, J. H., Eriksson, H. A., and Sjövall, J. (1981b). Estrogen binding in target tissues. A GC/MS method for assessing uptake, retention and processing of estrogens in target cell nuclei under *in vivo* conditions. *J. Steroid Biochem.* **14**, 1253–1260.

Axelson, M., Sahlberg, B.-L., and Sjövall, J. (1981c). *J. Chromatogr. Biomed. Appl.* **224**, 355–370.

Baba, S., Shinohara, Y., and Kasuya, Y. (1979). Determination of plasma testosterone by mass fragmentography using testosterone-19-d_3 as an internal standard. Comparison with radioimmunoassay. *J. Chromatogr. Biomed. Appl.* **162**, 529–537.

Baba, S., Shinohara, Y., and Kasuya, Y. (1980). Differentiation between endogenous and exogenous testosterone in human plasma and urine after oral administration of deuterium-labeled testosterone by mass fragmentography. *J. Clin. Endocrinol. Metab.* **50**, 889–894.

Bailey, E., Fenoughty, M., and Chapman, J. R. (1974). Evaluation of a gas–liquid chromatographic method for the determination of urinary steroids using high-resolution open-tubular glass capillary columns. *J. Chromatogr.* **96**, 33–46.

Baillie, T. A., Brooks, C. J. W., and Horning, E. C. (1972). O-butyloximes and O-pentyloximes as derivatives for the study of ketosteroids by gas chromatography. *Anal. Lett.* **5**, 351–361.

Baillie, T. A., Eriksson, H., Herz, J. E., and Sjövall, J. (1975a). Specific deuterium labelling and computerized gas chromatography–mass spectrometry in studies on the metabolism *in vivo* of a steroid sulphate in the rat. *Eur. J. Biochem.* **55**, 157–165.

Baillie, T. A., Sjövall, J., and Sjövall, K. (1975b). Origin of 5α-pregnane-3α,20α,21-triol 3-sulphate in pregnant women. *FEBS Lett.* **60**, 145–148.

Baillie, T. A., Anderson, R. A., Sjövall, K., and Sjövall, J. (1976). Identification and quantitation of 16α-hydroxy C_{21} steroid sulphates in plasma from pregnant women. *J. Steroid Biochem.* **7**, 203–209.

Baillie, T. A., Anderson, R. A., Axelson, M., Sjövall, K., and Sjövall, J. (1978). Pathways of steroid metabolism *in vivo* studied by deuterium labelling techniques. *In* "Stable Isotopes. Applications in Pharmacology, Toxicology and Clinical Research" (T. A. Baillie, ed.), pp. 177–188. Macmillan, New York.

Baillie, T. A., Curstedt, T., Sjövall, K., and Sjövall, J. (1980). Production rates and metabolism of sulphates of 3β-hydroxy-5α-pregnane derivatives in pregnant women. *J. Steroid Biochem.* **13**, 1473–1486.

Batra, S., and Bengtsson, L. P. (1976). A highly efficient procedure for the extraction of progesterone from uterus and its compatibility with subsequent radioimmunoassay. *J. Steroid Biochem.* **7**, 599–603.

Baty, J. D., and Wade, A. P. (1974). Analysis of steroids in biological fluids by computer-aided gas–liquid chromatography–mass spectrometry. *Anal. Biochem.* **57**, 27–37.

Beckey, H. D., and Schulten, H.-R. (1975). Felddesorptions-Massenspekrometrie. *Angew. Chem.* **87**, 425–460.

Bègue, R.-J., Desgres, J., Gustafsson, J.-Å., and Padieu, P. (1976). Analyse modulaire des steroides urinaires pendant la gestation humaine. *J. Steroid Biochem.* **7**, 211–221.

Bègue, R.-J., Brun, J.-M., Morinière, M., and Padieu, P. (1977). C_{19} steroids urinaries dans une luteose ovarienne gravidique. *J. Steroid Biochem.* **8**, 737–742.

Bègue, R.-J., Morinière, M., and Padieu, P. (1978a). Urinary excretion of 5β-pregnane-3α,20α,21-triol in human gestation. *Biomed. Mass Spectrom.* **5**, 184–187.

Bègue, R. J., Morinière, M., and Padieu, P. (1978b). Urinary excretion of 5β-pregnane-3α,6α,20α-tiol in human gestation. *J. Steroid Biochem.* **9**, 779–784.

Bègue, R.-J., Dumas, M., Morinière, M., Nivois, C., and Padieu, P. (1979a). Steroids and hypertension. 1—Gas–liquid chromatography and gas chromatography–mass spectrometry of 3,15- and 3,16-dihydroxy-17-oxosteroids. *Biomed. Mass Spectrom.* **6**, 476–481.

Bègue, R. J., Dumas, M., Losty, H., Morinière, M., Perrier, C., and Padieu, P. (1979b). Analysis of urinary steroids by liquid-gel chromatography and gas chromatography–mass spectrometry. Clinical applications. *Recent Dev. Mass Spectrom. Biochem. Med.* **2**, 355–376.

Berthou, F., Picart, D., Bardou, L., and Floch, H. H. (1976). Separation of C_{19} and C_{21}

dihydroxysteroids by open-hole tubular glass columns and lipophilic gel chromatography. *J. Chromatogr.* **118**, 135–155.

Bhaskar, A., Schulze, P. E., Acksteiner, B., and Laumas, K. R. (1979). Quantitative analysis of norethindrone in milk using deuterated carrier and gas chromatography–mass spectrometry. *J. Steroid Biochem.* **11**, 1323–1328.

Bicknell, D. C., and Gower, D. B. (1975). Separation of some 16-androstenes on hydroxyalkoxypropyl-Sephadex (Lipidex™). *J. Chromatogr.* **110**, 210–212.

Biemann, K. (1962). "Mass Spectrometry," pp. 204–250. McGraw-Hill, New York.

Biller, J. E., and Biemann, K. (1974). Reconstructed mass spectra, a novel approach for the utilization of gas chromatograph-mass spectrometer data. *Anal. Lett.* **7**, 515–528.

Björkhem, I. (1971). Isotope discrimination in steroid hydroxylations. *Eur. J. Biochem.* **18**, 299–304.

Björkhem, I. (1972). On the rate-limiting step in microsomal hydroxylation of steroids. *Eur. J. Biochem.* **27**, 354–363.

Björkhem, I. (1979). Selective ion monitoring in clinical chemistry. *CRC Crit. Rev. Clin. Lab. Sci.* **11**, 53–105.

Björkhem, I., and Holmberg, I. (1978). Assay and properties of a mitochondrial 25-hydroxylase active on vitamin D_3. *J. Biol. Chem.* **253**, 842–849.

Björkhem, I., and Karlmar, K.-E. (1975). A novel technique for assay of side-chain cleavage of exogenous and endogenous cholesterol in adrenal mitochondrial and submitochondrial preparations. *Anal. Biochem.* **68**, 404–414.

Björkhem, I., and Lewenhaupt, A. (1979). Preferential utilization of newly synthesized cholesterol as substrate for bile acid biosynthesis. An *in vivo* study using $^{18}O_2$-inhalation technique. *J. Biol. Chem.* **254**, 5252–5256.

Björkhem, I., Blomstrand, R., Lantto, O., Löf, A., and Svensson, L. (1974). Plasma cortisol determination by mass fragmentography. *Clin. Chim. Acta* **56**, 241–248.

Björkhem, I., Lantto, O., and Svensson, L. (1975a). Serum testosterone determination by mass fragmentography. *Clin. Chim. Acta* **60**, 59–66.

Björkhem, I., Blomstrand, R., Svensson, L., Tietz, F., and Carlström, K. (1975b). Validation of methods for determination of urinary estriol during pregnancy using mass fragmentography. *Clin. Chim. Acta* **62**, 385–392.

Björkhem, I., Blomstrand, R., and Lantto, O. (1975c). Validation of routine methods for serum progesterone determination using mass fragmentography. *Clin. Chim. Acta* **65**, 343–350.

Björkhem, I., Lantto, O., and Löf, A. (1980). Detection and quantitation of methandienone (Dianabol^R) in urine by isotope dilution–mass fragmentography. *J. Steroid Biochem.* **13**, 169–175.

Blair, I. A., and Phillipou, G. (1977), Evaluation of allyldimethylsilyl ethers as steroid derivatives for gas chromatography–mass spectrometry. *J. Chromatogr. Sci.* **15**, 478–479.

Blair, I. A., and Phillipou, G. (1978). Derivatisation of steroid hormones with *t*-butyldimethylsilyl imidazole. *J. Chromatogra. Sci.* **16**, 201–203.

Blaisdell, B. E., and Sweeley, C. C. (1980a). Determination in gas chromatography–mass spectrometry data of mass spectra free of background and neighboring substance contributions. *Anal. Chim. Acta* **117**, 1–15.

Blaisdell, B. E., and Sweeley, C. C. (1980b). Analysis of gas chromatography–mass spectrometry data by reverse library search and the detection of substances not in the library. *Anal. Chim. Acta* **117**, 17–33.

Blaisdell, B. E., Gates, S. C., Martin, F. E., and Sweeley, C. C. (1980). Comparison of two methods of detection, determination, and library search of the substances present in gas chromatography–mass spectrometry data. *Anal. Chim. Acta* **117**, 35–43.

Blakley, C. R., Carmody, J. J., and Vestal, M. L. (1980). Liquid chromatograph–mass spectrometer for analysis of nonvolatile samples. *Anal. Chem.* **52**, 1636–1641.

Blau, K., and King, G. S., eds. (1977). "Handbook of Derivatives for Chromatography." Heyden, London.

Blunt, J. W., and Stothers, J. B. (1977). ^{13}C N.m.r. spectra of steroids—A survey and commentary. *Org. Magn. Reson.* **9**, 439–464.

Boettger, H. G., Giffin, C. E., Norris, D. D., Dreyer, W. J., and Kuppermann, A. (1977). Electro-optical ion detection: A novel approach to the application of mass spectrometers in biomedical research and clinical analysis. *In* "Advances in Mass Spectrometry in Biochemistry and Medicine" (A. Frigerio, ed.), Vol. 2, pp. 513–524. Spectrum, New York.

Bokkenheuser, V. D., Winter, J., Honour, J. W., and Shackleton, C. H. L. (1979). Reduction of aldosterone by anaerobic bacteria: Origin of urinary 21-deoxy metabolites in man. *J. Steroid Biochem.* **11**, 1145–1149.

Boreham, D. R., Vose, C. W., Palmer, R. F., Books, C. J. W., and Balasubramaniam, V. (1978). Application of ion-exchange and lipophilic-gel chromatography to the purification and group fractionation of steroidal spirolactones, isolated from biological fluids. *J. Chromatogr.* **153**, 63–75.

Bournot, P., Prost, M., and Maume, B. F. (1975). Separation and characterization of the reduced metabolites of the 18-hydroxydeoxycorticosterone hormone by gas–liquid chromatography–mass spectrometry. Occurrence of stereoisomeric forms in rat adrenals and liver. *J. Chromatogr.* **112**, 617–630.

Bradlow, H. L. (1968). Extraction of steroid conjugates with a neutral resin. *Steroids* **11**, 265–272.

Bradlow, H. L. (1970). The hydrolysis of steroid conjugates. *In* "Chemical and Biological Aspects of Steroid Conjugation" (S. Bernstein and S. Solomon, eds.), pp. 131–181. Springer-Verlag, Berlin and New York.

Bradlow, H. L. (1977). Modified technique for the elution of polar steroid conjugates from Amberlite XAD-2^R. *Steroids* **30**, 581–582.

Braselton, W. E., Jr., Orr, J. C., and Engel, L. L. (1973). The twin ion technique for detection of metabolites by gas chromatography–mass spectrometry: intermediates in estrogen biosynthesis. *Anal. Biochem.* **53**, 64–85.

Braselton, W. E., Lin, T. J., Mills, T. M., Ellegood, J. O., and Mahesh, V. B. (1977). Identification and measurement by gas chromatography–mass spectrometry of norethindrone and metabolites in human urine and blood. *J. Steroid Biochem.* **8**, 9–18.

Breiter, J., Helger, R., and Lang, H. (1976). Evaluation of column extraction: A new procedure for the analysis of drugs in body fluids. *Forensic Sci.* **7**, 131–140.

Bremmelgaard, A., and Sjövall, J. (1979). Bile acid profiles in urine of patients with liver diseases. *Eur. J. Clin. Invest.* **9**, 341–348.

Breuer, H., and Siekmann, L. (1975). Mass fragmentography as reference method in clinical steroid assay. *J. Steroid Biochem.* **6**, 685–688.

Brooks, C. J. W., and Gaskell, S. J. (1980). Hormones. *In* "Biochemical Applications of Mass Spectrometry" (G. R. Waller and O. C. Dermer, eds.), pp. 611–659. Wiley, New York.

Brooks, C. J. W., and Harvey, D. J. (1970). Gas chromatographic and mass spectrometric studies of oximes derived from 20-oxosteroids. *Steroids* **15**, 283–301.

Brooks, C. J. W., and Harvey, D. J. (1971). Comparative gas chromatographic studies of corticosteroid boronates. *J. Chromatogr.* **54**, 193–204.

Brooks, C. J. W., and Middleditch, B. S. (1971). The mass spectrometer as a gas chromatographic detector. *Clin. Chim. Acta* **34**, 145–157.

Brooks, C. J. W., and Middleditch, B. S. (1972). Uses of chloromethyldimethylsilyl ethers as derivatives for combined gas chromatography–mass spectrometry of steroids. *Anal. Lett.* **5**, 611–618.

Brooks, C. J. W., and Middleditch, B. S. (1973a). Some aspects of mass spectrometry in steroid analysis. *In* "Modern Methods of Steroid Analysis" (E. Heftmann, ed.), pp. 139–198. Academic Press, New York.

Brooks, C. J. W., and Middleditch, B. S. (1973b). Gas chromatography–mass spectrometry. *In* "Mass Spectrometry," Vol. 2, pp. 302–335. Chemical Society, London.

Brooks, C. J. W., and Middleditch, B. S. (1975). Gas chromatography–mass spectrometry. *In* "Mass Spectrometry," Vol. 3, pp. 296–338. Chemical Society, London.

Brooks, C. J. W., and Middleditch, B. S. (1977). Gas chromatography–mass spectrometry. *In* "Mass Spectrometry," Vol. 4, pp. 146–185. Chemical Society, London.

Brooks, C. J. W., and Middleditch, B. S. (1979). Gas chromatography–mass spectrometry. *In* "Mass Spectrometry," Vol. 5, pp. 142–185. Chemical Society, London.

Brooks, C. J. W., and Smith, A. G. (1975). Cholesterol oxidase. Further studies of substrate specificity in relation to the analytical characterisation of steroids. *J. Chromatogr.* **112**, 499–511.

Brooks, C. J. W., Thawley, A. R., Rocher, P., Middleditch, B. S., Anthony, G. M., and Stillwell, W. G. (1971a). Characterization of steroidal drug metabolites by combined gas chromatography–mass spectrometry. *J. Chromatogr. Sci.* **9**, 35–43.

Brooks, C. J. W., Middleditch, B. S., and Harvey, D. J. (1971b). The mass spectra of some corticosteroid boronates. *Org. Mass Spectrom.* **5**, 1429–1453.

Brooks, C. J. W., Harvey, D. J., Middleditch, B. S., and Vouros, P. (1973). Mass spectra of trimethylsilyl ethers of some Δ^5-3β-hydroxy C_{19} steroids. *Org. Mass Spectrom.* **7**, 925–948.

Brown, F. J., and Djerassi, C. (1980). Elucidation of the course of the electron impact induced fragmentation of α,β-unsaturated 3-keto steroids. *J. Am. Chem. Soc.* **102**, 807–817.

Buchanan, B. G., Smith, D. H., White, W. C., Gritter, R. J., Feigenbaum, E. A., Lederberg, J., and Djerassi, C. (1976). Applications of artificial intelligence for chemical inference. 22. Automatic rule formation in mass spectrometry by means of the meta-DENDRAL program. *J. Am. Chem. Soc.* **98**, 6168–6178.

Budzikiewicz, H. (1972). Steroids *In* "Biomedical Applications of Mass Spectrometry" (G. R. Waller, ed.), pp. 251–289. Wiley (Interscience), New York.

Budzikiewicz, H. (1980). Steroids. *In* "Biochemical Applications of Mass Spectrometry" (G. R. Waller and O. C. Dermer, eds.), pp. 211–228. Wiley, New York.

Budzikiewicz, H., Djerassi, C., and Williams, D. H. (1964). "Structure Elucidation of Natural Products by Mass Spectrometry. Vol. II: Steroids, Terpenoids, Sugars, and Miscellaneous Classes." Holden-Day, San Francisco, California.

Burlingame, A. L., and Johanson, G. A. (1972). Mass spectrometry. *Anal. Chem.* **44**, 337 R-378 R.

Burlingame, A. L., Cox, R. E., and Derrick, P. J. (1974). Mass spectrometry. *Anal. Chem.* **46**, 248R–287R.

Burlingame, A. L., Kimble, B. J., and Derrick, P. J. (1976). Mass spectrometry. *Anal. Chem.* **48**, 368R–403R.

Burlingame, A. L., Shackleton, C. H. L., Howe, I., and Chizhov, O. S. (1978). Mass spectrometry. *Anal. Chem.* **50**, 346R–384R.

Burlingame, A. L., Baillie, T. A., Derrick, P. J., and Chizhov, O. S. (1980). Mass spectrometry. *Anal. Chem.* **52**, 214R-258R.

Burstein, S. (1976). Decomposition of 11-deoxycorticosterone and corticosterone in soda-lime glass. *Steroids* **27**, 493–496.

Burstein, S., and Middleditch, B. S. (1974). Enzymatic formation of (20R,22R)-20,22-

dihydroxycholesterol from cholesterol and a mixture of $^{16}O_2$ and $^{18}O_2$: Random incorporation of oxygen atoms. *Biochem. Biophys. Res. Commun.* **61,** 692–697.

Bush, I. E. (1961). "The Chromatography of Steroids." Pergamon, Oxford.

Carlström, K., and Sköldefors, H. (1977). Determination of total oestrone in peripheral serum from nonpregnant humans. *J. Steroid Biochem.* **8,** 1127–1128.

Carr, B. R., Mikhail, G., and Flickinger, G. L. (1971). Column chromatography of steroids on Sephadex LH-20. *J. Clin. Endocrinol.* **33,** 358–360.

Carroll, D. I., Dzidic, I., Stillwell, R. N., Horning, M. G., and Horning, E. C. (1974). Subpicogram detection system for gas phase analysis based upon atmospheric pressure ionization (API) mass spectrometry. *Anal. Chem.* **46,** 706–710.

Carroll, D. I., Dzidic, I., Stillwell, R. N., Haegele, K. D., and Horning, E. C. (1975). Atmospheric pressure ionization mass spectrometry: Corona discharge ion source for use in liquid chromatography–mass spectrometer–computer analytical system. *Anal. Chem.* **47,** 2369–2373.

Carroll, D. I., Nowlin, J. G., Stillwell, R. N., and Horning, E. C. (1981). Adduct ion formation in chemical ionization mass spectrometry of nonvolatile organic compounds. *Anal. Chem.* **53,** 2007–2013.

Caspi, E., and Wittstruck, Th. (1967). Outline of the application of nuclear magnetic resonance to the investigation of steroids. *In* "Steroid Hormone Analysis" (H. Carstensen, ed.), Vol. 1, pp. 93–133. Dekker, New York.

Chambaz, E. M., Madani, C., and Ros, A. (1972). TMS-enol-TMS: A new type of derivative for the gas phase study of dihydroxyacetone side chain saturated corticosteroid metabolites. *J. Steroid Biochem.* **3,** 741–747.

Chambaz, E. M., Defaye, G., and Madani, C. (1973). Trimethyl silyl ether-enoltrimethylsilyl ether—a new type of derivative for the gas phase study of hormonal steroids. *Anal. Chem.* **45,** 1090–1098.

Chan, T. H., Moreland, M., Hum, W.-T., and Birmingham, M. K. (1977). Quantitative determination of 18-hydroxydeoxycorticosterone and corticosterone by high pressure liquid chromatography. *J. Steroid Biochem.* **8,** 243–245.

Chapman, J. R. (1978). "Computers in Mass Spectrometry." Academic Press, New York.

Clark, S. J., and Wotiz, H. H. (1973). Gas chromatography of steroid hormones. *In* "Modern Methods of Steroid Analysis" (E. Heftmann, ed.), pp. 71–102. Academic Press, New York.

Cochran, R. C., and Ewing, L. L. (1979). Celite column chromatography followed by reversed-phase high-performance liquid chromatography: A simple, two-step method for separating 14 testicular steroids. *J. Chromatogr.* **173,** 175–181.

Cohen, S. L., Patric, H., Suzuki, Y., and Alspector, F. E. (1978). The preparation of pregnancy urine for an estrogen profile. *Steroids* **32,** 279–293.

Colby, B. N., and McCaman, M. W. (1979). A comparison of calculation procedures for isotope dilution determinations using gas chromatography–mass spectrometry. *Biomed. Mass Spectrom.* **6,** 225–230.

Coty, W. A. (1980). Reversible dissociation of steroid hormone–receptor complexes by mercurial reagents. *J. Biol. Chem.* **255,** 8035–8037.

Cronholm, T. (1969). Position of the sulfate group in steroid sulfates from human plasma. *Steroids* **14,** 285–296.

Cronholm, T. (1972). Steroid metabolism in rats given $[1\text{-}^2H_2]$ethanol. Biliary metabolites of corticosterone and administered 4-androstene-3,17-dione. *Eur. J. Biochem.* **27,** 10–22.

Cronholm, T., and Fors, C. (1976). Transfer of the 1-*pro*-R and the 1-*pro*-S hydrogen atoms of ethanol in metabolic reductions *in vivo. Eur. J. Biochem.* **70,** 83–87.

Cronholm, T., and Rudqvist, U. (1979). Coupling between steroid oxidoreductions *in vivo.*

Deuterium transfer from [17α-²H]estradiol to C_{19} steroids. *Eur. J. Biochem.* **96,** 605–611.

Cronholm, T., and Sjövall, J. (1970). Effect of ethanol metabolism on redox state of steroid sulphates in man. *Eur. J. Biochem.* **13,** 124–131.

Cronholm, T., Burlingame, A. L., and Sjövall, J. (1974). Utilization of the carbon and hydrogen atoms of ethanol in the biosynthesis of steroids and bile acids. *Eur. J. Biochem.* **49,** 497–510.

Cronholm, T., Sjövall, J., Wilson, D. M., and Burlingame, A. L. (1979). Exchange of methyl hydrogens in ethanol during incorporation in bile acids *in vivo. Biochim. Biophys. Acta* **575,** 193–203.

Curtius, H.Ch., Völlmin, J., Zagalak, M. J., and Zachmann, M. (1975). Gas chromatography of steroids and its clinical applications, including loading tests with deuterated compounds. *J. Steroid Biochem.* **6,** 677–684.

Dahlberg, E., Snochowski, M., and Gustafsson, J.-Å. (1980). Removal of hydrophobic compounds from biological fluids by a simple method. *Anal. Biochem.* **106,** 380–388.

Damen, H., Henneberg, D., and Weimann, B. (1978). SISCOM—A new library search system for mass spectra. *Anal. Chim. Acta* **103,** 289–302.

Daniel, C. P., Gaskell, S. J., Bishop, H., and Nicholson, R. I. (1979). Determination of tamoxifen and an hydroxylated metabolite in plasma from patients with advanced breast cancer using gas chromatography–mass spectrometry. *J. Endocrinol.* **83,** 401–408.

Dann, A. E., Davis, J. B., and Nagler, M. J. (1979). A rapid and convenient technique for converting ketones into their ethylenedioxy- or trimethylenedioxy-derivatives, and for making acetonides. *J.C.S. Perkin I,* 158–160.

Dawkins, B. G., and McLafferty, F. W. (1978). The mass spectrometer as a detector for high-performance liquid chromatography. *Chromatogr. Sci.* **9,** 259–275.

Deelder, R. S., Ramaekers, J. J. M., van den Berg, J. H. M., and Wetzels, M. L. (1969). Study on the efficiency of support-coated open-tubular columns for steroid analysis. *J. Chromatogr.* **119,** 99–107.

Dehennin, L., and Levisalles, J. (1976). Esterification des steroides par l'anhydride heptafluorobutanoique. *Bull. Soc. Chim. Belg.* **85,** 333–345.

Dehennin, L., and Scholler, R. (1975). A new derivative for the gas–liquid chromatography with electron capture detection of steroidal secondary alcohols. *J. Chromatogr.* **111,** 238–241.

Dehennin, L., Reiffsteck, A., and Scholler, R. (1974). A quantitative method for the estimation of testosterone and progesterone in human plasma, using the gas chromatograph/mass spectrometer combination with single ion monitoring. *J. Steroid Biochem.* **5,** 81–86.

Delaforge, M., Maume, B. F., Bournot, P., Prost, M., and Padieu, P. (1974). Use of gas–liquid chromatography with glass capillary columns for steroid trace analysis in tissues. *J. Chromatogr. Sci.* **12,** 545–549.

De Leenheer, A. P., and Cruyl, A. A. (1978). Vitamin D_3 in plasma: Quantitation by mass fragmentography. *Anal. Biochem.* **91,** 293–303.

De Leenheer, A. P., and Cruyl, A. A. (1980). Quantitative mass spectrometry. *In* "Biochemical Applications of Mass Spectrometry" (G. R. Waller and O. C. Dermer, eds.), pp. 1169–1207. Wiley, New York.

De Leenheer, A. P., and Roncucci, R. R., eds. (1977). "Quantitative Mass Spectrometry in Life Sciences." *Proc. Int. Symp., Ghent, 1st, 1976.*

De Leenheer, A. P., Roncucci, R. R., and van Peteghem, C. (eds). (1978). "Quantitative Mass Spectrometry in Life Sciences II." *Proc. Int. Symp., Ghent, 2nd, 1978.*

De Ridder, J. J., and van Hal, H. J. M. (1978). Automation of high-performance liquid chromatographic sample clean-up for mass fragmentographic assays. *J. Chromatogr. Biomed. Appl.* **146,** 425–432.

De Vries, C. P., Lomecky-Janousek, M., and Popp-Snijders, C. (1980). Rapid quantitative assay of plasma 11-deoxycortisol and cortisol by high-performance liquid chromatography for use in the metyrapone test. *J. Chromatogr. Biomed. Appl.* **183,** 87–91.

Derks, H. J. G. M., and Drayer, N. M. (1978a). Polar corticosteroids in human neonatal urine; synthesis and gas chromatography–mass spectrometry of ring A reduced 6-hydroxylated corticosteroids. *Steroids* **31,** 9–22.

Derks, H. J. G. M., and Drayer, N. M. (1978b). The identification and quantification of three new 6α-hydroxylated corticosteroids in human neonatal urine. *Steroids* **31,** 289–305.

Derks, H. J. G. M., and Drayer, N. M. (1978c). Improved methods for isolating cortisol metabolites from neonatal urine. *Clin. Chem.* **24,** 1158–1162.

Desgrès, J., Guiguet, M., Bègue, R. J., and Padieu, P. (1976). Study of progesterone metabolism in fetal and postnatal rat liver cells in culture. *In* "Advances in Mass Spectrometry in Biochemistry and Medicine" (A. Frigerio and N. Castagnoli, eds.), Vol. I, pp. 139–155. Spectrum, New York.

Devaux, P. G., Horning, M. G., and Horning, E. C. (1971a). Benzyloxime derivatives of steroids. A new metabolic profile procedure for human urinary steroids. *Anal. Lett.* **4,** 151–160.

Devaux, P. G., Horning, M. G., Hill, R. M., and Horning, E. C. (1971b). *O*-Benzyloximes: Derivatives for the study of ketosteroids by gas chromatography. Application to urinary steroids of the newborn humans. *Anal. Biochem.* **41,** 70–82.

Diczfalusy, E. (1969). Steroid metabolism in the foetoplacental unit. *In* "The Foetoplacental Unit" (A. Pecile and C. Finzi, eds.), pp. 65–109. Excerpta Medica, Amsterdam.

Doerr, P. (1971). Thin-layer chromatography and elution of picogram amounts of estradiol. *J. Chromatogr.* **59,** 452–456.

Dominguez, O. V. (1967). Chromatography of steroids on paper. *In* "Steroid Hormone Analysis" (H. Carstensen, ed.), Vol. 1, pp. 135–318. Dekker, New York.

Dreyer, W. J., Kuppermann, A., Boettger, H. G., Giffin, C. E., Norris, D. D., Grotch, S. L., and Theard, L. P. (1974). Automatic mass-spectrometric analysis: Preliminary report on development of a novel mass-spectrometric system for biomedical applications. *Clin. Chem.* **20,** 998–1002.

Dromey, R. G., Stefik, M. J., Rindfleisch, T. C., and Duffeld, A. M. (1976). Extraction of mass spectra free of background and neighboring component contributions from gas chromatography/mass spectrometry data. *Anal. Chem.* **48,** 1368–1375.

Duque, C., Morisaki, M., Ikekawa, N., Shikita, M., and Tamaoki, B-i. (1978). The final step of side-chain cleavage of cholesterol by adrenocortical cytochrome P-450(scc) studied with [22-^{18}O]20,22-dihydroxy-cholesterols, [^{18}O]isocaproaldehyde, [^{18}O]water and atmospheric [^{18}O]oxygen. *Biochem. Biophys. Res. Commun.* **85,** 317–325.

Dürbeck, H. W., Büker, I., and Leymann, W. (1978a). Ein neus Interface für die GC/MS-Kopplung von Glaskapillarsäulen. *Chromatographia* **11,** 295–300.

Dürbeck, H. W., Büker, I., and Leymann, W. (1978b). Ein modifiziertes Interface für die GC/MS-Kopplung von Glaskapillarsäulen. *Chromatographia* **11,** 372–375.

Dyfverman, A., and Sjövall, J. (1978). A novel liquid-gel chromatographic method for extraction of unconjugated steroids from aqueous solutions. *Anal. Lett. Ser. B* **11,** 485–499.

Dyfverman, A., and Sjövall, J. (1979). Liquid-gel extraction of bile acids. *In* "Biological Effects of Bile Acids" (G. Paumgartner, A. Stiehl, and W. Gerok, eds.), pp. 281–286. MTP Press, Lancaster.

Eberlein, W. R. (1969). The measurement of low levels of estrone and estradiol-17β in urine, employing ion-exchange, thin-layer, and gas-liquid chromatography. *Steroids* **14**, 553–573.

Edwards, R. W. H. (1978a). Prediction of the relative molar flame ionization response for steroids. *J. Chromatogr.* **153**, 1–6.

Edwards, R. W. H. (1978b). Temperature dependence of methylene-unit values of steroids in gas–liquid chromatography. *J. Chromatogr.* **154**, 183–190.

Egger, H.-J., Reiner, J. Spiteller, G., and Häffele, R. (1978). Harn-Steroidprofile hirsuter Frauen. *J. Chromatogr. Biomed. Appl.* **145**, 359–369.

Einarsson, K., Gustafsson, J.-Å., Ihre, T., and Ingelman-Sundberg, M. (1976). Specific metabolic pathways of steroid sulfates in human liver microsomes. *J. Clin. Endocrinol. Metab.* **43**, 56–63.

Ellingboe, J., Nyström, E., and Sjövall, J. (1968). A versatile lipophilic Sephadex derivative for "reversed-phase" chromatography. *Biochim. Biophys. Acta* **152**, 803–805.

Ellingboe, J., Nyström, E., and Sjövall, J. (1970a). Liquid-gel chromatography on lipophilic-hydrophobic Sephadex derivatives. *J. Lipid Res.* **11**, 266–273.

Ellingboe, J., Almé, B., and Sjövall, J. (1970b). Introduction of specific groups into polysaccharide supports for liquid chromatography. *Acta Chem. Scand.* **24**, 463–467.

Ende, M., and Spiteller, G. (1971). Massenspektren von 11-Hydroxypregnan-3,20-dionen und 3-Hydroxypregnan-11,20-dionen. Zur Lokalisierung funktioneller Gruppen in Steroiden mit Hilfe der Massenspektrometrie. *Monatsh. Chem.* **102**, 929–939.

Ende, M., and Spiteller, G. (1973). Zur Lokalisierung funktioneller Gruppen in Steroiden mit Hilfe der Massenspektrometrie—VII. 3,11-Dihydroxypregnan-20-one. *Tetrahedron* **29**, 2457–2463.

Ende, M., and Spiteller, G. (1975). Zum Mechanismus massenspektrometrischer Fragmentierungsreaktionen bei A/B-CIS-verküpften 3α-Hydroxysteroiden mit und ohne 11-Ketogruppe. *Org. Mass Spectr.* **10**, 200–214.

Ende, M., Pfeifer, P., and Spiteller, G. (1980). Über das Einschleppen von Verunreinigungen bei Verwendung von Extrelut^R-Fertigsäulen. *J. Chromatogr. Biomed. Appl.* **183**, 1–7.

Eneroth, P., and Nyström, E. (1967). A study on liquid-gel partition of steroids and steroid derivatives on lipophilic Sephadex gels. *Biochim. Biophys. Acta* **144**, 149–161.

Engel, L. L., and Orr, J. C. (1972). Hormones. *In* "Biochemical Applications of Mass Spectrometry" (G. R. Waller, ed.), pp. 537–572. Wiley (Interscience), New York.

Engel, L. L., Neville, A. M., Orr, J. C., and Raggatt, P. R. (1970). Quantitative gas chromatography of steroid methoxime-trimethylsilyl ethers. *Steroids* **16**, 377–386.

Ercoli, A., Vitali, R., and Gardi, R. (1964). Adsorbents for detection, isolation and evaluation of ethynyl steroids. *Steroids* **3**, 479–485.

Eriksson, H. (1976). Hepatic 15-hydroxylation of corticosteroids in the rat. Substrate specificity studied in the isolated perfused liver. *Eur. J. Biochem.* **64**, 573–581.

Eriksson, H., Gustafsson, J.-Å., and Sjövall, J. (1970). Excretion of steroid hormones in adults. C_{19} and C_{21} steroids in faeces from pregnant women. *Eur. J. Biochem.* **12**, 520–526.

Eriksson, H., Gustafsson, J.-Å., Sjövall, J., and Sjövall, K. (1972). Excretion of neutral steroids in urine and faeces of women with intrahepatic cholestasis of pregnancy. *Steroids Lipids Res.* **3**, 30–48.

Exley, D. (1979). Steroid immunoassay in clinical chemistry. *Pure Appl. Chem.* **52**, 33–44.

Fairclough, R. J., Rabjohns, M. A., and Peterson, A. J. (1977). Chromatographic separation of androgens, estrogens and progestogens on hydroxyalkoxypropyl-Sephadex (Lipidex[R]). *J. Chromatogr.* **133**, 412–414.

Fales, H. M., Milne, G. W. A., and Vestal, M. (1969). Chemical ionization mass spectrometry of complex molecules. *J. Am. Chem. Soc.* **91**, 3682–3685.

Fantl, V., and Gray, C. H. (1977). Automated urinary steroid profiles by capillary column gas–liquid chromatography and a computing integrator. *Clin. Chim. Acta* **79**, 237–253.

Farhi, R. L., and Monder, C. (1978). Analysis of steroidal carboxylic acids by high pressure liquid chromatography. *Anal. Biochem.* **90**, 58–68.

Felber, J. P. (1978). Radioimmunoassay in the clinical chemistry laboratory. *Adv. Clin. Chem.* **20**, 129–179.

Fels, J. P., Dehennin, L., Grenier, J., and Scholler, R. (1979). Quantitative estimation of urinary estrogens during the menstrual cycle by gas–liquid chromatography with a glass capillary column. *J. Steroid Biochem.* **11**, 1303–1308.

Fotherby, K., Warren, R. J., Shrimanker, K., Siekmann, L., Siekmann, A., and Breuer, H. (1979). Plasma levels of norethisterone measured by radioimmunoassay and gas chromatography–mass fragmentography. *J. Steroid Biochem.* **10**, 121–122.

Fotsis, T., Järvenpää, P., and Adlercreutz, H. (1980). Purification of urine for quantification of the complete estrogen profile. *J. Steroid Biochem.* **12**, 503–508.

Fotsis, T., Adlercreutz, H., Järvenpää, P., Setchell, K. D. R., Axelson, M., and Sjövall, J. (1981). Group separation of steroid conjugates by DEAE-Sephadex anion exchange chromatography. *J. Steroid Biochem.* **14**, 457–463.

Fransson, B., and Schill, G. (1975a). Isolation of acidic conjugates by ion pair extraction. I. Extraction of glycine, glucuronic and sulphuric acid conjugates. *Acta Pharm. Suec.* **12**, 107–118.

Fransson, B., and Schill, G. (1975b). Isolation of acidic conjugates by ion-pair extraction. II. Extraction of taurocholic and derivatives. *Acta Pharm. Suec.* **12**, 417–424.

Fransson, B., Wahlund, K.-G., Johansson, I. M., and Schill, G. (1976). Ion-pair chromatography of acidic drug metabolites and endogenic compounds. *J. Chromatogr.* **125**, 327–344.

Frey, F. J., Frey, B. M., and Benet, I. Z. (1979). Liquid-chromatographic measurement of endogenous and exogenous glucocorticoids in plasma. *Clin. Chem.* **25**, 1944–1947.

Gallant, S., Bruckheimer, S. M., and Brownie, A. C. (1978). The use of high-pressure liquid chromatography in the simultaneous assay of 11β-hydroxylase and 18-hydroxylase in zona fasciculata-reticularis tissue of the rat adrenal cortex. *Anal. Biochem.* **89**, 196–202.

Games. D. E. (1980). Mass spectroscopy coupled with chromatography. Combined high-performance liquid chromatography–mass spectrometry. *Anal. Proc.* 110–116.

Ganjam, V. K. (1976). Simultaneous ultramicroanalysis of both 17-keto and 17β-hydroxy androgens in biological fluids. *Steroids* **28**, 631–647.

Gardiner, W. L., and Horning, E. C. (1966). Gas–liquid chromatographic separation of C_{19} and C_{21} human urinary steroids by a new procedure. *Biochim. Biophys. Acta* **115**, 524–526.

Gaskell, S. J., and Brooks, C. J. W. (1976). *t*-Butyldimethylsilyl derivatives in the gas chromatography–mass spectrometry of steroids. *Biochem. Soc. Trans.* **4**, 111–113.

Gaskell, S. J., and Brooks, C. J. W. (1978). Studies of aldosterone 20,21-cyclic boronates by gas–liquid chromatography and mass spectrometry. *J. Chromatogr.* **158**, 331–336.

Gaskell, S. J., and Millington, D. S. (1978). Selected metastable peak monitoring: A new, specific technique in quantitative gas chromatography–mass spectrometry. *Biomed. Mass Spectrom.* **5**, 557–558.

Gaskell, S. J., and Pike, A. W. (1978). Gas chromatography–high resolution mass spectrometry in the analysis of steroids in physiological fluids. *Quant. Mass Spectrom. Life Sci.* **II**, 181–189.

Gaskell, S. J., Smith, A. G., and Brooks, C. J. W. (1975). Gas chromatography–mass spectrometry of trimethylsilyl ethers of sidechain hydroxylated Δ^4-3-ketosteroids. Long range trimethylsilyl group migration under electron impact. *Biomed. Mass Spectrom.* **2**, 148–155.

Gaskell, S. J., Edmonds, C. G., and Brooks, C. J. W. (1976). Cyclic boronate derivatives in combined gas chromatography–chemical ionisation mass spectrometry. *Anal. Lett.* **9**, 325–340.

Gaskell, S. J., Brooks, C. J. W., and Matin, S. B. (1977). The detection and quantification of an experimental steroid drug in dog plasma. *Biochem. Soc. Trans.* **5**, 1378–1380.

Gaskell, S. J., Pike, A. W., and Millington, D. S. (1979a). The fragmentation of stereoisomeric androstanediol *t*-butyldimethylsilyl ethers. A study by linked field scanning. *Biomed. Mass Spectrom.* **6**, 78–81.

Gaskell, S. J., Finney, R. W., and Harper, M. E. (1979b). The determination of testosterone in hamster prostate by gas chromatography–mass spectrometry with selected metastable peak monitoring. *Biomed. Mass Spectrom.* **6**, 113–116.

Gates, S. C., Smisko, M. J., Ashendel, C. L., Young, N. D., Holland, J. F., and Sweeley, C. C. (1978). Automated simultaneous qualitative and quantitative analysis of complex organic mixtures with a gas chromatography–mass spectrometry–computer system. *Anal. Chem.* **50**, 433–441.

Gelbke, H. P., Löffler, H., and Knuppen, R. (1976). Borate complexes of catecholestrogens: a new approach for the purification and isolation of 2- and 4-hydroxyestrogens. *Acta Endocrinol.* **82**, 36–38.

German, A. L., and Horning, E. C. (1972). Capillary column inlet system for the gas chromatography of biological samples. *Anal. Lett.* **5**, 619–628.

German, A. L., and Horning, E. C. (1973). Thermostable open tube cpillary columns for the high resolution gas chromatography of human urinary steroids. *J. Chromatogr. Sci.* **11**, 76–82.

Gips, H., Korte, K., Meinecke, B., and Bailer, P. (1980). Separation of C_{21}-, C_{19}- and C_{18}-steroids on Sephadex LH-20 microcolumns. *J. Chromatogr.* **193**, 322–328.

Gleispach, H. (1974). The use of different silylating agents for structure analyses of steroids. *J. Chromatogr.* **91**, 407–412.

Glencross, R. G., Abeywardene, S. A., Corney, S. J., and Morris, H. S. (1981). The use of oestradiol-17β antiserum covalently coupled to Sepharose to extract oestradiol-17β from biological fluids. *J. Chromatogr. Biomed. Appl.* **223**, 193–197.

Golder, W. A., and Sippell, W. G. (1976). Sephadex LH-20 multiple-column chromatography for the simultaneous separation of progesterone, deoxycorticosterone and 17α-hydroxyprogesterone from small plasma samples. *J. Chromatogr.* **123**, 293–299.

Goldzieher, J. W., de la Pena, A., and Aivaliotis, M. M. (1978). Radioimmunoassay of plasma androstenedione, testosterone and 11β-hydroxyandrostenedione after chromatography on Lipidex-5000 (Hydroxyalkoxypropyl Sephadex). *J. Steroid Biochem.* **9**, 169–173.

Graef, V., Furuya, E., and Nishikaze, O. (1977). Hydrolysis of steroid glucuronides with β-glucuronidase preparations from bovine liver, *Helix pomatia,* and *E. coli. Clin. Chem.* **23**, 532–535.

Gray, C. H., and James, V. H. T., eds. (1979). "Hormones in Blood," Vol. 3. Academic Press, New York.

Grob, K. (1978). Elastic fittings for glass capillary columns. *J. High Resol. Chromatogr.* **1,** 103–104.

Grob, K., and Grob, G. (1976). A new, generally applicable procedure for the preparation of glass capillary columns. *J. Chromatogr.* **125,** 471–485.

Grob, K., and Grob, K., Jr. (1978). On-column injection on to glass capillary columns. *J. Chromatogr.* **151,** 311–320.

Grob, K., Grob, G., and Grob, K., Jr. (1977). The barium carbonate procedure for the preparation of glass capillary columns; further informations and developments. *Chromatographia* **10,** 181–187.

Grob, K., Grob, G., and Grob, K., Jr. (1979a). Deactivation of glass capillary columns by silylation. Part 1: Principles and basic technique. *J. High Resol. Chromatogr.* **2,** 31–35.

Grob, K., Grob, G., and Grob, K., Jr. (1979b). Deactivation of glass capillaries by persilylation. Part 2: Practical recommendations. *J. High Resol. Chromatogr.* **2,** 677–678.

Grote, H., and Spiteller, G. (1976). Zur Lokalisierung funktioneller Gruppen mit Hilfe der Massenspektrometrie. XV—Massenspektren von Androstanen mit Hydroxylgruppen in den Positionen 3, 16 und 17. *Org. Mass Spectrom.* **11,** 1297–1307.

Grote, H., and Spiteller, G. (1977). Location of functional groups with the aid of mass spectrometry. XVI—Mass spectra of trimethylsilylated androstan-3,16-17β-triols. *Biomed. Mass Spectrom.* **4,** 216–219.

Grupe, A., and Spiteller, G. (1978). Zur Lokalisierung funktioneller Gruppen mit Hilfe *der Massenspektrometrie. XVII–Massenspektren von 3,6,20β*-Trihydroxypregnanen. *Org. Mass Spectrom.* **13,** 448–454.

Gudzinowicz, B. J. (1977). Integrated GC–MS analytical systems. Part I. Recent technological advances affecting integrated GC–MS system utilization. *Chem. Instrum.* **8,** 225–293.

Gustafsson, B. E., Gustafsson, J.-Å., and Sjövall, J. (1968). Steroids in germfree and conventional rats. 2. Identification of 3α,16α-dihydroxy-5α-pregnan-20-one and related compounds in faeces from germfree rats. *Eur. J. Biochem.* **4,** 568–573.

Gustafsson, J.-Å., and Ingelman-Sundberg, M. (1976). Multiple forms of cytochrome *P*-450 in rat-liver microsomes. Separation and some properties of different hydroxylases active on free and sulphoconjugated steroids. *Eur. J. Biochem.* **64,** 35–43.

Gustafsson, J.-Å., and Sjövall, J. (1968). Steroids in germfree and conventional rats. 6. Identification of 15α- and 21-hydroxylated C_{21} steroids in faeces from germfree rats. *Eur. J. Biochem.* **6,** 236–247.

Gustafsson, J.-Å., and Sjövall, J. (1969). Identification of 22-, 24- and 26-hydroxycholesterol in the steroid sulphate fraction of faeces from infants. *Eur. J. Biochem.* **8,** 467–472.

Gustafsson, J.-Å., Ryhage, R., Sjövall, J., and Moriarty, R. M. (1969). Migrations of the trimethylsilyl group upon electron impact in steroids. *J. Am. Chem. Soc.* **91,** 1234–1236.

Gustafsson, J.-Å., Shackleton, C. H. L., and Sjövall, J. (1970). Steroids in newborns and infants. A semiquantitative analysis of steroids in faeces from infants. *Acta Endocrinol.* **65,** 18–28.

Halket, J. M. (1979). Factor analysis of repetitively scanned spectra in gas chromatography–mass spectrometry. The number of components in partially resolved peaks. *J. Chromatogr.* **175,** 229–241.

Halket, J. M., and Lisboa, B. P. (1980). Simple mass chromatographic procedure for the detection and identification of sterols using derivative correlations. *J. Chromatogr.* **189,** 267–271.

Hammerschmidt, F. J., and Spiteller, G. (1973a). Zur Lokalisierung funktioneller Gruppen mit Hilfe der Massenspektrometrie—VIII. 6-Hydroxy-androstan-3,17-dione und 6,17β-dihydroxy-androstan-3-one. *Tetrahedron* **29,** 2465–2472.

Hammerschmidt, F. J., and Spiteller, G. (1973b). Zur Lokalisierung funktioneller Gruppen mit Hilfe der Massenspekrometrie—IX. 17β-hydroxy-androstan-3,6-dione, 3-hydroxy-androstan-6,17-dione und 3,17β-dihydroxy androstan-6-one. *Tetrahedron* **29**, 3995–4001.

Hammerum, S., and Djerassi, C. (1975). Mass spectrometry in structural and stereochemical problems—CCXLIV. The influence of substituents and stereochemistry on the mass spectral fragmentation of progesterone. *Tetrahedron* **31**, 2391–2400.

Hammond, G. L., Ruokonen, A., Kontturi, M., Koskela, E., and Vihko, R. (1977). The simultaneous radioimunoassay of seven steroids in human spermatic and peripheral venous blood. *J. Clin. Endocrinol. Metab.* **45**, 16–24.

Hara, A., and Radin, N. S. (1978). Lipid extraction of tissues with a low-toxicity solvent. *Anal. Biochem.* **90**, 420–426.

Harvey, D. J. (1977a). Allyldimethylsilyl ethers as derivatives for the characterization of steroids and cannabinoids by combined gas chromatography and mass spectrometry. *Biomed. Mass Spectrom.* **4**, 265–274.

Harvey, D. J. (1977b). Mass spectrometry of the triethylsilyl, tri-n-propylsilyl and tri-n-butylsilyl derivatives of some alcohols, steroids and cannabinoids. *Org. Mass Spectrom.* **12**, 473–474.

Harvey, D. J. (1978). Comparison of fourteen substituted silyl derivatives for the characterization of alcohols, steroids and cannabinoids by combined gas–liquid chromatography and mass spectrometry. *J. Chromatogr.* **147**, 291–298.

Harvey, D. J., and Vouros, P. (1979). Influence of the 6-trimethylsilyl group on the fragmentation of the trimethylsilyl derivatives of some 6 hydroxy- and 3,6 dihydroxy-steroids and related compounds. *Biomed. Mass Spectrom.* **6**, 135–143.

Hedfjall, B., and Ryhage, R. (1979). Electro-optical ion detector for capillary column gas chromatography/negative ion mass spectrometry. *Anal. Chem.* **51**, 1687–1690.

Heftmann, E. (1976). "Chromatography of Steroids." Elsevier, Amsterdam.

Heftmann, E., and Hunter, I. R. (1979). High-pressure liquid chromatography of steroids. *J. Chromatogr. Rev.* **165**, 283–299.

Henion, J. D., and Maylin, G. A. (1980). Drug analysis by direct liquid introduction micro liquid chromatography mass spectrometry. *Biomed. Mass Spectrom.* **7**, 115–121.

Henneberg, D., Henrichs, U., and Schomburg, G. (1975a). Special techniques in the combination of gas chromatography and mass spectrometry. *J. Chromatogr.* **112**, 343–352.

Henneberg, D., Henrichs, U., and Schomburg, G. (1975b). Open split connection of glass capillary columns to mass spectrometers. *Chromatographia* **8**, 449–451.

Henneberg, D., Henrichs, U., Husmann, H., and Schomburg, G. (1978). High-performance gas chromatograph–mass spectrometer interfacing: Investigation and optimization of flow and temperature. *J. Chromatogr.* **167**, 139–147.

Hermanasson, J. (1978). Reversed-phase liquid chromatography of steroid glucuronides. *J. Chromatogr.* **152**, 437–445.

Hermansson, J. (1980). Separation of steroid glucuronides by reversed-phase liquid column chromatography. *J. Chromatogr.* **194**, 80–84.

Hobkirk, R., and Davidson, S. (1971). Behaviour of dehydroisoandrosterone, testosterone and their conjugates on DEAE-Sephadex. *J. Chromatogr.* **54**, 431–432.

Hobkirk, R., and Nilsen, M. (1970). Separation of monoglucosiduronate conjugates of estrone and 17β-estradiol by DEAE-Sephadex chromatography. *Anal. Biochem.* **37**, 337–344.

Hoffmann, A. F. (1967). Efficient extraction of bile acid conjugates with tetraheptylammonium chloride, a liquid ion exchanger. *J. Lipid Res.* **8**, 55–58.

Holick, M. F., and DeLuca, H. F. (1971). A new chromatographic system for vitamin D₃ and its metabolites: resolution of a new vitamin D_3 metabolite. *J. Lipid Res.* **12**, 460–465.

Holmdahl, T., and Sjövall, J. (1971). Liquid-gel chromatography on hydrophobic Sephadex and competitive protein binding of 17α-hydroxyprogesterone in plasma. *Steroids* **18**, 69–76.

Honour, J. W., and Shackleton, C. H. L. (1977). Mass spectrometric analysis for tetrahydroaldosterone. *J. Steroid Biochem.* **8**, 299–305.

Honour, J. W., Tourniaire, J., Biglieri, E. G., and Shackleton, C. H. L. (1978). Urinary steroid excretion in 17α-hydroxylase deficiency. *J. Steroid Biochem.* **9**, 495–505.

Hoppen, H.-O., and Siekmann, L. (1974). Gas chromatography–mass spectrometry of catechol estrogens. *Steroids* **23**, 17–34.

Horning, E. C. (1968). Gas phase analytical methods for the study of steroid hormones and their metabolites. *In* "Gas Phase Chromatography of Steroids" (K. B. Eik-Nes and E. C. Horning, eds.), pp. 1–71. Springer-Verlag, Berlin and New York.

Horning, E. C., and Horning, M. G. (1971). Human metabolic profiles obtained by GC and GC/MS. *J. Chromatogr. Sci.* **9**, 129–140.

Horning, E. C., Carroll, D. I., Dzidic, I., Haegele, K. D., Horning, M. G., and Stillwell, R. N. (1974). Atmospheric pressure ionization (API) mass spectrometry. Solvent-mediated ionization of samples introduced in solution and in a liquid chromatograph effluent stream. *J. Chromatogr. Sci.* **12**, 725–729.

Horning, E. C., Carroll, D. I., Dzidic, I., and Stillwell, R. N. (1978). Development and use of bioanalytical systems based on mass spectrometry with ionization at atmospheric pressure. *Pure Appl. Chem.* **50**, 113–127.

Horning, M. G., Chambaz, E. M., Brooks, C. J. W., Moss, A. M., Boucher, E. A., Horning, E. C., and Hill, R. M. (1969). Characterization and estimation of urinary steroids of the newborn human by gas-phase analytical methods. *Anal. Biochem.* **31**, 512–531.

Hosoda, H., Yamashita, K., Sagae, H., and Nambara, T. (1975). Studies on dimethyl-*tert*-butylsilyl ethers of steroid. *Chem. Pharm. Bull.* **23**, 2118–2122.

Hosoda, H., Yamashita, K., Ikegawa, S., and Nambara, T. (1977). Blockage of coordination with shift reagent by *tert*-butyldimethylsilylation in nuclear magnetic resonance spectroscopy and its applications to deuterium-labeled steroids. *Chem. Pharm. Bull.* **25**, 2545–2553.

Ishii, D., Hibi, K., Asai, K., Nagaya, M., Mochizuki, K., and Mochida, Y. (1978). Studies of micro high-performance liquid chromatography. IV. Application of the micro precolumn method to the analysis of corticosteroids in serum. *J. Chromatogr.* **156**, 173–180.

Jacob, K., and Vogt, W. (1978). Dimethylthiophosphinic esters for the gas chromatographic determination of monohydroxy-steroids with the alkali flame detector. VI. Steroid phosphorus compounds. *J. Chromatogr.* **150**, 339–344.

Jänne, O. (1971). Urinary excretion of mono- and disulphates of C_{19} and C_{21} steroids with reference to the menstural cycle. *Acta Endocrinol.* **67**, 316–330.

Jänne, O., and Vihko, R. (1970). Neutral steroids in urine during pregnancy. I. Isolation and identification of dihydroxylated C_{19} and C_{21} steroid disulphates. *Acta Endocrinol.* **65**, 50–68.

Jänne, O., Vihko, R., Sjövall, J., and Sjövall, K. (1969). Determination of steroid mono- and disulfates in human plasma. *Clin. Chim. Acta* **23**, 405–412.

Jänne, O., Apter, D., and Vihko, R. (1974). Assay of testosterone, progesterone and 17α-hydroxyprogesterone in human plasma by radioimmunoassay after separation on hydroxyalkoxypropyl Sephadex. *J. Steroid Biochem.* **5**, 155–162.

Järvenpää, P., Fotsis, T., and Adlercreutz, H. (1979). Ion exchange purification of estrogens. *J. Steroid Biochem.* **11**, 1583–1588.

Jeannin, J. F., Bournot, P., Maume, G., and Maume, B. F. (1978). Détermination simultanée d'androgens plasmatiques chez le rat par fragmentographie de masse et dilution isotopique. *J. Steroid Biochem.* **9**, 615–622.

Jeffcoate, S. L. (1977). Recent developments in steroid radioimmunoassays. *J. Reprod. Fertil.* **51**, 267–272.

Johnson, D. W., Phillipou, G., Ralph, M. M., and Semark, R. F. (1979a). Specific quantitation of urinary progesterone by gas chromatography–mass spectrometry. *Clin. Chim. Acta* **94**, 207–208.

Johnson, D. W., Phillipou, G., Blair, I. A., and Seamark, R. F. (1979b). Measurement of urinary steroid production rates using stable-isotopes and GC–MS. *Experientia* **35**, 1261–1262.

Johnson, D. W., Phillipou, G., James, S. K., Seaborn, C. J., and Ralph, M. M. (1980). Specific quantitation of plasma dehydroepiandrosterone sulphate by GC–MS; comparison with a direct RIA. *Clin. Chim. Acta* **106**, 99–101.

Johnson, L. P., Rao, S. C. S., and Fenselau, C. (1978). Pyridine as a reagent gas for the characterization of glucuronides by chemical ionization mass spectrometry. *Anal. Chem.* **50**, 2022–2024.

Jones, P. R., and Yang, S. K. (1975). A liquid chromatograph/mass spectrometer interface. *Anal. Chem.* **47**, 1000–1003.

Kabra, P. M., Tsai, L.-L., and Marton, L. J. (1979). Improved liquid-chromatographic method for determination of serum cortisol. *Clin. Chem.* **25**, 1293–1296.

Kachel, C. D., and Mendelsohn, F. A. O. (1979). An automated multicolumn systems for chromatography of aldosterone on Sephadex LH-20 in water. *J. Steroid Biochem.* **10**, 563–567.

Karger, B. L., Kirby, D. P., Vouros, P., Foltz, R. L., and Hidy, B. (1979). On-line reversed phase liquid chromatography–mass spectrometry. *Anal. Chem.* **51**, 2324–2328.

Kautsky, M. P., and Hagerman, D. D. (1979). Purification of steroid hormones from ovarian tissue by high pressure liquid chromatography. *Chromatogr. Sci.* **10**, 123–135.

Kawahara, C., Kozbur, X., Geduld, S., and Parker, L. (1980). Magnesium oxide column chromatography: A novel and rapid method for steroid purification. *Anal. Biochem.* **102**, 310–312.

Kawasaki, T., Maeda, M., and Tsuji, A. (1979). Determination of plasma and urinary cortisol by high-performance liquid chromatography using fluorescence derivatization with dansyl hydrazine. *J. Chromatogr.* **163**, 143–150.

Kelly, R. W. (1971). The measurement by gas chromatography–mass spectrometry of oestra-1,3,5,-triene-3,15α, 16α,17β-tetrol (oestetrol) in pregnancy urine. *J. Chromatrogr.* **54**, 345–355.

Kelly, R. W., and Taylor, P. L. (1976a). *tert*-Butyl Dimethylsilyl ethers as derivatives for qualitative analysis of steroids and prostaglandins by gas phase methods. *Anal. Chem.* **48**, 465–467.

Kelly, R. W., and Taylor, P. L. (1976b). Gas chromatography–mass spectrometry of steroids and prostaglandins as *t*-butyldimethylsilyl ethers. *In* "Advances in Mass Spectrometry in Biochemistry and Medicine" (A. Frigerio and N. Castagnoli, eds.), Vol. 1, pp. 449–455. Spectrum, New York.

Kerebel, A., Morfin, R. F., Berthou, F. L., Picart, D., Bardou, L. G., and Floch, H. H. (1977). Analysis of $C_{19}O_3$ steroids by thin-layer and gas–liquid chromatography and mass spectrometry. *J. Chromatogr.* **140**, 229–244.

Kern, H., and Brander, B. (1979). Precision of an automated all-glass capillary gas chromatography system with an electron capture detector for the trace analysis of estrogens. *J. High Resol. Chromatogr.* **2**, 312–318.

Kirby, D. P., Vouros, P., and Karger, B. L. (1980). Ion pairing techniques: Compatibility with on-line liquid chromatography–mass spectrometry. *Science* **209**, 495–497.

Klein, E. R., and Klein, P. D. (1978, 1979). A selected bibliography of biomedical and environmental applications of stable isotopes. *Biomed. Mass Spectrom.* **5**, 91–111 (Pt. I), 321–330; (Pt II), 373–379; (Pt III), 425–432; (Pt. IV), **6**, 515–545 (Pt. V).

Klein, P. D., Haumann, J. R., and Hachey, D. L. (1975). Stable isotope ratiometer–multiple ion detector unit for quantitative and qualitative stable isotope studies by gas chromatography–mass spectrometry. *Clin. Chem.* **21**, 1253–1257.

Knuppen, R., Haupt, O., Schramm, W., and Hoppen, H.-O. (1979). Selected ion monitoring: A new approach for the specific determination of steroids in the lower picogram range. *J. Steroid Biochem.* **11**, 153–160.

Kornel, L., and Saito, Z. (1975). Studies on steroid conjugates—VIII: Isolation and characterization of glucuronide-conjugated metabolites of cortisol in human urine. *J. Steroid Biochem.* **6**, 1267–1284.

Kornel, L., Miyabo, S., and Saito, Z. (1975). New paper chromatographic systems for the separation of conjugated corticosteroids. *J. Chromatogr.* **111**, 200–205.

Koshy, K. T. (1976). Structure-gas chromatographic electron capture sensitivity relationships of some substituted 17α-acetoxyprogesterones. *J. Chromatogr.* **126**, 641–650.

Koshy, K. T., Kaiser, D. G., and VanDerSlik, A. L. (1975). O-(2,3,4,5,6-pentafluorobenzyl)hydroxylamine hydrochloride as a sensitive derivatizing agent for the electron capture gas–liquid chromatographic analysis of keto steroids. *J. Chromatogr. Sci.* **13**, 97–104.

Kruger, T. L., Kondrat, R. W., Joseph, K. T., and Cooks, R. G. (1979). Identification of individual steroids in biological matrices by mass-analyzed ion kinetic energy spectrometry. *Anal. Biochem.* **96**, 104–112.

Kulkarni, B. D., and Goldzieher, J. W. (1969). Isolation of 17α-ethynyl steroids by column chromatography on silver impregnated florisil. *Steroids* **13**, 467–475.

Laatikainen, T., and Karjalainen, O. (1972). Excretion of conjugates of neutral steroids in human bile during late pregnancy. *Acta Endocrinol.* **69**, 775–788.

Laatikainen, T., Perheentupa, J., Vihko, R., Makino, I., and Sjövall, J. (1972). Bile acids and hormonal steroids in bile of a boy with 3β-hydroxysteroid dehydrogenase deficiency. *J. Steroid Biochem.* **3**, 715–719.

Lambert, P. W., Syverson, B. J., Arnaud, C. D., and Spelsberg, T. C. (1977). Isolation and quantitation of endogenous vitamin D and its physiologically important metabolites in human plasma by high pressure liquid chromatography. *J. Steroid Biochem.* **8**, 929–937.

Landon, J., Hassan, M., Pourfarzaneh, M., and Smith, D. S. (1979). Non-isotopic immunoassay of hormones in blood. *In* "Hormones in Blood" (C. H. Gray and V. H. T. James, eds.), Vol. 3, pp. 1–40. Academic Press, New York.

Lawrence, R. H., Jr., Waller, G. R., and Kinneberg, K. F. (1974). An improved method of sample introduction in gas chromatography–mass spectrometry of biological materials. *Anal. Biochem.* **62**, 102–107.

Lawson, A. M., Leemans, F. A. J. M., and McCloskey, J. A. (1969). Oxygen-18 exchange reactions in steroidal ketones. Determination of relative rates of incorporation by gas chromatography–mass spectrometry. *Steroids* **14**, 603–615.

Lebel, M., Nowaczynski, W., and Genest, J. (1975). Efficient method for purifying progesterone for competitive protein-binding technique. *J. Steroid Biochem.* **6**, 1359–1361.

Leclercq, P. A. (1974). Mass spectrometry of 16,16'-O-permethylated 17-ketosteroids. *Biomed. Mass Spectrom.* **1**, 109–114.

Lehmann, W. D., and Schulten, H.-R. (1978). Quantitative Massenspekrometrie in Biochemie und Medizin. *Angew. Chem.* **90**, 233–250.

Leunissen, W. J. J., and Thijssen, J. H. H. (1978). Quantitative analysis of steroid profiles from urine by capillary gas chromatography. I. Accuracy and reproducibility of the sample preparation. *J. Chromatogr. Biomed. Appl.* **146**, 365–380.

Lin, J.-T., Heftmann, E., and Hunter, I. R. (1980). High-performance liquid chromatography of the reduction products of progesterone. *J. Chromatogr.* **190**, 169–174.

Lisboa, B. P. (1969). Thin-layer chromatography of steroids, sterols and related compounds. *In* "Methods of Enzymology" (R. B. Clayton, ed.), Vol. XV, pp. 3–157. Academic Press, New York.

Lisboa, B. P., and Strassner, M. (1975). Gel chromatography of steroid oestrogens on Sephadex LH-20. *J. Chromatogr.* **111**, 159–164.

Losty, H., Begue, R.-J., Moriniere, M., and Padieu, P. (1979). Analysis of the urinary steroids from a pathological pregnancy by liquid-gel chromatography and gas chromatography–mass spectrometry. *Recent Dev. Mass Spectrom. Biochem. Med.* **2**, 283–295.

Ludwig, H., Reiner, J., and Spiteller, G. (1977). Untersuchung der Steroide im Blut mit der Kombination Glaskapillargaschromatographie–Massenspekrometrie. *Chem. Ber.* **110**, 217–227.

Ludwig, H., Spiteller, G., Matthaei, D., and Scheler, F. (1978). Profile bei chronischen Erkrankungen. I. Steroidprofiluntersuchungen bei Uramie. *J. Chromatogr. Biomed. Appl.* **146**, 381–391.

Ludwig-Köhn, H., Messing, F., Spiteller, G., Matthaei, D., Henning, H. V., and Scheler, F. (1979). Profile bei chronischen Erkrankungen. II. Steroidprofile von Patienten mit Psoriasis vulgaris. *J. Chromatogr. Biomed. Appl.* **162**, 573–578.

Luyten, J. A., and Rutten, G. A. F. M. (1974). Analysis of steroids by high-resolution gas–liquid chromatography. II. Application to urinary samples. *J. Chromatogr.* **91**, 393–406.

McFadden, W. H. (1980). Liquid chromatography/mass spectrometry systems and applications. *J. Chromatogr. Sci.* **18**, 97–115.

McFadden, W. H., Schwartz, H. L., and Evans, S. (1976). Direct analysis of liquid chromatographic effluents. *J. Chromatogr.* **122**, 389–396.

McGinley, R., and Casey, J. H. (1979). Analysis of progesterone in unextracted serum: A method using danazol [17α-pregn-4-en-20-yno(2,3-d) isoxazol-17-ol] a blocker of steroid binding to proteins. *Steroids* **33**, 127–138.

McLafferty, F. W. (1980). Separation/identification systems applicable to complex mixtures. *In* "Biochemical Applications of Mass Spectrometry" (G. R. Waller and O. C. Dermer, eds.), pp. 1159–1168. Wiley, New York.

McLafferty, F. W., and Venkataraghavan, R. (1979). Computer techniques for mass spectral identification. *J. Chromatogr. Sci.* **17**, 24–29.

Madani, C., and Chambaz, E. M. (1978). Glass open-tubular capillary columns with chemically bonded methyl-phenyl siloxane stationary phases of tailor made polarity. *Chromatographia* **11**, 725–730.

Madani, C., Chambaz, E. M., Rigaud, M., Durand, J., and Chebroux, P. (1976). New method for the preparation of highly stable polysiloxane-coated glass open-tubular capillary columns and application to the analysis of hormonal steroids. *J. Chromatogr.* **126**, 161–169.

Makino, I., and Sjövall, J. (1972). A versatile method for analysis of bile acids in plasma. *Anal. Lett.* **5**, 341–349.

Matsui, M., and Hakozaki, M. (1978). Disulphates of 16-oxygenated ketonic C_{19} steroids as biliary metabolites of androsterone sulphate in female rats. *Steroids* **31**, 219–226.

Matsui, M., Hakozaki, M., and Kinuyama, Y. (1975). Extraction of steroid diconjugates using Amberlite XAD-2 resin. *J. Chromatogr.* **115**, 625–628.

Matthews, D. E., and Hayes, J. M. (1976). Systematic errors in gas chromatography–mass spectrometry isotope ratio measurements. *Anal. Chem.* **48**, 1375–1382.

Matthews, D. E., Ben-Galim, E., and Bier, D. M. (1979). Determination of stable isotopic enrichment in individual plasma amino acids by chemical ionization mass spectrometry. *Anal. Chem.* **51**, 80–84.

Mattox, V. R., and Litwiller, R. D. (1979). An evaluation of systems for paper chromatography of C_{21} steroids. *Steroids* **34**, 227–239.

Mattox, V. R., Litwiller, R. D., and Goodrich, J. E. (1972a). Extraction of steroidal glucosiduronic acids from aqueous solutions by anionic liquid ion-exchangers. *Biochem. J.* **126**, 533–543.

Mattox, V. R., Litwiller, R. D., and Goodrich, J. E. (1972b). Recovery of steroidal glucosiduronic acids from organic solvents containing anionic liquid ion-exchangers. *Biochem. J.* **126**, 545–552.

Mattox, V. R., Goodrich, J. E., and Litwiller, R. D. (1972c). Liquid ion exchangers for chromatography of steroidal glucosiduronic acids and other polar compounds. *J. Chromatogr.* **66**, 337–346.

Mattox, V. R., Goodrich, J. E., and Litwiller, R. D. (1975a). Liquid ion exchangers in paper chromatography of steroidal glucosiduronic acids, glucosiduronic esters and free steroids. *J. Chromatogr.* **108**, 23–35.

Mattox, V. R., Litwiller, R. D., and Goodrich, J. E. (1975b). Liquid ion exchangers in paper chromatography of steroidal glucosiduronic acids. Influence of different exchangers on the mobility in chloroform-formamide and correlation of chromatographic data. *J. Chromatogr.* **109**, 129–147.

Mattox, V. R., Litwiller, R. D., Goodrich, J. E., and Tan, W. C. (1976). Liquid ion exchangers in reversed-phase systems for chromatography of steroidal glucosiduronic acids. *J. Chromatogr.* **120**, 435–447.

Mattox, V. R., Litwiller, R. D., and Carpenter, P. C. (1979). Comparison of the resolving properties of a group of chromatography systems for a collection of compounds. *J. Chromatogr.* **175**, 243–260.

Maume, B. F., and Luyten, J. A. (1973). Evaluation of gas chromatographic–mass spectrometric and mass fragmentographic performance in steroid analysis with glass capillary columns. *J. Chromatogr. Sci.* **11**, 607–610.

Maume, B. F., Bournot, P., Lhuguenot, J. C., Baron, C., Barbier, F., Maume, G., Prost, P., and Padieu, P. (1973). Mass fragmentographic analysis of steroids, catecholamines and amino acids in biological materials. *Anal. Chem.* **45**, 1073–1082.

Maume, B. F., Prost, M., and Padieu, P. (1976). Steroid hormone biosynthesis in adrenal cell cultures from newborn rats. *In* "Advances in Mass Spectrometry in Biochemistry and Medicine" (A. Frigerio and N. Castagnoli, eds.), Vol. 1, pp. 525–540. Spectrum, New York.

Maume, B. F., Millot, C., Mesnier, D., Patouraux, D., Doumas, J., and Tomori, E. (1979). Quantitative analysis of corticosteroids in adrenal cell cultures by capillary column gas chromatography combined with mass spectrometry. *J. Chromatogr.* **186**, 581–594.

Maynard, P. V., Pike, A. W., Weston, A., and Griffiths, K. (1977). Analysis of dehydroepiandrosterone and androstenediol in human breast tissue using high resolution gas chromatography–mass spectrometry. *Eur. J. Cancer* **13**, 971–975.

Michnowicz, J., and Munson, B. (1974). Studies in chemical ionization mass spectrometry: Steroidal ketones. *Org. Mass Spectrom.* **8**, 49–60.

Mickan, H., and Zander, J. (1979). Pregnanolones and pregnenolone in human myometrium at term of pregnancy. *J. Steroid Biochem.* **11**, 1455–1459.

Middleditch, B. S., and Desiderio, D. M. (1973). Comparison of selective ion monitoring and repetitive scanning during gas chromatography–mass spectrometry. *Anal. Chem.* **45**, 806–808.

Middleditch, B. S., Vouros, P., and Brooks, C. J. W. (1973). Mass spectrometry in the analysis of steroid drugs and their metabolites: electron-impact-induced fragmentation of ring D. *J. Pharm. Pharmacol.* **25**, 143–149.

Milberg, R. M., and Cook, J. C., Jr. (1978). The mass spectrometer as a detector for gas–liquid chromatography. *Chromatogr. Sci.* **9**, 235–258.

Millard, B. J. (1978). "Quantitative Mass Spectrometry." Heyden, London.

Millington, D. S. (1975). Determination of hormonal steroid concentrations in biological extracts by high resolution mass fragmentography. *J. Steroid Biochem.* **6**, 239–245.

Millington, D. S. (1977). New techniques in quantitative mass spectrometry. *J. Reprod. Fertil.* **51**, 303–308.

Millington, D. S., Jenner, D. A., Jones, T., and Griffiths, K. (1974). Endogenous steroid concentrations in human breast tumors determined by high-resolution mass fragmentography. *Biochem. J.* **139**, 473–475.

Millington, D. S., Buoy, M. E., Brooks, G., Harper, M. E., and Griffiths, K. (1975). Thin-layer chromatography and high resolution selected ion monitoring for the analysis of C_{19} steroids in human hyperplastic prostate tissue. *Biomed. Mass Spectrom.* **2**, 219–224.

Milne, G. W. A. (1971). The application of mass spectrometry to problems in medicine and biochemistry. *In* "Mass Spectrometry. Techniques and Applications" (G. W. A. Milne, ed.), pp. 327–371. Wiley (Interscience), New York.

Miyabo, S., and Kornel, L. (1974). Corticosteroids in human blood—VI. Isolation, characterization and quantitation of sulfate conjugated metabolites of cortisol in human plasma. *J. Steroid Biochem.* **5**, 233–247.

Miyazaki, H., Ishibashi, M., Itoh, M., and Nambara, T. (1975). Use of new silylating agents for identification of hydroxylated steroids by gas chromatography–electron impact–mass spectrometry. *Chem. Pharm. Bull.* **23**, 3033–3035.

Miyazaki, H., Ishibashi, M., Itoh, M., Morishita, N., Sudo, M., and Nambara, T. (1976). Analysis of estrogen glucuronides. I—Characterization of estrogen glucuronides by gas chromatography–mass spectrometry. *Biomed. Mass Spectrom.* **3**, 55–59.

Miyazaki, H., Ishibashi, M., Itoh, M., Yamashita, K., and Nambara, T. (1977a). Use of silylating agents for the identification of hydroxylated steroids by gas chromatography and gas chromatography–mass spectrometry. Discrimination between phenolic and alcoholic hydroxyl groups. *J. Chromatogr.* **133**, 311–318.

Miyazaki, H., Ishibashi, M., Itoh, M., and Nambara. T. (1977b). Use of new silylating agents for identification of hydroxylated steroids by gas chromatography and gas chromatography–mass spectrometry. *Biomed. Mass Spectrom.* **4**, 23–35.

Miyazaki, H., Ishibashi, M., and Itoh, M. (1977c). Application of an ion-cluster technique to the analysis of endogenous hydroxylated compounds. I. Preparation of a doublet by use of a mixture of trimethylsilylimidazole (TSIM) and TSIM-d_3. *J. Chromatogr.* **135**, 109–116.

Miyazaki, H., Ishibashi, M., and Yamashita, K. (1979). Dimethylisopropylsilyl ether derivatives in gas chromatography–mass spectrometry of hydroxylated stteroids. *Biomed. Mass Spectrom.* **6**, 57–62.

Moneti, G., Pazzagli, M., Fiorelli, G., and Serio, M. (1980). Measurement of 5α-androstane-3α,17β-diol in human spermatic venous plasma by mass-fragmentography. *J. Steroid Biochem.* **13**, 623–627.

Morfin, R. F., Leav, I., Orr, J. C., Picart, D., and Ofner, P. (1980). C_{19}-Steroid metabolism by canine prostate, epididymis and perianal glands. *Eur. J. Biochem.* **109**, 119–127.

Morgan, E. D., and Poole, C. F. (1974). Preparation and assessment of fluorocarbonsilyl ethers as gas chromatography derivatives for steroids. *J. Chromatogr,* **89**, 225–230.

Morgan, E. D., and Poole, C. F. (1975). Formation of pentafluorophenyldimethylsilyl ethers and their use in the gas chromatographic analysis of sterols. *J. Chromatogr.* **104**, 351–358.

Mori, Y., and Sato, T. (1973). Retention indices of steroids and their group increment with temperature. *J. Chromatogr.* **76**, 133–139.

Morreal, C. E., and Dao, T. L. (1975). Protection of estrogenic hormones by ascorbic acid during chromatography. *Steroids* **25**, 421–426.

Mourey, T. H., and Siggia, S. (1980). Microparticulate bonded pyrrolidone for high performance liquid chromatographic separation of estrogenic steroids in urine. *Anal. Chem.* **52**, 881–885.

Müller, O. A., Braun, J., Fröhlich, R., and Scriba, P. C. (1974). Eine mechanisierte kompetitive Proteinbindungs analyse für Cortisol im Serum ohne vorherige Extraktion mit organischen Lösungsmitteln. *Z. Klin. Chem. Klin. Biochem.* **12**, 276–278.

Murphy, B. E. P. (1971). Sephadex column chromatography as an adjunct to competitive protein binding assays of steroids. *Nature (London) New Biol.* **232**, 21–24.

Murphy, B. E. P., and Diez D'Aux, R. C. (1975). The use of Sephadex LH-20 column chromatography to separate unconjugated steroids. *J. Steroid Biochem.* **6**, 233–237.

Murray, S., and Baillie, T. A. (1979). Direct derivatization of sulphate esters for analysis by gas chromatography–mass spectrometry. *Biomed. Mass Spectrom.* **6**, 82–89.

Musey, P. I., Collins, D. C., and Preedy, J. R. K. (1977). Isocratic separation of estrogen conjugates on DEAE-Sephadex. *Steroids* **29**, 657–668.

Musey, P. I., Collins, D. C., and Preedy, J. R. K. (1978). Separation of estrogen conjugates by high pressure liquid chromatography. *Steroids* **31**, 583–592.

Nambara, T., and Iwata, T. (1973). Analytical chemical studies on steroids. LXIII. Steroid numbers of androstanones and their oxime derivatives on gas chromatography. *Chem. Pharm. Bull.* **21**, 899–902.

Nambra, T., Bae, Y. H., Anjyo, T., and Goya, S. (1971). Analytical chemical studies on steroids. LII. Studies on steroid conjugates. VII. Gas chromatography of steroid *n*-acetylglucosaminides. *J. Chromatogr.* **62**, 369–372.

Nambara, T., Kigasawa, K., Iwata, T., and Ibuki, M. (1975). Studies on steroids. CIII. A new type of derivative for electron capture-gas chromatography of ketosteroids. *J. Chromatogr.* **114**, 81–86.

Nambara, T., Iwata, T., and Kigasawa, K. (1976). Studies on steroids. CIX. O-ω-haloalkyloximes, new derivatives for gas chromatography–mass spectrometry of oxosteroids. *J. Chromatogr.* **118**, 127–133.

Nice, E. C., and O'Hare, M. J. (1978). Selective effects of reversed-phase column packings in high-performance liquid chromatography of steroids. *J. Chromatogr.* **166**, 263–267.

Nicosia, S. Z., Galli, G., and Fiecchi, A. (1973). Base-catalyzed silylation. A quantitative procedure for the gas chromatographic–mass spectrometric analysis of neutral steroids. *J. Steroid Biochem.* **4**, 417–425.

Nilsson, B., Tejler, L., and Dymling, J.-F. (1979). Purification and quantitation of plasma protein bound vitamins and steroids by combined affinity and high-performance liquid chromatography techniques. *Chromatogra. Sci.* **2**, 349–358.

Nishikaze, O., and Kobayashi, T. (1977). Improved hydrolysis of urinary 17-hydroxycorticosteroid glucuronides with β-glucuronidase from Helix pomatia, on adding sodium sulfate. *Clin. Chem.* **23**, 2332–2334.

Novotny, M., and Zlatkis, A. (1970). High resolution chromatographic separation of steroids with open tubular glass columns. *J. Chromatogr. Sci.* **8**, 346–350.

Nowlin, J. G., Carroll, D. I., Dzidic, I., Horning, M. G., Stillwell, R. N., and Horning, E. C. (1979). Plasma desorption ionization mass spectra of unconjugated human steroids. *Anal. Lett.* **12**, 573–580.

Nystedt, L. (1980). On the mathematics of tracer kinetics when pools are not in steady-state. *J. Steroid Biochem.* **13**, 1487–1488.

Nyström, E., and Sjövall, J. (1968). Recycling and capillary column chromatography of steroids on lipophilic Sephadex. *Ark. Kem.* **29**, 107–115.

Obermann, H., Spiteller-Friedmann, M., and Spiteller, G. (1971a). Zur Lokalisierung funktioneller Gruppen in Steroiden mit Hilfe der Massenspektrometrie—IV 17β-Hydroxy-androstan-3,11-dione, 11-Hydroxy-androstan-3,17-dione und 3-Hydroxy-androstan-11,17-dione. *Tetrahedron* **27**, 1737–1746.

Obermann, H., Spiteller-Friedmann, M., and Spiteller, G. (1971b). Zur Lokalisierung funktioneller Gruppen in steroiden mit Hilfe der Massenspekrometrie—V 3,17β-Dihydroxy-androstan-11-one und 11,17-Dihydroxy-androstan-3-one. *Tetrahedron* **27**, 1747–1754.

Ögren, L., Csiky, I., Risinger, L., Nilsson, L. G., and Johansson, G. (1980). A post-column enzyme reactor for detection of oxidized cholesterols in H.P.L.C. separations. *Anal. Chim. Acta* **117**, 71–79.

O'Hare, M. J., Nice, E. C., Magee-Brown, R., and Bullman, H. (1976). High-pressure liquid chromatography of steroids secreted by human adrenal and testis cells in monolayer culture. *J. Chromatogr.* **125**, 357–367.

Pasqualini, J. R. (1967). Analysis and identification of steroid conjugates. *In* "Steroid Hormone Analysis" (H. Carstensen, ed.), Vol. 1, pp. 407–456. Dekker, New York.

Pellizzari, E. D., Liu, J., Twine, M. E., and Cook, C. E. (1973). A novel silver-sulfoethyl cellulose column for purification of ethynyl steroids from biological fluids. *Anal. Biochem.* **56**, 178–190.

Peltonen, J. I., Laatikainen, T. J., and Hesso, A. (1979). Determination of conjugated steroids in amniotic fluid. *J. Steroid Biochem.* **10**, 499–503.

Pesheck, P. S., and Lovrien, R. E. (1977). Cosolvent control of substrate inhibition in cosolvent stimulation of β-glucuronidase activity. *Biochem. Biophys. Res. Commun.* **79**, 417–421.

Pettit, B. R., and King, G. S. (1979). The electron impact mass spectra of some clinically important androsterones and androsterols as their formate derivatives. *Biomed. Mass Spectrom.* **6**, 162–164.

Pfaffenberger, C. D., and Horning, E. C. (1975). High-resolution biomedical gas chromatography. Determination of human urinary steroid metabolites using glass open tubular capillary columns. *J. Chromatogr.* **112**, 581–594.

Pfaffenberger, C. D., and Horning, E. C. (1977). Sex differences in human urinary steroid metabolic profiles determined by gas chromatography. *Anal. Biochem.* **80**, 329–343.

Pfaffenberger, C. D., Malinak, L. R., and Horning, E. C. (1978). High-resolution biomedical gas chromatography. Study of urinary steroid metabolite ratios of women with breast lesions using open-tubular glass cpillary columns. *J. Chromatogr.* **158**, 313–330.

Phillipou, G. (1976). Allyldimethylsilyl ethers. New derivatives for the analysis of steroids by gas chromatography–mass spectrometry. *J. Chromatogr.* **129**, 384–386.

Phillipou, G., and Frith, R. G. (1980). Specific quantitation of plasma medroxyprogesterone acetate by gas chromatography/mass spectrometry. *Clin. Chim. Acta* **103**, 129–133.

Phillipou, G., Bigham, D. A., and Seamark, R. F. (1975). Steroid *t*-butyldimethylsilyl ethers as derivatives for mass fragmentography. *Steroids* **26**, 516–524.

Phillipou, G., Seamark, R. F., and Cox, L. W. (1978). A procedure for comprehensive analysis of neutral urinary steroids in endocrine investigations. *Aust. N. Z. J. Med.* **8**, 63–68.

Pierrat, G., Prost, M., Lavoue, G., and Lumbroso, C. (1976). Utilisation d'un éxchangeur d'ions comme moyen rapide d'extraction appliqué au dosage des estrogènes et du pregnandiol urinaires de grossesse par colorimétrie ou par chromatographie en phase gazeuse. *Ann. Biol. Clin.* **34**, 423–430.

Pinkus, J. L., Charles, D., and Chattoraj, S. C. (1971). Deuterium-labeled steroids for study in humans. I. Estrogen production rates in normal pregnancy. *J. Biol. Chem.* **246**, 633–636.

Pinkus, J. L., Charles, D., and Chattoraj, S. C. (1979). Deuterium-labeled steroids for study in humans. II. Preliminary studies on estrogen production rates in pre- and post-menopausal women. *Horm. Res.* **10**, 44–56.

Poole, C. F., and Morgan, E. D. (1975). Electron-impact fragmentation of pentafluorophenyldimethylsilyl ethers of some sterols of biological importance. *Org. Mass Spectrom.* **10**, 537–549.

Poole, C. F., and Zlatkis, A. (1979). Trialkylsilyl ether derivatives (other than TMS) for gas chromatography and mass spectrometry. *J. Chromatogr. Sci.* **17**, 115–123.

Pratt, J. J. (1978). Steroid immunoassay in clinical chemistry. *Clin. Chem.* **24**, 1869–1890.

Pratt, J. J., and Woldring, M. G. (1977). Recent developments in radioimmunoassay. *J. Radioanal. Chem.* **35**, 45–54.

Privett, O. S., and Erdahl, W. L. (1978). Practical aspects of liquid chromatography–mass spectrometry (LC–MS) of lipids. *Chem. Phys. Lipids* **21**, 361–387.

Prost, M., and Maume, B. F. (1974). Hormones steroides de la surrénale de rat. Analyse des 18-hydroxycorticostéroides par chromatographie gaz-liquide couplée a la spectrométrie de masse et par fragmentographie de masse. *J. Steroid Biochem.* **5**, 133–144.

Quilliam, M. A., and Westmore, J. B. (1977). Mass spectra of sterically crowded trialkylsilyl ether derivatives of steroids. *Steroids* **29**, 579–611.

Quilliam, M. A., and Westmore, J. B. (1978). Sterically crowded trialkylsilyl derivatives for chromatography and mass spectrometry of biologically-important compounds. *Anal. Chem.* **50**, 59–68.

Quilliam, M. A., Templeton, J. F., and Westmore, J. B. (1977). Sterically crowded trialkylsilyl ether derivatives for the analysis of steroid metabolites. *Steroids* **29**, 613–626.

Radin, N. S. (1969). Preparation of lipid extracts. *In* "Methods in Enzymology" (J. M. Lowenstein, ed.), Vol. XIV, pp. 245–254. Academic Press, New York.

Rao, P. N., Purdy, R. H., Williams, M. C., Moore, P. H., Jr., Goldzieher, J. W., and Layne, D. S. (1979). Metabolites of estradiol-17β in bovine liver: Identification of the 17β-D-glucopyranoside of estradiol-17α. *J. Steroid Biochem.* **10**, 179–185.

Reardon, G. E., Caldarella, A. M., and Canalis, E. (1979). Determination of serum cortisol and 11-deoxycortisol by liquid chromatography. *Clin. Chem.* **25**, 122–126.

Reiffsteck, A., Dehennin, L., and Scholler, R. (1980). Experiments on the carrier effect in quantitative mass spectrometry of steroids. *In* "Advances in Mass Spectrometry" (A. Quayle, ed.), Vol. 8, pp. 295–304. Heyden, London.

Reimendal, R., and Sjövall, J. (1972). Analysis of steroids by off-line computerized gas chromatography–mass spectrometry. *Anal. Chem.* **44**, 21–29.

Reimendal, R., and Sjövall, J. (1973a). Computer evaluation of gas chromatographic–mass spectrometric analyses of steroids from biological materials. *Anal. Chem.* **45**, 1083–1089.

Reimendal, R., and Sjövall, J. (1973b). Computerized gas chromatography–mass spectrometry in steroid analysis. *In* "Organisation des Laboratoires-Biologie Prospective" (G. Siest, ed.), pp. 625–636. Expansion Scientifique Française, Paris.

Reiner, J., and Spiteller, G. (1975). Untersuchung der Steroidausscheidung im Neugeborenen-Urin mit der Kombination Glaskapillargaschromatograph-Massenspektrometer. *Monatsh. Chem.* **106**, 1415–1428.

Reynolds, W. D., Mitchum, R. K., Newton, J., Bystroff, R. I., Pomernacki, C., Brand, H. A., and Siegel, M. W. (1977). An ultra-sensitive mass spectrometer system for quantitative biological studies. *Chem. Instrum.* **8**, 63–98.

Richter, H., and Spiteller, G. (1976). Synthesen und Massenspektren von 3,17β-Dihydroxyandrostan-11,16-dionen   und   17β-Hydroxyandrostan-3,11,16-trionen. *Monatsh. Chem.* **107**, 459–572.

Rigaud, M., Chebroux, P., Durand, J., Maclouf, J., and Madani, C. (1976). Une nouvelle technique de frabrication de colonnes capillaires de verre, utilisant des chlorosilanes polymerises. Application a l'analyse des steroides et des prostaglandines. *Tetrahedron Lett.* **44**, 3935–3938.

Roginsky, M. S., Panetz, A. I., and Gordon, R. D. (1975). The use of Amberlite XAD-2 columns for the determination of plasma aldosterone by radioimmunoassay. *Clin. Chim. Acta* **63**, 303–308.

Romanoff, L. P., and Brodie, H. J. (1976). Quantification of urinary 3α,21-dihydroxy-5β-pregnan-20-one and 5-pregnene-3β,20α-diol by mass fragmentography. *J. Steroid Biochem.* **7**, 289–294.

Ros, A., and Sommerville, I. F. (1971). Gas–liquid chromatography with high resolution glass capillary columns for the simultaneous determination of urinary steroids. *J. Obstet. Gynaecol. Br. Comm.* **78**, 1096–1107.

Rose, J. Q., and Jusko, W. J. (1979). Corticosteroid analysis in biological fluids by high-performance liquid chromatography. *J. Chromatogr. Biomed. Appl.* **162**, 273–280.

Rosenfeld, J., and Taguchi, V. Y. (1978). Quantitative determination of catechol estrogens by mass spectrometry—a model study with 2-hydroxyestradiol. *Anal. Lett. Ser. B* **11**, 207–219.

Rotsch, T. D., and Pietrzyk, D. J. (1980). Ion-interaction in high performance liquid chromatography of benzenesulfonic acids on Amberlite XAD-2. *Anal. Chem.* **52**, 1323–1327.

Rotter, H., and Varmuza, K. (1978). Computer-aided interpretation of steroid mass spectra by pattern recognition methods. Part III. Computation of binary classifiers by linear regression. *Anal. Chim. Acta* **103**, 61–71.

Roy, T. A., Field, F. H., Lin, Y. Y., and Smith, L. L. (1979). Hydroxyl ion negative chemical ionization mass spectra of steroids. *Anal. Chem.* **51**, 272–278.

Ruokonen, A., and Vihko, R. (1974). Steroid metabolism in testis tissue: Concentrations of unconjugated and sulfated neutral steroids in boar testis. *J. Steroid Biochem.* **5**, 33–38.

Rutten, G. A. F. M., and Luyten, J. A. (1972). Analysis of steroids by high resolution gas–liquid chromatography. I. Preparation of apolar columns. *J. Chromatogr.* **74**, 177–193.

Ryhage, R. (1964). Use of a mass spectrometer as a detector and analyzer for effluents emerging from high temperature gas–liquid chromatography columns. *Anal. Chem.* **36**, 759–764.

Sahlberg, B.-L., Axelson, M., Collins, D. J., and Sjövall, J. (1981). Analysis of isomeric ethynylestradiol glucuronides in urine. *J. Chromatogr.* **217**, 453–461.

Samuelsson, B., Hamberg, M., and Sweeley, C. C. (1970). Quantitative gas chromatography of prostaglandin E_1 at the nanogram level. Use of deuterated carrier and multiple ion analyzer. *Anal. Biochem.* **38**, 301–304.

Sandra, P., Verzele, M., and Vanluchene, E. (1979). Polar phase glass capillary GC columns for hormonal steroid analysis: OV-17. *J. High Resol. Chromatogr.* **2**, 187–188.

Satyaswaroop, P. G., Lopez de la Osa, E., and Gurpide, E. (1977). High pressure liquid chromatographic separation of C_{18} and C_{19} steroids. *Steroids* **30**, 139–145.

Scandrett, M. S., and Ross, E. J. (1976). Polyamide thin-layer chromatography of corticosteroids: A substitute for column chromatography with LH-20. *Clin. Chim. Acta* **72,** 165–169.

Schill, G. (1974). Isolation of drugs and related organic compounds by ion-pair extraction. *In* "Ion Exchange and Solvent Extraction" (J. A. Marinsky and Y. Marcus, eds.), Vol. 6, pp. 1–57. Dekker, New York.

Schill, G. (1981). Recent advances in ion-pair chromatography. *Acta Pharm. Fennica* **90,** 43–56.

Schill, G., Modin, R., Borg, K. O., and Persson, B.-A. (1977). Ion-pair extraction and chromatography. *In* "Drug Fate and Metabolism. Methods and Techniques" (E. R. Garrett and J. Hirtz, eds.), pp. 135–185. Dekker, New York.

Schindler, A. E., and Sparke, H. (1975). Method for the quantitation of steroids in umbilical cord plasma. *Endocrinol. Exp.* **9,** 205–214.

Schmid, P. P., Muller, M. D., and Simon, W. (1979). A versatile all-glass GC/MS interface for capillary columns. *J. High Resol. Chromatogr.* **2,** 225–228.

Schmidt, G. J., Vandemark, F. L., and Slavin, W. (1978). Estrogen determination using chromatography with precolumn fluorescence labeling. *Anal. Biochem.* **91,** 636–645.

Schöneshöfer, M., and Dulce, H. J. (1979). Comparison of different high-performance liquid chromatographic systems for the purification of adrenal and gonadal steroids prior to immunoassay. *J. Chromatogr. Biomed. Appl.* **164,** 17–28.

Schöneshöfer, M., Fenner, A., and Dulce, H. J. (1981). Assessment of eleven adrenal steroids from a single serum sample by combination of automatic high-performance liquid chromatography and radioimmunoassay (HPLC–RIA). *J. Steroid Biochem.* **14,** 377–386.

Schramm, W., Schill, W., and Louton, T. (1979a). Simultaneous quantitative estimates of several isotopically labelled substances in the picogram range with selected ion monitoring. *Biomed. Mass Spectrom.* **6,** 335–339.

Schramm, W., Louton, T., and Schill, W. (1979b). Quantitative estimates for isotopic dilution analysis in mass spectrometry. *Fresenius Z. Anal. Chem.* **294,** 107–111.

Schulten, H.-R., and Games. D. E. (1974). High resolution field desorption mass spectrometry. II. Glycosides. *Biomed. Mass Spectrom.* **1,** 120–123.

Scott, N. R., and Dixon, P. F. (1979). Determination of cortisol in human plasma by reversed-phase high-performance liquid chromatography. *J. Chromatogr. Biochem. Appl.* **164,** 29–34.

Scott, R. P. W., Scott, C. G., Munroe, M., and Hess, J., Jr. (1974). Interface for on-line liquid chromatography-mass spectroscopy analysis. *J. Chromatogr.* **99,** 395–405.

Seamark, R. F., Phillipou, G., and McIntosh, J. E. A. (1977). Ovarian steroidogenesis studied by mass fragmentography. *J. Steroid Biochem.* **8,** 885–891.

Seki, T. (1967). Chromatographic separation of 17-hydroxycorticosteroids on Sephadex LH-20. *J. Chromatogr.* **29,** 246–247.

Seki, T., and Sugase, T. (1969). Chromatographic separation of 17-ketosteroids and 17-hydroxycorticosteroids on Sephadex LH-20. *J. Chromatogr.* **42,** 503–508.

Senciall, I. R., and Dey, A. C. (1976). Acidic steroid metabolites: Evidence for the excretion of C-21-carboxylic acid metabolites of progesterone in rabbit urine. *J. Steroid Biochem.* **7,** 125–129.

Setchell, K. D. R. (1979). Gas chromatography–mass spectrometry. *In* "Hormones in Blood" (C. H. Gray and V. H. T. James, eds.), Vol. 3, pp. 63–127. Academic Press, New York.

Setchell, K. D. R., and Shackleton, C. H. L. (1973). The group separation of plasma and urinary steroids by column chromatograhpy on Sephadex LH-20. *Clin. Chim. Acta* **47,** 381–388.

Setchell, K. D. R., Almé, B., Axelson, M., and Sjövall, J. (1976a). The multicomponent analysis of conjugates of neutral steroids in urine by lipophilic ion exchange chromatography and computerised gas chromatography–mass spectrometry. *J. Steroid Biochem.* **7**, 615–629.

Setchell, K. D. R., Axelson, M., Simarina, A. I., and Gontscharow, N. P. (1976b). Urinary steroid excretion and conjugation by the baboon (*Papio Hamadryas*)—A comprehensive study. *J. Steroid Biochem.* **7**, 809–816.

Setchell, K. D. R., Gontscharow, N. P., Axelson, M., and Sjövall, J. (1976c). The identification of $3\alpha,6\beta,11\beta,17,21$-pentahydroxy-$5\beta$-pregnan-20-one ($6\beta$-hydroxy-THF)—the major urinary steroid of the baboon (*Papio Papio*). *J. Steroid Biochem.* **7**, 801–808.

Setchell, K. D. R., Chua, K. S., and Himsworth, R. L. (1977). Urinary steroid excretion by the squirrel monkey (*Saimuri Sciureus*). *J. Endocrinol.* **73**, 365–375.

Setchell, K. D. R., Axelson, M., Sjövall, J., Kirk, D. N., and Morgan, R. E. (1978). The identification of 6α-hydroxytetrahydrocortisol ($3\alpha,6\alpha,11\beta,17\alpha,21$-pentahydroxy-$5\beta$-pregnan-20-one) in urine. *FEBS Lett.* **88**, 215–218.

Setchell, K. D. R., Taylor, N. S., Adlercreutz, H., Axelson, M., and Sjövall, J. (1979). The group separation of conjugates of oestrogens using lipophilic ion exchange chromatography. *In* "Research on Steroids" (A. Klopper, L. Lerner, H. J. Van der Molen, and F. Sciarra, eds.), Vol. VIII, pp. 131–135. Academic Press, New York.

Shackleton, C. H. L. (1974). Steroid excretion in the neo-natal period: A comparative study of the excretion of steroids by human, ape and rhesus monkey infants. *J. Steroid Biochem.* **5**, 113–118.

Shackleton, C. H. L. (1976). Congenital adrenal hyperplasia caused by defect in steroid 21-hydroxylase. Establishment of definitive urinary steroid excretion pattern during first weeks of life. *Clin. Chim. Acta* **67**, 287–298.

Shackleton, C. H. L. (1981). The analysis of steroids. *In* "Glass Capillary Gas Liquid Chromatography: Clinical and Pharmacological Analyses" (H. Jaeger, ed.), Dekker, New York.

Shackleton, C. H. L., and Honour, J. W. (1976). Simultaneous estimation of urinary steroids by semiautomated gas chromatography. Investigation of neo-natal infants and children with abnormal steroid synthesis. *Clin. Chim. Acta* **69**, 267–283.

Shackleton, C. H. L., and Honour, J. W. (1977). Identification and measurement of 18-hydroxycorticosterone metabolites by gas chromatography–mass spectrometry. *J. Steroid Biochem.* **8**, 199–203.

Shackleton, C. H. L., and Snodgrass, G. H. A. I. (1974). Steroid excretion by an infant with an unusual salt-losing syndrome: A gas chromatographic–mass spectrometric study. *Ann. Clin. Biochem.* **11**, 91–99.

Shackleton, C. H. L., and Taylor, N. F. (1975). Identification of the androstenetriolones and androstenetetrols present in the urine of infants. *J. Steroid Biochem.* **6**, 1393–1399.

Shackleton, C. H. L., and Whitney, J. O. (1980). Use of Sep-pak^R cartridges for urinary steroid extraction: Evaluation of the method for use prior to gas chromatographic analysis. *Clin. Chim. Acta* **107**, 231–243.

Shackleton, C. H. L., Gustafsson, J.-Å., and Sjövall, J. (1970). The identification of epimeric 5-androstene-3,16,17-triols in plasma from the umbilical cord and in meconium, faeces and urine from infants. *Steroids* **15**, 131–137.

Shackleton, C. H. L., Gustafsson, J.-Å., and Sjövall, J. (1971). Steroids in newborns and infants. Identification of steroids in urine from newborn infants. *Steroids* **17**, 265–280.

Shackleton, C. H. L., Gustaffson, J.-Å., and Mitchell, F. L. (1973). Steroids in newborns and infants. The changing pattern of urinary steroid excretion during infancy. *Acta Endocrinol.* **74**, 157–167.

Shackleton, C. H. L., Honour, J. W., Dillon, M., and Milla, P. (1976). Multicomponent gas chromatographic analysis of urinary steroids excreted by an infant with a defect in aldosterone biosynthesis. *Acta Endocrinol.* **81**, 762–773.

Shackleton, C. H. L., Swift, P. G. F., Savage, D. C. L., and Honour, J. W. (1979a). Deficient 3β-hydroxy-5-ene steroid secretion by newborn infants. *J. Clin. Endocrinol. Metab.* **49**, 247–251.

Shackleton, C. H. L., Honour, J. W., Winter, J., and Bokkenheuser, V. D. (1979b). Urinary metabolites of 18-hydroxylated corticosteroids: Microbial preparation of reference compounds. *J. Steroid Biochem.* **11**, 1141–1144.

Shackleton, C. H. L., Honour, J. W., Dillon, M. J., Chantler, C., and Jones, R. W. A. (1980a). Hypertension in a four-year-old child: Gas chromatographic and mass spectrometric evidence for deficient hepatic metabolism of steroids. *J. Clin. Endocrinol. Metab.* **50**, 786–792.

Shackleton, C. H. L., Roitman, E., Monder, C., and Bradlow, H. L. (1980b). Gas chromatographic and mass spectrometric analysis of urinary acidic metabolites of cortisol. *Steroids* **36**, 289–298.

Shimada, K., Tanaka, T., and Nambara, T. (1979). Separation of catechol estrogens by high-performance liquid chromatography with electrochemical detection. *J. Chromatogr.* **178**, 350–354.

Shimizu, K. (1978). Formation of 5-[17β-^{2}H]androstene-3β, 17α-diol from 3β-hydroxy-5-[17,21,21,21-^{2}H]-pregnen-20-one by the microsomal fraction of boar testis. *J. Biol. Chem.* **253**, 4237–4241.

Shimizu, K. (1979). Metabolism of [17-^{2}]pregnenolone into 5-[17β-^{2}H,17α-^{18}O] androstene-3β,17α-diol and other products by incubation with the microsomal fraction of boar testis under $^{18}O_2$ atmosphere. *Biochim. Biophys. Acta* **575**, 37–45.

Siekmann, L. (1979). Determination of steroid hormones by the use of isotope dilution–mass spectrometry: A definitive method in clinical chemistry. *J. Steroid Biochem.* **11**, 117–123.

Siekmann, L., Hoppen, H.-O., and Breuer, H. (1970). Zur gas-chromatographisch-massenspektrometrischen Bestimmung von Steroidhormonen in Körperflüssigkeiten unter Verwendung eines Multiple Ion Detectors (Fragmentographie). *Z. Anal. Chem.* **252**, 294–298.

Siekmann, L., Martin, S., Siekmann, A., and Breuer, H. (1976). Determination of testosterone and 5α-dihydrotestosterone in human plasma by isotopic dilution–mass fragmentography. *Acta Endocrinol. Suppl.* **82**, 65–67.

Siekmann, L., Siekmann, A., and Breuer, H. (1978). Monitoring of the oral contraceptive 17α-ethinyloestradiol-17β in human plasma by isotopic-dilution mass spectrometry. *Fresenius Z. Anal. Chem.* **290**, 159–160.

Siekmann, L., Disse, B., and Breuer, H. (1980). Biosynthesis and metabolism of 16α,17-epoxy-C_{21}-steroids in rat liver microsomes. *J. Steroid Biochem.* **13**, 1181–1205.

Siggia, S., and Dishman, R. A. (1970). Analysis of steroid hormones using high resolution liquid chromatography. *Anal. Chem.* **42**, 1223–1229.

Siiteri, P. K. (1963). The isolation of urinary estrogens and determination of their specific activities following the administration of radioactive precursors to humans. *Steroids* **2**, 687–712.

Siiteri, P. K. (1970). The isolation of steroid conjugates. *In* "Chemical and Biological Aspects of Steroid Conjugation" (S. Bernstein and S. Solomon, eds.), pp. 182–218. Springer-Verlag, Berlin and New York.

Sippell, W. G., Lehmann, P., and Hollmann, G. (1975). Automation of multiple Sephadex LH-20 column chromatography for the simultaneous separation of plasma corticosteroids. *J. Chromatogr.* **108**, 305–312.

Sippell, W. G., Putz, G., and Scheuerecker, M. (1978). Convenient system for the simultaneous separation of 11-deoxycortisol and aldosterone by Sephadex LH-20 multiple column chromatography. *J. Chromatogr. Biomed. Appl.* **146,** 333–336.

Sjövall, K. (1970). Gas chromatographic determination of steroid sulphates in plasma during pregnancy. *Ann. Clin. Res.* **2,** 393–408.

Sjövall, J., and Sjövall, K. (1968). Identification of 5α-pregnane-3α,20α,21-triol in human pregnancy plasma. *Steroids* **12,** 359–366.

Sjövall, J., and Sjövall, K. (1970). Steroid sulphates in plasma from pregnant women with pruritus and elevated plasma bile acid levels. *Ann. Clin. Res.* **2,** 321–337.

Sjövall, J., and Vihko, R. (1966a). Identification of 3β,17β-dihydroxyandrost-5-ene, 3β,20α-dihydroxypregn-5-ene and epiandrosterone in human peripheral blood. *Steroids* **7,** 447–458.

Sjövall, J., and Vihko, R. (1966b). Chromatography of conjugated steroids on lipophilic Sephadex. *Acta Chem. Scand.* **20,** 1419–1421.

Sjövall, J., and Vihko, R. (1968). Analysis of solvolyzable steroids in human plasma by combined gas chromatography–mass spectrometry. *Acta Endocrinol.* **57,** 247–260.

Sjövall, J., Sjövall, K., and Vihko, R. (1968a). Steroid sulfates in human pregnancy plasma. *Steroids* **11,** 703–715.

Sjövall, J., Nyström, E., and Haahti, E. (1968b). Liquid chromatography on lipophilic Sephadex: Column and detection techniques. *In* "Advances in Chromatography" (J. C. Giddings and R. A. Keller, eds.), pp. 119–170. Dekker, New York.

Smith, A. G., and Brooks, C. J. W. (1976). Mass spectra of Δ⁴- and 5α-3-ketosteroids formed during the oxidation of some 3β-hydroxysteroids by cholesterol oxidase. *Biomed. Mass Spectrom.* **3,** 81–87.

Smith, A. G., Gaskell, S. J., and Brooks, C. J. W. (1976). Trimethylsilyl group migration during electron impact and chemical ionization mass spectrometry of the trimethylsilyl ethers of 20-hydroxy-5α- pregnan-3-ones and 20-hydroxy-4-pregnen-3-ones. *Biomed. Mass Spectrom.* **3,** 161–165.

Smith, A. G., Joannou, G. E., Mák, M., Uwajima, T., Terada, O., and Brooks, C. J. W. (1978). Oxidation of 3β-hydroxyandrostenes by the 3β-hydroxysteroid oxidase (cholesterol oxidase) from *Brevibacterium Sterolicum* prior to their analysis by gas-liquid chromatography–mass spectrometry. *J. Chromatogr.* **152,** 467–474.

Smith, D. H., Buchanan, B. G., Engelmore, R. S., Adlercreutz, H., and Djerassi, C. (1973a). Applications of artificial intelligence for chemical inference. IX. Analysis of mixtures without prior separation as illustrated for estrogens. *Am. Chem. Soc.* **95,** 6078–6084.

Smith, D. H., Buchanan, B. G., White, W. C., Feigenbaum, E. A., Lederberg, J., and Djerassi, C. (1973b). Applications of artificial intelligence for chemical inference—X. INTSUM. A data interpretation and summary program applied to the collected mass spectra of estrogenic steroids. *Tetrahedron* **29,** 3117–3134.

Smith, D. H., Achenbach, M., Yeager, W. J., Anderson, P. J., Fitch, W. L., and Rindfleisch, T. C. (1977). Quantitative comparison of combined gas chromatographic/mass spectrometric profiles of complex mixtures. *Anal. Chem.* **49,** 1623–1632.

Smith, M. D. (1979). High-performance liquid chromatographic determination of hydrocortisone and methylprednisolone and their hemisuccinate estares in human serum. *J. Chromatogr. Biomed. Appl.* **164,** 129–137.

Smyth, M. R., and Frischkorn, C. G. B. (1980). Trace determination of some phenolic growth-promoting hormones in meat by high-performance liquid chromatography with voltametric detection. *Fresenius Z. Anal. Chem.* **301,** 220–223.

Snedden, W., and Parker, R. B. (1971). Determination of volatile constituents of human blood and tissue specimens by quantitative high resolution mass spectrometry. *Anal. Chem.* **43,** 1651–1656.

Snedden, W., and Parker, R. B. (1976). The direct determination of oestrogen and progesterone in human ovarian tissue by quantitative high resolution mass spectrometry. *Biomed. Mass Spectrom.* **3**, 295–298.

Spiegelhalder, B., Röhle, G., Siekmann, L., and Breuer, H. (1976). Mass-spectrometry of steroid glucuronides. *J. Steroid Biochem.* **7**, 749–756.

Spiteller, G., Spiteller, M., Ende, M., and Hoyer, G.-A. (1978). Identifikation der Partialstrukturen von unbekannter Steroiden mit einer Schlüsselionenkarte und einem recherunterstützten Retrieval-System. *Org. Mass Spectrom.* **13**, 646–652.

Spiteller-Friedman, M., and Spiteller, G. (1969). Massenspektren von Steroiden. *Fortschr. Chem. Forsch.* **12**, 440–537.

Stan, H.-J., and Abraham, B. (1978). All-glass open-split interface for gas chromatography–mass spectrometry. *Anal. Chem.* **50**, 2161–2164.

Stenhagen, E. (1964). Jetziger Stand der Massenspektrometrie in der organischen Analyse. *Zeitschr. Anal. Chem.* **205**, 109–124.

Stillwell, W. G., Horning, E. C., Horning, M. G., Stillwell, R. N., and Zlatkis, A. (1972). Characterization of metabolites of steroid contraceptives by gas chromatography and mass spectrometry. *J. Steroid Biochem.* **3**, 699–706.

Stillwell, W. G., Hung, A., Stafford, M., and Horning, M. G. (1973). A new procedure for the extraction of unconjugated steroids from plasma and urine. *Anal. Lett.* **6**, 407–419.

Stillwell, W. G., Stillwell, R. N., and Horning, E. C. (1974). Analysis of nanogram quantities of norethisterone in plasma using a GC–MS–COM selective ion detection procedure. *Steroids Lipids Res.* **5**, 79–90.

Stock, B., and Spiteller, G. (1974). Zur Lokalisierung funktioneller Gruppen in Steroiden mit Hilfe der Massenspektrometrie. XIII. Massenspektren von 3,7,17-trihydroxyandrostanen und 7,17-dihydroxyandrostan-3-onen. *Org. Mass Spectrom.* **9**, 888–902.

Sweeley, C. C., Young, N. D., Holland, J. F., and Gates, S. C. (1974). Rapid computerized identification of compounds in complex biological mixtures by gas chromatography–mass spectrometry. *J. Chromatogr.* **99**, 507–517.

Takeuchi, T., Hirata, Y., and Okumura, Y. (1978). On-line coupling of a micro liquid chromatograph and mass spectrometer through a jet separator. *Anal. Chem.* **50**, 659–660.

Taylor, N. F., and Shackleton, C. H. L. (1977). Identification and measurement of estetrols and estriolones in pregnancy urine. *In* "Research on Steroids" (A. Vermeulen, A. Klopper, F. Sciarra, P. Jungblut, and L. Lerner, eds.), pp. 497–511. Elsevier, Amsterdam.

Taylor, N. F., and Shackleton, C. H. L. (1979). Gas chromatographic steroid analysis for diagnosis of placental sulfatase deficiency: A study of nine patients. *J. Clin. Endocrinol. Metab.* **49**, 78–86.

Taylor, N. F., Curnow, D. H., and Shackleton, C. H. L. (1978). Analysis of glucocorticoid metabolites in the neonatal period: Catabolism of cortisone acetate by an infant with 21-hydroxylase deficiency. *Clin. Chim. Acta* **85**, 219–229.

Taylor, P. J., and Sherman, P. L. (1979). Liquid crystals as stationary phases for high performance liquid chromatography. *J. Liquid Chromatogr.* **2**, 1271–1290.

Taylor, P. J., and Sherman, P. L. (1980). Liquid crystals as stationary phases for high performance liquid chromatography. *J. Liquid Chromatogr.* **3**, 21–40.

Tetsuo, M., Axelson, M., and Sjövall, J. (1980). Selective isolation procedures for GC/MS analysis of ethynyl steroids in biological material. *J. Steroid Biochem.* **13**, 847–860.

Thenot, J.-P., and Horning, E. C. (1972a). MO–TMS derivatives of human urinary steroids for GC and GC–MS studies. *Anal. Lett.* **5**, 21–33.

Thenot, J.-P., and Horning, E. C. (1972b). GC behavior of 3-ketosteroid methoximes.

Application to GC studies of adrenocortical steroid hormone MO–TMS deriatives. *Anal. Lett.* **5**, 801–814.

Thenot, J.-P., and Horning, E. C. (1972c). GC–MS derivatization studies: The formation of dexamethasone MO–TMS. *Anal. Lett.* **5**, 905–913.

Thenot, J.-P., Nowlin, J., Carroll, D. I., Montgomery, F. E., and Horning, E. C. (1979). Coated glass probe tips for the determination of thermally labile compounds by mass spectrometry. *Anal. Chem.* **51**, 1101–1104.

Thomas, B. S. (1980). Steroid analysis by gas chromatography with SCOT and wide-bore WCOT columns. *J. High Resol. Chromatogr.* **3**, 241–247.

Thomas, M. J., Danutra, V., Read, G. F., Hillier, S. G., and Griffiths, K. (1977). The detection and measurement of D-norgestreol in human milk using Sephadex LH-20 chromatography and radioimmunoassay. *Steroids* **30**, 349–361.

Thome, F. A., and Young, G. W. (1976). Direct coupling of glass capillary columns to a mass spectrometer. *Anal. Chem.* **48**, 1423–1424.

Thompson, R. M. (1976). Gas chromatographic and mass spectrometric analysis of per-methylated estrogen glucuronides. *J. Steroid Biochem.* **7**, 845–852.

Thompson, R. M., and Desiderio, D. M. (1972). Permethylation and mass spectrometry of intact ether glucuronides at the low nanomolar level. *Biochem. Biophys. Res. Commun.* **48**, 1303–1310.

Tikkanen, M. J., and Adlercreutz, H. (1970). Separation of estriol conjugates on Sephadex. *Acta Chem. Scand.* **24**, 3755–3757.

Tökés, L., and Throop, L. J. (1972). Introduction of deuterium into the steroid system. *In* "Organic Reactions in Steroid Chemistry" (J. Fried and J. A. Edwards, eds.), Vol. 1, pp. 145–221. Van Nostrand-Reinhold, Princeton, New Jersey.

Touchstone, J. C., and Dobbins, M. F. (1975). Direct determination of steroidal sulfates. *J. Steroid Biochem.* **6**, 1389–1392.

Tsuge, S., Hirata, Y., and Takeuchi, T. (1979). Vacuum nebulizing interface for direct coupling of micro-liquid chromatograph and mass spectrometer. *Anal. Chem.* **51**, 166–169.

Tymes, N. W. (1977). The determination of corticoids and related steroid analogs by high-performance liquid chromatography. *J. Chromatogr. Sci.* **15**, 151–155.

Ulick, S., Ramirez, L. C., and New, M. I. (1977). An abnormality in steroid reductive metabolism in a hypertensive syndrome. *J. Clin. Endocrinol. Metab.* **44**, 799–802.

van den Berg, J. H. M., Mol. Ch. R., Deelder, R. S., and Thijssen, J. H. H. (1977). A quantitative assay of cortisol in human plasma by high performance liquid chromatography using a selective chemically bonded stationary phase. *Clin. Chim. Acta* **78**, 165–172.

van den Berg, P. M. J., and Cox, T. P. M. (1972). An all-glass solid sampling device for open tubular columns. *Chromatographia* **5**, 301–304.

van der Wal, Sj., and Huber, J. F. K. (1974). High-pressure liquid chromatography with ion-exchange celluloses and its application to the separation of estrogen glucuronides. *J. Chromatogr.* **102**, 353–374.

van der Wal, Sj., and Huber, J. F. K. (1977). Separation of estrogen glucuronides, sulphates and phosphates on ion-exchange cellulose by high-pressure liquid chromatography. *J. Chromatogr.* **135**, 305–321.

van der Wal, Sj., and Huber, J. F. K. (1978). Comparative study of several phase systems for the separation of estrogen conjugates by high-pressure liquid chromatography. *J. Chromatogr.* **149**, 431–453.

Vandenheuvel, F. A. (1974). Gas–liquid chromatographic studies of reactions and structural relationships of steroids. Part I. Positions 3, 11 and 17 in the androstane series. *J. Chromatogr.* **96**, 47–78.

Vandenheuve, F. A. (1975a). Gas–liquid chromatographic studies of reactions and structural relationships of steroids. II. Positions 3, 11 and 20 in this pregnane series. *J. Chromatogr.* **103,** 113–134.

Vandenheuvel, F. A. (1975b). Gas–liquid chromatographic studies of reactions and structural relationships of steroids. Part III. 11α-hydroxysteroids of the androstane and pregnane series. *J. Chromatogr.* **105,** 359–375.

Vandenheuvel, F. A. (1975c). Gas–liquid chromatographic studies of reactions and structural relationships of steroids. IV. Substitution in the pregnane side-chain. *J. Chromatogr.* **115,** 161–175.

Vandenheuvel, F. A. (1977). Gas–liquid chromatographic studies of reactions and structural relationships of steroids. V. Concurrent substitution in the pregnane side-chain and position 11. *J. Chromatogr.* **133,** 107–125.

Varmuza, K. (1976). Vergleich von Bibliothekssuchverfahren für Steroidmassenspektren. Wiedererkennung verrauschter Spektren in einer Bibliothek. *Z. Anal. Chem.* **282,** 129–134.

Vestergaard, P. (1973). Liquid column chromatography of hormonal steroids. *In* "Modern Methods of Steroid Analysis" (E. Heftmann, ed.), pp. 1–35. Academic Press, New York.

Vestergaard, P. (1978). The hydrolysis of conjugated neutral steroids in urine. *Acta Endocrinol. Suppl. 217,* **88,** 96–120.

Vestergaard, P., Sayegh, J. F., and Mowat, J. H. (1975). Mass-fragmentographic assay for testosterone in blood using high specific activity tritiated testosterone as an internal standard. *Clin. Chim. Acta* **62,** 163–168.

Vestergaard, P., Sayegh, J. F., Mowat, J. H., and Hemmingsen, L. (1978). Estimation after multi-column liquid chromatography of common urinary neutral steroids with an application to the assay of plasma 17-oxosteroids. *Acta Endocrinol. Suppl. 217,* **88,** 1–245.

Viinikka, L., and Jänne, O. (1973). Urinary excretion of neutral steroid glucuronides with reference to the menstrual cycle. *Clin. Chim. Acta* **49,** 277–285.

Viinikka, L., Jänne, O., Perheentupa, J., and Vihko, R. (1973). Congenital adrenal hyperplasia. Plasma and urinary steroid conjugates in seven children with steroid 21-hydroxylase deficiency. *Clin. Chim. Acta* **48,** 359–365.

Vogt, W., Jacob, K., and Knedel, M. (1974). A high sensitive and selective gas chromatographic determination of monohydroxy steroids as phosphinic esters with the alkali flame detector. *J. Chromatogr. Sci.* **12,** 658–661.

von Unruh, G., and Spiteller, G. (1970a). Tabellen zur massenspekrometrischen Strukturaufklärung von Steroiden—III. Schlüsseldifferenzen von Freien Steroiden. *Tetrahedron* **26,** 3289–3301.

von Unruh, G., and Spiteller, G. (1970b). Tabellen zur massenspekrometrischen Strukturaufklärung von Steroiden—IV. Schlüsselbruchstücke und Schlüsseldifferenzen von Steroidderivaten. *Tetrahedron* **26,** 3303–3311.

von Unruh, G., and Spiteller, G. (1970c). Tabellen zur massenspektrometrischen Strukturaufklärung von Steroiden—II.Schlüsselbruchstücke von freien Steroiden. *Tetrahedron* **26,** 3329–3346.

Vouros, P. (1973). Silyl derivatives of steroids. Evidence for intramolecular silylation processes and electron impact induced reciprocal exchange of trimethylsilyl groups. *J. Org. Chem.* **38,** 3555–3560.

Vouros, P., and Harvey, D. J. (1972a). Specificity of trimethylsilanol elimination in the mass spectra of the trimethylsilyl derivatives of di- and tri-hydroxy-steroids. *J.C.S. Chem. Comm.* 765–766.

Vouros, P., and Harvey, D. J. (1972b). Factors influencing the formation of some characteristic fragment ions in the mass spectra of 16-trimethylsilyloxy androstanes. *Org. Mass Spectrom.* **6,** 953–962.

Vouros, P., and Harvey, D. J. (1973a). Method for selective introduction of trimethylsilyl and perdeuterotrimethylsilyl groups in hydroxy steroids and its utility in mass spectrometric interpretations. *Anal. Chem.* **45**, 7–12.

Vouros, P., and Harvey, D. J. (1973b). Influence of 11-trimethylsilyloxy- or 11-hydroxy-substituents on the electron-impact-induced fragmentation of trimethylsilyl derivatives of some androstanols. *J. Chem. Soc. Perkin Trans.* **I**, 727–732.

Ward, R. J., Shackleton, C. H. L., and Lawson, A. M. (1975). Gas chromatographic–mass spectrometric methods for the detection and identification of anabolic steroid drugs. *Br. J. Sports Med.* **9**, 93–97.

Ward, R. J., Lawson, A. M., and Shackleton, C. H. L. (1977). Metabolism of anabolic steroid drugs in man and the marmoset monkey (*Callithrix Jacchus*)—I. Nilevar and orabolin. *J. Steroid Biochem.* **8**, 1057–1063.

Watson, J. T., and Biemann, K. (1964). High-resolution mass spectra of compounds emerging from a gas chromatograph. *Anal. Chem.* **36**, 1135–1137.

Wegmann, A. (1978). Variations in mass spectral fragmentation produced by active sites in a mass spectrometer source. *Anal. Chem.* **50**, 830–832.

Wehner, R., and Handke, A. (1979). An improved extraction method for plasma steroid hormones. *Clin. Chim. Acta* **93**, 429–431.

Westphal, U. (1971). "Steroid-Protein Interactions." Springer-Verlag, Berlin and New York.

Williams, M. C., and Goldzieher, J. W. (1979). The metabolism of the ethynyl estrogens. Preparative HPLC profiling of radiolabeled urinary estrogens. *Chromatogr. Sci.* **2**, 395–409.

Wilson, D. M., Burlingame, A. L., Cronholm, T., and Sjövall, J. (1974). Deuterium and carbon-13 tracer studies of ethanol metabolism in the rat by ^{2}H,^{1}H-decoupled ^{13}C nuclear magnetic resonance. *Biochem. Biophys. Res. Commun.* **56**, 828–835.

Wilson, D. M., Burlingame, A. L., Hazelby, D., Evans, S., Conholm, T., and Sjövall, J. (1977). Analysis of stable isotope incorporation in bile acids. Separation of complex ^{12}C^{2}H *vs.* ^{13}C^{2}H-type multiplets employing ultra-high resolution mass spectrometry. *Annu. Conf. Mass Spectrom. Allied Top., 25th, Washington, D.C.* pp. 357–359.

Wilson, D. W., John, G. M., Groom, G. V., Pierrepoint, C. G., and Griffiths, K. (1977). Evaluation of an oestradiol radioimmunoassay by high-resolution mass fragmentography. *J. Endocrinol.* **74**, 503–504.

Yamamoto, H., and McCloskey, J. A. (1977). Calculations of isotopic distribution in molecules extensively labeled with heavy isotopes. *Anal. Chem.* **49**, 281–283.

Yapo, E. A., Barthelemy-Clavey, V., Racadot, A., and Mizon, J. (1978). Le comportement du 16α-glucuronide d'oestriol sur resine Amberlite XAD-2. *J. Chromatogr. Biomed. Appl.* **145**, 478–482.

Zamecnik, J., Armstrong, D. T., and Green, K. (1978). Serum estradiol-17β as determined by mass fragmentography and by radioimmunoassay. *Clin. Chem.* **24**, 627–630.

Zaretskii, Z. V. (1976). "Mass Spectrometry of Steroids." Wiley, New York.

Zielinski, W. L., Jr., Johnston, K., and Muschik, G. M. (1976). Nematic liquid crystal for gas–liquid chromatographic separation of steroid epimers. *Anal. Chem.* **48**, 907–911.

Zietz, E., and Spiteller, G. (1974). Zur Lokalisierung funktioneller Gruppen mit Hilfe der Massenspektrometrie —XI. 3,12,17β-Trihydroxy-androstane, 12,17β-Dihydroxy-androstan-3-one, 3,12-Dihydroxy-androstan-17-one und 12-Hydroxy-androstan-3,17-dione. *Tetrahedron* **30**, 585–596.

VITAMINS AND HORMONES, VOL. 39

Insulin: The Effects and Mode of Action of the Hormone

RACHMIEL LEVINE

*Department of Metabolism and Endocrinology,
City of Hope Medical Center and Research Institute, Duarte, California*

I. Introduction

There have been so many reviews on hormone action in general and on insulin in particular that a word of explanation seems necessary for yet another exposition on the subject.

The time is fast approaching when it will become possible to describe the sequential steps in the biochemistry of insulin action in great detail.

The more recent reviews have concentrated mainly on the molecular biological aspects, such as receptor binding, internalization, enzyme modulation, and receptor antibodies. The physiological aspects of the integrative role of the hormone in the whole organism need to be considered in the light of the data obtained by the biochemical approaches.

There is, finally, a need to view this subject in its historical perspective in order to understand the origin and the progressive development of the ideas that we now work with.

This writer has been involved in the field for some 45 years and has shared in the joys as well as in the disappointing moments of the insulin Odyssey. He would like to apologize from the start for any inadvertent omissions of one or another contribution to the literature, and he accepts the responsibility for the interpretations of the data and deductions therefrom.

145

The ultimate aim of all the work on insulin action is to be able to describe the sequential chemical changes that occur as a result of the initial contact of the insulin molecule with its specific receptor in the membrane. This has not yet been achieved, but recent work indicates that the time may not be far off. Of particular relevance are the findings, beginning in about 1979, that specific second messengers for insulin action do exist. These may include *the* mediator, or one of the mediators, of many of the effects of insulin on intracellular, enzymatic activities, spatially distant from the initial point of action at the membrane (Larner *et al.*, 1979; Jarett and Seals, 1979).

Over the last 10–15 years much has been learned of the control of enzyme properties and modifications of enzyme activity produced by phosphorylation of key enzymes important in the metabolism of foodstuffs. This is, therefore, an auspicious time to review the present status of the nature of insulin action in the light of the older data and in the light of presently accumulating evidence regarding changes in enzymatic activity brought about by second messengers, produced as a result of the initial interaction between insulin and its receptor.

II. DEVELOPMENT OF THE FIELD (1891–1970)

Over the years, many excellent reviews have appeared detailing the effects of lack of insulin or the effects of insulin administration on the metabolism of foodstuffs (Naunyn, 1898; Cori, 1931; De Duve, 1945; Soskin and Levine, 1946; Stadie, 1954; Levine and Goldstein, 1955; Krahl, 1961; Fritz, 1972). It is, therefore, not necessary to review the older information in any detail. What is needed is a succinct summary of the several stages undergone by the field, in order to understand the present approaches and the expectations of future events.

The story begins many years ago, long before the successful extraction of insulin from the pancreas. It was Minkowski, Hedon, and Laguesse who, between 1889 and 1893, demonstrated that the pancreas contains within its substance cells producing an internal secretion. Surgical excision of the pancreas resulted in a fatal syndrome consisting of the inability to retain and store the three major foodstuffs. Glycogen disappeared from the liver and muscles; the fat depots decreased progressively, and β-keto acids derived from fat were rapidly produced and excreted. Endogenous and exogenous proteins were broken down with the formation of sugar and urea. The nitrogen balance became negative. Exogenous carbohydrate was to a large extent simply excreted as urinary glucose. The total syndrome could be prevented by the subcutaneous implantation of a small portion of the freshly removed pancreas. The severe metabolic disturbances, however, began to develop as soon as the subcutaneous pancreatic implant had degenerated. Hence, it was correctly deduced that pancreatic diabetes was due to the loss of an internal secretion, not to the lack of digestive ferments secreted by the gland. The antidiabetic material was postulated to be elaborated and secreted by the cells of the islets of Langerhans, which formed a diffuse endocrine gland within the pancreas (Mering and Minkowski, 1889; Minkowski, 1893; Hedon, 1898; Laguesse, 1893).

These well known facts are presented here to demonstrate that, at the very beginning of the quest, it was seen that the pancreatic antidiabetic factor (later called insulin), must exert its effects on the metabolism of *all* three foodstuffs, in the direction of favoring their *anabolism*.

In the 25 years between the successful extraction of insulin and the late 1940s, the accumulated body of evidence could be summarized as follows (for details, consult the reviews referred to above).

1. Insulin reversed the catabolism of all of three foodstuffs.
2. It favored their synthetic buildup and storage.

Because the details of intermediary metabolism of carbohydrates became known earlier than those of fat and of protein metabolism, the bulk of the work concentrated on glucose and its derivatives. It was shown that insulin favored the storage of glucose as glycogen in both muscles and liver, that it inhibited the output of glucose by the liver, and that tissues supplied by carbohydrate and insulin derived their energy mainly from carbohydrate and decreased the proportion previously derived from fats and proteins. As a result, fat stores were not mobilized, and, therefore, ketosis was inhibited. Muscle protein was also preserved, probably by inhibition of its breakdown in the periphery as well as by inhibition of gluconeogenesis from the amino acids derived from the peripheral tissues.

It was also observed that glucose itself (in large amounts) favored anabolism not only by promoting its own retention, but also by an inhibition of protein and fat breakdown. Glucose did not do it as efficiently as when insulin was also present, but it was striking enough to suggest that perhaps insulin acted anabolically on all three foodstuffs *because* of its action in promoting glucose uptake by the tissues. On the other hand, up to the late 1940s it was not possible to demonstrate convincingly a direct effect of insulin on any one of the key enzymatic reactions of carbohydrate metabolism.

In the years between 1945 and 1949, the search for the possible major effect of insulin on the key enzymatic step of carbohydrate metabolism narrowed down to the phosphorylation of glucose by hexokinase. The failure to prove that thesis was a turning point in thinking about the nature of regulation of intermediary metabolism and the effects of hormones thereon.

It was in 1948 and 1949 that attention shifted in the whole field of insulin action from attempting to demonstrate an effect of insulin on intracellular enzymatic activity, to considerations that insulin may act and exert its effects via the cell membrane. Stadie and co-workers demonstrated (Stadie et al., 1949, 1952) that native and radioactively labeled insulin became bound to tissues and exerted effects most probably by being bound first to the cell surface. At the same time, Levine, Goldstein, and co-workers showed that insulin increased the rate of inward transport of sugars into many cell systems. This was first demonstrated with nonmetabolizable hexoses and pentoses and by measuring the volume of distribution of such sugars in the tissues of the eviscerated animal (Levine et al., 1949, 1950; Goldstein et al. 1953a).

It was shown at that time, also, that in many tissues sugars were taken up by means of specific systems (transport protein carriers), and that insulin speeded up the activity of these carriers leading to the faster inward movement of sugar molecules. The facilitation by insulin of the transmembrane transport of sugars was first demonstrated in the case of galactose, d-xylose, and l-arabinose. This work was confirmed very readily, and the concept was extended to striated muscle, cardiac muscle, and fibroblasts in vitro. Most important, Park and his co-workers established that the phenomenon applied to glucose as well as to nonutilizable sugars (Park et al., 1955, 1959).

It was then found that in adipose tissue, as well as in muscle, glucose transport is rate-limiting and that insulin exerts an accelerating effect on the glucose transport system of the fat cell (Renold et al., 1965).

Because of the consideration that the facilitation of glucose uptake could also inhibit the breakdown of proteins and fats, it was then proposed that all other effects of the hormone were consequences of this membrane transport action. Theoretically, it was possible to account for increases in glucose oxidation, glycogen synthesis, protein sparing, fat sparing, etc. On this basis it was difficult however, to account for any action on liver metabolism, since glucose transport was found not to be rate-limiting in the hepatic cell (Levine and Goldstein, 1955).

It was soon shown that the view that all the effects of insulin could be traced to its stimulation of membrane transport was entirely too simplistic. Larner and co-workers pointed out that the fast rate of glucose entry caused by insulin favored the glycogen storage pathway when compared with the proportional rates of glucose entry into the cell by diffusion from a high extracellular concentration. It was postulated and found that there was a more direct effect of insulin on the activity of glycogen synthase (Villar-Palasi and Larner, 1961). The effect on transport and the separate effect on glycogen synthase, taken together, accounted for the high activity of the glycogen storage mechanism.

The influx into cells of substances not chemically related to the sugars is also stimulated by insulin even in the absence of added external glucose. These materials include nonutilizable amino acids, some of the natural amino acids, potassium, etc. It was also observed that insulin changed the membrane potential of some tissue systems in the absence of sugar in the medium, and that the inhibition of lipolysis by insulin was expressed fully in the absence of glucose in the medium. [For detailed references, consult Krahl (1961).]

It would seem, therefore, that all the effects of the hormone could not be simply secondary to an action of insulin on glucose transport. It was reasonable, however, to suppose that insulin affected the cell membrane and that the resulting modification of structure accounted for the transport effects both on sugar and nonsugar materials.

Insulin was also found to increase the incorporation of labeled amino acids into tissue proteins in the absence of glucose in the medium. This was independent of the influence on amino acid transport. Wool and his co-workers pointed out that the effect is probably due to an action on the activity and aggregation of the ribosomes. They showed that ribosomal activity was enhanced by the prior injection of insulin to the intact animal, but that insulin *in vitro* did not have such an effect (Wool *et al.,* 1966).

The insulin-sensitive barrier to free glucose diffusion in the chick embryo heart arises only after the eighth or ninth day of embryonic life. Prior to this time, glucose diffuses rapidly inward at a rate unaffected by insulin (Guidotti and Foa, 1961). However, even when insulin did not exert any effect on glucose entry into the young embryonic heart fiber, it did enhance incorporation of acetate into fat and of amino acids into protein. One could interpret such data in favor of the existence of a variety of intracellular actions of insulin in addition to its membrane effects. It could also have been argued that insulin primarily affects the cell membrane; the initial chemical changes produced thereby then would serve as signals affecting glucose transport, amino acid incorporation, fatty acid esterification, etc.

The effect on glucose transport in the early embryo was not seen, perhaps because the glucose transporters were not yet incorporated into the membrane. The other mechanisms were present and hence were affected by the membrane signal.

It was shown by many investigators that perturbation of membrane structure, by the use of appropriate amounts of certain hydrolytic enzymes, could mimic the action of insulin (Kono, 1969; Kuo *et al.,* 1967;

Rieser and Rieser, 1964; Blecher, 1965; Rodbell, 1966). Kono, Kuo, and Rieser used proteolytic systems. Rodbell and Blecher demonstrated by the use of isolated dispersed fat cells that phospholipase affects the cells in a manner similar to insulin, not only in respect to the inward transport of glucose, but also that it exerts an antilipolytic effect, presumably by a signal transmitted from the perturbed membrane to the enzymes governing lipolysis.

By about 1970, one could arrive at the following conclusions about insulin action. The hormone is recognized by the cells on which it acts because the membranes of those cells contain a material that specifically binds insulin. This primary event, the interaction of the hormone with its specific receptor, initiated changes that result in activation of certain transport processes in the membrane. The transport itself is due to the presence in the membrane of specific proteins that presumably were the system by which the substrate molecules gain access into the cell. It was probable that these transport systems were specific carrier proteins. In addition to the transport effects, insulin, in some manner requiring intactness of the cell, activated some enzyme systems located in the interior. One such system is glycogen synthase, which is the last step by which UDPglucose attaches to preformed glycogen and thereby increases the storage of the material. The storage of glycogen then is governed by insulin in two ways: by the stimulation of the final step in its synthesis and by the greater entry of glucose molecules that are the precursors of the glycogen (Larner and Palasi, 1971).

Another enzymatic step that is stimulated by the exhibition of insulin to intact cells involves pyruvate dehydrogenase, which was shown to operate more rapidly in the presence of the hormone (Jungas, 1971). A third enzymatic step, which was modified by exhibition of insulin or certain insulin-mimicking agents (proteases and phospholipases), is the triglyceride lipase step. Insulin inhibits the activity of the hormone-sensitive lipase that breaks down triglycerides to fatty acids (Fain et al., 1966).

Another effect that again requires cell intactness is the increase in the activity and aggregation of ribosomes, which catalyze the initiation and elongation of proteins, thereby stimulating amino acid incorporation. In addition, insulin also exerts a transport-enhancing effect on the uptake of some of the amino acids (Wool et al., 1968).

One could interpret these findings in one of two ways. One was to suppose that in addition to its interaction with a specific receptor at the membrane, which was responsible for the transport effects of insulin, the insulin molecule could enter the cell interior and interact with the enzymes, the activity of which it affects, in some direct fashion. Or, one could suppose that the membrane interaction was the only one in which insulin participated directly, and that this interaction, in some manner, released a signal or signals in the form of second messengers, which then would affect the enzyme systems located in the cell interior.

The brilliantly successful concept of a second messenger for hormonal activity began with the analysis of the cellular events initiated by epinephrine and glucagon (Sutherland and Robinson, 1966). Since insulin could counteract many of the effects of glucagon and of the β-adrenergic agonists, it was eminently logical to inquire whether insulin did so by modulating cyclic AMP (cAMP). The "message" evoked by insulin would simply be a weakening or destruction of the "message" sent by its physiological antagonists. There is no doubt that in many instances it can be shown that insulin opposes, for example, the glycogenolytic and/or lipolytic actions of glucagon and simultaneously lowers the tissue levels of cAMP. This effect could be due to an inhibition of the activity of adenyl cyclase or to an increased activity of a phosphodiesterase (Hepp, 1977).

The effect on tissue levels of cAMP is not an invariable result of insulin action. In addition, the stimulation of glycogenolysis via the α-adrenergic route is not caused by a cAMP rise, yet insulin does counteract it (Park et al., 1972; Exton et al., 1980).

It seems more probable that insulin via its own specific second messenger influences adenyl cyclase or phosphodiesterase, or both. The insulin effect follows whether or not the cAMP level is changed.

III. Role of the Insulin Receptor

We shall now examine in more detail what has been learned in the last decade about the details of the interaction of insulin with cell membranes and the present evidence for secondary messengers.

Much has been uncovered concerning the nature of the insulin receptor, especially about the specificity and behavior of the interaction between insulin and the receptor molecule. The receptor has not yet been completely purified, but sufficient evidence exists to consider that it is a compound glycoprotein molecule of apparent molecular weight of about 350,000, consisting of two heavy and two light chains interconnected by disulfide bonds (Cuatrecasas and Hollenberg, 1976; Kahn, 1976; Czech, 1977; Pilch and Czech, 1980; Jacobs et al., 1980). Evidence from Czech's laboratory favors the view that insulin receptors may represent a related but heterogeneous population of disulfide-linked complexes (M_r 350,000, 320,000, and 290,000) (Massague et al. 1980).

According to Kahn et al. (1981); and Harmon and Kahn (1981), the insulin receptor is composed of two units: (a) the binding component (M_r ca 115,000); and (b) the affinity regulator (M_r ca 260,000). The reaction with insulin causes a decrease in the size of the binding component to a molecular weight of 76,000. It will be of great interest to know how this finding relates to the suggestion that the insulin receptor complex activates a proteolytic system in the membrane (Kikuchi *et al.*, 1981; Larner *et al.*, 1982).

The specificity of binding has been definitely demonstrated by the finding that the characteristics of the binding reaction and of the biological activity go hand in hand. That is, when one compares the binding characteristics of the native, fully active insulin with the binding characteristics of modified insulins that have less biological activity, the affinity of the binding is directly related to the degree of biological activity (Roth, 1979; Kahn, 1976).

This work came primarily from the laboratories of Cuatrecasas, Kono, and Roth, now joined by many other groups. By utilizing the kinetic studies of the ligand interaction, it has been shown that the affinity and the number of ligand sites determine the degree of biological activity (Kono and Barham, 1971; Kahn, 1976) and that those cells that were known previously not to be affected by insulin in regard to either transport, glucose oxidation, or other parameters of insulin action, contain less ligand capacity for the hormone. That is, they tend to have fewer insulin receptors. It has also been demonstrated that the number of receptors is governed by many environmental conditions in which the cell finds itself. For example, the concentration of the hormone in tissue fluids determines the number of insulin receptors available. This has been called "down regulation," and it has been shown that if tissues or organs are subjected, for a period, to high insulin levels, the number of receptors diminishes. Because of that, resistance develops not only to binding, but to the expected actions of insulin (Gavin *et al.*, 1974; Freychet, 1976; Olefsky, 1976, 1981; Kobayashi and Olefsky, 1978; Kahn *et al.*, 1981).

The process of down regulation is more complex than would appear on first glance. Ordinarily, one would think that the increased occupancy of receptors by insulin increases internalization, and therefore destruction, of insulin and perhaps destruction of the receptor. Thus, fewer receptors are present in the membrane after the membrane has been exposed to a high hormone level. But it has been shown that insulin-mimicking agents, such as hydrogen peroxide, spermine, vitamin K_5, do not exert any effects on insulin binding but do decrease the degree of binding after a cell system has been incubated with them for 12–18 hours. This leads to a decrease in the number of receptors without a change in affinity. There is no similar effect on glucagon binding or on other functions of the cell. Therefore, down regulation may also be related to some steps in the pathway of biological effects of insulin ahead of the receptor, in one or more of the postreceptor reactions.

The problem of spare receptors is another rather complex issue. The notion of spare receptors is derived from the fact that maximal biological effects are obtained in various tissues after the occupancy of only 5% to, at most, 35% of the available receptor number. Tissues differ in the number or percentage of spare receptors. The greater the number of spare receptors, the more sensitive is the action at low hormone concentrations; however, the less sensitive is the biological activity at high insulin levels. It has been supposed that the lesser number of spare receptors in liver, 65% as against 90–95% in adipose tissue, allows continued response at high portal insulin levels. The biological significance of spare receptors has not yet been completely clarified.

It had been known for many years that the utilization and oxidation of glucose by the brain, *in situ,* is not interfered with by complete removal of insulin from the body. When one examines the insulin-binding capacity of brain, by techniques that visualize the insulin receptor complex, it is seen that the receptors are concentrated on the vascular endothelium of the brain capillaries, and very sparsely on the surfaces of the neurons (van Houten *et al.,* 1979). There have been indications that while the bulk of neuronal tissue may not require insulin, there may be individual cells or nuclei that react to insulin in a physiologically significant manner and that the hormone plays a role in the regulation of centers for food ingestion, appetite, etc. (Porte and Woods, 1979; Szabo, 1981). Insulin has been localized and demonstrated on the surfaces of certain hypothalamic neurons (Baskin *et al.,* 1981), and blood-borne ^{125}I-labeled insulin was bound to dendrites and cell bodies in the area postrema, and internalized after binding (Van Houten and Posner, 1981). Thus, although the overwhelming bulk of the central nervous system neurons seem not to be affected by the metabolic activities of insulin, the hormone may exert a regulatory effect on some specific functions especially of autonomic centers.

Mature red blood cells do not require insulin for sugar transport or for its breakdown to lactate. They have relatively few binding sites for insulin. However, when a precursor of the normal adult red cell is examined, insulin promotes glucose entry and utilization. Such cells as erythroblasts and other precursors of red blood cells contain many more sites to which insulin is specifically bound (Gambhir *et al.,* 1978; Eng *et al.,* 1980; Galbraith *et al.,* 1980).

While there is a general correlation between degrees of binding and the biological effects of insulin, it had been demonstrated that in the case of red blood cells insulin fails to show effects on glucose uptake irrespective of the number of specific receptors (Sinha et al., 1981). Evidently, a transducing step is missing in these cells.

Individuals with acanthosis nigricans may have severe insulin resistance with intense hyperglycemia. Such individuals possess antibodies to the insulin receptor. However, such antibodies, when added to an insulin-responsive tissue, may stimulate the tissue in the same fashion as does insulin. This is presumed to occur because of the combination of the antibody with the receptor, thereby, crosslinking it. It provides some presumptive evidence that one of the results of the interaction of the hormone with its receptor is to make it prone to aggregation and that this action is part of the cavalcade of processes necessary for the biological insulin effects (Kahn et al., 1978; Kahn, 1979).

Studies utilizing the antibody to the insulin receptor (antireceptor antibody) are beginning to clarify very important points that are basic to the understanding of the action of peptide hormones. The structurally specific key (insulin) fits snugly into the slot of the lock (the attachment site on the receptor). This fit induces the proper movements of the tumblers to activate (open) the lock mechanism. When the attachment site on the receptor is already occupied by an antireceptor antibody, the key cannot enter (insulin resistance). The fact, however, that the "plug" (antireceptor antibody) can itself activate the lock poses the question: Which of the two participants (hormone or receptor) elicits the full program of the biological responses? Work thus far has shown that the antireceptor antibody binds specifically to the receptor and elicits a full program of biological responses that include transport, enzyme modulation, and enzyme biosynthesis (Kahn et al., 1977; Belsham et al., 1980; Kahn and Harrison, 1981; Roth, 1981; Baldwin et al., 1980).

Phylogenetically the receptor seems to antedate the appearance of the hormone (Czaba, 1980), and it is a very highly conserved protein among all the vertebrates studied (Muggeo et al., 1979).

It would appear then that the receptor possesses the full biological program for the events ordinarily attributed to the hormone. In primitive organisms this may be the cellular regulatory apparatus. In the more complex organisms there is a need to integrate biochemical events occurring in the separate organs and tissues, especially the metabolic demands brought about by the influx and efflux of nutrients during food absorption and in times of food scarcity. The hormone (insulin) is the integrative messenger that coordinates the myriad of separately acting membrane receptors.

Elegant studies have shown that, after the interaction between insulin and its receptor, the insulin receptor combination is internalized by endocytosis and migrates via the Golgi apparatus into the lysosomal area of the cell, and that insulin and perhaps its receptor are destroyed within the lysosome (Terris and Steiner, 1975; Gorden *et al.*, 1980). In the course of these studies it was shown that the internalization and the insulin-destroying processes are not part of the biological action of insulin, since interference with lysosomal incorporation of the insulin receptor complex has no effect on the biological activities of the hormone (Suzuki and Kono, 1979; Hammons and Jarett, 1979; Marshall and Olefsky, 1979).

The process of insulin receptor complex formation, and probably internalization, has effects beyond that step, because it can be shown that in many insulin-resistant states that are presumably due to losses in the number of receptors, there is also evidence of inhibition of other steps, such as glucose transport and oxidation. In other words, the resistance is finally manifest not only by the lack of insulin receptor complex formation, but also by postreceptor difficulties. The relief of the inhibition by various means also slowly reverses the postreceptor inhibitions so that resistance to the biological activity is then completely removed (Olefsky, 1981; Le Marchand-Brustel *et al.*, 1978; Marshall and Olefsky, 1980).

How the insulin receptor combination reflects positively on the maintenance of postreceptor combination steps is not yet known.

The majority of workers in the field do not feel that there exist biologically significant insulin receptors in the cell interior, such as those on the surfaces of cell organelles, for example, the nucleus. However, insulin can be identified in the cell interior, and specific binding to internal membranes has been demonstrated (Goldfine, 1977; Horvat, 1980). It has not been completely resolved whether these findings are related to hormonal action or to its internalization and degradation (Posner *et al.*, 1980).

We know from the work of Kono and others that the insulin receptor is synthesized continuously. For example, when trypsin is allowed to act on the cell surfaces in certain concentrations, it will abolish completely the specific binding with insulin. When such a tissue is then transferred to a non-trypsin-containing vessel and allowed to "rest," the specific binding activity will again be seen within several hours (Kono and Barham, 1971). We do not as yet know fully whether the migration of insulin plus its receptor via endocytosis to the lysosomes serves to destroy the insulin and release the receptor for reincorporation into the membrane or whether the receptor is also destroyed by proteolysis in the same location (Gorden *et al.*, 1979; Krupp and Lane, 1981; Marshall and Olefsky, 1981).

IV. Transduction of the Insulin Signal

How does the brief period in which insulin receptor complexes are formed and the insulin receptor is complex internalized affect the transport of glucose and other molecules into the cell? The glucose transport system consists, presumably, of a specific protein carrier for the sugar. As such, it exists in the membrane. What happens to it after it has transported the molecule to the internal surface of the membrane? Is it reincorporated, or is it destroyed and resynthesized? Second, does the insulin receptor combination activate the rate at which the glucose carrier operates and leave the number of glucose carriers the same as it was, or does the insulin receptor combination result in the production or mobilization of more carrier molecules?

Independent work from two laboratories (Suzuki and Kono, 1980; Cushman and Wardzala, 1980) demonstrated the presence of specific glucose transporters in the cytoplasm (Golgi-rich fraction), identical to those found in the cell membrane.

Insulin seems to mobilize the internal glucose carriers and incorporate them into the membrane, thus speeding the entry of sugar (Suzuki and Kono, 1980; Cushman and Wardzala, 1980; Kono *et al.*, 1981; Ciaraldi, 1981).

The recycling of glucose transporters between the membrane and the cell interior does not depend upon new protein synthesis but does require metabolic energy (Kono *et al.*, 1981).

Work from Czech's laboratory cautions against this concept as the only action of insulin on glucose transport. Their data point also to an effect of insulin on the rate at which each carrier moves in its work of transport (Carter-Su and Czech, 1980).

The same group has adduced evidence from which they conclude that insulin may influence glucose transport by affecting membrane fluidity and thus increasing the activity of the glucose transporter systems. (Pilch *et al.*, 1980).

Clausen (1975) has written a comprehensive review of insulin and sugar transport in which the membrane effects are related to the distribution of electrolytes, especially the role of calcium ions on the state of the membrane.

An intriguing relationship between the glucose transporter and the insulin-sensitive phosphodiesterase (PDE) has been found in Froesch's laboratory. Both of these activities (in rat fat cells) are increased by hypophysectomy, and both then become insensitive to insulin. Inhibitors of PDE also decrease glucose transport rates. Growth hormone administration (long-term) decreases transport, which then becomes again sensitive to insulin (Schoenle et al., 1981). In view of the more recent data on the effect of insulin on translocating glucose transporters from the Golgi area to the membrane, the effects of growth hormone, and the relation of PDE to the glucose transporter are of great interest.

In the case of amino acids, very little is known about the character of the carrier; but, in the case of potassium, the work of Guidotti and co-workers would seem to implicate sodium-potassium ATPase as the potassium carrier that is activated by the insulin receptor interaction (Resh et al., 1980).

V. Protein Phosphorylation as a Modulator of Enzyme Action

It was demonstrated some years ago that intracellular enzyme systems operative in intermediary metabolism may exhibit varying activity depending upon the presence or the absence of covalently bound phosphate. This was first demonstrated for the enzyme glycogen phosphorylase, which can be isolated in two forms. The fully phosphorylated form is the most active in producing glucose 1-phosphate from glycogen. When the phosphate is removed by the action of a phosphatase, glycogen phosphorylase becomes very much less active.

When glucagon attaches to its receptor it activates the membrane enzyme adenyl cyclase, which then produces cAMP from ATP. The cAMP attaches to the "regulatory unit" of the enzyme protein kinase and causes its dissociation from the "catalytic unit." Protein kinase catalyzes the phosphorylation of several enzyme proteins, especially phosphorylase kinase and glycogen synthase. Finally, the phosphorylase kinase leads to the addition of phosphate to glycogen phosphorylase. By this means glycogen phosphorylation is activated and glycogenolysis ensues.

On the other hand, glycogen synthesis is promoted by the UDPglucose glycogen synthase, which is most active in its dephosphorylated form. Glucagon, therefore, via the adenyl cyclase system, at one end and the same time activates glycogenolysis via the phosphorylated form of glycogen phosphorylase and, by promoting phosphorylation of the glycogen synthase, it inhibits the formation of glycogen. Insulin has the reverse effect. The activity imparted by insulin leads to dephosphorylation of these enzyme proteins, thereby inactivating the glycogenolytic pathway and activating the final step in glycogen synthesis (Fisher *et al.*, 1971; Larner *et al.*, 1971; Cohen and Nimmo, 1978; Van de Werwe *et al.*, 1977; Hems and Whitton, 1980).

It had been known for 40 or more years that a rise in the level in blood glucose inhibits glycogenolysis and promotes the uptake of glucose into the liver in the normal animal (Soskin *et al.*, 1938). This autoregulation of liver sugar output has been confirmed by the use of the perfused rat liver (McCraw *et al.*, 1967; Glinsmann *et al.*, 1969). More recently, mainly through the work of the laboratories of Hers in Belgium and Hems in England, it has been shown that the glucose effect is not exerted by glucose as a substrate, but with glucose acting as a regulator. Phosphorylase, *a*, the fully active glycogenolytic system, combines with glucose, and this combination seems to be a better substrate for the phosphatase by which phosphorylase *a* is converted to phosphorylase *b*, the less active form (Hers, 1976; Stalmans, 1976; Hems, 1978).

In turn, this releases the activity of glycogen synthase phosphatase, which converts the synthase to its active form. The glucose molecule itself, acting as a regulator, can initiate the inhibition of glycogenolysis and the promotion of the last step in glycogen synthesis. We do not as yet know the exact relationship between the effect of insulin on glycogen synthase and the effect of glucose itself (Hems, 1977). This relationship seems to vary depending on the tissue examined. Thus, in liver, adipose tissue, and heart muscle, glucose has a major effect of stimulation of glycogen synthase activity, while in skeletal muscle insulin itself appears to play the principal regulatory role (Chiasson *et al.*, 1980). But it is the work on glycogen synthase, primarily by Larner and his co-workers, that has finally led to the detection of a factor produced by insulin in the tissues, a "mediator," which seems to activate the phosphatase that removes phosphate from the inactive glycogen synthase, thereby changing it into its active form (Larner *et al.*, 1974, 1979; Roach and Larner, 1976; Cheng *et al.*, 1980).

This is the so-called factor II of Larner, isolated from muscle after its exposure to insulin. The factor has a presumed molecular weight of about 1000, and it is assumed, but not proved, to be a peptide liberated by the action of insulin on muscle. There is no definitive proof as yet that this reasonably small molecule is a peptide. However, Larner and his co-workers have shown that it is probably not a portion of the insulin molecule that could be liberated by the proteolysis of the hormone within the cell.

Jarett and his co-workers utilized the Larner factor II to demonstrate, in elegant fashion, that it was a mediator of insulin action. It had been known for some time that the enzyme pyruvate dehydrogenase, located within the mitochondria, is activated by insulin. Jarett showed that in a preparation containing both mitochondria and the membrane fraction of fat cells, insulin activated pyruvate dehydrogenase within the mitochondria. Presumably insulin binds to the membrane portion and secondarily affects an enzyme within the mitochondria in this mixture of organelles (Jarett and Seals, 1979; Seals and Jarett, 1980; Popp et al., 1980).

In the absence of the membrane fraction, insulin added to isolated mitochondria from fat cells had no effect on the activity of pyruvate dehydrogenase. On the other hand, factor II of Larner will activate this enzyme in the absence of the membrane fraction by a direct effect on mitochondria. Pyruvate dehydrogenase is another example of a system that changes activity depending upon the degree of phosphorylation of the enzyme protein. It is inactive in the phosphorylated form and is fully active when the phosphate is removed by a phosphatase.

The evidence of Jarett and of others now indicates that factor II of Larner (whether or not it is a peptide) acts on the phosphatase that leads to the activation of pyruvate dehydrogenase (Kiechle et al., 1981).

Larner and co-workers (Kikuchi and Larner, 1981a,b; Kikuchi et al., 1981) have added interesting data comparing insulin with "insulin mimicking" agents (such as H D, GSSG, and trypsin) on membrane transport, glucose oxidation, and activation of glycogen synthase. Their tentative conclusions are as follows:

The insulin receptor complex evokes, in the membrane, proteolytic activity. As a result, two glycopeptides (?) are released into the cell interior. One of them mediates the dephosphorylation of certain enzyme proteins; the other seems to favor phosphorylation. At present, dephosphorylation (and hence activation) of two systems has been shown (synthase and pyruvate dehydrogenase).

Of the substances that are known to mimic insulin action, only trypsin activates glycogen synthase in the same manner as does the hormone itself (via a mediator). [See also a fuller account by Larner et al. (1982) presented at the Laurentian Hormone Conference, September 1981.]

The "mediator" aspect of the field of insulin action is of great interest and potential importance. It requires careful confirmatory data, extension to other anabolic enzymes, and interpretive restraint.

VI. ROLE IN PROTEIN METABOLISM

It was first demonstrated by Minkowski, during his initial experiments with pancreatectomy that in diabetes there is intense destruction of protein and the formation of sugar from the resulting amino acids. When insulin became available for experimentation, the reversal of the negative nitrogen balance was one of the first metabolic phenomena observed. It was also noted that insulin in the presence of a sufficient quantity of amino acids and energy would lead to the synthesis of additional body protein. In more recent years, it has been shown that insulin affects the transport of amino acids. But it was demonstrated by Wool and co-workers that insulin enhances amino acid incorporation directly from an intracellular pool, independent of the influx from outside the cell, either of glucose or of amino acids (Wool *et al.*, 1968; Wool, 1972).

Wool and his co-workers also observed a phenomenon that has been repeatedly confirmed—that there is a defect (in the absence of insulin) in the aggregation of ribosomes into polysomes. And, hence, there is a defect in the initiation of peptide formation from amino acids by the ribosomes. This could be repaired by the administration of insulin to the organism as a whole or in an intact cell system. The work has been confirmed and extended by Jefferson, Manchester, Lyons, and other workers. It has been shown, however, that the defect in initiation and elongation of peptides and the change in polysome versus ribosome percentage is not uniformly seen in every tissue, even though thre is an effect on the retention and production of protein. Thus, mixed fiber muscles differ from cardiac and from red muscle, and the liver does not show the same type of impairment. In liver, especially in relation to the synthesis of excretory proteins like albumin, it was shown that the diabetic state suffers a loss in the amount of mRNA, a defect that is restored by the administration of insulin to the intact animal (Jefferson, 1980; Jefferson *et al.*, 1980; Lyons *et al.*, 1980).

It would be tempting to speculate that some of the factors involved in the ribosomal process of protein synthesis may also be modified by covalent phosphorylation and dephosphorylation (Jackson and Hunt, 1980), in that insulin would then have an analogous effect on such factors as it does on glycogen synthase, pyruvate dehydrogenase, acetyl-CoA carboxylase, and most probably on other enzymes. However, since there is such variation from one muscle type to another and from muscle and heart to liver, it does not seem directly evident that the mechanism of insulin action on synthesis involves the simple process of changing the covalent phosphorylation of an initiation or an elongation factor, or both.

It may well be that in the case of protein synthesis the situation is far more complex than in glycogen storage or in lipogenesis. However, there is also another analogy possible between the effects of insulin on lipids and glycogen and its effects on protein buildup. And that is that a major part of the action may be exerted on restraining breakdown (Mortimore and Mondon, 1970; Hider *et al.*, 1971; Fulks *et al.*, 1975).

Unfortunately, not enough is known about the details of protein catabolism in such tissues as muscle, which, during starvation or diabetes, provide a major portion of the amino acids used in gluconeogenesis. Is the proteolytic process always lysosomal in nature, and does insulin inhibit proteolysis by stabilizing effects on the lysosome? If it does, by what type of action does it affect lysosomal proteolytic activity?

The present evidence is in conformity with an action of insulin on the proteolytic systems in the lysosomal apparatus. By what mechanism? As in the case of the two other foodstuffs, there is evidence for a concerted action of insulin in favor of synthesis by a pull mechanism on the synthetic reactions and an inhibition of the catabolic side of protein metabolism.

VII. Role in Fat Metabolism

Just as in the case of carbohydrates and proteins, the effect of insulin on the synthesis and storage of fats is exerted by a combination of stimulation of synthetic steps and simultaneous inhibition of fat breakdown.

Insulin had been known for many years to favor and stimulate the production of triglycerides from carbohydrates or any other metabolite that yields acetyl-CoA (Stetten and Boxer, 1944; Renold and Cahill, 1965). The predominent precursor is glucose. The action of insulin in relation to lipogenesis expresses itself first through its effect on glucose entry into the cell that forms the fat. This provides the initial substrate. In the course of the reactions from glucose to triglyceride, there are a number of enzymes that exert key roles in lipogenesis. Many of these enzymes are affected by covalent modulation of their activity via phosphorylation and dephosphorylation (Denton *et al.*, 1977; Geelen *et al.*, 1980). Insulin, as we have seen in the case of glycogen synthase, favors the dephosphorylated form. In most instances, this is probably affected by favoring protein phosphatases that remove phosphate from the phosphorylated form of the enzyme.

Although we have no hard evidence for each one of these enzymes, we can draw a probable analogy to what we know about glycogen synthase and pyruvate dehydrogenase (Hardie, 1981). In those cases, insulin favors the dephosphorylated form and probably acts by way of the second messenger or factor II of Larner and Jarett. Among the key enzymes involved are phosphofructokinase, pyruvate dehydrogenase, acetyl-CoA carboxylase. Let us recall the pathway of lipogenesis. The intermediate most important for lipogenesis is acetyl-CoA. Acetyl-CoA arises in the following manner: glucose is broken down to pyruvate. One of the steps in glycolysis that promotes the generation of pyruvate is the phosphorylation of fructose 6-phosphate to fructose 1,6-diphosphate.

Before pyruvate is formed, fructose diphosphate splits to dihydroxyacetone phosphate, from which glycerol phosphate is formed. Therefore, the combination of the inward transport of glucose and the stimulation of glycolysis, producing pyruvate, is very important in promoting lipogenesis.

Once pyruvate is formed, acetyl-CoA is produced by the action of pyruvate dehydrogenase in the mitochondrion. This enzyme is active in its dephosphorylated form, and for it we have very good evidence that insulin promotes the dephosphorylation of the enzyme protein. Hence, insulin will speed up the formation of acetyl-CoA. In the mitochondria, acetyl-CoA combines with oxaloacetate to form citrate. Citrate can and does diffuse out of the mitochondria. The citrate in the cytosol has two effects. It will itself stimulate acetyl-CoA carboxylase, but equally important is the fact that acetyl-CoA carboxylase is an enzyme that is also active in its dephosphorylated form. We may expect to find that the insulin "mediator" will act on this system as it does on pyruvate dehydrogenase. Acetyl-CoA carboxylase forms malonyl-CoA from acetyl-CoA.

Seven moles of malonyl-CoA and one of acetyl-CoA in the presence of NADPH form a mole of palmitic acid. Palmityl-CoA and phosphoglycerol combine to become triglyceride.

Glucagon depresses lipogenesis, most probably via cAMP; this leads to the phosphorylation of enzyme proteins (Beynen et al., 1979).

By inhibiting acylcarnitine transferase, malonyl-CoA favors the production of triglycerides. It also inhibits the entry of acetyl-CoA into the mitochondrion, where it could readily produce ketone bodies. When malonyl-CoA is low, ketone production is high (McGarry et al., 1978; Zammit, 1981).

A third way by which lipogenesis is favored is the decrease in the process by which triglycerides are broken down into fatty acids. The hormonally sensitive lipase is activated by glucagon, epinephrine, and certain pituitary hormones, by means of cyclic adenylate. This is counteracted by insulin. This step is probably modulated by the insulin "mediator," through an inhibition of the lipase.

We have known for many years that carbohydrate in its metabolism suppresses the production of ketones. But it is only within recent years that we have finally begun to express it in terms of enzymatic control and found the key in the production of malonyl-CoA by the carboxylase system. Production of malonyl-CoA immediately begins to interfere with the entry of fatty acyl-CoA for oxidation by the mitochondria. Malonyl-CoA strengthens the synthetic pathway and inhibits the oxidative ketogenic pathway (McGarry et al., 1978; McGarry and Foster, 1980).

VIII. The "Slow" Effects of Insulin

All the effects of insulin discussed above occur rapidly after administration *in vivo* and *in vitro*, in a matter of minutes or within 1 hour after the exhibition of the hormone. There exists, in addition, a set of insulin effects that becomes evident only some hours or even days after hormone administration. These effects consist of the induction of certain enzyme systems, primarily in the liver, and the enhancement of the growth and proliferation of cells.

Insulin administration to diabetic animals over a period of days decreases the levels of the gluconeogenic enzymes, for example, pyruvate carboxylase and glucose-6-phosphatase, and increases the levels of the glycolytic systems, glucokinase, aldolase, pyruvate kinase, etc. (Weinhouse, 1976; Weber et al., 1965). Protein and RNA syntheses are required for such hormone effects. Thre is no evidence that insulin acts directly as an inducer or repressor of specific enzyme syntheses. It is possible that these slow changes in enzyme amounts are a result of altered levels of substrates caused by insulin, which then protect the enzymes against degradation or promote their induction.

The "growth" effects are not as yet understood on the cellular or molecular levels. They are accompanied by an increased synthesis of the nucleic acids. Insulin shares these effects with a group of peptides, many of which are structurally related to the insulin molecule [nonsuppressible insulin-like activity (NSILA), the somatomedins, nerve growth factor, etc.] (Pastan, 1975; Hall et al., 1975; Froesch et al., 1975).

Recent work suggests that the cell membrane possesses a separate specific receptor for the "growth" effects. The insulin receptor proper has the greatest affinity for insulin itself and low affinity for the insulin-like growth factors. On the other hand, the "growth" receptor possesses high affinity for the various growth factors and lower affinity for the insulin.

It would seem, therefore, that the rapid, metabolic effects of insulin are processed via the high-affinity metabolic receptor for the hormone; while the growth effects (which may also include enzyme induction) proceed via the "growth" receptor (Roth, 1979; King *et al.*, 1979; Rosenfeld and Hintz, 1980).

Comparison of the effects of different insulins and of insulin analogs on "metabolic" and "growth" effects (thymidine incorporation) suggests that these major divisions of the activity of this hormone may involve separate functional regions of the molecule (King and Kahn, 1981).

Despite the rapid progress in this field, many outstanding questions remain unanswered. Thus nothing is known concerning the existence of second messengers for the more delayed "growth" effects of the hormone. There is as well a set of seemingly contradictory data with respect to the effects of insulin on protein phosphorylation. As we have seen, the second messenger generated by insulin leads to the stimulation of enzyme dephosphorylation of many systems. In the main, this leads to higher activity of many enzymes in the anabolic pathways. On the other hand, it has been shown repeatedly that insulin can and does induce, by some means, the phosphorylation of certain membrane proteins, probably by way of a cAMP-dependent process (Walaas *et al.*, 1977; Benjamin and Singer, 1975; Avruch *et al.*, 1976).

The puzzle presented by the effects of insulin on inducing the dephosphorylated state of certain intracellular enzyme proteins and also leading to the incorporation of phosphate in some membrane proteins is beginning to be resolved. Marchmont and Houslay have presented evidence that insulin may lead to simultaneous phosphorylation of certain membrane proteins and the inhibition of phosphorylation of other membrane proteins. Interestingly enough, the membrane proteins in which insulin induces the phosphorylated state are peripheral proteins, that is those that are bound to the external surface of the plasma membrane by predominantly electrostatic interactions. Insulin leads to the inhibition of the phosphorylation of integral proteins that go through the membrane and bind to it by extensive hydrophobic interaction. The peripheral proteins are affected by insulin modulating a cAMP-dependent phosphorylation while the integral proteins also phosphorylated by a cAMP dependent process are inhibited. It might appear, therefore, that the insulin receptor combination triggers peripherally a cAMP-dependent process by which these enzymes are phosphorylated and that the "second messenger" inhibits the phosphorylation of the deeper integral proteins as it does in the case of glycogen synthase and pyruvate dehydrogenase. One of the peripheral proteins, phosphorylated by insulin action, is a 52,000 M_r species that is a phosphodiesterase (Marchmont and Houslay, 1980).

On the basis of experiments in their laboratory, Larner and co-workers postulated that there are two mediators of insulin action. One works by promoting dephosphorylation, the other by phosphorylation of catalytic proteins. Such a postulate accounts for the biphasic responses obtained in glycogen synthase phophatase activity with increasing amounts of insulin and for the findings that insulin action leads to the addition of phosphate to certain proteins and to the dephosphorylation of others (Larner et al., 1979; Cheng et al., 1980; Seals and Jarett, 1980; Seals and Czech, 1981).

Marchmont and Houslay speculated that one of the integral proteins, the phosphorylation of which is inhibited by insulin, may be a component of the sodium-potassium ATPase, another may be a protein that is responsible for calcium fluxes. It might also be speculated that one of the peripheral proteins phosphorylated under the influence of insulin may be the source of the second messenger, if that is a peptide.

IX. Transduction by Ions

The finding that insulin action at the membrane may lead to the production of one or possibly two mediators that carry the hormonal message to intracellular enzyme systems does not signify that there are no other transducing elements in the totality of insulin effects. In the area of the known transport effects there are gaps in our understanding of the means by which hormone binding is signaled to the specific transporter molecules for the passage of glucose, potassium, and amino acids.

During the period from 1960 to 1972, much work and extensive speculation concerned the possible role of sodium and potassium fluxes as signals for insulin effects. No firm, confirmable conclusions could be drawn as to the role of the monovalent cations. Czech reviewed the relevant literature in 1977 (Czech, 1977).

More recently, more attention has been paid to the calcium ion as a possible messenger for insulin action. This hypothesis grew out of the work of several laboratories and states essentially that insulin causes the release of membrane-bound Ca^{2+}, which proceeds by way of the cytoplasm to the mitochondria and the endoplasmic reticulum, where it affects enzymes in the direction of glycogenesis and lipogenesis and inhibits glycogenolysis and lipolysis (Clausen, 1975; Bihler, 1972; Kissebah *et al.*, 1975). The hypothesis is based on the need for Ca^{2+} for optimal responsiveness to insulin or the demonstration that conditions that mimic insulin action on hexose transport seem to increase intracellular calcium levels (Clausen, 1975; Czech, 1977). Many of the data relating calcium flux and insulin action are not in accord with a second-messenger role for many of the insulin effects except perhaps for membrane transport of hexoses. The review by Czech, referred to above, lists all the work in this area and examines the data critically.

In many ways related to the role of electrolytes is the hypothesis put forward by Zierler that the electrical field through the membrane may act as a transducer of certain insulin signals. It was Zierler who showed, in 1957, that insulin hyperpolarized the muscle membrane (Zierler, 1957). This was confirmed and extended to other tissues (adipose, heart, bladder, stomach). The hyperpolarization does not depend upon the presence of K^+. To test whether it can mimic insulin action (in its absence), Zierler and Rogus induced hyperpolarization in muscle *in vitro* and measured its influence on the uptake of 2-deoxyglucose. It had the postulated effect to the same degree as did 10 mU per milliliter of insulin (Zierler and Rogus, 1980). It will be of interest to determine whether other known insulin effects are also achieved by such means. It may well be that the induced hyperpolarization may have perturbed the insulin receptor sufficiently to have evoked the hypothetical mediator molecule and thus mimicked insulin action.

Some doubt as to the physiological significance of hyperpolarization has been expressed on the basis that neither electrical changes nor changes in intracellular sodium and potassium were found in association with insulin effects on sugar transport (Stark *et al.*, 1980).

X. INSULIN DISSOCIATION

An aspect of insulin action requiring further study is the question whether insulin needs to be continuously present for one or another of its effects to persist. It has been shown that insulin dissociates from the membrane and is also degraded after internalization. If one measures the rates of glucose transport with time, the decay of that function is slower than the rate of dissociation of the hormone from the bound state. The dissociation of transport activity takes longer than the dissociation of insulin from its receptor. The same can be said about glucose oxidation. In other words, these postreceptor effects of insulin are activated by the insulin receptor combination and continue to exert their activities after insulin is no longer being bound, or has completely dissociated. This is not surprising, because the association and dissociation of binding need not be the same as the processes that are secondarily set in motion by the insulin receptor complex (Bliziotes *et al.*, 1979; Ciaraldi and Olefsky, 1980).

In the light of the present work on the possible peptide nature of an insulin mediator (Czech, 1981), one should recall a series of papers in the 1970s by Rieser and Rieser, in which it was shown that trypsin and chymotrypsin could mimic the action of insulin on glucose transport and that chymotrypsin injected into diabetic rats had a hypoglycemic effect in 4–6 hours. In addition, Rieser showed that insulin had a weak proteolytic action on hemoglobin as a substrate.

Looked at in the light of present-day events, these findings would fit in with the present concept that after insulin combines with its specific receptor it may itself exert or cause to be exerted a proteolytic effect on a membrane constituent with the liberation of a second messenger for insulin action.

Because of the typically curvilinear Scatchard plots of insulin binding, several theories to explain that feature have been proposed. Originally it was interpreted as evidence for two distinct populations of insulin receptors, one of high affinity and low capacity and another of low affinity and high capacity. However, DeMeyts and co-workers proposed that the curvilinearity of the plot is explicable by negative cooperativity. However, the older notion of two distinct receptors varying in capacity and affinity has emerged again from the work of Pollett, of Glieman, and of Olefsky with adipocytes.

Olefsky's interpretation is that in addition to negative cooperativity the adipocyte insulin receptors behave functionally as two types, the high-affinity, low-capacity and the low-affinity, high-capacity binding sites. We do not know as yet whether this refers to two distinct systems in the membrane or represents changes after translocation of receptors to another site (Olefsky and Chang, 1979).

XI. Insulin-Mimicking Factors

Over the years, an increasingly large group of substances and conditions have been observed to mimic one or another of the known effects of insulin. Such phenomena have quite naturally been used as possible probes into the mechanisms of the effect (transport, antilipolysis) or into the transduction of insulin action. Oxidizing agents (H_2O_2, vitamin K_5, methylene blue), proteolytic enzymes, phospholipases, inhibitors of oxidative phosphorylation, hyperosmolarity, anoxia, ouabain, vanadium derivatives—all have had effects on sugar transport, antilipolysis, protein formation, etc., resembling those of insulin. While such data have provided some insights into the regulation of certain metabolic events, they have not, thus far, led to critical insights into mechanisms of hormonal action. Czech (1980) has reviewed many of these data, and there are some later relevant papers of interest (Debyak and Kleinzeller, 1980; Little and de Haen, 1980).

Muscular exercise enhances the inward transport of sugars. On the basis of cross-circulation experiments *in vivo,* it was postulated that exercising muscle liberates a material that mimics the insulin effect on transport (Goldstein *et al.,* 1953a; Goldstein, 1961; Havivi and Wertheimer, 1964). This has been questioned because muscular contraction seems also to hasten insulin absorption. The whole subject has been reviewed extensively (Vranic and Berger, 1979).

XII. Present Status of the Problem

The role of insulin in the organism is to promote cell anabolism and growth. It does so primarily by combining with specific cell membrane complex proteins (the "metabolic" and "growth" receptors). It has not yet been clearly established whether the hormone molecule has meaningful, biologically active receptors in the cell interior.

The anabolic activity of insulin consists of two major processes: (*a*) transport of the metabolites and ions; and (*b*) modulation of the phosphorylation of enzyme proteins. The latter process seems to proceed through the generation in the cell membrane of mediators that are, at present, presumed to be of peptide nature.

The transduction of the insulin signal to activate the various transport systems is not known at present. In the case of glucose transport, the data support the novel proposal that the hormone causes the mobilization of "internal" transport proteins and their temporary incorporation into the cell membrane. It is also not known whether the "mediators" now under investigation also play that same role for the "growth" effects (enzyme induction, RNA synthesis, cell growth) or whether an additional set of transducers will emerge in the future. These "unknowns" represent the major areas that require fresh, new insights on both the physiological and molecular levels.

REFERENCES

Avruch, J., Leone, G. R., and Martin, D. B. (1976). *J. Biol. Chem.* **251,** 1511–1515.

Baldwin, D., Terris, S., and Steiner, D. F. (1980). *J. Biol. Chem.* **225,** 4028–4034.

Baskin, D. G., Woods, S. C., Van Houten, M., and Posner, B. I. (1981). *Diabetes* **30** (Suppl. 1), 54A.

Belsham, G. J., Brownsey, R. W., Hughes, W. A., and Denton, R. M. (1980). *Diabetologia* **18,** 307–312.

Benjamin, W. A., and Singer, I. (1975). *Biochemistry* **15,** 3301–3310.

Beynen, A. C., Vaartjes, W. J., and Geelen, M. J. H. (1979). *Diabetes* **28,** 828–835.

Bihler, I. (1972). *In* "Role of Membranes in Metabolic Regulation" (M. A. Melhorn and R. W. Hanson, eds.), pp. 411–421. Academic Press, New York.

Blecher, M. (1965). *Biochem. Biophys. Res. Commun.* **21,** 202–209.

Blioziotes, M. M., Lewis, S. B., Schultz, T. A., and Daniels, E. L. (1979). *Diabetes* **28,** 391.

Carter-Su, C., and Cezch, M. P. (1980). *J. Biol. Chem.* **255,** 10382.

Cheng, K., Galasko, G., Huang, L., Kellogg, J., and Larner, J., (1980). *Diabetes* **29,** 659–661.

Chiasson, J. L., Dietz, M. R., Shikama, H., Wootten, M., and Exton, J. H. (1980). *Am. J. Physiol.* **239,** E70–73.

Ciaraldi, T. P. (1981). *Diabetes* **30** (Suppl 1), 109A.

Ciaraldi, T. P., and Olefsky, J. M. (1980). *J. Biol. Chem.* **255,** 327–330.

Clausen, T. (1975). *Curr. Top. Membr. Transp.* **6,** 169–226.

Cohen, P. (1976). *Trends Biochem. Sci.* **1,** 38.

Cohen, P., and Nimmo, G. A. (1978). *Biochem. Soc. Trans.* **6,** 17–20.

Cori, C. F. (1931). *Physiol. Rev.* **11,** 234.

Cuatrecasas, P., and Hollenberg, M. D. (1976). *Adv. Prot. Chem.* **30,** 252–451.

Cushman, S. W., and Wardzala, L. J. (1980). *J. Biol. Chem.* **255,** 4758–4762.

Czaba, G. (1980). *Biol. Rev.* **55,** 47–63.

Cezch, M. P. (1977). *Annu. Rev. Biochem.* **46,** 359–384.

Czech, M. P. (1980). *Diabetes* **29,** 399–409.

Czech, M. P. (1981). *Fed. Proc. Fed. Am. Soc. Exp. Biol.* **40,** 1737.

Cheng, K., Galasko, G., Huang, L., Kellogg, J., and Larner, J. (1980). *Diabetes* **29,** 659–661.

Debyak, G. R., and Kleinzeller, A. (1980). *J. Biol. Chem.* **255,** 5306–5312.

De Duve, C. (1945). "Glucose, Diabète et Insuline." Masson, Paris.

DeMeyts, P., Bianco, A. R., and Roth, J. (1976). *J. Biol. Chem.* **251,** 1877–1878.

Denton, R., Bridges, B., Brownsey, R., Evans, G., Hughes, W., and Stansbie, D. (1977). *Biochem. Soc. Trans.* **5,** 894–900.

Eng, J., Lee, L., and Yalow, R. S. (1980). *Diabetes* **29,** 164–166.

Exton, J. H., Dehaye, J. P., El-Refai, M. F., and Blackmore, P. F. (1980). *In* "Diabetes 1979" pp. 302–307. Excerpta Medica, Amsterdam.

Fain, J. N., Kovacev, V. P., and Scow, R. O. (1966). *Endocrinology* **78,** 773–778.

Fisher, E. H., Heilmeyer, L. M. G., and Haschke, R. H. (1971). *Curr. Top. Cell Regul.* **4,** 211–251.

Freychet, P. (1976). *Diabetologia* **12,** 83–100.

Fritz, I., ed. (1972). "Insulin Action." Academic Press, New York.

Froesch, E. R., Zapf, J., Meuli, C., Mader, M., Waldvogel, M., Kaufmann, U., and Morell, B. (1975). *Adv. Metab. Dis.* **5,** 211–236.

Fulks, R. M., Li, J. B., and Goldberg, A. L. (1975). *J. Biol. Chem.* **250,** 290–298.

Galbraith, R. A., Wise, C., and Buse, M. G. (1980). *Diabetes* **29,** 571–578.

Gambhir, K. K., Archer, J. A., and Bradley, C. J. (1978). *Diabetes* **27**, 701–708.

Gavin, J. R., Roth, J., Neville, D. M., de Meyts, P., and Buell, D. N. (1974). *Proc. Natl. Acad. Sci. U.S.A.* **71**, 842—88.

Geelen, M. J. H., Harris, R. A., Beynen, A. C., and McCune, S. A. (1980). *Diabetes* **29**, 1006–1022.

Glinsmann, W. H., Hern, E. P., and Lynch, A. (1969). *Am. J. Physiol.* **216**, 698–703.

Goldfine, I. D. (1977). *Diabetes* **26**, 148–55.

Goldstein, M. S. (1961). *Diabetes* **10**, 232–234.

Goldstein, M. S., Henry, W. L., Huddlestun, B., and Levine, R. (1953a). *Am. J. Physiol.* **173**, 207–211.

Goldstein, M. S., Mullick, V., Huddlestun, B., and Levine, R. (1953b). *Am. J. Physiol.* **173**, 212–216.

Gorden, P., Carpentier, J. L., Van Obberghen, E., Barazzone, P., Roth, J., and Orci, L. (1979). *J. Cell Sci.* **39**, 77–88.

Gorden, P., Carpentier, J. L., Freychet, P., and Orci, L. (1980). *Diabetologia* **18**, 263–274.

Guidotti, G., and Foa, P. P. (1961). *Am. J. Physiol.* **201**, 869–872.

Guidotti, G., Kanameishi, D., and Foa, P. P. (1961). *Am. J. Physiol.* **201**, 863–868.

Hall, K., Takano, K., Fryklund, L., and Sievertsson, H. (1975). *Adv. Metab. Dis.* **8**, 19–46.

Hammons, G. T., and Jarett, L. (1979). *Diabetes* **28**, 389.

Hardie, G. (1981). *Trends Biochem. Sci.* **6**, 75–77.

Harmon, J. T., and Kahn, C. R. (1981). *J. Biol. Chem.* **256**, 771g–24.

Havivi, E., and Wetheimer, H. E. (1964). *J. Physiol. (London)* **172**, 342–352.

Hedon, E. (1898). "Travaux de Physiologie" Doin, Paris.

Hems, D. A. (1977). *Trends Biochem. Sci.* **2**, 241–244.

Hems, D. A. (1978). *Biochem. Soc. Trans.* **6**, 33–39.

Hems, D. A., and Whitton, P. D. (1980). *Physiol. Rev.* **60**, 1–50.

Hepp, K. D. (1977). *Diabetologia* **13**, 177–186.

Hers, H. G. (1976). *Annu. Rev. Biochem.* **45**, 167–188.

Hider, R. C., Fern, E. B., and London, D. R. (1971). *Biochem. J.* **125**, 751–756.

Horvat, A. (1980). *Nature (London)* **286**, 906–908.

Jackson, R. J., and Hunt, T. (1980). *Biochem. Soc. Trans.* **8**, 457.

Jacobs, S., Hazum, E., and Cuatrecasas, P. (1980). *J. Biol. Chem.* **255**, 6937–6940.

Jarett, L., and Seals, J. R. (1979). *Science* **206**, 1407–1408.

Jefferson, L. S. (1980). *Diabetes* **29**, 487–496.

Jefferson, L. S., Boyd, T. A., Flaim, K. E., and Peavy, D. E. (1980). *Biochem. Soc. Trans.* **8**, 282–285.

Jungas, R. L. (1971). *Metabolism* **20**, 43–53.

Kahn, C. R. (1976). *J. Cell Biol.* **70**, 261–286.

Kahn, C. R. (1979). *Fed. Proc. Fed. Am. Soc. Exp. Biol.* **38**, 2607–2609.

Kahn, C. R., and Harrison, L. C. (1981). *In* "Carbohydrate Metabolism and its Disorders" (P. J. Randle, I. D. Steiner and W. T. Whelan, eds.). Academic Press, New York.

Kahn, C. R., Baird, K. L., Flier, J. S., and Jarrett, D. B. (1977). *J. Clin. Invest.* **60**, 1094–1106.

Kahn, C. R., Baird, K. L., Jarrett, D. B., and Flier, J. S. (1978). *Proc. Natl. Acad. Sci. U.S.A.* **75**, 4209–4213.

Kahn, C. R., Baird, K. L., Flier, J. S., Grunfeld, C., Harmon, J. T., Harrison, L. C., Karlsson, F. A., Kasuga, M., King, G. L., Lang, U. C., Podskalny, J. M., and Van Obberghen, E. (1981). *Recent Prog. Horm. Res.* **37**, 477–538.

Karnieli, E., Zarnowski, M. J., Hissin, P. J., Simpson, I. A., Salans, L. B., and Cushman, S. W. (1981). *J. Biol. Chem.* **256**, 4772–4777.

Kiechle, F. L., Jarett, L., Kotagal, N., and Popp, D. A. (1981). *J. Biol. Chem.* **256,** 2945–2951.

Kikuchi, K., and Larner, J. (1981a). *Mol. Cell. Biochem.* **37,** 109–k5m.

Kikuchi, K., and Larner, J. (1981b). *Mol. Cell. Biochem.* **37,** 117–123.

Kikuchi, K., Schwartz, C., Creacy, S., and Larner, J. (1981). *Mol. Cell. Biochem.* **37,** 125–130.

King, G. L., and Kahn, C. R. (1981). *Nature (London)* **292,** 644–646.

King, G. L., Kahn, C. R., Rechler, M. M., and Nissley, S. P. (1979). *Clin. Res.* **47,** 486.

Kissebah, A. H., Hope-Gill, H., Vydelingum, N., Tulloch, B. R., Clarke, P. V., and Fraser, T. R. (1975). *Lancet* **1,** 144–147.

Kobayashi, M., and Olefsky, J. M. (1978). *Am. J. Physiol.* **4**(1), E53–62.

Kono, T. (1969). *J. Biol. Chem.* **244,** 1772–1778.

Kono, T., and Barham, F. W. (1971). *J. Biol. Chem* **246,** 6210.

Kono, T., Suzuki, K., Dansey, L. E., Robinson, F. W., and Blevins, T. L. (1981). *J. Biol. Chem.* **256,** 6400–6407.

Krahl, M. E. (1961). "The Action of Insulin on Cells." Academic Press, New York.

Krupp, M. N., and Lane, M. D. (1981). *Diabetes* **30** (Suppl. 1), 7A.

Kuo, J. F., Holmlund, C. E., and Dill, I. K. (1967). *J. Biol. Chem.* **242,** 3659–3664.

Laguesse, M. E. (1893). *C. R. Soc. Biol.* **45,** 819–920.

Larner, J., and Palasi, C. V. (1971). *Curr. Top. Cell. Reg.* **3,** 196–233.

Larner, J., Galasko, G., *et al.* (1979). *Science* **206,** 1408–1410.

Larner, J., Cheng, K., Schwartz, C., Kikuchi, K., Tamura, S., Creacy, S., Dubler, R., Galasko, G., Pullin, C., and Katz, M. (1982). *Rec. Prog. Horm. Res.,* **38,** 511–556.

Le Marchand-Brustel, Y., Jeanrenaud, B., and Freychet, P. (1978). *Am. J. Physiol.* **234,** E348–358.

Levine, R., and Goldstein, M. S. (1955). *Rec. Prog. Horm. Res.* **11,** 343.

Levine, R., Goldstein, M. S., Klein, S., and Huddlestun, B. (1949). *J. Biol. Chem.* **179,** 985–986.

Levine, R., Goldstein, M. S., Huddlestun, B., and Klein, S. (1950). *Am. J. Physiol.* **163,** 70–76.

Little, S. A., and de Haen, C. (1980). *J. Biol. Chem.* **255,** 10888–10895.

Lyons, R. T., Nordeen, S. K., and Young, D. A. (1980). *J. Biol. Chem.* **255,** 6330–6334.

McCraw, E. F., Peterson, M. J., and Ashmore, J. (1967). *Proc. Soc. Exp. Biol. Med.* **126,** 232–236.

McGarry, J. D. (1979). *Diabetes* **28,** 517–523.

McGarry, J. D., and Foster, D. W. (1980). *Annu. Rev. Biochem.* **49,** 395–420.

McGarry, J. D., Takabayashi, Y., and Foster, D. W. (1978). *J. Biol. Chem.* **253,** 8294–8300.

Marchmont, R. J., and Houslay, M. D. (1980). *FEBS Lett.* **118,** 18–24.

Marshall, S., and Olefsky, J. M. (1979). *J. Biol. Chem.* **254,** 10153–10160.

Marshall, S., and Olefsky, J. M. (1980). *J. Clin. Invest.* **66,** 763–772.

Marshall, S., and Olefsky, J. M. (1981). *Diabetes* **30** (Suppl. 1), 8A.

Massague, J., Pilch, P. F., and Czech, M. P. (1980). *Proc. Natl. Acad. Sci. U.S.A.* **77,** 7137–7141.

Mering, V., and Minkowski, O. (1889). *Arch. Exp. Pathol. Pharmacol.* **26,** 371–376.

Minkowski, O. (1893). *Arch. Exp. Pathol. Pharmacol.* **31,** 85–132.

Mortimore, G. E., and Mondon, C. E. (1970). *J. Biol. Chem.* **245,** 2375–2383.

Muggeo, M., Ginsberg, B. H., Both, J., Kahn, C. R., de Meyts, P. and Neville, D. M. (1979). *Endocrinology* **104,** 1393–1402.

Naunyn, A. (1898). "Der Diabetes Mellitus." W. Hoelder, Vienna.

Olefsky, J. M. (1976). *Diabetes* **25,** 1154–1165.

Olefsky, J. M. (1981). *Diabetes* **30,** 148–162.

Olefsky, J. M., and Chang, H. (1979). *Diabetes* **27,** 946–958.

Park, C. R., Bornstein, J., and Post, R. L. (1955). *Am. J. Physiol.* **182,** 12–16.

Park, C. R., Reinwein, D., Henderson, M. J., Cadenas, E., and Morgan, H. E. (1959). *Am. J. Med. Sci.* **26,** 674–684.

Park, C. R., Lewis, S. B., and Exton, J. H. (1972). *Diabetes* **21** (Suppl. 2), 439–446.

Pastan, I. (1975). *Adv. Metab. Dis.* **8,** 7–18.

Pilch, P. F., and Czech, M. P. (1980). *J. Biol. Chem.* **255,** 1722–1731.

Pilch, P. F., Thompson, P. A., and Czech, M. P. (1980). *Proc. Natl. Acad. Sci. U.S.A.* **77,** 915–918.

Pollett, R. J., Standaert, M. L., and Haase, B. A. (1977). *J. Biol. Chem.* **252,** 5828–5834.

Popp, D. A., Kiechle, F. L., Kotagal, N., and Jarett, L. (1980). *J. Biol. Chem.* **255,** 7540–7543.

Porte, D., and Woods, S. C. (1979). *In* "Diabetes 1979," pp. 64–69. Excerpta Medica, Amsterdam.

Posner, B. I., Verma, A. K., Patel, B., and Bergeron, J. J. M. (1980). *In* "Diabetes 1979," pp. 92–97. Excerpta Medica, Amsterdam.

Renold, A. E., and Cahill, G. F. eds. (1965). "Adipose Tissue" (Handbook of Physiology, Section 5). Amer. Physiol. Soc., Washington, D.C.

Renold, A. E., Crofford, O. B., Stauffacher, W., and Jeanrenaud, B. (1965). *Diabetologia* **1,** 4–12.

Resh, M. D., Nemenoff, R. A., and Guidotti, G. (1980). *J. Biol. Chem.* **255,** 10938–10945.

Rieser, P. (1967). "Insulin, Membranes and Metabolism." Williams & Wilkins, Baltimore, Maryland.

Rieser, P., and Rieser, C. H. (1964). *Proc. Soc. Exp. Biol. Med.* **116,** 669–673.

Roach, P. J., and Larner, J. (1976). *Trends Biochem. Sci.* **1,** 110–112.

Rodbell, M. (1966). *J. Biol.Chem.* **241,** 130–136.

Rosenfeld, R. G., and Hintz, R. L. (1980). *Endocrinology* **107,** 1841–1848.

Roth, J. (1979). *In* "Endocrinology," Vol. 3, pp. 2037–2054. Grune & Stratton, New York.

Roth, J. (1981). *Diabetes Care* **4,** 27–32.

Schoenle, E., Zapf, J., and Froesch, E. R. (1981). *Endocrinology* **109,** 561–566.

Seals, J. R., and Czech, M. P. (1981). *J. Biol. Chem.* **256,** 2894–2899.

Seals, J. R., and Jarett, L. (1980). *Proc. Natl. Acad. Sci. U.S.A.* **77,** 77–81.

Sinha, M. K., Ganguli, S., and Sperling, M. A. (1981). *Diabetes* **30,** 411–415.

Soskin, S., and Levine, R. (1946). "Carbohydrate Metabolism." Univ. of Chicago Press, Chicago, Illinois.

Soskin, S., Essex, H. E., Herrick, J. F., and Mann, F. C. (138). *Am. J. Physiol.* **124,** 558–567.

Stadie, W. C. (1954). *Physiol. Rev.* **34,** 52.

Stadie, W. C., Haugaard, N., Hills, A. G., and Marsh, J. B. (1949). *Am. J. Med. Sci.* **218,** 265–274.

Stadie, W. C., Haugaard, N., and Vaughan, M. (1952). *J. Biol. Chem.* **199,** 792.

Stalmans, W. (1976). *Curr. Top. Cell. Reg.* **11,** 51–90.

Stark, R. J., Read, P., and O'Doherty, J. (1980). *Diabetes* **29,** 1040–1049.

Stetten, D. W., and Boxer, G. E. (1944). *J. Biol. Chem.* **156,** 271–278.

Sutherland, E. W., and Robinson, G. A. (1966). *Pharmacol. Rev.* **18,** 145–161.

Suzuki, K., and Kono, T. (1979). *J. Biol. Chem.* **254,** 9786–9794.

Szabo, A. (1981). *Diabetes* **30** (Suppl. 1), 107A.

Terris, S., and Steiner, D. F. (1975). *J. Biol. Chem.* **250,** 8389–8398.

van Houten, M., and Posner, B. I. (1981).

van Houten, M., Posner, B. I., Kopriwa, B. M., and Brawer, J. R. (1979). *Endocrinology* **105,** 666–673.

Van de Werwe, G. W., Stalmans, W., and Hers, H. G. (1977). *Biochem. J.* **162,** 143–146.

Villar-Pallasi, C., and Larner, J. (1961). *Arch. Biochem.* **94,** 436–442.

Vranic, M., and Berger, M. (1979). *Diabetes* **28,** 147–167.

Wallaas, O.,Wallaas, E., Lystad, E., Alertsen, A. R., Horn, R. S., and Fossum, S. (1977). *FEBS Lett.* **80,** 417–422.

Weber, G., Singhal, R. L., and Srivastava, S. K. (1965). *Proc. Natl. Acad. Sci. U.S.A.* **53,** 96–104.

Weinhouse, S. (1976). *Current Top. Cell. Reg.* **11,** 1–97.

Wool, I. G. (1972). *In* "Insulin Action" (I. Fritz, ed.), pp. 201–215. Academic Press, New York.

Wool, I. G., Rampersad, O. R., and Moyer, A. N. (1966). *Am. J. Med.* **40,** 716–723.

Wool, I. G., Stirewalt, W. S., Kurihara, K., Low, R. B., Bailey, P., and Oyer, D. (1968). *Rec. Prog. Horm. Res.* **24,** 139–208.

Zammit, V. A. (1981). *Trend. Biochem. Sci.* **6,** 46–49.

Zierler, K. L. (1957). *Science* **126,** 1067–1068.

Zierler, K. L., and Rogus, E. M. (1980). *Am. J. Physiol.* **239,** E21–29.

VITAMINS AND HORMONES, VOL. 39

Formation of Thyroid Hormones

J. NUNEZ AND J. POMMIER

*Unité de Recherche sur la Glande Thyroide et la Régulation Hormonale,
I.N.S.E.R.M. Bicetre Paris, France*

I. Introduction

The metabolic pathway that allows the synthesis of thyroid hormones from inorganic iodide has been extensively documented at the physiological level, the investigations being greatly facilitated by the use of the iodine isotopes. However, only the phenomenology of this process can be easily studied in these conditions, not the mechanism. *In vivo* the situation is complicated by the asymmetry of the thyroid cell (with its apical and basal membranes); by the morphology of the thyroid vesicles and their variability in size and in activity; by large variations in iodide fluxes, which depend not only on changes in dietary intake but also on the regulatory status of the gland; by the secretion process, which seems to remove preferentially from the colloid either the newly iodinated thyroglobulin or older molecules depending on

175

the physiological situation, etc. (for reviews, see Van Der Hove-Vandenbroucke, 1980; Wollman, 1980). *In vitro,* with the isolated and purified enzyme, these difficulties are eliminated: the system that can be used consists only of a mixture of the enzyme, thyroid peroxidase, H_2O_2, iodide, and thyroglobulin. The concentrations of iodide and thyroglobulin can be modified, but the thyroglobulin must be prepared under such conditions that it is not (or very poorly) iodinated. Studies could be conducted with this simplified system on (a) the chemical mechanism of the enzymatic reaction and its specificity; (b) the role of the structure of thyroglobulin, which is not only the iodine acceptor but also the matrix of thyroid hormone synthesis (coupling reaction); (c) the kinetic properties of the enzyme in performing these two reactions; (d) the role of different ligands in the activity of the enzyme; (e) the origin of some thyroid diseases, which are probably dependent on some defect in the activity of their peroxidase; and (f) the mechanism of action of antithyroid drugs or other chemicals (e.g., thiocyanate) that are suspected to act by modifying the activity of this enzyme.

Some of these aspects of the subject were considered in the earlier review by Taurog (1970b); in this chapter we will examine the successive attempts to solve these problems. Reviews on thyroglobulin have appeared (Ui, 1974; Salvatore and Edelhoch, 1973), and therefore the problems related to the properties of this protein will be summarized only briefly as necessary.

Chemical and enzymatic iodination being also widely used in other fields of research (radioimmunology—methodology of polypeptide hormone and neurotransmitter receptors, labeling of membrane proteins, etc.), the sections related to the iodination reaction will not be restricted to the problems of thyroid interest: some discussion will be included on the chemical mechanisms involved depending on the conditions of iodination.

II. The Enzymatic System

A. Thyroid Peroxidase

Electron microscopic studies (Strum and Karnovsky, 1970; Morrison *et al.,* 1971; Strum *et al.,* 1971; Tice and Wollman, 1974) and differential centrifugation studies (De Groot and Carvalho, 1960; Klebanoff *et al.,* 1962; Ljunggren and Akeson, 1968; Hosoya *et al.,* 1971a; Valenta *et al.,* 1973) have shown that thyroid peroxidase is a membrane-bound enzyme associated with the endoplasmic reticulum and the apical membrane of the thyroid cell. By differential centrifugation studies it was found that the enzyme distributes equally between the mitochondrial and microsomal fraction with no activity detectable in the soluble fraction. Thyroid peroxidase, being tightly bound to the membranes, has proved to be difficult to purify. The methods of extraction of the enzyme activity have varied and involved proteolysis, treatments with ionic or nonionic detergents, or treatment with detergent associated with proteolysis. Depending on the procedure, two types of preparations were obtained: (a) the completely solubilized enzyme obtained by the methods using mild proteolysis (De Groot et al., 1965; Coval and Taurog, 1967; Hosoya and Morrison, 1967; Taurog et al., 1970; Pommier et al., 1972; Alexander, 1977); and (b) the "pseudosolubilized" peroxidase obtained with the nonproteolytic methods (Ljunggren and Akeson, 1968; Davidson et al., 1973; Neary et al., 1973, 1976). In general, the former preparation can be purified further, whereas the "pseudopurified" enzyme aggregates and resists purification. It is likely that the native enzyme is altered by the proteolytic procedure, although the fragment obtained is extremely active and has from experiment to experiment the same hydrodynamic and enzymatic properties.

Alexander (1977) described a highly purified preparation obtained by the use of trypsin only, but the extract contained a heterogeneous mixture of components with peroxidase activity and different molecular sizes; this preparation loses its activity within a few days. In contrast, the enzyme obtained by Taurog (1970a) and Pommier et al. (1972) is exceedingly stable for several years. Taurog's enzyme is prepared by simultaneous use of trypsin and deoxycholate. In our preparation, the thyroid particulate material is pretreated with trypsin under conditions that do not release the enzyme; further treatment of the washed particulate material with digitonin releases the activity in a soluble form. The purity estimated, based on disc electrophoresis, for Taurog's preparation is 80–95%. In our case a similar degree of purity has been achieved, but the enzyme becomes less stable on purification; in contrast, enzyme preparations of 50% purity are stable for years, and the method is easily reproducible.

Table I summarizes the physicochemical properties of the different enzyme preparations. The main conclusions are that thyroid peroxidase is a hemoprotein (one heme per mole) and probably also a glycoprotein (Neary et al., 1977). There is some controversy concerning the nature of the heme, a ferriprotoporphyrin IX, according to Hosoya and Morrison (1967) and Krinsky and Alexander (1971), or a different porphyrin, according to Rawitch et al. (1979).

TABLE I

PHYSICOCHEMICAL PROPERTIES OF ENZYME PREPARATIONS

Enzyme preparation	$A_{410}:A_{280}$	Molecular weight	Sedimentation Coefficient (S)	Carbohydrate Composition (%)	Subunits
Alexander (1977)	0.55	92,000	—	—	—
Hosoya-Morrison (1967)	—	104,000	—	—	—
Pommier (1972)	0.43	103,000	5.2	—	—
Taurog (1979)	0.54	90,000	5.7	10	$2\begin{cases} 60,000 \\ 24,000 \end{cases}$

Most authors have reported a molecular weight of 90,000–100,000. According to Rawitch et al. (1979), the enzyme is composed of two polypeptide chains crosslinked by disulfide bonds with molecular weights of ~60,000 and 24,000, respectively.

B. THE H_2O_2 GENERATING SYSTEM

Little is known about the H_2O_2 generating system that operates in the thyroid gland.

General systems may generate H_2O_2 in cells. For instance, Fischer et al. (1966) proposed that H_2O_2 is formed in the thyroid gland through oxidation of tyramine by monoamine oxidase (MAO). However, the best described H_2O_2 generating system is the NADPH oxidase of the polymorphonuclear leukocytes, where it is associated with myeloperoxidase (Babior, 1977; Ross, 1977). NADPH oxidase catalyzes one-electron reduction of O_2 to the superoxide anion O_2^-.

$$2\ O_2 + NADPH \xrightarrow[\text{oxidase}]{\text{NADPH}} 2\ O_2^- + NADP^+ + H^+$$

H_2O_2 is then produced from the spontaneous or enzymatic dismutation of O_2^-. The enzyme that catalyzes this reaction, the superoxide dismutase, is ubiquitous; it is a metalloenzyme that contains Cu^{2+}, Mn^{2+}, or Zn^{2+} and is either mitochondrial or microsomal.

$$O_2^- + O_2^- + 2\ H^+ \xrightarrow[\text{dismutase}]{\text{superoxide}} H_2O_2 + O_2$$

The existence of superoxide dismutase in the thyroid gland has been reported by Alexander (1972), but the presence of NADPH oxidase has not yet been demonstrated. Other authors (De Groot and Davis, 1961; Schussler and Ingbar, 1961; Klebanoff et al., 1962; Suzuki, 1966;

Ohtaki *et al.,* 1973) found that iodination by a mitochondrial–microsomal system was markedly augmented by addition of reduced pyridine nucleotides and by flavin nucleotides. Based on these observations, Suzuki (1966), Nagasaka *et al.* (1971), and Hati and De Groot (1973) proposed that H_2O_2 formation in the thyroid occurs through NADPH oxidation by a flavoprotein. De Groot reported an iodination of tyrosine in a system including NADPH, NADPH–cytochrome *c*-reductase, cytochrome *c,* and thyroid peroxidase (stimulated by vitamin K_3) (Yamamoto and De Groot, 1975).

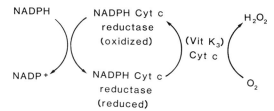

Although Aust *et al.* (1972) reported that NADPH–cytochrome *c* reductase can produce superoxide anion, studies performed in our laboratory were unable to confirm this role for the enzyme.

Our results with thyroid NADPH cytochrome *c* reductase confirmed the results obtained by Auclair *et al.* (1978). These authors had shown that the formation of O_2^- with NADPH-cytochrome P-450 reductase is an artifact when Nitro Blue Tetrazolium (NBT) or epinephrine is used to measure this anion. On the other hand, De Groot observed that superoxide dismutase has no effect on iodination supported by NADPH Cytochrome *c* reductase (Yamamoto and De Groot, 1975).

Although it is likely that NADPH plays a role in generating H_2O_2, none of these schemes can be considered of physiological significance.

Progress in this field is of utmost importance not only because the H_2O_2 generating system is essential in the iodination and coupling reactions catalyzed by thyroid peroxidase, but also because it is possible that it is an important substrate for TSH and cAMP regulation (Ahn and Rosenberg, 1970).

III. The Iodination Reaction

A. General Aspects

Protein iodination can be achieved under enzymatic and nonenzymatic conditions. It has long been known that several purified peroxidases, including horseradish peroxidase (Nunez *et al.,* 1965b), lactoperoxidase (Morrison and Sisco-Bayse, 1970), myeloperoxidase (Klebanoff *et al.*, 1962), chloroperoxidase (Taurog and Howells, 1966), and thyroid peroxidase, when supplemented with H_2O_2 or a H_2O_2 generating system, catalyze very efficiently the iodination of free tyrosine or of tyrosine residues of different proteins. Chemical iodination can also be achieved under a variety of conditions, i.e., with molecular iodine, I_2, with iodide in the presence of chloramine-T, with ICl, etc. We will see below that the conditions of iodination as well as the products vary markedly depending on the enzyme, the protein that is iodinated, or the chemical procedure used. However, the basic chemical mechanism appears to be similar under all conditions: an oxidized species of iodine reacts with the ortho position of the tyrosine phenolic ring to yield successively a mono and a diiodo derivative, monoiodo-(MIT) and diiodo-(DIT)tyrosine:

$$I_{ox} + Tyr \rightarrow MIT + H^+ \qquad\qquad (1)$$
$$MIT + I_{ox} \rightarrow DIT + H^+ \qquad\qquad (2)$$

The peroxidases are also able to catalyze the oxidation of a variety of other substrates. For instance, in the absence of a protein acceptor, iodide is oxidized to I_2, which, in the presence of excess I^-, forms I_3^-. The formation of I_3^- can be followed by spectrometry at 353 nm (Alexander, 1962), and this reaction is often used to measure the activity of the peroxidases. In addition, various phenolic substrates are oxidized by all the peroxidases tested; with free tyrosine the product is bityrosine, and this reaction can be followed by spectrofluorimetry (Bayse *et al.*, 1972; Michot *et al.*, 1979); with guaiacol, tetraguaiacol is formed, which can be measured by spectrometry (Chance and Maehly, 1955). Thus the peroxidases appear as a class of relatively unspecific enzymes, since they are able to oxidize a variety of substrates having in common only the fact that they all are hydrogen and electron donors.

For theoretical and practical reasons this view needs, however, to be amended, since with the same enzyme, for instance, the pH optimum of oxidation varies for each substrate. For example, iodide oxidation to I_2 is generally catalyzed at a slightly more acidic pH than tyrosine iodination, whereas bityrosine formation occurs at a much more and distinct alkaline pH. In addition, and this is less surprising, the optimum pH for each substrate varies with the peroxidase. One may therefore speculate that the lack of specificity seen with the peroxidase is only apparent, since at a given pH a given enzyme performs mainly one type of reaction. We will see below that two sequential reactions, protein iodination and thyroid hormone synthesis, may even be dissociated by using the same enzyme, horseradish peroxidase, at two different pH levels.

As far as the protein acceptor is concerned, all the peroxidases so far tested show a complete lack of specificity: probably the only requirement is that one or more tyrosine residues must be exposed at the surface of the protein so that they can interact with the enzyme. Several lines of information suggest that both the oxidized iodine species and the tyrosine residue of the protein are bound to the enzyme and that the iodination reaction proceeds inside this ternary complex, i.e. before the release of the products.

$$E + I^- + Tyr - protein \rightarrow (E - I - Tyr - protein) \rightarrow E + \text{iodinated protein} \quad (3)$$

In contrast, under chemical conditions of iodination, the iodide-oxidized species (I_2 or I^+) is free in the medium and can penetrate more or less easily inside the protein, thus iodinating tyrosine residues that are not accessible to the peroxidases. This probably explains why the levels of iodination reached under chemical conditions are always much higher than those obtained by enzymatic iodination. The complete incubation system for *in vitro* studies of protein iodination requires, therefore, well defined pH conditions, a protein acceptor, the enzyme, iodide, and a source of H_2O_2.

The amount of H_2O_2 that is introduced into the medium is critical for several reasons. The first reaction catalyzed by the peroxidase is the formation of an addition compound with H_2O_2. This reaction has been extensively studied but remains essentially at the level of knowledge reached by Chance and George (Chance, 1952; Theorell *et al.*, 1952; George, 1952, 1953). The first enzymatic derivative that is formed contains the two equivalents of oxidation of H_2O_2 (compound I). These equivalents of oxidation are removed stepwise to produce successively compound II and then the native enzyme.

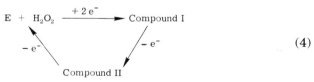

$$(4)$$

More sophisticated models (Yokota and Yamazaki, 1965) have been proposed for such a reaction, but practically this scheme remains operational. The two equivalents of oxidation contained in compound I are thus used to oxidize two molecules of monohydrogen donor, or one molecule of bihydrogen donor.

$$E - H_2O_2 + 2 AH \rightarrow 2 A^. + 2 H_2O \quad (5)$$
$$E - H_2O_2 + AH_2 \rightarrow A^. + 2 H_2O \quad (6)$$

Since the rate of the iodination reaction depends on the presence of enough H_2O_2 in the medium, maximal rates of this reaction can be achieved only in the presence of nonlimiting amounts of hydrogen peroxide. This is why, in principle, one may add a great excess of H_2O_2 to start the reaction. However, such a procedure may be misleading, since an inactive peroxidase complex may be formed with excess H_2O_2 (compound IV) (Keilin and Hartree, 1951). A range of H_2O_2 concentrations that are neither limiting nor inhibitory must be chosen, but, depending on the pH, the substrate, etc., this range varies widely; for instance, thyroid peroxidase is rapidly inactivated in the presence of slight excesses of H_2O_2 at alkaline pH values (8–9); iodide oxidation to I_2 is catalyzed with a much higher turnover than protein iodination at pH 7.4 with the same enzyme, and greater amounts of H_2O_2 are therefore required to obtain maximal rates of iodide oxidation. It is possible to adjust the proper amount of H_2O_2 either by adding it in small portions during the time course of the reaction or by continuous infusion or by producing it continuously with an H_2O_2 generating system, usually glucose–glucose oxidase; with this latter solution it is easy to obtain a steady-state production of H_2O_2 suited for each reaction, pH level, substrate concentration, etc.

To be assured that H_2O_2 is neither limiting nor inhibitory, the simplest method is to measure the initial rate of a reaction with a constant amount of both the substrate and the H_2O_2 generating system and in the presence of varying amounts of enzyme; if the rates are proportional to the enzyme concentration, one may conclude that a correct steady-state production of H_2O_2 has been obtained (Fig. 1).

B. The Oxidized Iodine Species in the Iodination Reaction

It is well established that all the peroxidases so far tested are able to catalyze the oxidation of I^- to I_2. Since I_2 is itself a good iodinating species of tyrosine and of tyrosine residues present in proteins, it has been believed for a long time that the sole role of the peroxidases is to produce I_2, I_2, once released in the medium, would subsequently iodinate the protein in a nonenzymatic substitution reaction.

$$\text{Tyr} - \text{protein} + I_2 \rightarrow \text{MIT} - \text{protein} + \text{IH} \tag{7}$$

However, enzymatic iodination can be performed, depending on the peroxidase, at acidic or neutral pH levels, whereas chemical iodination by I_2 is efficient only above pH 7 (Mayberry $et~al.$, 1964). In contrast, I^+ is an efficient iodinating species at acidic or neutral pH levels. The

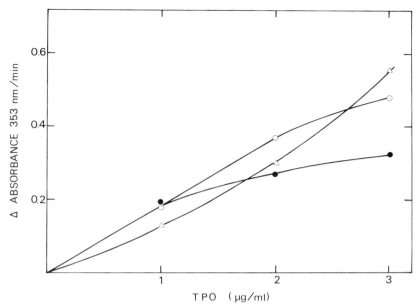

F<small>IG</small>. 1. Relationship between initial velocities of iodide oxidation and thyroid peroxidase (TPO) concentrations obtained for three glucose oxidase concentrations: 5 μg/ml ($\bullet$——$\bullet$), 7.5 μg/ml ($\bigcirc$——$\bigcirc$), and 15 μg/ml ($\triangle$——$\triangle$). The oxidation of iodide (10^{-2} M) was measured at 353 nm in 0.05 M phosphate buffer, pH 7.4, with 6 mM glucose. Reprinted from Pommier *et al.* (1976).

possibility existed therefore that I_2 is formed from I^+ in the absence of a protein acceptor whereas in its presence I^+ reacts immediately with a tyrosine residue.

Iodide is in fact a two-electron donor that can be oxidized stepwise by the peroxidase, yielding successively the iodide atom $I^{\cdot}$ and then the iodinium ion I^+.

$$I^- \xrightarrow{-e^-} I^{\cdot} \xrightarrow{-e^-} I^+ \qquad (8)$$

Both $I^{\cdot}$ and I^+ may produce I_2 when released into the medium.

$$2I^{\cdot} \rightarrow I_2 \qquad (9)$$
$$I^+ + I^- \rightarrow I_2 \qquad (10)$$

In addition, both iodine oxidized species, I^+ and $I^{\cdot}$, may react at neutral or acidic pH with a tyrosine. I^+ can react directly with a reduced tyrosine residue.

$$I^+ + \text{tyrosine} \rightarrow \text{MIT} + H^+ \qquad (11)$$

whereas the formation of MIT from $I^{\cdot}$ is possible only if the tyrosine residue is also oxidized to the free radical $Tyr^{\cdot}$.

$$I^{\cdot} + Tyr^{\cdot} \rightarrow MIT + H^{\cdot} \tag{12}$$

The oxidation of Tyr to $Tyr^{\cdot}$ is actually catalyzed by the peroxidases, since tyrosine is a phenolic monohydrogen donor, i.e., a good substrate for these enzymes.

Three oxidized iodine species might therefore be involved in the enzymic iodination reaction: I_2, $I^{\cdot}$, and I^+.

I_2 is probably not the iodinating species, since, as indicated above, tyrosine iodination with molecular iodine occurs only at alkaline pH levels. Mayberry et al. (1964) have shown that the rate of the chemical iodination with I_2 depends on the amount of phenoxide formed, which itself increases with the pH; at neutral pH very little phenoxide is formed. In addition, a second alkaline catalysis is required for the removal of the hydrogen present in position 3.

$$\text{(13)}$$

Thus, at pH 7.4 with thyroid peroxidase, and a fortiori at pH 5 with the horseradish enzyme, the rate of the iodination reaction with I_2 is very slow, since it depends on such a double alkaline catalysis. Chemical iodination by I_2 requires 15–20 hours of incubation, whereas similar maximal levels of thyroglobulin iodination (70–80 iodine atoms per mole of protein), are obtained in less than 15 minutes under enzymatic conditions. The production of I_2 being very fast, whatever the enzyme used, this oxidized species of iodine cannot be involved in the enzymatic reaction.

Actually there is competition between I_2 formation and protein iodination. For instance, Fig. 2 shows the results of one experiment comparing the rates of I_2 formation and of thyroglobulin iodination at different iodide concentrations (0.01 to 4 mM) and under identical conditions of pH and with identical H_2O_2 and peroxidase concentrations (Pommier et al., 1973a). It is clear that at low iodide concentrations no I_2 is produced, at high iodide concentrations I_2 is formed and protein iodination is inhibited. Similar results have been obtained by Taurog (1970a). They reveal that I_2 is not the iodinating species and that the enzyme is able to catalyze two possible competitive pathways from I^-,

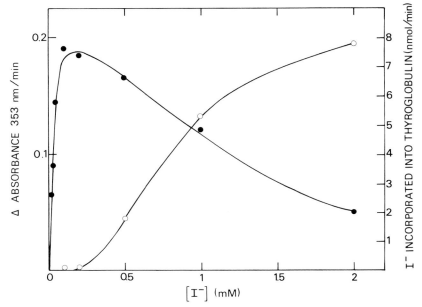

FIG. 2. Relationship between initial rates of I_2 formation ($\bigcirc$——$\bigcirc$) or of thyroglobulin iodination ($\bullet$——$\bullet$) and iodide concentration. Reprinted from Pommier *et al.* (1973a).

one resulting in the formation of I_2 the other in the iodination of thyroglobulin.

$$E_{H_2O_2} + 2\ I^- \to I_{ox} \begin{array}{l} \nearrow I_2 \\[6pt] \searrow \text{iodination} \end{array} \tag{14}$$

Other lines of evidence against the view that I_2 is the active intermediate in enzymatically catalyzed iodination are also that (*a*) when thyroglobulin is iodinated either enzymatically or chemically with I_2, the number of MIT and DIT residues formed is different depending on the procedure (Dème *et al.*, 1978); (*b*) the lack of correlation between the formation of I_2 and protein iodination was directly demonstrated with a pathological thyroid peroxidase; this defective enzyme catalyzed iodide oxidation to I_2 efficiently but was not able to iodinate proteins (see below) (Pommier *et al.*, 1976).

It is much more difficult to decide whether I^- or I^+ is the oxidized species involved in protein enzymatic iodination. Free tyrosine is a good substrate for the peroxidases and is oxidized by these enzymes to 3,3'-bi(tyrosine) [Eq. (15)]; however, the pH optimum for this reaction is, whatever the enzyme, much more alkaline than that of the iodination reaction. It is very difficult, in addition, to devise unequivocal experiments to prove that free tyrosine or tyrosine-protein is oxidized during the iodination reaction and that the free radical, Tyr·, is the iodinated species.

$$2 \text{ Tyr} \xrightarrow{-\text{H·}} \text{bityrosine} \qquad (15)$$
$$\text{Tyr·} + \text{I·} \rightarrow \text{MIT} \qquad (16)$$

What can be shown in contrast (Nunez and Pommier, 1969) is that the protein interacts with the enzyme during the iodination reaction; as indicated above, an intermediary ternary complex is probably formed, with the protein and iodide both being bound to the enzyme.

C. THE TWO-SUBSTRATE SITE MODEL

The first evidence that peroxidases have two binding sites for the substrate comes from kinetic studies on I_2 formation performed with horseradish peroxidase. If I_2 is formed from $I^+ + I^-$ or from 2 I· previously released into the medium, the kinetic data would fit a first-order mechanism. Actually the results obtained at pH 6.9 are consistent with a second-order reaction (Pommier et al., 1973a). This means that 2 mol of substrate are bound to the enzyme, oxidized, and then dimerized inside the enzyme; the product I_2 is then released into the medium.

$$E + 2\,I \rightarrow E \Big\langle{}^{I}_{I} \quad E - I_2 \rightarrow E + I_2 \qquad (17)$$

Maguire and Dunford (1972) found that lactoperoxidase exhibits both a first- and a second-order dependence on the concentration of iodide ion. However, it is again difficult to know from the kinetic data whether the two oxidation equivalents contained in compound I are used to remove two electrons from only one of the two iodide molecules, thus yielding the ternary complex $E \Big\langle{}^{I^+}_{I^-}$, or if only one electron is removed from each of the two moles of substrate, yielding $E \Big\langle{}^{I·}_{I·}$. This second ternary complex is more likely to be formed, but again no proof can be obtained from these kinetic studies.

A second piece of evidence is provided by the competition between I_2 formation and protein iodination reported above (Fig. 2). Since I_2 is not the iodinating species, this competition also suggests a two-site model, one iodide being bound to the first site and the second site being able to bind either a second molecule of iodide or a tyrosine residue.

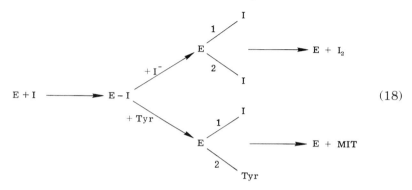

(18)

This model is further supported by the fact that the K_m of iodide differs by two orders of magnitude depending on the reaction that is studied. In the iodination reaction catalyzed by thyroid peroxidase, K_m of iodide is 0.08 mM (K_1), whereas for iodide oxidation it is equal to 6.0 mM (K_2). K_1 and K_2 may reflect the affinity of iodide for site 1 and site 2 of the enzyme, respectively.

Since two different substrates bind to the substrate sites, one may raise the question whether the binding is ordered or at random (Pommier *et al.*, 1973a). This question has been answered for horseradish peroxidase: both substrates may be bound at random, but when iodide is first bound the rate of formation of the products is faster. The data fit a random-order sequence of substrate fixation, but with one of the two sequences kinetically preferred.

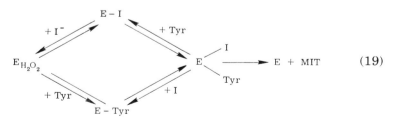

(19)

Actually, in the presence of an excess of protein (versus iodide) the reaction is so slow that the iodination is inhibited. This finding provides further evidence for the existence of an intermediary ternary complex between the enzyme and the two substrates, iodide and a tyrosine residue of the protein. It also has a practical interest, since it explains why horseradish peroxidase cannot be used to prepare proteins labeled with iodide at high specific activity and low iodine content. However, neither thyroid nor lactoperoxidase seem to follow the same mechanism of iodination and thus may be used for such purposes.

Finally the two-site model enables a decision to be made between I^+ and I^- as an iodinating species. As indicated above, I^+ reacts easily at neutral pH with nonoxidized tyrosine, whereas with I^-, tyrosine must be oxidized to Tyr$^.$; with I^+, the mechanism of the reaction is very similar to that involving I_2, but no alkaline catalysis is required since I^+ is already charged positively and can attack directly the ortho position of tyrosine. With I^-, the mechanism is quite different, since iodination results from the radical addition between two unshared electrons, one from I^- and other from Tyr$^.$. However, Roman and Dunford (1972) observed that, in the presence of iodide, native peroxidase was directly produced from compound I without any detectable amount of compound II. On the basis of these spectrophotometric results, they concluded that 1 mol of compound I (1 mol of H_2O_2 per mole of peroxidase) oxidizes only 1 mol of iodide producing I^+. Such a conclusion would be valid only if no iodination of the enzyme occurred. Using the experimental conditions of Roman and Dunford (pH 5.9, high horseradish peroxidase concentration), we have found evidence that horseradish peroxidase behaves not only as an enzyme but also as a protein substrate for iodination. Indirect proof has been provided (Yip and Hadley, 1966, 1967; Bjorksten, 1970; Pommier et al., 1973a, 1976) suggesting that I^- is the oxidized species involved in these enzymatic reactions. More direct proof was provided by a defective peroxidase prepared from a congenital goiter (Pommier et al., 1976). As reported below, this enzyme oxidized I^- to I_2 with the same K_m as a normal enzyme but was almost unable to iodinate tyrosine; further experiments revealed that it oxidizes phenols very poorly (guaiacol, for instance, or tyrosine).

To explain this result one may assume that the enzyme defect concerns site 2, i.e., the site that binds tyrosine in the normal enzyme. If this site still binds iodide efficiently, I_2 formation will be unchanged. If, on the contrary, the same site binds tyrosine less efficiently, protein iodination will be impaired.

Actually, above pH 8 with thyroid peroxidase, I_2 production is completely abolished as well as protein iodination; in contrast, the enzyme catalyzes very efficiently tyrosine oxidation to bityrosine. If one assumes that raising the pH increases the affinity of the second tyrosine for site 1, 2 mol of this substrate will be bound to the intermediary complex and bityrosine may be formed. Similarly lowering the pH with horseradish peroxidase favors I_2 formation at the expense of protein iodination. Thus, although the two sites seem to be relatively nonspecific since they may bind several types of substrates, some sort of specificity may be demonstrated by changing the pH of the medium. This conclusion was used to explain why horseradish peroxidase is not able, under usual conditions, to iodinate free tyrosine. According to the two-site model and to the expected changes in affinity of the two sites, depending on the pH, it was postulated that free tyrosine cannot be iodinated because it is dimerized readily at the pH previously used (5.5); lowering the pH to 4.8 resulted actually in low dimer formation and high MIT and DIT synthesis. Further decrease of the pH to ~4 inhibits tyrosine iodination since the affinity of site 2 for iodide increases; I_2 is formed, and iodination is suppressed.

$$E\begin{smallmatrix} \text{site 1} \\[6pt] \text{site 2} \end{smallmatrix} \quad + \quad 2\ \text{Tyr} \longrightarrow E\begin{smallmatrix} \text{Tyr} \\[6pt] \text{Tyr} \end{smallmatrix} \longrightarrow E\ +\ \text{bityrosine} \quad (20)$$

In conclusion, as to the mechanism of iodination, it is seen that (a) both iodide and tyrosine are bound to the enzyme, each one of these two substrates occupying one of the two substrate sites; (b) both substrates undergo a monoelectron oxidation yielding the free radicals I· and Tyr· (or MIT), respectively; (c) these radicals undergo radical addition while still bound to the enzyme in a ternary complex; (d) the product (MIT or DIT) is released into the medium.

$$E_{H_2O_2} + I^- \longrightarrow E\begin{smallmatrix} I^\circ \\[6pt] \ \end{smallmatrix} + \text{Tyr} \longrightarrow E\begin{smallmatrix} I^\circ \\[6pt] \text{Tyr}^\circ \end{smallmatrix} \longrightarrow E + \text{MIT}$$

$$(21)$$

$$E_{H_2O_2} + \text{MIT} + I^- \longrightarrow E\begin{smallmatrix} I^\circ \\[6pt] \text{MIT}^\circ \end{smallmatrix} \longrightarrow E + \text{DIT}$$

Although several lines of evidence suggest that I· is the iodinating species, this conclusion might be valid only for thyroid and lacto- and horseradish peroxidases (and at pH 5 to 7). With chloroperoxidase, Morris and Hager (1966) have reported that the iodinating species is I^+. However, chloroperoxidase works at very acidic pH levels and oxidizes not only iodide, but also chloride.

D. RELATIVE PROPERTIES OF THE DIFFERENT PEROXIDASES

As we have seen above, the optimum pH for the oxidation of the different substrates of a given peroxidase varies markedly depending on the enzyme. Thus, most of the comparative data in the literature must be taken with reservations, since the experiments were often performed at the same pH and without taking into account the optimal iodide or H_2O_2 concentration. Since the protein is involved in the reaction, its concentration must also be carefully controlled. At pH 7.4, for instance, the rates of iodination are dependent on protein concentration; with $\sim 2 \times 10^{-4} M$, iodide maximal rates are observed with $\sim 10^{-6}$ M noniodinated thyroglobulin when thyroid peroxidase is used.

Once these precautions are taken, a comparison can be made between the K_m of iodide for iodide oxidation and protein iodination, respectively, with three enzymes, thyroid and lacto- and horseradish peroxidases. Table II shows that the efficiency in catalyzing the iodination reaction follows the order: thyroid > lacto > horseradish peroxidases. In contrast, for iodide oxidation the affinity decreases in the opposite order: horseradish > lacto- > thyroid peroxidases. If the K_m oxidation (K_1) represents the affinity of the first site in the two-site model discussed above and K_2 that of the second site, it is clear that the largest difference between these two parameters is found with thyroid peroxidase ($K_2/K_1 = \sim 75$), whereas it is also different for the other two enzymes ($K_2/K_1 = 17$ and 6, respectively). This means that, with thyroid peroxidase, maximal rates of iodination are obtained with much lower iodide concentrations; similarly, the inhibition of the iodination reaction in the presence of an excess of iodide occurs at higher iodide concentrations than with the two other enzymes. The thyroid enzyme appears, therefore, to be the best adapted to perform protein iodination at high rates and in a larger range of iodide concentrations.

Taurog et al. (1974), comparing lacto- and thyroid peroxidase in the iodination of bovine serum albumin observed similarly that thyroid peroxidase is more efficient than lactoperoxidase at low iodide concentrations.

We will see below that the distribution of iodine between MIT and DIT also differs depending on the enzyme, thyroid peroxidase being

TABLE II

COMPARISON OF THE IODIDE CONCENTRATION GIVING HALF-MAXIMAL RATES ("K_m IODIDE")
MEASURED FOR BOTH REACTIONS: IODIDE OXIDATION AND PROTEIN IODINATION, WITH
THYROID, LACTO-, AND HORSERADISH PEROXIDASES

Peroxidase	"K_m" iodination (K_1)	"K_m" oxidation (K_2)	K_2/K_1
Thyroid	0.8×10^{-4}	6×10^{-3}	75
Lacto	2.0×10^{-4}	3.5×10^{-3}	17
Horseradish	4×10^{-4}	2.5×10^{-3}	6

best adapted to synthesize iodotyrosine residues potentially able to couple to thyroid hormones.

IV. THE COUPLING REACTION

Thyroid hormones are formed from some of the iodotyrosine residues that are present in the iodinated thyroglobulin molecule. This process includes several aspects that can be analyzed separately: (a) the mechanism of the coupling reaction; (b) the role of the structure of the thyroglobulin molecule; (c) the relationship between iodination and coupling and the role of thyroid peroxidase in these two processes.

A. MECHANISM OF THE COUPLING REACTION

Johnson and Tewkesbury (1942) proposed a model to explain the conversion of two diiodotyrosine residues of thyroglobulin to thyroxine. This model includes four steps: (a) the oxidation of two iodotyrosyl residues to iodotyrosyl radicals; (b) the formation of an unstable quinol ether by radical addition of these two iodotyrosyl radicals; and (c) the decomposition of the quinol intermediate to 1 mol of thyroid hormone and 1 mol of dehydroalanine; (d) the decomposition of the unstable dehydroalanine residue to pyruvic acid and ammonia during the hydrolysis of the protein.

Step 1 is very likely to occur since the coupling reaction is an enzymatic process and, on the other hand, peroxidases are known to catalyze free radical oxidations. However, coupling can also be achieved under purely chemical conditions, though at a very slow rate; thus it seems likely that the first step is not very critical and that diiodotyrosine residues may react to yield thyroid hormone without being oxidized to free radicals. It seems likely that in such a case these residues are ionized in a reaction similar to that demonstrated for the chemical iodination with I_2 [see Eq. (13)].

Little is known about step 2, i.e., the quinol ether intermediate postulated by Johnson and Tewkesbury (1942). It is even possible that this intermediate does not form and that coupling is a concerted mechanism in which the two diiodotyrosine residues couple, yielding immediately the thyroid hormone residue and a three-carbon fragment. This fragment is derived from the aliphatic side chain of one of the two diiodotyrosine residues. The side chain, which has been for many years a matter of controversy, has been named the "lost side chain" (Cahnmann and Matsuura, 1960). Johnson and Tewkesbury predicted that the lost side chain would be split off from the quinol ether intermediate as dehydroalanine, but Harington (1944), in a critical review of their work, argued that it might be converted either to dehydro-alanine or to serine. On the other hand, if dehydroalanine residues were formed within the polypeptide chain of thyroglobulin they would appear in the protein hydrolyzate as pyruvic acid and ammonia, since free dehydroalanine undergoes spontaneous hydrolysis.

Pyruvic acid as well as serine have been reported as reaction products in nonenzymatic model reactions carried out under non-physiological conditions. Other nonenzymatic model reactions carried out at pH 7.5 by Pitt-Rivers and James (1958) gave rise to hydroxy-pyruvic acid.

Thus, with model reactions, different results have been reported: dehydroalanine and pyruvate (Johnson and Tewkesbury, 1942), hy-droxpyruvate (Pitt-Rivers and James, 1958), and serine (Sela and Sarid, 1956), respectively, seemed to be good candidates for the products de-rived from the "lost side chain."

The availability of thyroid peroxidase and of ^{14}C-labeled noniodin-ated thyroglobulin allowed a reexamination of the mechanism of the coupling reaction and the identification of the side chain in physiologi-cal and nonphysiological conditions.

With Gavaret and Cahnmann (Gavaret *et al.,* 1979), experiments were conducted using [^{14}C]tyrosine-labeled thyroglobulin prepared by incubating thyroid slices with [^{14}C]tyrosine; as previously reported (Nunez *et al.,* 1965a), the neosynthesized thyroglobulin obtained in these *in vitro* conditions is not iodinated and thus does not contain ^{14}C-labeled iodotyrosine or ^{14}C-labeled thyroid hormones. *In vitro,* en-zymatic iodination of this purified protein yields ^{14}C-labeled hormones and a ^{14}C-labeled derivative of the side chain. After enzymatic hydro-lysis, this fragment has been identified as pyruvic acid, whereas after acidic hydrolysis labeled acetic acid was formed. In both cases serine or hydroxypyruvic acid were absent whatever the amount of thyroxine formed. During enzymatic iodination of ^{14}C-labeled thyroglobulin, the radioactivity of the acidic compound was always one-fifth of that of the hormone. Therefore pyruvate or acetic acid could be the products de-rived from the side chain after hydrolysis of thyroglobulin. Both pyru-vate and acetic acid are likely to be formed upon the decomposition, during the proteolysis, of a dehydroalanine residue present in the nonhydrolyzed protein; free dehydroalanine decomposes to pyru-vate + ammonia under enzymatic conditions and to acetic acid, CO_2, and ammonia under acidic conditions.

Direct proof of dehydroalanine being present before hydrolysis was provided by treating the native iodinated protein either with sodium borohydride or with benzylmercaptan (Gavaret *et al.*, 1980). As expected, ^{14}C-labeled alanine was formed with the first reagent and *S*-benzylcysteine with the second. Again, for each hormone residue synthesized, one dehydroalanine residue was formed.

Scheme 1 summarizes the different results obtained in the identification of the "lost side chain" depending on the analytical procedure used.

Thus two final steps of the model proposed by Johnson and Tewkesbury (1942) are likely to occur under physiological conditions. Scheme 2 summarizes the two possible mechanisms of the coupling reaction (free radical or ionic oxidation) as demonstrated by Gavaret *et al.* (1981).

B. Role of Thyroglobulin in the Iodination and the Coupling Reactions

Extensive studies of the properties of thyroglobulin have been performed in the past few years (for review, see Ui, 1974; Salvatore and Edelhoch, 1973), and the data accumulated show that this protein

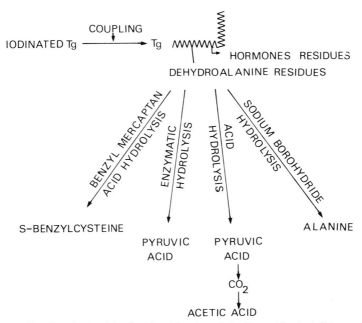

SCHEME 1. Results obtained in the identification of the "lost side chain" depending on the analytical procedure used. Tg, thyroglobulin. Reprinted from Gavaret *et al.* (1980).

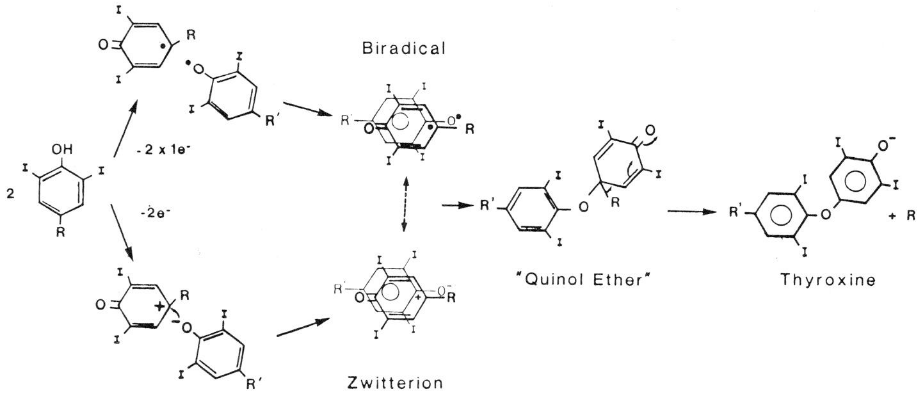

SCHEME 2. Coupling reaction.

plays a central role in the physiology of the thyroid gland and particularly in (a) the trapping and storage of iodine: more iodine is present in thyroglobulin in the form of iodotyrosine residues that never undergo coupling than in the form of thyroid hormones; (b) the storage of hormones: large amounts of thyroglobulin are present in the colloid follicle, thus providing a stored form of thyroid hormones sufficient to maintain euthyroidism for long periods of time; and (c) the process of iodination and coupling.

Only this latter aspect will be discussed in this chapter.

1. *The Iodine Content of Thyroglobulin*

Thyroglobulin is a glycoprotein with a molecular weight of 660,000 and a sedimentation coefficient of ~19 S. It may be dissociated into two 12 S subunits under a variety of conditions, but the amino acid sequence of the elementary chains remains unknown. The amino acid composition of this protein is not unusual, and ~140 tyrosine residues per mole of protein are present. Thus, though a great effort has been made in the past few years (Salvatore and Edelhoch, 1973), little is known about the structure of this protein. More data are available on its iodine content and on the iodoamino acid distribution. However, here again a major difficulty is encountered, which depends on the variability of the iodine content and on the heterogeneity of iodination of this protein.

In most mammals the iodine content of thyroglobulin varies between 0.2 and 1% of the protein weight, i.e., between 10 and 50 iodine atoms per molecule. Most of this variability depends on environmental factors such as the availability of iodine in the diet. However, thyroglobulin, even if isolated from a single gland, is highly heterogeneous as far as its iodine content is concerned (Ingbar et al., 1959; Roche et al., 1960; Ui et al., 1961; Assem et al., 1964). Such heterogeneity has been observed by determination of the iodine content after fractionation by column chromatography or by density gradient ultracentrifugation. For instance, Gavaret et al. (1977), with rats kept on a well controlled diet containing a constant amount of iodine, still found very extensive iodine heterogeneity of thyroglobulin. This heterogeneity is illustrated in Figure 3, where a preparation of rat thyroglobulin labeled at isotopic equilibrium with ^{125}I was fractionated by isopycnic centrifugation in RbCl. It is clear that iodine distribution is quite heterogeneous and that the number of iodine atoms per molecule of the thyroglobulin sample used for this analysis was only an average; this considerably weakens the studies of iodine distribution in thyroglobulin and precludes any speculation on the reactivity of the tyrosine residues of this protein. The only numbers that might be significant are those obtained for thyroglobulin samples containing maximal iodine contents; such samples contain, respecitvely, ~20 mol of MIT, ~10 of DIT, ~3 of thyroxine (T_4), and ~0.3 of triiodothyronine (T_3) per mole of protein. This means that a total of ~40 tyrosine residues out of ~140 undergo iodination in vivo in the rat and that only ~7–10 of the iodotyrosines thus formed are able to couple. However, even at these highest levels of iodination there is still heterogeneity.

This has prevented several studies, for instance those related to the structure of the protein in the region of the sequence containing the hormone residues. Because of this heterogeneity, and also because the thyroglobulin structure remains largely unknown, peptide analysis of iodine-containing peptides has been unsuccessful so far. Progress in this respect has occurred (Gavaret et al., 1977); when very poorly iodinated thyroglobulin was iodinated in vitro with thyroid peroxidase, no sign of heterogeneity was found whatever the level of iodination (Fig. 3b). Thus, neither the iodinating enzyme nor the molecular structure of the thyroglobulin are of importance in the heterogeneity of iodination. The only possibilities left to explain the large variability in the iodine content of native thyroglobulin are those related to anatomical or functional properties of the thyroid gland. For instance, variations in the iodide flux or in the thyroglobulin availability at the level of the iodination site might generate such heterogeneity.

In addition, the finding that in vitro iodinated thyroglobulin is ho-

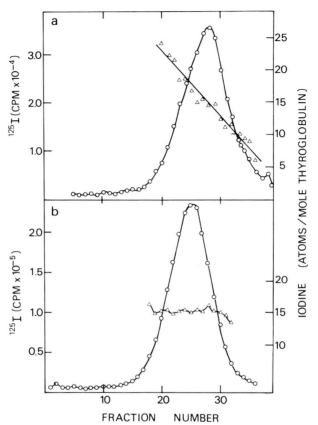

Fig. 3. (a) Iodine distribution in equilibrium density gradient (33.7% RbCl) of rat thyroglobulin labeled at isotopic equilibrium with [125]I. The average iodine content of thyroglobulin was 14.3 atoms per mole. O——O, ^{125}I cpm; △——△, iodine (atoms) per mole of thyroglobulin. (b) Equilibrium density gradient (33.7% RbCl) of human goiter thyroglobulin after iodination *in vitro* by thyroid peroxidase at an average iodine content of 15 iodine (atoms per mole of thyroglobulin). O——O, ^{125}I cpm; △——△, iodine (atoms) per mole of thyroglobulin. Reprinted from Gavaret *et al.* (1977).

mogeneous as far as its iodine content is concerned allowed a renewal of the studies on the iodoamino acid distribution and on the relationship between the level of iodination and the level of coupling.

2. The Reactivity of the Tyrosine Residues of Thyroglobulin

In native thyroglobulin, as well as in many other proteins, only a fraction of the tyrosyl residues are available to iodination, most likely those residues exposed to the solvent and having phenolic groups with normal ionization behavior. When the thyroglobulin molecule is noniodinated it contains a group of tyrosine residues not available to the enzyme, whereas a second group undergoes only monoiodination, and a third group diiodination. This depends on the structure of thyroglobulin and hence on the availability of the tyrosine residues. In addition, as has been reported above, the tyrosine residues are probably oxidized during the iodination reaction; thus the sequence of iodination might depend not only on the availability, but also on the reactivity, of the tyrosyl residues that are potentially capable of being iodinated. If their reactivity is identical the iodination reaction would proceed at random. If each tyrosyl residue differs in its reactivity from the others the iodination would occur sequentially. To decide between these possibilities Gavaret et al. (1977) have performed double labeling experiments. Very poorly iodinated thyroglobulin was first iodinated with ^{125}I-labeled iodine and then mixed with an equal amount of noniodinated protein. This mixture was then further iodinated with ^{131}I-labeled iodide and then analyzed by isopycnic ultracentrifugation in RbCl (Fig. 4). It was found that all the molecules had the same final iodine content at the end of the second incubation i.e., no heterogeneity of iodination could be detected. These results indicated that after the second iodination the heterogeneous mixture of the two proteins became homogeneous. Evidently during the second iodination the iodine first reacted with the tyrosyl residues of the uniodinated protein. This means that the reactivity of the tyrosine residues that are exposed and available to the enzyme are so different from each other that iodination of this protein takes place in a rigid sequential order. Even at low levels of iodination, when a large proportion of the tyrosyl residues is still uniodinated, the iodination takes place in a sequence that is predetermined by the microenvironment of each residue and hence by the structure of the protein.

However, the iodoamino acid distribution greatly varies depending on the peroxidase used (thyroid, lacto- or horseradish peroxidase) or when performed under purely chemical conditions. This introduces the idea that the sequential order of iodination also depends on the enzyme.

3. The Iodoamino Acid Distribution

Higher levels of iodination may be obtained in vitro (70–90 iodine atoms per mole of thyroglobulin) than in vivo (50 atoms) (Gavaret et al., 1975). Further iodination is possible in vitro, but after denaturation of the protein. In vitro, as in vivo, the iodotyrosine content is similar

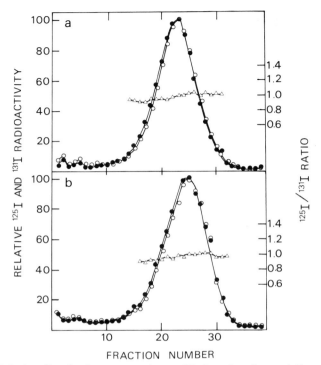

FIG. 4. Relative distribution pattern in equilibrium density centrifugation (33.7% RbCl) of a labeled thyroglobulin sample iodinated by thyroid peroxidase and containing 4 iodine atoms (labeled with ^{125}I) per mole of protein. (a) This thyroglobulin sample was mixed with an equal amount of noniodinated thyroglobulin. The mixture was then iodinated again with 8 iodine atoms (labeled with ^{131}I) per mole of protein. (b) The same experimental procedure was used as in (a), but during the first iodination 8 atoms of iodine (labeled with ^{131}I) per mole of protein were introduced. Relative radioactivity: ^{131}I (●——●), ^{125}I (○——○) ^{125}I: ^{131}I ratio (△——△). Reprinted from Gavaret *et al.* (1977).

(Dème *et al.*, 1976a). For instance, when 50 iodine atoms have been introduced, ~20 MIT residues and ~10 DIT residues are formed in both cases (Fig. 5b). Significant amounts of DIT are already formed at very low levels of iodination, whereas with free tyrosine DIT appears only when the formation of MIT levels off. This shows that the MIT residues that are formed at low levels of iodination are readily diiodinated before the enzyme interacts with other tyrosine residues to produce additional MIT residues. This confirms the sequential reactivity of the Tyr residues of thyroglobulin not only for the first iodination step yielding MIT but also for the second one producing DIT.

Another observation clearly obtained during the *in vitro* iodination is

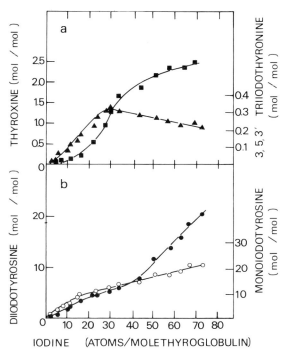

FIG. 5. Iodoamino acid distribution. (a) Thyroxine (■——■) and triiodothyronine (▲——▲) contents of various samples of *in vitro* iodinated human goiter thyroglobulin as a function of the number of iodine atoms introduced into one molecule of thyroglobulin. (b) Monoiodotyrosine (○——○) and diiodotyrosine (●——●) contents of various samples of *in vitro* iodinated human goiter thyroglobulin as a function of the number of iodine atoms introduced into one molecule of thyroglobulin. Reprinted from Déme *et al.* (1976a).

that a number of tyrosine residues undergo only monoiodination. A similar finding has been reported *in vivo* (Simon and Lissitzky, 1964; Inoue and Taurog, 1968; Chevillard *et al.*, 1972), and this again signifies that the distribution of iodine between MIT and DIT greatly depends on the structure of thyroglobulin (Fig. 5b).

The coupling reaction also occurs readily as soon as a very low level of iodination is achieved (Fig. 5a). The enzyme probably interacts with two iodotyrosine residues that belong to the same molecule of thyroglobulin, and it is therefore an intramolecular reaction. Only a fraction of the iodotyrosine residues can couple to the thyroid hormones, thyroxine and triiodothyronine.

Previous studies have demonstrated that the degree (or level) of iodination is of utmost importance in determining the thyroxine content of iodinated thyroglobulin. Since the iodination of the different tyrosyl residues takes place in a rigid sequential order and since only a small fraction of these residues undergoes coupling, the first problem was to determine the minimal level of iodination compatible with some coupling. It was also interesting to know the maximal number of iodotyrosine residues that can be coupled in one molecule of thyroglobulin.

The relationship between the iodine content and the distribution of T_4 and T_3 after *in vivo* iodination is shown in Fig. 5a. The shape of the curve is clearly sigmoid, and significant amounts of thyroxine are formed at very low levels of iodination; for 10 iodine atoms per mole of thyroglobulin, 0.1 mol of T_4 was found. Maximal T_4 contents were found in thyroglobulin samples containing ~70 iodine atoms per mole. The curve for T_3 is different from that for T_4; at low iodine contents the amount of T_3 is slightly higher than that of T_4, but the maximal T_3 content never exceeds 0.3 mol.

From the data reported in Fig. 5a, the efficiency of thyroid hormone formation as a function of the degree of iodination can be calculated (Fig. 6); the efficiency of coupling is defined as the amount of T_4 formed in successive 5-iodine-atom intervals introduced into thyroglobulin. Although T_4 formation already occurs at very low levels of iodination, the highest efficiency is always observed in a very narrow range of iodination. For instance, after the first 25 atoms of iodine were incorporated the next 5 atoms were converted to T_4 with an efficiency of 40%. Similar high efficiencies in coupling are observed *in vivo* in a narrow range of iodination, but the highest values are observed at lower levels of iodine content than *in vitro*. This difference may be due to the heterogeneity of *in vivo* iodinated thyroglobulin.

These results suggest that two DIT residues that are able to couple to T_4 are located in a very precise sequence of the protein. In addition, the efficiency of coupling decreases very rapidly after 50 atoms of iodine have been introduced, and this suggests that the last mole of T_4 is not coupled as readily as the first two. The reasons for this difference are unknown, but these observations suggest that the structure of thyroglobulin changes with the level of iodination; some transitions would be fast and some slow; above 50 iodine atoms, only one fraction of the thyroglobulin molecules present in the incubation medium would contain two hormonogenic DIT residues properly aligned in the tertiary structure of the protein to be able to couple, the proportion of such a type of conformation increasing with the iodine content.

Similar assumptions might also explain the "preferential synthesis" described by Lamas *et al.* (1974). These authors have shown that some

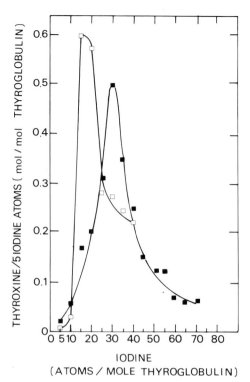

FIG. 6. Efficiency of thyroxine formation as a function of the different iodine atoms incorporated *in vitro* in human thyroglobulin (■——■) or *in vivo* (□——□) in rat thyroglobulin. Reprinted from Dème *et al.* (1976a).

DIT residues that are precursors of T_4 are the first to be iodinated, but are not readily coupled. This observation might signify either that these hormonogenic DIT are not completely iodinated at low levels of iodination so that they do not couple readily or that their coupling is possible only after the "maturation" of the thyroglobulin molecule itself, which would depend on further iodination. In other words, since the *in vitro* iodination yields homogeneous thyroglobulin molecules in terms of iodine content, and since some T_4 already do couple at low iodine contents, one may assume either a functional heterogeneity in the primary structure of the thyroglobulin molecules or a heterogeneity in the maturation process of this protein.

Another observation is that odd or fractional maximal numbers of thyroid hormone residues are obtained (Fig. 5a) after *in vitro* iodination, ~3 mol of T_4 and 0.3 mol of T_3 (Dème *et al.*, 1976a). If the two 12 S subunits of thyroglobulin (19 S) are identical, both of them should contain the same number of thyroxine residues. An explanation might be that the two 12 S subunits are different, as suggested by Van Der Walt et al. (1978). However this possibility does not provide an explanation for the fractional number of T_3 residues. Odd values for thyroxine have frequently been reported for in vivo iodinated thyroglobulin (Rolland et al., 1970, 1972; Sorimachi and Ui, 1974a,b). However, this situation was not surprising, since thyroglobulin iodinated in vivo is heterogeneous as far as its iodine content is concerned. Another possibility that might be considered is that thyroglobulin is heterogeneous in its protein portion, and some data are not against this idea (Dunn and Ray, 1975; Haeberli et al., 1975).

4. Structural Conditions Required for the Coupling Reaction

The importance of thyroglobulin structure in the formation of thyroid hormones has been emphasized by investigations in various laboratories (Van Zyl and Edelhoch, 1967; Lamas et al., 1971; Dème et al., 1976a; Lamas and Taurog, 1977). The concepts of "sequentiality of iodination," "preferential synthesis," and the findings related to the efficiency of coupling imply that the native structure of thyroglobulin plays an important role in facilitating intramolecular conversion of DIT to T_4. On the other hand, because only a small fraction of the iodotyrosine residues in thyroglobulin couples, the spatial alignment of the interacting residues is probably of utmost importance. The report by Dunn (1970), who analyzed the composition of thyroxine-containing small peptide fractions, states that only a few particular amino acids are present in close association with thyroxine. He suggested that thyroxine is located in a unique sequence and that the primary structure around certain tyrosine residues in thyroglobulin may be essential to the formation of thyroxine. Two lines of evidence were presented by Lamas et al. (1970) in favor of the view that the conformation of thyroglobulin is important for TPO-catalyzed coupling. The first evidence was based on comparison of T_4 yields in thyroglobulin and other proteins. The second involved the effect of guanidine pretreatment on T_4 yield in thyroglobulin; disruption of secondary and tertiary thyroglobulin structures by prior exposure to guanidine significantly reduced the efficiency of TPO-catalyzed coupling.

However, thyroglobulin, primary sequence unknown, is much too complex a molecule, and Cahnmann et al. (1977) searched for simple models for thyroglobulin containing, besides tyrosine, only one or a few other amino acids. A number of tyrosine-containing synthetic di- and tripeptides, oligopeptides, and copolymers were investigated for their ability to produce thyroid hormone. In the simplest model, free tyrosine is iodinated, but the diiodotyrosine formed does not undergo self-coupling nor does it couple with diiodotyrosine residues in thyroglobulin. Di- and tripeptides of tyrosine also did not form thyroxine, showing that in the absence of a tertiary structure no thyroxine can be formed. Results obtained with the synthetic copolymers of tyrosine (linear random, linear ordered, and multichain) are shown in Table III. Of all these polymers, with only one of them, the linear random copolymer of tyrosine and lysine, are all the tyrosine residues converted to diiodotyrosine residues. This polymer had an average molecular weight of 29,500 and contained 2.1% tyrosine. The same polymer was the only one in which coupling proceeded with an appreciable yield (15%).

The good coupling yield given by the Tyr-Lys copolymer, together with the lack of thyroxine formation by di- and tripeptides containing a

TABLE III

ENZYMATIC IODINATION OF COPOLYMERS WITH LACTOPEROXIDASE (LPO) AND WITH THYROID PEROXIDASE (TPO)

Copolymer	Type of copolymer[a]	Iodination, iodine incorporation (% of maximal incorporation		Coupling amount of thyroxine formed (% of incorporated iodine)	
		LPO	TPO	LPO	TPO
(LTyr,LAla,LGlu)$_n$ (33 mol % Tyr)	LR	27	0.74	0	0
(LTyr-LAla-LGlu)$_n$ (33 mol % Tyr)	LO	33	2.7	2	0
(LTyr,LGlu)$_n$ (2.5 mol % Tyr)	LR	100	37	2	1
(LTyr,LLys)$_n$ (2.1 mol % Tyr)	LR	100	100	11	15
poly(LLys) poly(LTyr)-poly(LGlu)-poly(DLAla) (15 wt % Tyr)	M	44	3.1	0	0
poly(LLys) poly(LTyr)-poly(LGlu)-poly(DLAla) (21 wt % Tyr)	M	37	3.4	0	0
poly(LLys) poly(LGlu)-poly(DLAla)-poly(LTyr) (10 wt % Tyr)	M	27	8.6	0	0

[a] LR, linear random; LO, linear ordered; M, multichain.

single tyrosine residue, confirmed the hypothesis that efficient coupling requires interaction of two diiodotyrosine residues within the same peptide chain. The polymer must be able to assume a configuration in which the two interacting diiodotyrosine residues come close together and align themselves in such a way that coupling can proceed. The distance between the two diiodotyrosine residues along the polypeptide chain would therefore be of utmost importance. This distance could not be determined in the random copolymer. Two oligopeptides of known sequence Lys-Tyr-(Lys)$_n$-Tyr-Lys (I: $n = 3$; II: $n = 5$) that contained two differently spaced tyrosine residues were synthesized. Both peptides, in which the tyrosine residues were separated by three or five lysine residues, respectively, were almost completely iodinated and both formed triiodothyronine and thyroxine. However, peptide II produced twice as much hormone as peptide I, and peptide I produced more triiodothyronine than peptide II.

Atom models of these peptides showed that the polypeptide chain of both could easily be arranged in such a way that they formed a semicircle with all Lys side chains pointing toward the outside and the aromatic rings of Tyr sandwiched in the center (Fig. 7). However, while

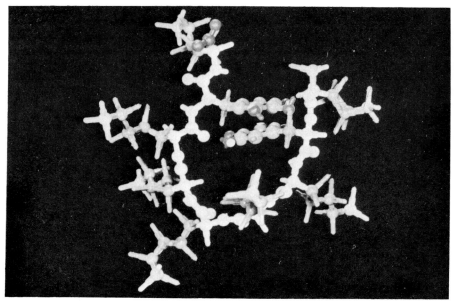

FIG. 7. Atom model of peptide I showing a conformation in which coupling can take place. Reprinted from Cahmann *et al.* (1977).

it is easy to align these rings in peptide II, this is less probable with peptide I where, at best, the alignment can be made without exerting strain. These results showed that not only the nature of the amino acid residues in the vicinity of the coupling sites is important, but also the distance between the two diiodotyrosine residues that couple, all these factors influencing the spatial alignment.

It appears that thyroglobulin, whose function is to form hormones at low levels of iodination, possesses specifically all these structural requirements for its function.

5. Comparative Efficiency of Different Peroxidases in Catalyzing the Coupling Reaction

As indicated above, the iodoamino acid distribution found in thyroglobulin after *in vitro* iodination with thyroid peroxidase greatly depends on the native structure of the thyroglobulin molecule. However, depending on the conditions of iodination, variations are observed in such a composition. For instance, the number of MIT and DIT residues, respectively, formed with three different peroxidases (Dème *et al.*, 1978) (thyroid, lacto- and horseradish enzymes) and in chemical conditions is different. Lactoperoxidase catalyzes the formation of DIT as efficiently as the thyroid enzyme, whereas with horseradish peroxidase and chemical iodination, monoiodination is favored. Krinsky and Fruton (1971), studying the iodination by thyroid, lacto-, and horseradish peroxidases of a series of synthetic di- and tripeptides containing tyrosine also observed differences in the specificity of these enzymes. Thus the iodination process depends not only on the properties of the thyroglobulin molecule, but also on the interaction of the enzyme with the different tyrosine residues that undergo iodination. In addition, more tyrosine residues can react (and are iodinated) with the horseradish enzyme than with the thyroid or lactoperoxidases.

As far as the coupling reaction is concerned, the differences between the three enzymes and chemical iodination are even more marked. Lactoperoxidase and thyroid peroxidase again perform the coupling reaction very similarly. However, thyroid peroxidase has almost the same optimum pH for both iodination and coupling whereas with lactoperoxidase there is a clear shift (Fig. 8) in the optimum pH between these two reactions. With the horseradish enzyme, the coupling reaction is very rare at the optimum pH for iodination. We will see below that, with this enzyme, a clear dissociation between iodination and coupling can be demonstrated. Finally, under chemical conditions of iodination, coupling occurs only when the iodine content reaches 30–40 atoms, clearly showing that the choice of the residues that undergo

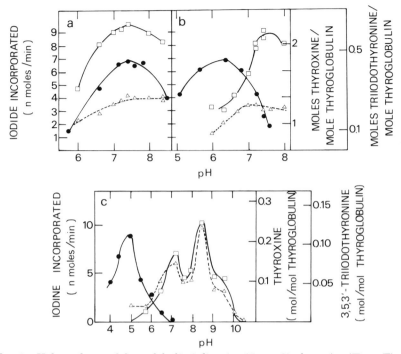

FIG. 8. pH dependency of thyroglobulin iodination (●——●), thyroxine (□——□), and triiodothyronine (△---△) formation catalyzed by (a) thyroid peroxidase, (b) lactoperoxidase, (c) horseradish peroxidase. (a and b) Reprinted from Déme *et al.* (1978); (c) reprinted from Virion *et al.* (1979).

iodination is quite different from that occurring in the enzymatic reaction.

C. THE KINETICS OF THE COUPLING REACTION

We have shown above that, with a given enzyme, the amount of thyroxine formed depends greatly on the structure of the thyroglobulin molecule: the same number of T_4 and T_3 residues is always measured from experiment to experiment for the same level of iodination, provided the thyroglobulin molecule is maintained in its native form and the time course of incubation is long enough to ensure complete coupling of the iodotyrosine residues potentially capable of being converted to thyroid hormones.

The situation is completely different if one measures the hormone content during the time course of the reaction; T_4 and T_3 begin to accumulate only when the iodination reaction and DIT formation reach a plateau (Fig. 9) Dème *et al.*, 1976b). These data also reveal that T_3 accumulates for a further 5–10 minutes and thereafter levels off, whereas T_4 content continues to increase almost linearly between 5 and 15 minutes of incubation. This suggests that T_3 is not the precursor of T_4. In addition, the dashed line on Fig. 9 represents the values of DIT (theoretical) that would have been found if none of this iodoamino acid had been transformed into T_4. The difference between the value of DIT (theoretical) and that of DIT experimentally found was in good agreement with the amount of T_4 determined experimentally (Table IV). This proves unequivocally that DIT is the precursor of T_4. This conclusion is also supported by the evolution of the MIT/DIT ratio during the time-course of incubation; this ratio is initially high, falls

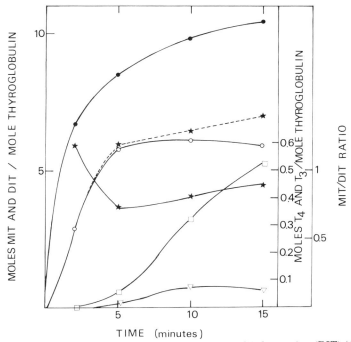

FIG. 9. Kinetics of monoiodotyrosine (MIT) (●——●), diiodotyrosine (DIT) (○——○), 3,5,3'-triiodothyronine (T_3) (▽——▽), and thyroxine (T_4) (□——□) synthesis during human goiter thyroglobulin iodination. (★——★) MIT/DIT ratios; (-----) calculated number of DIT residues that would have been found in the absence of coupling reaction. Reprinted from Pommier *et al.* (1973a).

TABLE IV

IODINE ATOMS INCORPORATED INTO THYROGLOBULIN DURING THE 5–15-MINUTES
INCUBATION INTERVAL AS TOTAL IODINE (Δ TOTAL), MONOIODOTYROSINE
(Δ MONOIODOTYROSINE), DIIODOTYROSINE (Δ DIIODOTYROSINE),
AND THYROXINE (Δ THYROXINE)[a]

I⁻ (mM)	Δ Total	Δ Monoiodo-tyrosine	Δ Diiodo-tyrosine	Δ Thyroxine Actual	Δ Thyroxine Theoretical
0.05	4.1	1.87	0.24	1.88	1.99
0.1	9.4	3.82	2.22	3.24	3.36
0.2	18.3	7.97	5.42	4.18	4.91
0.5	26.8	10.67	11.26	4.17	4.78

[a] Δ Diiodotyrosine (actual) is compared with Δ diiodotyrosine (theoretical) calculated from the formula

$$\Delta \text{ Diiodotyrosine (theoretical)} = \Delta \text{ Total} - \Delta \text{ Monoiodotyrosine}$$

Diiodotyrosine (theoretical) represents the number of diiodotyrosine residues that would have been found if none had been transformed into thyroxine. Δ Thyroxine (theoretical) is therefore equal to Δ diiodotyrosine (theoretical) minus Δ diiodotyrosine (actual).

rapidly as MIT is converted to DIT, and then rises again as DIT in turn is coupled to T_4.

As indicated above, T_4 and T_3 begin to accumulate only when the iodination levels off. This observation is true whatever the iodide concentration, i.e., whatever the rate of iodination, and thus the iodine content reached during the first minutes of incubation (Fig. 10). Iodination always proceeds during the first minutes at a fast rate and then for longer periods of time at a much slower rate, with T_4 accumulating only during this second period of time. In other words, thyroxine accumulates only after a constant lag period that is independent of the extent of iodination.

Similarly varying the enzyme or thyroglobulin concentration did not modify the length of the lag period. The existence of a lag between iodination and coupling might be expected, since it is obvious that enough hormonogenic iodotyrosine residues must be formed before they can be coupled to thyroid hormones; thus a precursor–product relationship should appear in the kinetics of iodination. However, it is also obvious that the length of the lag should decrease with the extent of iodination, i.e., should not be constant as observed. Another explanation would be that competition exists between iodination and coupling such that, as long as iodide and tyrosine residues are available, only iodination should occur. This would mean, since the same enzyme cata-

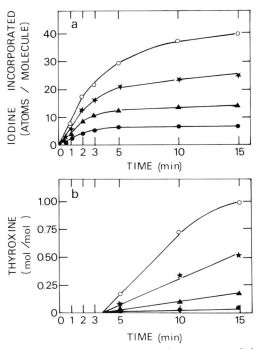

FIG. 10. Comparative kinetics of thyroglobulin iodination (a) and thyroxine formation (b) at four iodide concentrations: 10 μM (●——●), 25 μM (▲——▲), 50 μM (★——★), and 100 μM (○——○). Reprinted from Déme *et al.* (1976b).

lyzes both reactions, that thyroid peroxidase has a higher affinity for the substrates of the iodination reaction, iodide and tyrosine, than for the substrate of the coupling reaction, the hormonogenic DIT residues. However, this explanation does not hold because in several experiments sufficient amounts of iodide and of reactive tyrosine residues were still present at the end of the lag period when coupling began to occur. A third possibility would be that, at the end of the lag period, the hormonogenic iodotyrosine residues are partly but not completely iodinated, but this explanation does not allow for a constant lag being observed whatever the number of iodine atoms incorporated during the first period of incubation. In addition, we will see below that it can be shown that the hormonogenic tyrosine residues are actually fully iodinated before the end of the lag period. A more complicated but possibly more valid explanation might be postulated in terms of changes in conformation of the enzyme or of thyroglobulin, these changes occuring during the lag period. Several data suggest that structural changes occur in the thyroglobulin molecule when this protein is exposed to thyroid peroxidase. Two types of changes have been described. The first one results in a decrease in dissociability in the presence of sodium dodecyl sulfate (SDS) to the two 12 S subunits (Nunez *et al.*, 1966a,b; Gavaret *et al.*, 1971; Pommier *et al.*, 1973a; Sorimachi and Ui, 1974a). The second one, described by Ekholm and Berg (Berg, 1973; Berg and Ekholm, 1975), is a change in shape. It is interesting in this respect to indicate that the change in dissociability by SDS also occurs with a constant lag period similar to that observed for T_4 formation (J. M. Gavaret, J. Pommier, and J. Nunez, unpublished results).

On the other hand, the changes in conformation might depend on the enzyme; recent results (unpublished) have shown that the length of the lag can be modified by changing the H_2O_2 concentration or the H_2O_2/iodide ratio. These data suggest the existence of two conformations for thyroid peroxidase, one that favors iodination, the other one coupling with a slow and constant transition period between these two forms.

This latter explanation is largely hypothetical, but the existence of a constant lag had a practical interest; it made it possible to prepare thyroglobulin samples with different iodide contents but little or no hormone. Thus iodination and coupling could be studied separately.

D. Dissociation between Iodination and Coupling

Dissociation between these two reactions could be studied under several conditions. With thyroid peroxidase, for instance, thyroglobulin was iodinated for a short period of time with ^{125}I-labeled iodide and then purified. It was then incubated again with fresh enzyme in the presence and in the absence of ^{131}I-labeled iodide and with or without an H_2O_2 generating system (Fig. 11). These experiments made it possible to show (*a*) that no T_4 is synthesized in the absence of H_2O_2, thus the coupling reaction requires the oxidation of the iodotyrosine precursors; and (*b*) that iodide is required for coupling; increasing the iodide concentration results in an increased efficiency of coupling (Fig. 12). In contrast with these conclusions, Lamas *et al.* (1972) have reported that significant coupling occurs when chemically iodinated thyroglobulin containing no hormone was incubated with thyroid peroxidase in the absence of iodide. However, it is well known that chemically iodinated thyroglobulin releases iodide when incubated with thyroid peroxidase. This observation suggests that iodide is not only a substrate for the reaction catalyzed by thyroid peroxidase, but is also a regulatory ligand of the enzyme. Similar findings were also found with lac-

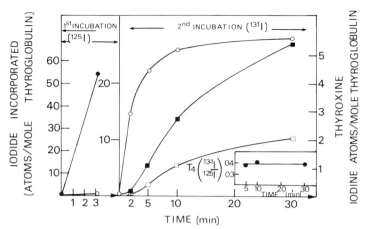

F$_{IG}$. 11. Time course of thyroglobulin iodination and thyroxine formation during a double incubation experiment. During the first incubation (left) noniodinated thyroglobulin was incubated for 3 minutes with the enzyme and 2×10^{-4} M KI labeled with ^{125}I. The iodinated thyroglobulin obtained was purified and incubated a second time in the presence of 5×10^{-5} M iodide labeled with ^{131}I (right). Both the incorporation of iodide into thyroglobulin and the thyroxine labeled with ^{125}I and ^{131}I contents were determined; (●———●) iodination with ^{125}I labeled iodide; (○———○) iodination with ^{131}I-labeled iodide; (■———■) thyroxine formed from ^{125}I-labeled iodide (first iodination); (□———□) T$_4$ formed from ^{131}I-labeled iodide (second incubation). *Inset:* The evolution of the ^{131}I/^{125}I ratio of thyroxine during the second incubation. Reprinted from Déme *et al.* (1976b).

toperoxidase: a constant lag exists between iodination and coupling, and iodide is required for the coupling reaction to occur. In contrast, coupling occurs with horseradish peroxidase in the absence of iodide (Virion *et al.*, 1979). This suggests that iodide stimulates the coupling reaction by interacting with thyroid (and lacto-) peroxidase, but not with horseradish peroxidase; it is also clear that thyroglobulin is not the target of this regulatory effect of iodide. We will also see below that SCN$^-$ mimics this stimulatory effect of iodide on the coupling reaction.

Lacto- and thyroid peroxidases appear, on the other hand, to be very similar in their iodinating and coupling properties. This was already shown by the data on iodine distribution between the different iodoamino acids (see Section III,B,3). Taurog *et al.* (1974), comparing these two peroxidases in their ability to catalyze T$_4$ formation, also concluded that thyroid peroxidase possesses no marked specificity at pH 7.0; however, they observed that although iodination with lactoperoxidase at pH 5.6 was extremely rapid, T$_4$ formation at a compar-

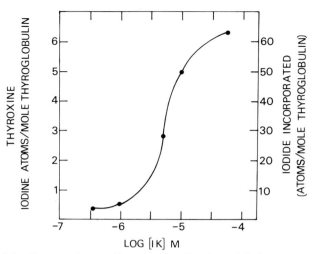

FIG. 12. Iodide effects on the coupling reaction. The thyroglobulin iodinated *in vitro* in the conditions described in Fig. 11 (left panel) and containing no thyroxine was incubated again with and without iodide in the presence of fresh enzyme and H_2O_2-generating system. Reprinted from Déme *et al.* (1976b).

able degree of iodination was considerably lower than that observed at pH 7.0. These results were confirmed by Dème *et al.* (1978) (Fig. 8), who showed in addition that thyroid peroxidase is the only enzyme that catalyzes, with the best efficiency, iodination and coupling in the same broad range of physiological pH levels. Thus some specificity has been acquired for thyroid peroxidase; it is also difficult to imagine how in the thyroid gland the optimum pH might change to perform with the highest efficiency iodination and coupling successively.

In contrast, with horseradish peroxidase very little hormone is made at the optimum pH (~5–5.5) for iodination. Results obtained with Virion (Virion *et al.*, 1979) (Fig. 8c) allowed us to show that horseradish peroxidase actually catalyzes the coupling, but at a pH quite different from that required for the iodination reaction. The experiments were performed in two ways. In the first, Thyroglobulin, iodinated but containing no hormone, was prepared at pH 7.0 with thyroid peroxidase as indicated above, purified, and then subjected at different pH levels to a second incubation with the horseradish enzyme. Clearly this latter enzyme catalyzed very efficiently the coupling reaction, but at much more alkaline pH levels (7.5–8.5) than that required for the iodination reaction (Fig. 8c). By the second method, iodination was performed at pH 5.5 with the horseradish enzyme. As expected, the coupling reaction was very rare if the pH was maintained low during all the incubation; in contrast, changing the pH to 8.5 after a given period of time resulted in normal T_4 content. Thus, this finding provided the first complete dissociation between iodination and coupling. One may speculate that iodination is catalyzed by one form of horseradish peroxidase that is favored at ~pH 5, whereas coupling occurs efficiently only at more alkaline pH because it is catalyzed by a different form of the same enzyme; actually it has been reported that horseradish peroxidase contains two heme-linked ionizable groups with $pK_i = 6.0$ and 8.5, respectively (Morishima and Ogawa, 1979). This analogy supports the idea that the thyroid enzyme exists in two forms that catalyze iodination and coupling differently.

V. REGULATORY EFFECTS OF IODIDE

A. IODIDE EFFECTS ON THE COUPLING REACTION

We have seen (Sections III,B and III,C) that when iodide is in great excess (above $2 \times 10^{-4} M$ for thyroid peroxidase), I_2 is produced and the iodination is inhibited (Fig. 2). This effect of iodide very likely implies the interaction of excess iodide with the substrate site and might be one explanation of the well-known Wolff–Chaikoff effect (Wolff and Chaikoff, 1948).

Other effects of iodide cannot be ascribed to a competition with the substrate site; we have seen (Section IV,D), for instance, that iodide stimulates the coupling reaction with both thyroid peroxidase and lactoperoxidase, but not with the horseradish enzyme.

However, a regulatory role of iodide is difficult to study, since during the coupling step some iodination occurs after the lag period (Section IV,C) (though at a much slower rate than before the end of the lag). In work with A. Virion, it has been found that thiocyanate (Virion et al., 1980) mimics the stimulatory effect of iodide on the coupling reaction. The concentration of this pseudohalide required for half-maximal stimulation is very low, $\sim 10^{-6} M$, with both the thyroid enzyme and lactoperoxidase. In contrast, no effect of SCN$^-$ was seen with horseradish peroxidase or under purely chemical coupling conditions.

Several other data suggest that SCN$^-$ binds to the enzyme and to a site distinct from the substrate site: Since no effect is seen with horseradish peroxidase a possible interaction of SCN^- with thyroglobulin can be eliminated; SCN^- also behaves as a competitive inhibitor of iodide oxidation, but at a much higher concentration than that required to stimulate the coupling reaction.

It is probable that SCN^- exerts its inhibitory effects by interacting with the substrate site, whereas the stimulation of the coupling reaction depends on the existence of another binding site, with regulatory properties and much higher affinities. Maximal stimulation of the coupling reaction is observed with 10^{-6} M SCN^- for thyroid peroxidase; this demonstrates that the enzyme contains a limited number of high-affinity regulatory sites for SCN^- (and iodide).

B. IODIDE EFFECTS ON BITYROSINE FORMATION

Similar effects of SCN^- and iodide have been found with another reaction catalyzed by the peroxidases. As indicated in Section III,C, all the peroxidases so far tested catalyze the formation of bityrosine from free tyrosine at a pH much more alkaline than that required to iodinate this amino acid or to oxidize iodide to I_2. Thus the effects of iodide and SCN^- could be studied in the absence of iodination or of iodide oxidation (and also in the absence of thyroglobulin) (Michot et $al.$, 1980). Under such conditions it was seen that iodide greatly stimulates the rate of bityrosine formation in the presence of thyroid peroxidase (Fig. 13). No effect was seen with horseradish or lactoperoxidases. K_{iodide} was equal to 2.8×10^{-5} M, suggesting that thyroid peroxidase contains a simple class of regulatory binding sites for iodide. SCN^- mimics iodide effects with a K_{SCN^-} equal to $10^{-4}M$.

The effects of SCN^- and iodide were not additive, and no effect of SCN^- was seen with lacto- and horseradish peroxidases. ClO_4^-, another anion with the same molecular size as iodide and SCN^-, neither had an effect on the oxidation of tyrosine to bityrosine, nor did it prevent the stimulatory effect of iodide on this reaction.

C. IODIDE EFFECTS AND THE MECHANISMS OF ACTION OF ANTITHYROID DRUGS

Maloof and Soodak (1965) showed that thiourea-like compounds, i.e., thioamides and thiourylenes, are oxidized by different peroxidases only in the presence of iodide. Since these compounds are used as antithyroid drugs in the treatment of hyperthyroidism, other authors have

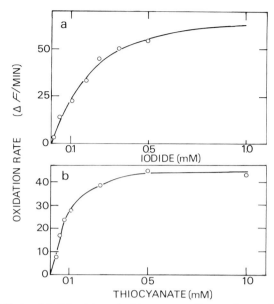

Fɪɢ. 13. Effect of iodide (a) and thiocyanate (b) on the oxidation of N^{α}-acetyl-tyrosinamide by thyroid peroxidase. Reprinted from Michot et al. (1980).

tried to understand the mechanism of this iodide effect. Morris and Hager (1966), for instance, proposed that inhibition of the iodination reaction depends on "a competition between the drug and tyrosine" toward a "complex formed between the enzyme and an oxidized form of iodide." Taurog (1976) also accepted such a pathway but concluded that it applies only when the drug-to-iodide ratio is low. At higher ratios no oxidation of the drug was noticed and the enzyme remained inactive, suggesting that the drug "inhibits the formation of the enzyme-oxidized iodide complex." However, since iodide also prevents inhibition by the antithyroid drug of the oxidation of guaiacol, none of these explanations seems to hold.

With Michot and Edelhoch (Michot et al., 1979), similar studies were undertaken, but taking as an assay the oxidation of tyrosine to bityrosine at alkaline pH, i.e., under conditions in which no competition can exist between the drug and tyrosine toward an enzyme-oxidized iodide complex. It was found at this pH that in the absence of iodide the enzyme is rapidly and irreversibly inactivated (Fig. 14). In the presence of iodide the drug is oxidized (Fig. 15); when all the drug

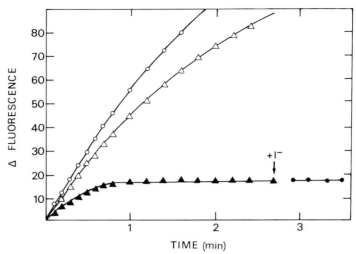

FIG. 14. Effect of methylthiouracil on N^α-acetyltyrosynamide oxidation catalyzed by lactoperoxidase with (▲——▲, △——△) and without (○——○), methylthiouracil. Iodide was introduced at time zero (△——△) or after 3 minutes (●——●) of incubation. Reprinted from Michot *et al.* (1979).

has disappeared the enzyme is available again to oxidize tyrosine. The data are therefore consistent with the existence of an enzyme–iodide complex in which the iodide is bound not to the substrate site, but to a regulatory site. Such a site has been characterized by its association

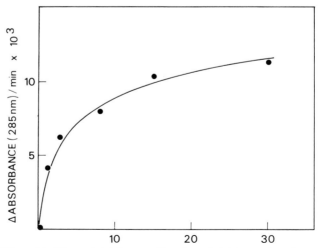

FIG. 15. Effect of iodide on initial rates (V_i) of methylthiouracil oxidation. Reprinted from Michot *et al.* (1979).

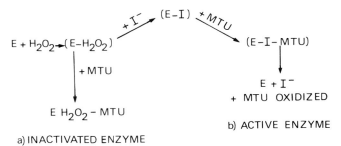

SCHEME 3. Mechanism of action of the antithyroid drug on peroxidases. (a) Action in the absence of iodide. (b) In the presence of iodide, the enzyme activates the oxidation of the drug. J. L. Michot and J. Nunez, unpublished results.

constant, which was found to be equal to $2 \times 10^{-5} M$. The identification of the enzyme–drug dead-end complex, obtained in the absence of iodide, was also achieved by differential spectroscopy in the Soret region.

The existence of such a site for iodide was found with both lacto- and thyroid peroxidases. However, with the thyroid enzyme the calculations of the association constant were difficult to establish, since iodide stimulates not only the oxidation of the drug, but also that of tyrosine (see Section V,B).

Finally, in other work (unpublished), also carried out in collaboration with Edelhoch *et al.*, a systematic study was performed with a series of antithyroid drugs. It was found that the iodide stimulatory effect on drug oxidation is not observed with all the thiourylene compounds tested. In addition, the relative importance of drug oxidation and enzyme inactivation greatly depends on the chemical structure of the drug, i.e. on the structure of the ternary complex formed between the enzyme, iodide, and drug. Scheme 3 summarizes the above results and shows that, depending on the presence or the absence of iodide, the peroxidase is either inactivated irreversibly or used to oxidize the drug, thus preventing the iodination reaction from proceeding until all the drug has disappeared.

VI. DIIODOTYROSINE EFFECTS ON THE IODINATION AND COUPLING REACTIONS

With Dème and Fimiani (Dème *et al.*, 1975), we showed that free diiodotyrosine has two opposite effects on thyroglobulin iodination and coupling. Inhibition of thyroglobulin iodination is observed when DIT concentration is higher than $5 \times 10^{-3} M$. This effect is competitive, and it is probable therefore that DIT interacts with the substrate site of the enzyme. The mechanism has been elucidated: the iodide present in the DIT molecule exchanges with the free iodide (Fig. 16) present in the medium; thus, DIT is not consumed and the reaction never stops, H_2O_2 being continuously consumed. When present at very low concentrations ($5 \times 10^{-8} M$), DIT has an opposite, stimulatory, effect on the coupling reaction (Fig. 17).

This latter observation suggests that the enzyme contains a regulatory site for DIT. Since maximal stimulatory effects of DIT are ob-

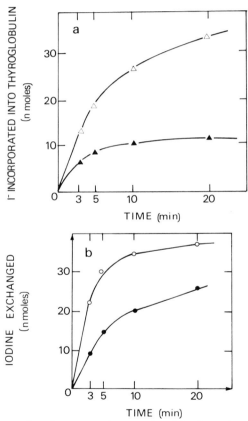

FIG. 16. Iodination and exchange reactions catalyzed by thyroid peroxidase. (a) Kinetics of thyroglobulin iodination in the presence (▲——▲) or in the absence (△——△) of free tyrosine. (b) Kinetics of exchange reaction between iodide and free diiodotyrosine in the presence (●——●) and in the absence (○——○) of thyroglobulin. Reprinted from Déme et al. (1975).

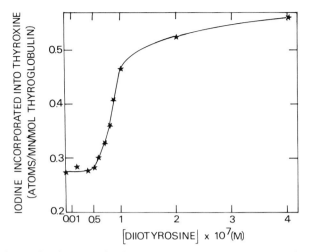

FIG. 17. Relationship between diiodotyrosine concentration and initial rate of thyroid hormone synthesis. Reprinted from Déme *et al.* (1975).

tained with $10^{-7}M$ DIT, it may also be excluded that this ligand stimulates the coupling reaction by interacting with thyroglobulin, as suggested by Taurog (Taurog and Nakashima, 1978); thyroglobulin was actually present at a much higher concentration $(10^{-6}M)$ than was DIT $(10^{-7}M)$, which produces maximal activation.

Taurog objected that DIT stimulates the coupling reaction by interacting with thyroid peroxidase and proposed thyroglobulin as a target for this ligand because (*a*) DIT effects were seen when the coupling reaction was performed with thyroglobulin under purely chemical conditions; and (*b*) DIT effects were not seen when fibrinogen was used instead of thyroglobulin to study the coupling reaction in chemical conditions.

We have confirmed that the stimulation of the coupling reaction by DIT is fairly unspecific, since it can be observed not only with thyroid peroxidase, but also with lacto and horseradish enzymes and under chemical conditions (unpublished results). However, DIT also stimulates tyrosine oxidation to bityrosine by thyroid peroxidase, a reaction occurring in the absence of thyroglobulin (unpublished results).

The finding that DIT stimulates coupling both under enzymatic and nonenzymatic conditions does not necessarily exclude the possibility that under enzymatic conditions DIT binds to a site on the peroxidase. Coupling is obtained under both conditions, but with large differences in rates. Complete coupling takes 30 minutes with the enzyme; in contrast, more than 15 hours and a great excess of iodine are required under chemical conditions.

Nevertheless, the mechanism by which DIT stimulates the coupling reaction and the physiological significance of this effect remain matters of speculation. It is, however, clear that free DIT does not stimulate the coupling reaction by being incorporated into the thyroid hormone that is formed (intermolecular coupling), as shown by experiments performed with ^{14}C-labeled DIT. This latter conclusion has been confirmed also by Taurog (Taurog and Nakashima, 1978).

VII. DEFECTIVE PEROXIDASES

A series of investigations has been carried out to find out whether goitrous patients with a decrease in iodide organification have abnormalities of the peroxidase molecule in performing one or more than one of the reactions catalyzed by this enzyme. Such a possibility is likely in the type of goiter that is referred to as "goiter with iodine organification defect." In general, this type of goiter is characterized only exceptionally by clear hypothyroidism but is detected by a positive perchlorate discharge test. A partial or total discharge by ClO_4^- of the radioactive iodide administered to the patient indicates that some limiting factor, which is involved in the iodination reaction, is not operating in the gland of the patient. In some cases an associated deafness is present, and this class of disease is referred to as Pendred syndrome.

Two types of enzyme preparations have been used to study the peroxidase of this type of goiter, the completely solubilized and the pseudo-solubilized enzymes (see Section II). Simultaneously, thyroglobulin was isolated and analyzed; it was found that the thyroglobulin of these goiters is always very poorly iodinated, confirming the iodide organification defect detected by the perchlorate discharge test. In a few cases, thyroglobulin was absent or present only in minute amounts. When present, the thyroglobulin of the goiter could be iodinated in $vitro$ with a hog enzyme; normal iodination and normal iodoamino acid distribution (including the hormone content) were always found.

As far as the peroxidase is concerned, all the theoretical possibilities were encountered.

1. The enzyme was completely absent (Pommier et $al.$, 1976); in general this situation corresponds to patients having also mental retardation.

2. The enzyme was present whatever the reaction tested (Pommier et $al.$, 1974),—iodide oxidation ($I^- \rightarrow I_2$), thyroglobulin iodination, and

coupling. The enzyme appeared thus to be normal; in some of these patients with normal enzyme, the iodination defect was attributable to the absence of thyroglobulin (or to a very low level of this protein) (Niepomniczcze *et al.*, 1977). In two cases, a brother and a sister, no clear defect of both the thyroglobulin and the enzyme could be detected.

3. Another type of situation was found in some cases: all the enzymatic parameters appeared to be normal when tested with the completely solubilized preparation, whereas a clear defect was found with the "pseudo-solubilized" enzyme (Pommier *et al.*, 1974). This suggested the presence of a defect at the level of the membranous structure to which the enzyme is normally bound.

The last category appeared to be very interesting; the enzyme was present when tested by the iodide oxidation test ($I^- \rightarrow I_2$), but defective as far as the iodination reaction was concerned (Pommier *et al.*, 1974; Abdelmoumene *et al.*, 1978) (Fig. 18a). This was true both for the solubilized and the pseudo-solubilized enzyme. In one case of Pendred syndrome, the pseudosolubilized enzyme was even more defective than the solubilized one. In another case the iodination reaction was slightly reduced, but the coupling reaction was severely impaired, suggesting the existence of a real "coupling defect" (Fig. 18b). Conversely, in two cases the enzyme was only poorly able to iodinate thyroglobulin, but, surprisingly, its ability to catalyze the coupling reaction was normal. This was shown with thyroglobulin samples iodinated with hog normal thyroid peroxidase during the lag period but containing no hormone (see Section III,C). The pathological enzymes that were defective in the catalysis of the iodination reaction were able to couple normally performed hormonogenic iodotyrosine residues.

These data therefore suggest that the classification based on a positive perchlorate test does not cover a homogeneous population of diseases. The two cases of Pendred syndrome studied were also heterogeneous, since in one case the enzyme was defective and the thyroglobulin normal whereas in the second case the opposite situation was detected. Actually, the perchlorate discharge test cannot be considered to be more than a preliminary indication; clear positive responses were also found with cases that were revealed to be adenomas or cancers (and were also characterized by a lack of peroxidase).

Since thyroglobulin from these goiters is always very poorly iodinated and does not contain hormone, a second problem raised by these studies is to know why these patients in most cases are euthyroid. This problem remains unsolved, and only speculations may be proposed.

Finally, one of the most interesting conclusions of these studies is that they contribute to a direct understanding of the mechanism of the iodination and coupling reaction. The finding of enzymes that perform

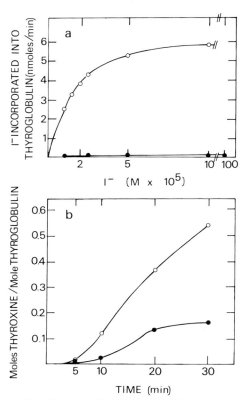

Fɪɢ. 18. Defective iodination (a) and defective coupling (b) found in two peroxidases prepared from two goiters with "iodide organification defect." (a) Relationship between initial velocities of thyroglobulin iodination and iodide concentration catalyzed by the same amount of enzymatic activity (0.8 U/ml iodide oxidation activity) of hog (○——○) and a goiter preoxidase (●——●). Reprinted from Pommier *et al.* (1976). (b) Kinetics of thyroxine formation catalyzed by hog (○——○) and (●——●) peroxidase during the iodination of thyroglobulin. Reprinted from Pommier *et al.* (1974).

quite normally the iodide oxidation reaction, but not iodination, are in good agreement with the two-site model [Section III,C, Eq. (18)], the interpretation being that some change in the structure of the peroxidase maintains the affinity of site 2 for iodide unchanged whereas it decreases its affinity for the tyrosyl residues. Similarly, the finding of an enzyme that does not iodinate thyroglobulin but is able to perform the coupling reaction normally is consistent with the hypothesis (Section IV,C) that thyroid peroxidase may exist in two forms, one adapted to perform iodination, the second to catalyze coupling.

REFERENCES

Abdelmoumene, N., Gavaret, J. M., Pommier, J., and Nunez, J. (1978). A defective thyroid peroxidase in a case of Pendred syndrome. *J. Mol. Med.* **3**, 305–318.

Ahn, C. S., and Rosenberg, I. N. (1970). Iodine metabolism in thyroid slices: effects of TSH, dibutyryl cyclic $3',5'$-AMP, NaF and prostaglandin E_1. *Endocrinology* **86**, 396–405.

Alexander, N. M. (1962). A spectrophotometric assay for iodide oxidation by thyroid peroxidase. *Anal. Biochem.* **4**, 341–345.

Alexander, N. M. (1972). Program of the Forty-eighth Meeting of the American Thyroid Association, Chicago, p. 66 (Abstract).

Alexander, N. M. (1977). Purification of bovine thyroid peroxidase. *Endocrinology* **100**, 610–1620.

Assem, E. S. K., Trotter, W. R., and Belyavin, G. (1964). The heterogeneity of human thyroglobulin. *Biochim. Biophys. Acta* **100**, 163–178.

Auclair, C., Torres, M., and Hakim, J. (1978). Superoxide anion involvement in NBT reduction catalyzed by NADPH–cytochrome P450 reductase: a pitfall. *FEBS Lett.* **89**, 26–28.

Aust, S. D., Roerig, L., and Pederson, T. C. (1972). Evidence for superoxide generation by NADPH–cytochrome C reductase of rat liver microsomes. *Biochem. Biophys. Res. Commun.* **47**, 1133–1137.

Babior, B. M. (1977). Recent studies on oxygen metabolism in human neutrophil: superoxide and chemiluminescence. *In* "Superoxide and Superoxide Dismutases" (A. M. Michelson, J. M. McCord, and I. Fridovich, eds.), pp. 271–281. Academic Press, New York.

Bayse, G. S., Michaels, A. W., and Morrison, M. (1972). The peroxidase catalyzed oxidation of tyrosine. *Biochim. Biophys. Acta* **284**, 34–42.

Berg, G. (1973). An electron microscopic study of the thyroglobulin molecule. *J. Ultrastruct. Res.* **42**, 324–336.

Berg, G., and Ekholm, R. (1975). Electron microscopy of low iodinated thyroglobulin molecules. *Biochim. Biophys. Acta* **386**, 422–431.

Bjorksten, F. (1970). The horse-radish peroxidase-catalyzed oxidation of iodide. Outline of the mechanism. *Biochim. Biophys. Acta* **212**, 396–406.

Cahnmann, H. J., and Matsuura, T. (1960). Model reactions for the biosynthesis of thyroxide. II. The fate of the aliphatic side chain in the conversion of 3,5-diiodophloretic acid to 3,5,3',5'-tetraiodothyropropionic acid. *J. Am. Chem. Soc.* **82**, 2050–2055.

Cahnmann, H. J., Pommier, J., and Nunez, J. (1977). Spatial requirement for coupling of iodotyrosine residues to form thyroid hormone. *Proc. Natl. Acad. Sci. U.S.A.* **74**, 5333–5335.

Chance, B. (1952). The kinetics and stoichiometry of the transition from the primary to the secondary peroxidase peroxide complexes. *Arch. Biochem. Biophys.* **41**, 416–424.

Chance, B., and Maehly, A. C. (1955). Assay of catalases and peroxidases A. The guaiacol test. *Methods Enzymol.* **2**, 770–773.

Chevillard, L., Gavaret, J. M., Julien, M. F., and Nunez, J. (1972). Regulation par l'iodure de l'halogénation de la thyroglobuline et de la thyroxinogénèse. *C. R. Hebd. Seances Acad. Sci.* **274**, 2782–2785.

Coval, M. L., and Taurog, A. (1967). Purification and iodinating activity of hog thyroid peroxidase. *J. Biol. Chem.* **242**, 5510–5523.

Davidson, B., Neary, J. T., Schwartz, S., Maloof, F., and Soodak, M. (1973). Partial purification and some properties of thyroid peroxidase solubilized by extraction with n-butanol. *Prep. Biochem.* **3**, 473–493.

De Groot, L. J., and Carvalho, E. (1960). Iodide binding in thyroid cellular fractions. *J. Biol. Chem.* **235**, 1390–1397.

De Groot, L. J., and Davis, A. M. (1961). Studies on the biosynthesis of iodotyrosines. *J. Biol. Chem.* **236**, 2009–2014.

De Groot, L. J., Thompson, J. E., and Dunn, A. D. (1965). Studies on an iodinating enzyme from calf thyroid. *Endocrinology* **76**, 632–645.

Dème, D., Fimiani, E., Pommier, J., and Nunez, J. (1975). Free diiodotyrosine effects on protein iodination and thyroid hormone synthesis catalyzed by thyroid peroxidase. *Eur. J. Biochem.* **51**, 329–336.

Dème, D., Gavaret, J. M., Pommier, J., and Nunez, J. (1976a). Maximal number of hormonogenic iodotyrosine residues in thyroglobulin iodinated by thyroid peroxidase. *Eur. J. Biochem.* **70**, 7–13.

Dème, D., Pommier, J., and Nunez, J. (1976b). Kinetics of thyroglobulin iodination and hormone synthesis catalyzed by thyroid peroxidase. Role of iodide in the coupling reaction. *Eur. J. Biochem.* **70**, 435–440.

Dème, D., Pommier, J., and Nunez, J. (1978). Specificity of thyroid hormone synthesis. The role of thyroid peroxidase. *Biochim. Biophys. Acta* **540**, 73–82.

Dunn, J. T. (1970). Amino acid neighbors of thyroxine in thyroglobulin. *J. Biol. Chem.* **245**, 5954–5961.

Dunn, J. T., and Ray, S. C. (1975). Changes in the structure of thyroglobulin following the administration of thyroid stimulating hormone. *J. Biol. Chem.* **250**, 5801–5807.

Fischer, A. G., Schulz, A. R., and Oliner, L. (1966). The possible role of thyroid moamine oxidase in iodothyronine synthesis. *Life Sci.* **5**, 995–1002.

Gavaret, J. M., Julien, M. F., Cadot, M., Nunez, J., and Chevillard, L. (1971). Relation entre teneur en iode et propriétés de thyroglobulines obtenues par la méthode d'équilibrage isotopique. *Biochim. Biophys. Acta* **236**, 706–717.

Gavaret, J. M., Pommier, J., Dème, D., Julien, M. F., and Nunez, J. (1975). In vivo and in vitro regulation by iodide of thyroglobulin iodination and thyroxine synthesis. *Horm. Metab. Res.* **7**, 166–172.

Gavaret, J. M., Dème, D., Nunez, J., and Salvatore, G. (1977). Sequential reactivity of tyrosyl residues of thyroglobulin upon iodination catalyzed by thyroid peroxidase. *J. Biol. Chem.* **252**, 3281–3285.

Gavaret, J. M., Cahnmann, H. J., and Nunez, J. (1979). The fate of the "lost side chain" during thyroid hormonogenesis. *J. Biol. Chem.* **254**, 11218–11222.

Gavaret, J. M., Nunez, J., and Cahnmann, H. J. (1980). Formation of dehydroalanine residues during thyroid hormone synthesis in thyroglobulin. *J. Biol. Chem.* **255**, 5281–5285.

Gavaret, J. M., Cahnmann, H. J., and Nunez, J. (1981). Formation of dehydroalanine residues during thyroid hormone synthesis in thyroglobulin. *J. Biol. Chem.* **256**, 9167–9172.

George, P. (1952). Chemical nature of the secondary hydrogen peroxide compound formed by cytochrome C peroxidase and horse-radish peroxidase. *Nature (London)* **169**, 612–613.

George, P. (1953). The chemical nature of the second hydrogen peroxide compound formed by cytochrome C peroxidase and horse-radish peroxidase. *Biochem. J.* **54**, 267–276.

Haeberli, A., Salvatore, G., Edelhoch, H., and Rall, J. E. (1975). Relationship between iodination and the polypeptide chain composition of thyroglobulin. *J. Biol. Chem.* **250**, 7836–7841.

Harington, C. R. (1944). Newer knowledge of the biochemistry of the thyroid gland. *J. Chem. Soc.* **193**, 193–201.

Hati, R., and De Groot, L. J. (1973). Studies on the mechanism of iodination supported by thyroidal NAPDH–cytochrome C reductase. *Acta Endocrinol.* **74**, 271–282.

Hosoya, T., and Morrison, M. (1967). The isolation and purification of thyroid peroxidase. *J. Biol. Chem.* **242**, 2828–2836.

Hosoya, T., Kondo, Y., and Ui, N. (1971a). Peroxidase activity in thyroid gland and partial purification of the enzyme. *J. Biochem. (Tokyo)* **52**, 180–189.

Hosoya, T., Matsusaki, S., and Nagai, Y. (1971b). Localization of peroxidase and other microsomal enzymes in thyroid cells. *Biochemistry* **10**, 3086–3092.

Ingbar, D. H., Askonas, B. A., and Work, T. S. (1959). Observations concerning the heterogeneity of ovine thyroglobulin. *Endocrinology* **64**, 110–122.

Inoue, K., and Taurog, A. (1968). Acute and chronic effects of iodide on thyroid radioiodine metabolism in iodine-deficient rats. *Endocrinology* **83**, 279–290.

Johnson, T. B., and Tewkesbury, L. B. (1942). The oxidation of 3,5-diiodo-tyrosine to thyroxine. *Proc. Natl. Acad. Sci. U.S.A.* **28**, 73–77.

Keilin, D., and Hartree, F. F. (1951). Purification of horse-radish peroxidase and comparison of its properties with those of catalase and methaemoglobin. *Biochem. J.* **49**, 88–104.

Klebanoff, S. J., Yip, C., and Kessler, D. K. (1962). The iodination of tyrosine by beef thyroid preparations. *Biochim. Biophys. Acta* **58**, 563–574.

Krinsky, M. M., and Alexander, N. M. (1971). The specificity of thyroid peroxidase toward tyrosine peptides. *J. Biol. Chem.* **246**, 4755–4758.

Krinsky, M. M., and Fruton, J. S. (1971). Thyroid peroxidase. *Biochem. Biophys. Res. Commun.* **43**, 935–940.

Lamas, L., and Taurog, A. (1977). Relationship between structure of thyroglobulin and synthesis of thyroxine. *Endocrinology* **100**, 1129–1136.

Lamas, L., Covelli, I., Edelhoch, H., Corteze, F., and Salvatore, G. (1971). Evidence for a catalytic role for thyroid peroxidase in the conversion of diiodotyrosine to thyroxine. *Further Adv. Thyroid. Res., Trans. Int. Thyroid Conf. 6th 1970*, **1**, 209–291.

Lamas, L., Morris, M. L., and Taurog, A. (1972). Preferential synthesis of thyroxine from early iodinated tyrosyl residues in thyroglobulin. *Endocrinology* **90**, 1417–1425.

Lamas, L., Taurog, A., Salvatore, G., and Edelhoch, H. (1974). The importance of thyroglobulin structure in thyroid peroxidase-catalyzed conversion of diiodotyrosine to thyroxine. *J. Biol. Chem.* **249**, 2732–2737.

Ljunggren, J. G., and Akeson, A. (1968). Solubilisation, isolation and identification of a peroxidase from the microsomal fraction of beef thyroid. *Arch. Biochem. Biophys.* **127**, 346–353.

Maguire, R. J., and Dunford, H. B. (1972). Kinetics of the oxidation of iodide ion by lactoperoxidase compound II. *Biochemistry* **11**, 937–941.

Maloof, F., and Soodak, M. (1965). The oxidation of thiourea, a new parameter of thyroid function. *Curr. Top. Thyroid Res. Proc. Int. Thyroid Conf. 5th 1965*, pp. 277–290.

Mayberry, W. E., Rall, J. P., and Bertoli, D. (1964). Kinetics of iodination. I. A comparison of the kinetics of iodination of N-acetyl-L-tyrosine and N-acetyl-3-iodo-L-tyrosine. *J. Am. Chem. Soc.* **86**, 5302–5305.

Michot, J. L., Nunez, J., Johnson, M. L., Irace, G., and Edelhoch, H. (1979). Iodide binding and regulation of lactoperoxidase activity toward thyroid goitrogens. *J. Biol. Chem.* **254**, 2205–2209.

Michot, J. L., Osty, J., and Nunez, J. (1980). Regulatory effects of iodide and thiocyanate on tyrosine oxidation catalyzed by thyroid peroxidase. *Eur. J. Biochem.* **107**, 297–301.

Morishima, I., and Ogawa, S. (1979). Nuclear magnetic resonance studies of hemoproteins. *J. Biol. Chem.* **254**, 2814–2820.

Morris, D. R., and Hger, L. P. (1966). Mechanism of the inhibition of enzymatic halogenation by antithyroid agents. *J. Biol. Chem.* **241**, 3582–3589.

Morrison, M., and Sisco-Bayse, G. (1970). Catalysis of iodination by lactoperoxidase. *Biochemistry* **9**, 2996–3000.

Morrison, M., Danner, D. J., and Sisco-Bayse, G. (1971). Subcellular distribution and control of thyroid peroxidase. *Further Adv. Thyroid Res., Trans. Int. Thyroid Conf. 6th, 1970,* Vol. 2, pp. 741–748.

Nagasaka, A., De Groot, L. J., Hati, R., and Liu, C. (1971). Studies on the biosynthesis of thyroid hormone: reconstruction of a defined in vitro iodinating system. *Endocrinology* **88**, 486–490.

Neary, J. T., Davidson, B., Armstrong, A., Maloof, F., and Soodak, M. (1973). Partial purification and some properties of thyroid peroxidase solubilized by alkaline treatment. *Prep. Biochem.* **3**, 495–508.

Neary, J. T., Davidson, B., Armstrong, A., Strout, H. V., and Maloof, F. (1976). Solubilization of thyroid peroxidase by nonionic detergents. *J. Biol. Chem.* **251**, 2525–2529.

Neary, J. T., Loepsell, D., Davidson, B., Armstrong, A., Strout, H. V., Soodak, M., and Maloof, F. (1977). Interaction of thyroid peroxidase with concanavalin A covalently coupled to agarose. *J. Biol. Chem.* **252**, 1264–1271.

Niepomniczcze, H., Medeiros-Neto, G. A., Refetoff, S., De Groot, L. J., and Frang, V. S. (1977). Familial goiter with partial iodine organification defect, lack of thyroglobulin and high levels of thyroid peroxidase. *Clin. Endocrinol.* **6**, 27–39.

Nunez, J., and Pommier, J. (1969). Iodation des protéines par voie enzymatique. (3) complexe intermédiaire enzyme-protéine et mécanisme de la réaction. *Eur. J. Biochem.* **7**, 286–296.

Nunez, J., Mauchamp, J., Macchia, V., and Roche, J. (1965a). Biosynthèse in vitro d'hormones doublement marquées dans des coupes de corps thyroide. II. Biosynthèse d'une préthyroglobuline non iodée. *Biochim. Biophys. Acta* **107**, 247–256.

Nunez, J., Pommier, J., El Hilali, M., and Roche, J. (1965b). Iodation enzymatique des protéines (I). *J. Labelled Compd.* **1**, 128–134.

Nunez, J., Mauchamp, J., Pommier, J., Circovik, T., and Roche, J. (1966a). Relationship between iodination and conformation of thyroglobulin. *Biochem. Biophys. Res. Commun.* **23**, 761–768.

Nunez, J., Mauchamp, J., Pommier, J., Circovik, T., and Roche, J. (1966b). Biogénèse de la thyroglobuline: les transitions d'halogénation. *Biochim. Biophys. Acta* **127**, 112–127.

Ohtaki, S., Mashimo, K., and Yamazaki, I. (1973). Hydrogen peroxide generating system in hog thyroid microsomes. *Biochim. Biophys. Acta* **292**, 825–833.

Pitt-Rivers, R., and James, A. T. (1958). Further observations on the oxidation of diiodotyrosine derivatives. *Biochem. J.* **70**, 173–176.

Pommier, J., De Prailauné, S., and Nunez, J. (1972). Peroxidase particulaire thyroidienne. *Biochimie* **54**, 483–492.

Pommier, J., Déme, D., and Nunez, J. (1973a). Effect of iodide concentration on thyroxine synthesis catalyzed by thyroid peroxidase. *Eur. J. Biochem.* **37**, 406–414.

Pommier, J., Déme, D., and Nunez, J. (1973b). Dissociation into subunits of thyroglobulin iodinated by thyroid and horse-radish peroxidase. *Biochimie* **55**, 263–267.

Pommier, J., Sokoloff, L., and Nunez, J. (1973c). Enzymatic iodination of protein. Kinetics of iodine formation and protein iodination catalyzed by horse-radish peroxidase. *Eur. J. Biochem.* **38**, 497–506.

Pommier, J., Tourniaire, J., Dème, D., Chalendar, D., Bornet, H., and Nunez, J. (1974). A defective thyroid peroxidase solubilized from a familial goiter with iodine organification defect. *J. Clin. Endocrinol. Metab.* **39**, 69–79.

Pommier, J., Tourniaire, J., Rahmoun, B., Dème, D., Pallo, D., Bornet, H., and Nunez, J. (1976). Thyroid iodine organification defects: a case with lack of thyroglobulin iodination and a case without any peroxidase activity. *J. Clin. Endocrinol. Metab.* **42**, 319–329.

Rawitch, A. B., Taurog, A., Chernoff, S. B., and Morris, M. L. (1979). Hog thyroid peroxidase: physical, chemical and catalytic properties of the highly purified enzyme. *Arch. Biochem. Biophys.* **194**, 244–257.

Roche, J., Nunez, J., and Gruson, M. (1960). Sur l'hétérogénéité de la thyroglobuline. *C. R. Seances Soc. Biol. Ses. Fil.* **154**, 2194–2201.

Rolland, M., Aquaron, R., and Lissitzky, S. (1970). Thyroglobulin iodoamino acids estimation after digestion with pronase and leucylaminopeptidase. *Anal. Biochem.* **33**, 307–317.

Rolland, M., Montfort, M. F., Valenta, L., and Lissitzky, S. (1972). Iodoamino acid composition of the thyroglobulin of normal and diseased thyroid glands. *Clin. Chim. Acta* **39**, 95–108.

Roman, R., and Dunford, H. B. (1972). pH dependence of the oxidation of iodide by compound I of horse-radish peroxidase. *Biochemistry,* **11**, 2076–2082.

Roos, D. (1977). Superoxide generation in relation to other oxidative reactions in human polymorphonuclear leukocytes. *In* "Superoxide and Superoxide Dismutases (A. M. Michelson, J. M. McCord, and I. Fridovich, eds.), pp. 307–311. Academic Press, New York.

Salvatore, G., and Edelhoch, H. (1973). Chemistry and biosynthesis of thyroid iodoproteins. *In* "Hormonal Proteins and Peptides" (C. H. Li, ed.), Vol. 1, pp. 201–241. Academic Press, New York.

Schussler, G. C., and Ingbar, S. H. (1961). The role of intermediary carbohydrate metabolism in regulating organic iodinations in the thyroid gland. *J. Clin. Invest.* **40**, 1394–1412.

Sela, M., and Sarid, S. (1956). Appearance of serine upon alkaline incubation of iodinated polytyrosine. *Nature (London)* **178**, 540–541.

Simon, C., and Lissitzky, S. (1964). Etude quantitative par la méthode d'équilibre isotopique avec le radioisotope ^{125}I. *Biochim. Biophys. Acta* **53**, 494–508.

Sorimachi, K., and Ui, N. (1974a). Comparison of the iodoamino acid distribution in thyroglobulines obtained from various animal species. *Gen. Comp. Endocrinol.* **24**, 38–43.

Sorimachi, K., and Ui, N. (1974b). Comparison of the iodoamino acid distribution in various preparations of hog thyroglobulin with different iodine content and subunit structure. *Biochim. Biophys. Acta* **342**, 30–40.

Strum, J. M., and Karnovski, M. J. (1970). Cytochemical localization of endogenous peroxidase in thyroid follicular cells. *J. Cell Biol.* **44**, 655–666.

Strum, J. M., Wicken, J., Stanbury, J. R., and Karnovski, M. J. (1971). Appearance and function of endogenous peroxidase in fetal rat thyroid. *J. Cell Biol.* **51**, 162–175.

Suzuki, M. (1966). Pyridine nucleotide and iodination reaction in the thyroid gland. *Gunma Symp. Endocrinol.* **3**, 81–94.

Taurog, A. (1970a). Thyroid peroxidase-catalyzed iodination of thyroglobulin, inhibition by excess iodide. *Arch. Biochem. Biophys.* **139**, 212–220.

Taurog, A. (1970b). Thyroid peroxidase and thyroxine biosynthesis. *Recent Prog. Horm. Res.* **26**, 189–247.

Taurog, A. (1976). The mechanism of action of the thioureylene antithyroid drugs. *Endocrinology* **98**, 1031–1046.

Taurog, A., and Howells, W. M. (1966). Enzymatic iodination of tyrosine and thyroglobulin with chloroperoxidase. *J. Biol. Chem.* **241**, 1329–1339.

Taurog, A., and Nakashima, T. (1978). Dissociation between degree of iodination and iodoamino acid distribution in thyroglobulin. *Endocrinology* **103**, 632–640.

Taurog, A., Lothrop, M. L., and Estabrook, R. W. (1970;). Improvements in the isolation procedure for thyroid peroxidase: nature of the heme prosthetic group. *Arch. Biochem. Biophys.* **139**, 221–229.

Taurog, A., Morris, M. L., and Lamas, L. (1974). Comparison of lactoperoxidase and thyroid peroxidase-catalyzed iodination and coupling. *Endocrinology* **94**, 1286–1294.

Theorell, H., Ehrenberg, A., and Chance, B. (1952). Electronic structure of the peroxidase peroxide complexes. *Arch. Biochem. Biophys.* **37**, 237–239.

Tice, L. W., and Wollman, S. H. (1974). Ultrastructural localization of peroxidase on pseudopods and other structures of the typical thyroid epithelial cell. *Endocrinology* **94**, 1555–1567.

Ui, N. (1974). Synthesis and chemistry of iodoproteins. *In* "Handbook of Physiology," pp. 55–79. Williams & Wilkins, Baltimore, Maryland.

Ui, N., Tarutani, O., Kondo, Y., and Tamura, H. (1961). Chromatographic fractionation of hog thyroglobulin. *Nature (London)* **191**, 1199–1201.

Valenta, L. J., Valenta, V., Wang, C. A., Vickery, A. L., Caulfields, J., and Maloof, F. (1973). Subcellular distribution of peroxidase activity in human thyroid tissue. *J. Clin. Endocrinol. Metab.* **37**, 560–569.

Van Der Hove-Vanderbroucke, M. F. (1980). Secretion of thyroid hormones. *In* "The Thyroid Gland (M. De Visscher, ed.), pp. 61–79. Raven, New York.

Van Der Walt, B., Kotze, B., Van Jaarsweld, P. P., and Edelhoch, H. (1978). Evidence that thyroglobulin contains nonidentical half molecule subunits. *J. Biol. Chem.* **253**, 1853–1858.

Van Zyl, A., and Edelhoch, H. (1967). The properties of thyroglobulin. (XV) The function of the protein in the control of diiodotyrosine synthesis. *J. Biol. Chem.* **242**, 2423–2427.

Virion, A., Pommier, J., and Nunez, J. (1979). Dissociation of thyroglobulin iodination and hormone synthesis catalyzed by peroxidases. *Eur. J. Biochem.* **102**, 549–554.

Virion, A., Dème, D., Pommier, J., and Nunez, J. (1980). Opposite effects of thiocyanate on tyrosine iodination and thyroid hormone synthesis. *Eur. J. Biochem.* **112**, 1–7.

Wolff, J., and Chaikoff, I. L. (1948). Plasma inorganic iodide as a hemostatic regulator of thyroid function. *J. Biol. Chem.* **174**, 555–564.

Wollman, S. H. (1980). Structure of the thyroid gland. *In* "The Thyroid Gland" (M. De Visscher, ed.), pp. 1–19. Raven, New York.

Yokota, K., and Yamazaki, I. (1965). Reaction of peroxidase with reduced nicotinamide-adenine dinucleotide and reduced nicotinamide dinucleotide phosphate. *Biochim. Biophys. Acta* **105**, 301–312.

Yamamoto, K., and De Groot, L. J. (1975). Participation of NADPH–cytochrome C reductase in thyroid hormone biosynthesis. *Endocrinology* **96**, 1022–1029.

Yip, C. C., and Hadley, L. D. (1966). The iodination of tyrosine by myeloperoxidase and beef thyroids. The possible involvement of free radicals. *Biochim. Biophys. Acta* **122**, 406–412.

Yip, C. C., and Hadley, L. D. (1967). Involvement of free radicals in the iodination of tyrosine and thyroglobulin by myeloperoxidase and a purified beef thyroid peroxidase. *Arch. Biochem. Biophys.* **120**, 533–536.

NOTE ADDED IN PROOF

Since the submission of this manuscript important results have been obtained on the enzymatic mechanism of the iodination and coupling reaction [Courtin, F., Dème, D., Virion, A., Michot, J. L., Pommier, J., and Nunez, J. (1982). *Eur. J. Biochem.*, in press]. Spectroscopic studies performed with lactoperoxidase have shown that (*a*) the iodination reaction is catalyzed exclusively by the enzyme–H_2O_2 species Compound I; (*b*) the coupling reaction is catalyzed by Compound II (which was shown by titration with ferrocyanide to contain two oxidizing equivalents above the native state); (*c*) free diiodotyrosine acts as a cofactor of Compound II by increasing the yield of electron transfer to stoichiometry; and (*d*) iodide and SCN apparently stimulate the coupling reaction by preventing the formation of the inactive enzyme species Compound III when the H_2O_2 enzyme ratio is higher than 1. These conclusions are summarized in a scheme of the enzymatic mechanism of iodination and coupling shown below.

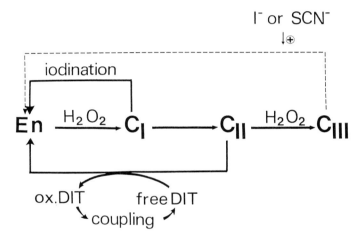

Chemistry of the Gastrointestinal Hormones and Hormone-like Peptides and a Sketch of Their Physiology and Pharmacology

VIKTOR MUTT

Department of Biochemistry II, Karolinska Institutet, Stockholm, Sweden

I. Historical Background and Some Problems with Definitions

Toward the end of the nineteenth century, physiological investigations were concerned with the role nerves played in various physiological activities. The effects of the stimulation or of the severance of individual nerves were investigated. However, not everyone was investigating nerves. At the Physiological Laboratory of University College in London, Oliver and Schäfer, and others, investigated the effects of injection of extracts of various organs into the blood stream of experimental animals. This led to the discovery of the blood pressure-

231

raising properties of extracts of the pituitary (Oliver and Schäfer, 1895b) and the suprarenal glands (Oliver and Schäfer, 1894) and that the effect of the suprarenal extracts was due to some substance(s) produced in the medulla, not in the cortex (Oliver and Schäfer, 1895a). The effect of the pituitary on blood pressure was localized to its posterior lobe by Howell at Johns Hopkins University in Baltimore (Howell, 1898).

Bayliss and Starling continued in this tradition at University College when in January 1902 they prepared an extract of the mucosa of the upper intestine of a dog and showed that, on intravenous injection, it stimulated the secretion of pancreatic juice and bile in the dog. They named the active substance secretin (Bayliss and Starling, 1902a,b). The discovery of secretin explained at once a physiological mystery, namely, that acidification of the upper intestine resulted in secretion of pancreatic juice. This had been clearly, although cursorily, described much earlier by Leuret and Lassaigne (1825), but their observations had evidently been forgotten and the effect was rediscovered in Pavlov's laboratory, where it was thoroughly studied (Becker, 1893; Dolinsky, 1894). According to the thinking of the time, the stimulation and inhibition of gastrointestinal organ functions had to take place via nerve impulses, despite elaborate work that had not disclosed any nerves mediating the stimulating effect of intestinal acidification on pancreatic secretion (Popielski, 1901; Wertheimer and Lepage, 1901). Bayliss and Starling correctly assumed that secretin was "probably a body of very definite composition" and, more important, that it was probably not the only "body" that acted as a blood-borne chemical messenger between different organs and that others would soon be discovered (Bayliss and Starling; 1902a). They therefore considered it expedient to create a new word to describe such messengers. At the suggestion of W. B. Hardy, they settled on the word hormone, from the Greek Ορμαω̄, "I arouse to activity" (Starling, 1905; Bayliss, 1920). For most endocrinologists, and even more so for chemists, typical hormones were for many decades to be substances, such as steroids, iodothyronines, and possibly biogenic amines, that could be isolated in crystalline form, the chemical structures precisely described, and replicates of which could be synthesized. In the background were the poorly characterized polypeptide and protein hormones, all, with the exception of the crystallizable insulin, amorphous, of doubtful purity, and, including insulin, seemingly out of reach of precise chemical characterization. This situation prevailed until the late 1940s and early 1950s, when du Vigneaud and co-workers isolated the peptide hormone oxytocin (Livermore and du Vigneaud, 1949), determined its amino acid sequence (du Vigneaud *et al.*, 1953a), in parallel with the independent work of Tuppy (1953), synthesized its replicate (du Vigneaud *et al.*, 1953b), and showed that the synthetic and natural products were indistinguishable in a variety of chemical and physiological tests. This finally dispelled the lingering suspicions that a peptide hormone could not be composed of amino acid residues only, but that the peptide structure was merely a carrier for some unrecognized functional prosthetic group.

The elucidation of the primary structure of bovine insulin by Sanger and co-workers (Sanger, 1945; Ryle *et al.*, 1955) then definitely placed the peptide and protein hormones into the range of chemical comprehensiblity.

As for the gastrointestinal hormones, the discovery of secretin was followed by that of gastrin (Edkins, 1905), of cholecystokinin (Ivy and Oldberg, 1928), and of pancreozymin (Harper and Raper, 1943). For years these substances were to be known through their actions, not by their structure, all being used by physiologists and pharmacologists in the form of more or less crude extracts. Nevertheless, important information concerning their actions was obtained. In particular, secretin soon had quite extensive clinical applications, mainly through the work of Lagerlöf (1942), who used pharmacologically acceptable preparations of the hormone prepared by methods devised by Hammarsten and co-workers (Hammarsten *et al.*, 1933), Diamond *et al.* (1939), and Dreiling and co-workers (Dreiling and Janowitz, 1962), who used either the same type of secretin preparations or else preparations based on the work of Ivy and co-workers (Greengard and Ivy, 1938) or of Crick *et al.* (1950). Defined only in a functional sense were "factors" such as villikinin (Kokas and Ludány, 1930), enterogastrone (Kosaka and Lim, 1930), and enterocrinin (Nasset, 1938).

A change took place in the first half of the 1960s when the application of efficient methods, developed in other areas of biochemistry for the purification of peptides, led to the essentially simultaneous isolation of (porcine) secretin (Jorpes *et al.*, 1962), (porcine) gastrin, or rather the gastrins (Gregory, 1962a), and soon thereafter of (porcine) cholecystokinin-pancreozymin (Jorpes *et al.*, 1964), a substance having the combined physiological properties assigned by their respective discoverers to cholecystokinin and to pancreozymin. The gastrins were subsequently isolated from several other mammalian species including man (Grossman, 1970b). Analyses of the isolated hormones confirmed their long suspected peptide nature, and their amino acid sequences were determined by the methods then known, among which the phenylisothiocyanate method of Edman (1950) in its various modifications played an important part, as it continues to do. Replicates of the gastrins (Anderson *et al.,* 1964), secretin (Bodanszky *et al.,* 1966), and the C-terminal, hormonally active part of CCK (Ondetti *et al.,* 1970a) were synthesized. This intense activity made it appear, for a time, as though the whole field of the gastrointestinal hormones had been brought into open view. Admittedly, there were areas in this field that required further work. It was of interest, as it always is with naturally occurring peptides, to isolate gastrin, secretin, and CCK from additional species so as to gain insight into evolutionary relationships and relations between structure and activity. Also those hormones that still remained known only as physiological "principles" had to be isolated. All this could be expected to be carried out with methods similar to those used for porcine gastrin, secretin, and CCK. Soon, however, unexpected findings started to change the picture so that the field today in many respects appears substantially different from that of the 1960s. The classic hormones enterogastrone and incretin have been redefined as physiological concepts rather than distinctive chemical substances (pp. 310 and 337). Instead, several candidate hormones (Grossman, 1974, 1975) for which names had to be invented were isolated, and there is no reason to believe that we now know all the gastrointestinal peptides with physiological or pharmacological properties (Snyder, 1980).

With the aid of a variety of morphological techniques, among which the indirect immunofluorescence technique of Coons *et al.* (1955) played a prominent part, the cells that biosynthesize and/or store the gastrointestinal hormones, or at least that contain substances reacting with antibodies to these hormones, were identified (Solcia *et al.,* 1978; Grube and Forssmann, 1979). This morphological work was stimulated by the unifying hypothesis of Pearse (1968) for peptide hormone-producing cells. Unexpectedly, hormonal peptides were found not only in endocrine types of cells, but also in both the peripheral and central nervous system (Snyder, 1980). The invention of the competitive ligand method of radioimmunoassay by Berson and Yalow (Berson and Yalow, 1958, 1959) made it possible to detect and quantitate peptide hormones in the circulating blood or in certain tissue extracts in amounts far too low to be detected previously by other methods. The use of region-specific antibodies has further increased the scope of the immunological techniques, and the evidence for the occurrence of gastrointestinal hormonal peptides in both intestinal tissue and the central nervous system became convincing (Snyder, 1980). It was shown completely independently of any immunological method that a peptide existed in both these locations. In 1936 v. Euler demonstrated the peptide nature of the "substance P" that he and Gaddum had discovered and shown to be present in horse brain and intestine (v. Euler, 1936; v. Euler and Gaddum, 1931). Substance P isolated from bovine collicular (Chang and Leeman, 1970a) or hypothalamic tissue (Carraway and Leeman, 1979) and from horse intestine by Studer *et al.* (1973) are identical. However, substance P could have been an isolated special case.

Radioimmunoassays, in combination with various separation procedures, showed that peptide hormones often, possibly always, occur in blood and tissues in different-sized forms, the smaller forms being derivable from the larger ones. Such heterogeneity had been known earlier in a few cases and suspected in others, but the extent to which it occurred was unexpected (pp. 262). In many cases, the different forms of a particular peptide were found to show different (mostly quantitatively) patterns of activity, and this complicated the description of the activities of the various hormones. Another complication was the finding that all the hormones had an unexpected variety of different actions. Eleven different actions had been described for gastrin by 1968 (Gregory, 1968) and still more have been described since then (p. 319). The picture was further complicated by the interactions of these hormones with each other and with the activities of nerves—an interaction between gastrin and the vagus nerves had been suspected early in the 1940s (Uvnäs, 1942)—and by various effects of some of the hormones on the release of other hormones.

There has never been a generally accepted definition of a gastrointestinal hormone. It was until recently probably believed by most workers in the field that such hormones were biosynthesized exclusively in cells of the gastrointestinal tract and that their release, by some appropriate physiological stimulus, into the blood influenced the state of activity of some organ of digestion in a physiologically meaningful way, without having any direct effects outside of the gastrointestinal area. Obviously this is not so. Not only are at least some gastrointestinal hormonal peptides also biosynthesized elsewhere in the organism than in the tissues of the gastrointestinal tract, but some may, irrespective of their place of synthesis, have effects outside of the gastrointestinal area. It has also become probable that some of these substances do not act, exclusively or even at all, in the classic blood-borne endocrine fashion, but in a paracrine manner (Feyrter, 1952) on cells in the immediate vicinity of their cells of origin or storage. In other cases "neurocrine" actions seem probable.

This new information has inevitably led to discussions of how to define a gastrointestinal hormone. In view of experiments suggesting that these hormones, either those known or those not yet isolated, may exert trophic effects on the hypothalamus and the thyroid, and as other extragastrointestinal actions have been described for several of the known hormones, Ugolev (1975) suggested the common name enterins for all these hormones, which would signify their site of origin while deemphasizing the gastrointestinal location of their target organs. The name is suggestive and should be considered in future discussions of nomenclature, although findings that some gastrointestinal hormones are also synthesized outside of the tissues of the gastrointestinal tract would seem to make it somewhat less attractive. Another suggestion (Wingate, 1976) goes further and proposes that the gastrointestinal hormones should not be classified as hormones at all because their cells of origin, unlike those of the hormones regulating growth, metabolism, and reproduction, are not aggregated in glands but dispersed over considerable areas of the gastrointestinal mucosa and because in their mode of action they also differ in various ways from those other hormones. Instead they could be called "eupeptides," the term uniting "the idea of eupeptic, or good digestive, function (which these substances clearly promote) with a reminder of the common chemical structure of these substances." It may be asked why specifically the gastrointestinal hormones, the discovery of which led to the creation of the word hormone—and at any rate several of which seem to act just as the chemical messengers envisaged by the meaning of the word—should be called something else. If a change should indeed be necessary it would seem more appropriate to create a new word to classify the substances, known today as hormones, that regulate growth, metabolism, and reproduction. Linguistically "eupeptide" is an interesting construction, the more so as the word peptide itself also is in part derived from the Greek word for digestion (Fischer, 1906).

Grossman (1979a) has pointed out that certain cells, which might be called regulator cells, have as their sole function the regulation of the activity of other cells that do the actual work of the body. He further suggests that if the regulator cells were to designate the neural, endocrine, and paracrine cells as a group, the chemical messengers they produce could be called regulins. An alternative term would be "chemitter," as a contraction of chemical transmitter (Grossman, 1979b). The concept of regulator cells is undoubtedly didactically useful. Regulins, however, would run the obvious risk of vernacularization into, for instance, "regulatory peptides," which in biochemistry have long been associated with the intracellular regulation of the functions of the genetic apparatus or of metabolic processes rather than with intercellular communication. One possibility would be to consider hormones as the messengers of the regulator cells, whether they exert their actions via endocrine, paracrine, or neurocrine mediators. After all, it is not uncommon for word usage to change with time. The once vivid discussions of what to name hormones that inhibited rather than stimulated physiological processes (Ivy, 1930) seem rather remote today. In this review, a gastrointestinal hormone is defined as a peptide that is biosynthesized, although not exclusively, in cells of some part of the wall of the gastrointestinal canal, and which, whatever else it may do, influences in either an endocrine, paracrine, or neurocrine manner the physiological activity of some organ or organs of digestion. This definition may be criticized for claiming that a gastrointestinal hormone is necessarily a peptide, since substances that belong to other chemical categories, like biogenic amines and prostaglandins, are also known to have hormone-like actions on gastrointestinal organs, a fact repeatedly pointed out in the review. It is indeed a somewhat arbitrary definition, but it follows common practice. However, the hormonal effects of several of the peptides to be discussed have as yet been observed only on parenteral administration of the peptides to experimental animals, and, in such cases, the true hormonal status of the candidate hormones (Grossman, 1974) remains to be established.

II. The Substances

The gastrointestinal hormones may be grouped as follows:

Group 1: Those isolated from one or more species and with the complete amino acid sequences disclosed. At the time of writing (1981), this group consists of gastrin, cholecystokinin-pancreozymin (CCK), secretin, the vasoactive intestinal polypeptide (VIP), motilin, the gastric inhibitory polypeptide (GIP), the bombesin-related gastrin-releasing polypeptide (GRP), somatostatin-28, Substance P, neurotensin, and glicentin.

Group 2: Those stated as isolated but for which sequence data are either not published or incomplete. To this group belong chymodenin, PHI PYY and oxyntomodulin. (For an explanation of the acronyms PHI and PYY see Section II,B,1.)

Group 3: Those that have not been isolated from gastrointestinal tissues. These peptides fall into two subgroups. Subgroup 3a contains known peptides with immunological and/or pharmacological evidence for their occurrence in gastrointestinal tissues, but that have not yet been isolated and chemically characterized from these tissues. Examples are glucagon, corticotropin, thyroliberin, urogastrone, perhaps physalaemin. Subgroup 3a may also contain as yet uncharacterized variant forms of some of these peptides, such as glucagon-related peptides, other than glicentin and oxyntomodulin of the "gut glucagon" complex and of peptides in groups 1 and 2. Subgroup 3b contains structurally completely uncharacterized peptides the existence of which is probable only on physiological or pharmacological evidence. Such hypothetical peptides are discussed in Section X. It is, however, obvious that several of the functions described for different peptides in this subgroup may turn out to be the properties of the same substance, and in some cases possibly even unrecognized properties of one or other of the already known hormones.

Finally there are peptides like the "pancreatic polypeptide" (Kimmel et al., 1975; Lin and Chance, 1974), coherin (Goodman and Hiatt, 1972), bombesin (Anastasi et al., 1971), cerulein (Anastasi et al., 1968a), and others that have not been isolated from gastrointestinal tissues and for which there is no evidence that they occur there but which show functional or structural similarities to gastrointestinal hormonal peptides. Such peptides will be discussed where appropriate, but not under a separate heading.

A. (GROUP 1) PEPTIDES WITH KNOWN AMINO ACID SEQUENCES

1. Gastrin

Edkins (1905, 1906) found that extracts of the pyloric mucosa of cats or pigs, on intravenous injection into anesthetized cats, stimulated the secretion of gastric acid, and he named the active substance gastrin (Edkins, 1905) or "gastric secretin" (Edkins, 1906). Extracts of fundic mucosa were inactive, but extracts of the cardiac mucosa of pigs were approximately as active as those of the pyloric mucosa. Porcine gastrin was isolated from stomach antral mucosa by Gregory and Tracy early in 1962. A preliminary amino acid analysis suggested that it was composed of eight different kinds of amino acid residues, some of which occurred repeatedly (Gregory, 1962a). No "wrong" amino acids were present, indicating purity of the preparation. Tryptophan had been overlooked but was soon recognized to be present. Further work led to the isolation of an additional gastrin (Gregory and Tracy, 1963, 1964). Both gastrins were found to be heptadecapeptides with identical amino acid sequences:

Glp-Gly-Pro-Trp-Met-Glu-Glu-Glu-Glu-Glu-Ala-Tyr-Gly-Trp-Met-Asp-Phe-NH₂*

* In this review the amino acid residues are designated by the three-letter [Eur. J. Biochem. **1**, 375–378 (1967)] or one-letter [Eur. J. Biochem. **5**, 151–153

The difference between the heptadecapeptides was explained by the finding that, although in "gastrin I" the phenolic group of the tyrosine residue was free, it was esterified with sulfuric acid in "gastrin II" (Gregory *et al.,* 1964). Corresponding pairs of heptadecapeptide gastrins (G-17 for either G-17-I or G-17-II, or both) were soon thereafter isolated from human (Gregory *et al.,* 1966), bovine and ovine (Agarwal *et al.,* 1968b), canine (Gregory *et al.,* 1969a), and feline (Gregory, quoted by Agarwal *et al.,* 1969b) antral mucosa. The human heptadecapeptides, identical to those isolated from the antral mucosa, also were isolated from tumor tissue from patients with the Zollinger–Ellison syndrome (Gregory *et al.,* 1969b). The amino acid sequence of human G-17 was determined by Bentley *et al.* (1966), that of ovine and bovine G-17 by Agarwal *et al.* (1968b), that of canine G-17 by Agarwal *et al.* (1969a), and that of feline G-17 by Agarwal *et al.* (1969b). Compared with porcine G-17, only small species differences were found. Human G-17 differed from porcine G-17 only by having a residue of leucine instead of one of methionine in position 5. In ovine and bovine G-17 a residue of valine was found in position 5 and, in addition, there was a residue of alanine in position 10 instead of the glutamic acid found there in porcine and in human G-17. Canine G-17 differed from porcine only by the substitution of the glutamic acid residue in position 8 by one of alanine, and feline G-17 differered from porcine by having Leu-5 and Ala-10. There also appeared to be some species differences in the ratio of the nonsulfated to the sulfated forms of G-17. This ratio was about 2 : 1 in man (Gregory *et al.,* 1966) and dog (Gregory *et al.,* 1969a), but about 3 : 4 in hog (Gregory and Tracy, 1964); also in bovine and ovine G-17 the sulfated form predominated in quantity over the nonsulfated (Agarwal *et al.,* 1968b).

(1968)] notations recommended by the IUPAC–IUB Commission on Biochemical Nomenclature.

Alanine	Ala or A	Glycine	Gly or G	Proline	Pro or P
Arginine	Arg or R	Histidine	His or H	Serine	Ser or S
Asparagine	Asn or N	Isoleucine	Ile or I	Threonine	Thr or T
Aspartic acid	Asp or D	Leucine	Leu or L	Tryptophan	Trp or W
Cysteine	Cys or C	Lysine	Lys or K	Tyrosine	Tyr or Y
Glutamine	Gln or Q	Methionine	Met or M	Valine	Val or V
Glutamic acid	Glu or E	Phenylalanine	Phe or F		

If a residue is either aspartic acid or asparagine, this is indicated by Asx or B; and similarly for glutamic acid and glutamine, Glx or Z. In addition, Glp or *Q are used for pyroglutamyl, and the symbol ■ if the C-terminal residue of a peptide has the α-amide structure.

In addition to the heptadecapeptides, pairs of larger gastrins were subsequently isolated from Zollinger–Ellison tumor tissue and from hog antral mucosa by Gregory and Tracy (1972). It was found that they consisted of the heptadecapeptides extended from their N termini by additional heptadecapeptides, with quite different amino acid compositions from the G-17's but identical in each species for G-17-I and G-17-II. There were, however, some species variations. For such N-terminal extension to be possible, the pyroglutamyl residue of G-17 was replaced by glutaminyl and the amino group of the latter was acylated by the C-terminal lysine residue of the extending peptide. The amino acid sequences of the human and porcine G-34's were determined by Ieuan Harris and were disclosed by Gregory and Tracy (1975). Further work led to a slight revision of the proposed structures—a transposition of His-7 and Pro-9 in the porcine peptide (Dockray *et al.*, 1979a) and the replacement of His-7 by Pro and of Ser-9 by His in the human (Choudhury *et al.*, 1980). The sequence of the N-terminal heptadecapeptide of porcine G-34 is

Glp-Leu-Gly-Leu-Gln-Gly-Pro-Pro-His-Leu-Val-Ala-Asp-Leu-Ala-Lys-Lys

and the corresponding sequence of human G-34 is

Glp-Leu-Gly-Pro-Gln-Gly-Pro-Pro-His-Leu-Val-Ala-Asp-Pro-Ser-Lys-Lys

Obviously this differs from the porcine by having Pro-4, Pro-14, and Ser-15 instead of Leu-4, Leu-14, and Ala-15. The above sequence information for the gastrins is summarized in Table I, and the formula structure of nonsulfated hG-34 is shown in Fig. 1. A pair of gastrins, shorter instead of longer than the G-17's, were also isolated from Zollinger–Ellison tumor tissue by Gregory and Tracy (1974). These "minigastrins" were first believed to constitute the C-terminal tridecapeptides of the G-17's, but more recently it was shown that they are C-terminal tetradecapeptides instead (Gregory *et al.*, 1979).

2. *Cholecystokinin (-Pancreozymin) (CCK)*

Ivy and Oldberg showed in 1928 that the intravenous administration of certain secretin preparations to anesthesized cats or dogs or to conscious dogs resulted in gallbladder contraction. They referred to work, published later (Ivy *et al.*, 1929a), suggesting that the causative agent was not secretin itself and postulated that the mucosa of the upper intestine contained a specific hormone for gallbladder contraction. They named this hormone cholecystokinin (Ivy and Oldberg, 1928). Harper and Raper (1943) showed that extracts of porcine, canine, or feline upper small intestinal mucosa contained a substance, distinct

TABLE I

Amino Acid Sequences of Six Mammalian Gastrins[a]

Human	*Q	L	G	P	Q	G	P	P	H	L	V	A	D	P	S	K	K	Q	G	P	W	L	E	E	E	E	E	A	Y[b]	G	W	M	D	F	■
Porcine	*Q	L	G	*L*	Q	G	P	P	H	L	V	A	D	*L*	A	K	K	Q	G	P	W	*M*	E	E	E	E	E	A	Y[b]	G	W	M	D	F	■
Bovine and ovine																		*Q	G	P	W	*V*	E	E	E	E	E	A	Y[b]	G	W	M	D	F	■
Canine																		*Q	G	P	W	*M*	E	E	*A*	E	E	A	Y[b]	G	W	M	D	F	■
Feline																		*Q	G	P	W	L	E	E	E	E	*A*	A	Y[b]	G	W	M	D	F	■

[a] Residues that in a certain position differ from those of the human form are shown in italics.

[b] The tyrosine residue may in each case be sulfated (II or s) or not sulfated (I or ns).

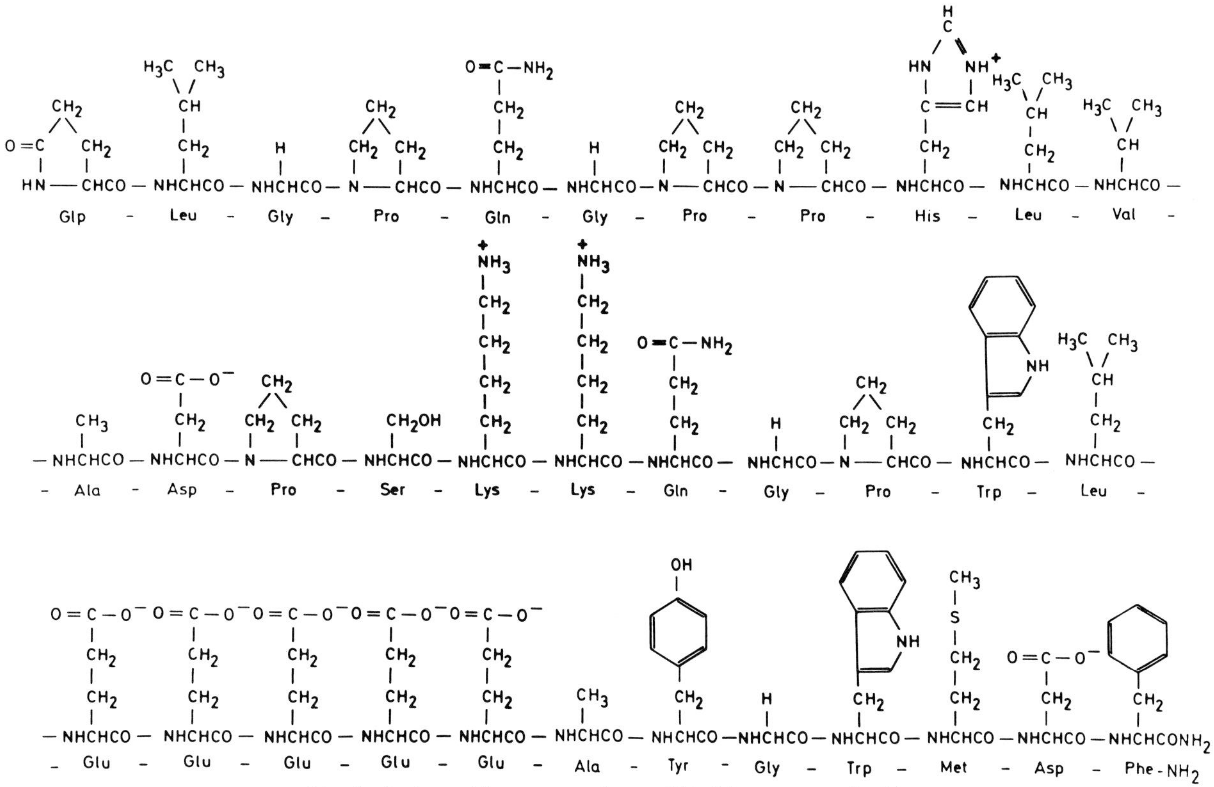

Fig. 1. Amino acid sequence of nonsulfated human gastrin-34.

from secretin, that, on intravenous injection into anesthetized cats, stimulated the secretion of pancreatic enzymes. They named this hormone pancreozymin.

Since the purification of cholecystokinin and of pancreozymin unexpectedly resulted in the isolation of a single hormone that exhibited the different activities ascribed to cholecystokinin and to pancreozymin (Jorpes and Mutt, 1966), it was originally referred to as cholecystokinin-pancreozymin (CCK-PZ) (Mutt and Jorpes, 1968). Since this name was somewhat cumbersome, Grossman (1970a) suggested that, in view of the 15-year antecedence in discovery of cholecystokinin over that of pancreozymin, the term cholecystokinin (CCK) be used instead of cholecystokinin-pancreozymin, it being understood that cholecystokinin had both cholecystokinetic and pancreozyminic activities. This suggestion has been widely followed, also in this review. Some workers, however, who are primarily interested in the pancreozyminic activity of the hormone still use the term cholecystokinin-pancreozymin, or even simply pancreozymin. Porcine cholecystokinin was isolated in highly purified form from hog upper intestinal tissue by Jorpes et al. (1964), and work with this type of material led to the recognition that (porcine) CCK did not contain threonine or cysteine/cystine. However, attempts at elucidation of its amino acid sequence ran into difficulties that were not overcome before an additional purification step, a chromatography on carboxymethyl cellulose, was introduced. With thus purified material, the correct amino acid composition of acid hydrolyzates of the peptide was determined and the peptide was shown to have N-terminal lysine and, like gastrin (Gregory et al., 1964), C-terminal aspartylphenylalanine amide (Mutt and Jorpes, 1967a). The determination of the amino acid sequence of the peptide, a tritriacontapeptide, did not present any particular difficulties. A partial sequence was described in 1968 (Mutt and Jorpes, 1968), and the following complete sequence was disclosed in 1971 (Mutt and Jorpes, 1971).

Lys-Ala-Pro-Ser-Gly-Arg-Val-Ser-Met-Ile-Lys-Asn-Leu-Gln-Ser-Leu-Asp-Pro-
Ser-His-Arg-Ile-Ser-Asp-Arg-Asp-Tyr(SO_3)-Met-Gly-Trp-Met-Asp-Phe-NH_2

Chromatography on carboxymethyl cellulose, mentioned above, revealed that a considerable quantity of CCK-like bioactive material remained on the column after the CCK used for structural studies had eluted, and it could be displaced from the column by drastically increasing the molarity of the ammonium bicarbonate used as the eluent (Mutt and Jorpes, 1968). This was first believed to be due to some technical inadequacy of the chromatographic system, such as secondary adsorption of CCK to peptides adsorbed to the column. However, it was soon recognized that the CCK retained on the column was different from the 33-amino acid residue molecule that had been sequenced. The difference was that the retained CCK consisted of 39 rather than of 33 amino acid residues, the additional 6 residues constituting an N-terminal extension of the tritriacontapeptide by the sequence, Tyr-Ile-Gln-Gln-Ala-Arg- (Mutt, 1976). The sequence of 39-CCK is shown in formula form in Fig. 2. It was shown that the C-terminal octapeptide of CCK and various longer peptides incorporating it at their C termini exhibited the cholecystokinetic and pancreozyminic activities of the whole molecule of CCK (Mutt and Jorpes, 1968). Subsequently, immunochemical analyses of variously fractionated extracts of intestinal (Harvey et al., 1974; Dockray, 1977; Rehfeld, 1977, 1978a,b; Straus and Yalow, 1978) and of brain (Dockray, 1976; del Mazo, 1977; Muller et al., 1977; Rehfeld, 1978a,b; Straus and Yalow, 1978) tissue from various species provided evidence for the occurrence of the free octapeptide in these tissues. This was supported by the finding of Robberecht et al. (1978) that material extracted from a 100,000 g pellet of human cortical gray matter released amylase from rat pancreatic fragments in vitro and reacted like CCK-8 in a radioreceptor assay. Final confirmation of the existence of the free octapeptide in brain tissue was provided by its direct chemical isolation from sheep brain by Dockray et al. (1978a).

The existence of gastrin and CCK in forms of different sizes, the larger being N-terminal extensions of the shorter, has raised questions of nomenclature. It has been pointed out (Walsh et al., 1974) that a gastrin peptide is defined by (a) the number of amino acids in its peptide chain; (b) the species; and (c) whether or not its tyrosine (in position 6 from the C terminus) is sulfated. The latter does not apply to the C-terminal pentapeptide and still shorter peptides. The same factors apply to CCK, although no unsulfated (in position 7 from the C terminus) form has yet been isolated from tissues.

In peptide chemistry, the amino acid residues of peptides are as a rule numbered from the N termini of the peptides. However, since the (known) biological activities of gastrin (Tracy and Gregory, 1964) and of CCK (Mutt and Jorpes, 1968) are dependent on the presence of the C-terminal parts of the peptide chains of these hormones, it is customary to name as gastrins or CCKs only such peptides as contain these C-terminal parts. The active octapeptide of CCK, for instance, is referred to as CCK-8, not CCK_{26-33} as it would have been if the first isolated CCK (CCK-33) had been used as the reference peptide for other forms of CCK. Gregory and Tracy originally referred to the non-

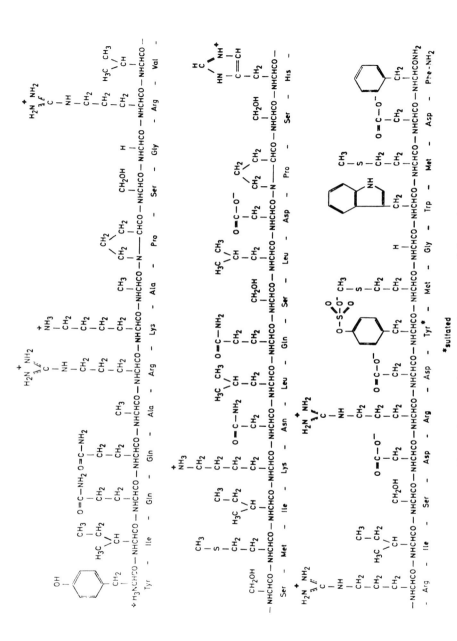

FIG. 2. Amino acid sequence of porcine 39-cholecystokinin.

*sulfated

sulfated and sulfated forms of gastrin with the Roman numerals I and II, respectively (Gregory and Tracy, 1964, 1975). An alternative suggestion is to use the lowercase postscript ns for the nonsulfated forms and s for the sulfated forms (Rehfeld, 1973; Dockray *et al.*, 1979b), G-17 ns, for instance, thereby becomes synonymous with G-17-I. Since gastrin and CCK have identical C-terminal pentapeptide amide sequences and since this sequence was known earlier for gastrin than for CCK, it has been suggested that this pentapeptide and shorter fragments of it be referred to as gastrin(s) irrespective of their origin (Dockray *et al.*, 1979b); thus Trp-Met-Asp-Phe-NH$_2$ is G-4, not CCK-4. An alternative nomenclature, however, is G/CCK-4 (Rehfeld *et al.*, 1980). It has also been suggested that the species from which a gastrin or CCK has been isolated, or in which it occurs endogenously, could, if necessary, be indicated by an appropriate abbreviation preceding G or CCK as a lowercase letter, for instance pG-17 s for the sulfated form of the porcine heptadecapeptide gastrin and hG-34 for human tetratriacontapeptide gastrin. This is reasonable except that the language for the species designation has not been agreed on and variability here may lead to confusion. Also if, as seems highly probable, C-terminally extended forms of the gastrins and cholecystokinins and of other gastrointestinal hormones are discovered, placing the residue numbers before the peptide designation rather than after might be reasonable, thus 8-CCK rather than CCK-8 (see p. 276).

3. Secretin

Bayliss and Starling (1902a,b) discovered that the intravenous injection into anesthetized dogs of extracts of the upper intestinal mucosa from various vertebrate species resulted in a stimulation of pancreatic secretion and of hepatic bile flow. They named the active substance secretin. The method that led to the isolation of secretin from porcine upper intestinal tissue was outlined in 1961 (Jorpes and Mutt, 1961a). The preparation of secretin described in that publication was presumably essentially pure since only traces of the "wrong" amino acids were found in acid hydrolyzates of the material. However, something had obviously gone wrong with the quantitative determination of the amino acids, since two acids, histidine and phenylalanine, later shown to be present in secretin, were lost somehow during the analysis, and the relative proportions in which the other amino acids were found to occur were also wrong in several cases. The correct amino acid composition of (porcine) secretin, its N-terminal His-Ser-Asx- sequence, and the amino acids present in two of its tryptic peptides, one of which was the C terminus, were disclosed in 1962 (Jorpes *et al.*, 1962). Soon thereafter it was found that valine was situated C-terminally in secretin and that its carboxyl group was amidated (Jorpes and Mutt, 1964). The complete amino acid sequence of (porcine) secretin was disclosed in 1966 (Mutt and Jorpes, 1966; Bodanszky *et al.,* 1966), although a detailed account of how it had been elucidated was not published until 1970 (Mutt *et al.,* 1970). The amino acid sequence of porcine secretin is

His-Ser-Asp-Gly-Thr-Phe-Thr-Ser-Glu-Leu-Ser-Arg-Leu-Arg-Asp-
$\qquad$ Ser-Ala-Arg-Leu-Gln-Arg-Leu-Leu-Gln-Gly-Leu-Val-NH$_2$

This is shown in formula form in Fig. 3. Bovine secretin has the same amino acid sequence as porcine secretin (Carlquist *et al.,* 1981a), whereas chicken secretin (Nilsson *et al.,* 1980) is remarkably different:

His-Ser-Asp-Gly-Leu-Phe-Thr-Ser-Glu-Tyr-Ser-Lys-Met-Arg-Gly-
$\qquad$ Asn-Ala-Gln-Val-Gln-Lys-Phe-Ile-Gln-Asn-Leu-Met-NH$_2$

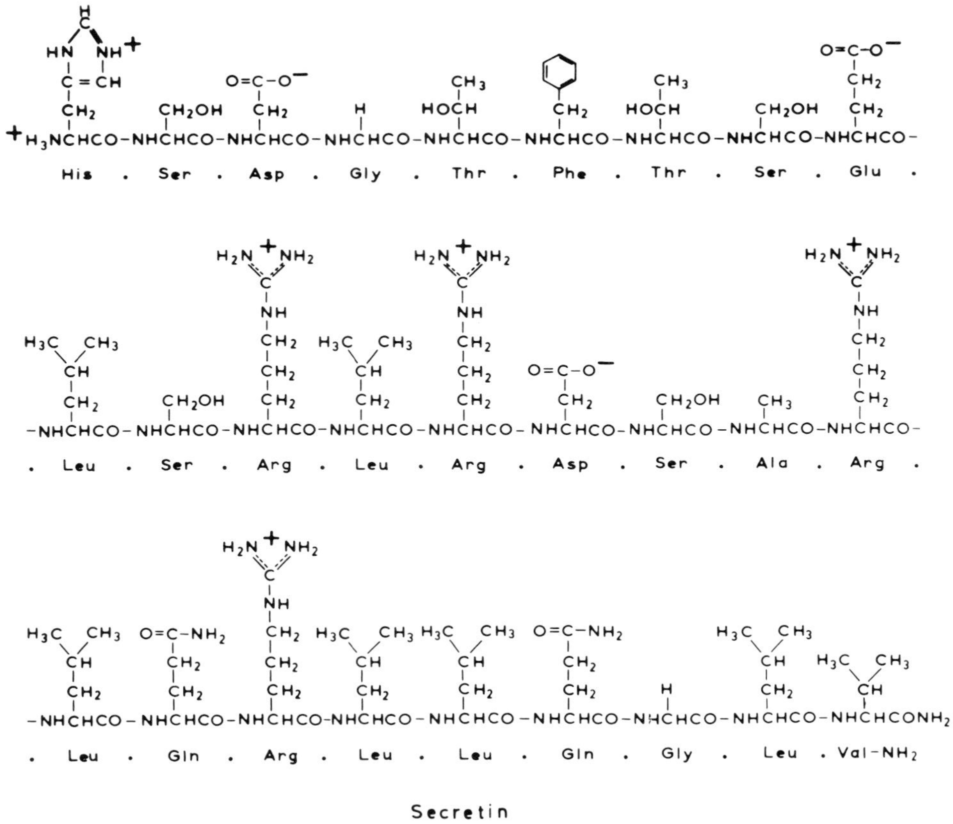

Secretin

FIG. 3. Amino acid sequence of porcine secretin.

4. *The Vasoactive Intestinal Polypeptide (VIP)*

The vasodepressor activities described by Bayliss and Starling (1902a,b) for extracts of upper intestinal tissue may in part have been due to VIP, but an interpretation is difficult since those extracts almost certainly contained histamine, among many other substances. It is more likely that Ivy *et al.* (1929b) may have observed the actions of VIP when they found that material precipitated from intestinal extracts by saturation of the extracts with NaCl had vasodepressor activities of a nonhistamine type. These observations do not, however, seem to have led to attempts to isolate the depressor substance(s) in question, and VIP was isolated (Said and Mutt, 1970a, 1972) under the name "vasoactive intestinal octacosapeptide" after the finding of intense peripheral and splanchnic vasodilator activities in a peptide side fraction from the isolation of secretin from hog upper intestinal tissue (Said and Mutt, 1970b). The amino acid sequence of porcine VIP is

His-Ser-Asp-Ala-Val-Phe-Thr-Asp-Asn-Tyr-Thr-Arg-Leu-Arg-Lys-
Gln-Met-Ala-Val-Lys-Lys-Tyr-Leu-Asn-Ser-Ile-Leu-Asn-NH$_2$

(Mutt and Said, 1974); it is shown in formula form in Fig. 4. Bovine (Carlquist *et al.*, 1979) and (presumably) human (Carlquist *et al.*, 1981b) VIP are identical to the porcine, whereas chicken VIP (Nilsson, 1975)

His-Ser-Asp-Ala-Val-Phe-Thr-Asp-Asn-Tyr-Ser-Arg-Phe-Arg-Lys-
Gln-Met-Ala-Val-Lys-Lys-Tyr-Leu-Asn-Ser-Val-Leu-Thr-NH$_2$

differs from it by having Ser-11, Phe-13, Val-26, and threonine amide-28 instead of Thr-11, Leu-13, Ile-26, and asparagine amide-28.

5. *Motilin*

According to Popielski (1909), motilin was the name given in 1903 by Enriquez and Hallion to a hypothetical hormone of the intestinal mucosa with the physiological function of stimulating intestinal peristalsis. Brown *et al.* (1966) reviewed earlier work showing that acidification of the upper intestine inhibits gastric motor activity and some observations suggesting that alkalinization might have the opposite effect. They found that, in dogs with vagally denervated or transplanted fundic pouches, introduction of a buffer solution of pH 9 or of pig pancreatic juice into the duodenum increased motor activity in the denervated pouches. The buffer solution, but not the pancreatic juice, with its lower pH, stimulated motor activity also in the transplanted pouches. They concluded that the alkalinization of the duodenum either inhibited the release from the duodenal mucosa of some substance with

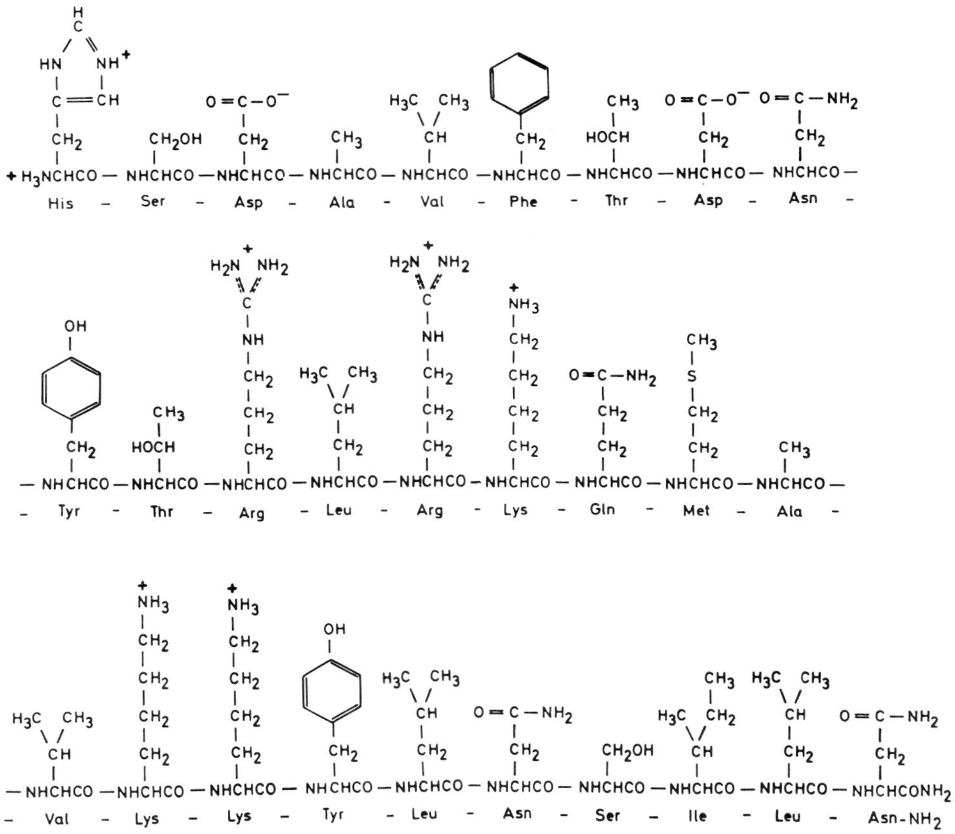

FIG. 4. Amino acid sequence of porcine vasoactive intestinal polypeptide.

gastric motor activity-inhibiting properties, or else released a humoral agent that stimulated this activity. Brown (1967) then showed that certain preparations of partially purified pancreozymin (CCK) obtained from porcine intestinal tissue stimulated gastric motor activity and that this stimulating activity was not due to the CCK content of the preparation. Further work by Brown and associates (Brown and Parkes, 1967; Brown et al., 1971) led to a highly purified peptide with N-terminal phenylalanine and lacking histidine, tryptophan, and cysteine/cystine. This peptide was named motilin. The relationship between the motilin isolated by Brown et al. and that described by Enriquez and Hallion is not known. Two further steps of purification by chromatography in acetic acid on Sephadex G-25 were added (Brown et al., 1972), and the sequence of the 22 amino acid residues of motilin was determined (Brown *et al.*, 1973). Later a form of motilin was isolated in which the residue in position 14 was found to be glutamine instead of glutamic acid, as first found (Schubert and Brown, 1974). The sequence of this form of porcine motilin is

Phe-Val-Pro-Ile-Phe-Thr-Tyr-Gly-Glu-Leu-Gln-
                    Arg-Met-Gln-Glu-Lys-Glu-Arg-Asn-Lys-Gly-Gln

and is shown in formula form in Fig. 5.

6. *The Gastric Inhibitory Peptide (GIP)*

Jordan and Peterson (1962) noted that the administration of a partially purified preparation of CCK to dogs with Heidenhain pouches inhibited the secretion of gastric acid in response to feeding. Gillespie and Grossman (1964b) investigated, also in Heidenhain pouch dogs, the effects of a similar preparation of CCK on gastric acid secretion that had been stimulated by either exogenous gastrin or histamine and found that the secretion in response to gastrin was strongly inhibited and the secretion in response to histamine was weakly inhibited. Since then many workers have studied the effects of CCK on basal and on variously stimulated gastric secretion in different species (p. 309). Brown and Pederson (1970a) compared various effects of two preparations of partially purified CCK in dogs with vagally denervated pouches of the body of the stomach. One of these preparations was about 10% pure on the basis of activity, and the other had been obtained from this "10% pure" material by additional purification and was about 40% pure. Doses of the two preparations that resulted in similar degrees of gallbladder contraction also stimulated antral motor activity to the same degree. However, their effects on gastric acid and pepsin secretion were distinctly different, the more highly purified preparation stimulating these secretions to a much greater extent then the less purified one. Brown and Pederson suggested that the less purified preparation contained some inhibitory substance for acid and possibly for pepsin secretion. In later work Brown and co-workers directly showed that such an inhibitory substance for acid and also for pepsin secretion and for motor activity in vagally denervated antral and fundic pouches could be separated from the "10% pure" CCK (Brown *et al.*, 1969). Further purification resulted in the isolation, in essentially pure form, of a polypeptide showing these inhibitory properties, and lacking cysteine and proline (Brown *et al.*, 1970). It had at first been referred to as "enterogastrone" (Brown *et al.*, 1969), but since enterogastrone had turned out to be a physiological property of several intestinal inhibitors of gastric secretion and motility (p. 310), the term

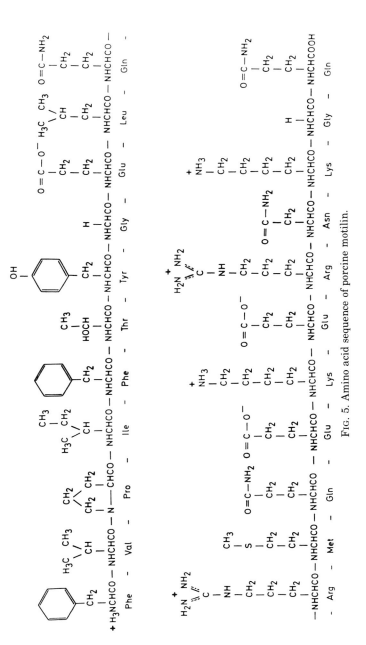

Fig. 5. Amino acid sequence of porcine motilin.

gastric inhibitory polypeptide (GIP) came into use. The amino acid sequence of GIP was determined by Brown and Dryburgh (1971). According to this, GIP was found to consist of 43 amino acid residues. Later the sequence was redetermined (Jörnvall *et al.,* 1981a), and a single mistake in the previous determination was discovered: GIP is composed of 42, not 43, amino acid residues, and the -Gln-Gln- in the 29–30 sequence had to be corrected to -Gln-. The revised sequence is

Tyr-Ala-Glu-Gly-Thr-Phe-Ile-Ser-Asp-Tyr-Ser-Ile-Ala-Met-
Asp-Lys-Ile-Arg-Gln-Gln-Asp-Phe-Val-Asn-Trp-Leu-Leu-Ala-Gln-Lys-
Gly-Lys-Lys-Ser-Asp-Trp-Lys-His-Asn-Ile-Thr-Gln

which is shown in formula form in Fig. 6. A peptide lacking the two N-terminal residues of GIP has also been isolated from a highly purified preparation of GIP (Jörnvall *et al.,* 1981a).

7. *The Bombesin-Related Gastrin-Releasing Polypeptide (GRP)*

Bombesin is a tetradecapeptide amide that was isolated from the skin of the European discoglossid frogs *Bombina bombina* and *Bombina variegata variegata* (Anastasi *et al.,* 1971). Its amino acid sequence is

Glp-Gln-Arg-Leu-Gly-Asn-Gln-Trp-Ala-Val-Gly-His-Leu-Met-NH$_2$

(Anastasi *et al.,* 1971). Soon after the isolation of bombesin, several reports appeared describing bombesin-like immunoreactivity and bioactivity in extracts of tissues of the mammalian gastrointestinal tract (Erspamer and Melchiorri, 1975; Polak *et al.,* 1976; Walsh and Holmquist, 1976; Melchiorri, 1980). McDonald *et al.* (1978) did not initially attempt to isolate a substance with bombesin-like properties from porcine gastric nonantral tissue. Their work started from the assumption that the target organ area for gastrin could, perhaps, contain some substance effecting a negative feedback regulation on the release of gastrin. Unexpectedly, extracts of nonantral gastric tissue, on administration to dogs, increased plasma levels of immunoreactive gastrin. The peptide nature of the active factor(s) was suggested by destruction of the activity by chymotrypsin. Since bombesin was known to release gastrin under these conditions, some similarity between the active peptide(s) and bombesin seemed probable, and this was confirmed when a heptacosapeptide was isolated in a form sufficiently pure for sequence analysis. Its amino acid sequence (McDonald *et al.,* 1979) is

Ala-Pro-Val-Ser-Val-Gly-Gly-Gly-Thr-Val-Leu-Ala-Lys-Met-
Tyr-Pro-Arg-Gly-Asn-His-Trp-Ala-Val-Gly-His-Leu-Met-NH$_2$

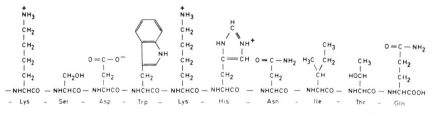

FIG. 6. Amino acid sequence of porcine gastric inhibitory peptide.

and this is shown in formula form in Fig. 7. It is evident that the C-terminal decapeptide of this heptacosapeptide is, with one exception, the substitution of histidine for glutamine in position 20, identical with the C-terminal decapeptide of bombesin.

The corresponding heptacosapeptide has been isolated from chicken proventricular tissue (McDonald *et al.*, 1980) after the demonstration

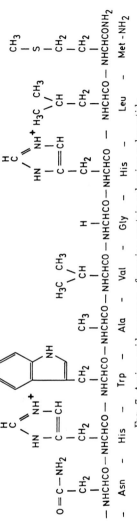

FIG. 7. Amino acid sequence of porcine gastrin-releasing polypeptide.

of bombesin-like immunoreactivity in this tissue (Erspamer *et al.*, 1978; Timson *et al.*, 1979; Vaillant *et al.*, 1979). Its amino acid sequence is

Ala-Pro-Leu-Gln-Pro-Gly-Gly-Ser-Pro-Ala-Leu-Thr-Lys-Ile-Tyr-
Pro-Arg-Gly-Ser-His-Trp-Ala-Val-Gly-His-Leu-Met-NH₂

It may be seen that this sequence differs from that of the porcine peptide in positions 3–5, 8–10, 12, 14, and 19. The C-terminal tridecapeptides of the porcine and chicken GRPs are consequently identical except in position 19, where the porcine peptide has a residue of asparagine and the chicken peptide has a residue of serine. The C-terminal decapeptide of the chicken peptide differs from bombesin in positions 19 and 20 by having serylhistidine instead of asparginylglutamine. Indeed the C-terminal decapeptide of the chicken proventricular heptacosapeptide is slightly more similar to the corresponding decapeptide sequence of alytesin, a polypeptide from the skin of the frog *Alytes obstetricans* isolated and sequenced by Anastasi *et al.* (1971), than it is to that of bombesin (McDonald *et al.*, 1980).

8. *Somatostatin-28*

After the isolation of the tetradecapeptide somatostatin from ovine hypothalamic tissue and the determination of its amino acid sequence (Brazeau *et al.*, 1973), an identical tetradecapeptide was isolated from porcine hypothalamic tissue (Schally *et al.*, 1976). Immunochemical evidence was soon presented for the occurrence of somatostatin outside of the hypothalamic area. It was found to be present in other areas of the brain (Brownstein *et al.*, 1975), but also in the islet cells of the pancreas (Luft *et al.*, 1974) and in the mucosa of the stomach, duodenum, and jejunum (Arimura *et al.*, 1975; Rufener *et al.*, 1975; Polak *et al.*, 1975; McIntosh *et al.*, 1978). Somatostatin was isolated from angler fish pancreatic islet tissue (Noe *et al.*, 1979), pigeon pancreas (Spiess *et al.*, 1979), and rat pancreas (Benoit *et al.*, 1980) and in all three cases found to be a tetradecapeptide identical with ovine and porcine somatostatin. However, several reports appeared describing the presence of immunoreactive somatostatin of larger molecular form(s) than the tetradecapeptide in hypothalamic (Schally *et al.*, 1975, 1976; Lauber *et al.*, 1979; Rorstad *et al.*, 1979; Spiess and Vale, 1980), extrahypothalamic brain (Rorstad *et al.*, 1979; Zingg and Patel, 1979; Zyznar *et al.*, 1979), pancreatic (Arimura *et al.*, 1975; McIntosh *et al.*, 1978; Goodman *et al.*, 1980a,b), and gastrointestinal (Arimura *et al.*, 1975; McIntosh *et al.*, 1978; Zyznar *et al.*, 1979) tissues from various species; one such peptide, somatostatin-28 or prosomatostatin, in which somatostatin-14 is lengthened from its N terminus by an additional tetradecapeptide, of different sequence than somatostatin-14, has been isolated from porcine intestinal (Pradayrol *et al.*, 1980), porcine hypothalamic (Schally *et al.*, 1980), and ovine hypothalamic (Böhlen *et al.*, 1980) tissues. The amino acid sequence of somatostatin-28 is

Ser-Ala-Asn-Ser-Asn-Pro-Ala-Met-Ala-Pro-Arg-Glu-Arg-Lys-
Ala-Gly-Cys-Lys-Asn-Phe-Phe-Trp-Lys-Thr-Phe-Thr-Ser-Cys

shown in formula form in Fig. 8. In addition, Böhlen *et al.* (1980) have isolated from ovine hypothalamic tissue somatostatin-25, which is identical to somatostatin-28 except that it lacks the three N-terminal amino acid residues of the latter. From catfish pancreatic islets, Oyama *et al.* (1980) have isolated two somatostatins, I and II, and determined the amino acid sequence of I, the shorter of the two. This catfish somatostatin consists of 22 amino acid residues in the sequence D N T V R S K P L N C M N Y F W K S S T A C. The sequence of its C-terminal tetradecapeptide shows 7 positional identities to mammalian somatostatin-14 and consequently to the corresponding sequence of somatostatin-28, whereas there is only one additional such identity to somatostatin-28 in its N-terminal extension. From work with the DNA coding for preprosomatostatin, Goodman *et al.* (1980a) have concluded that angler fish somatostatin-14 is identical to its mammalian counterpart and that the sequence of the hexapeptide preceding it in precursor form(s) is identical to the corresponding sequence of mammalian somatostatin-28. Hobart *et al.* (1980) came to the same conclusion but in addition found evidence for the existence of an additional angler fish somatostatin-like peptide with two amino acid replacements in the tetradecapeptide moiety, Tyr-7 for Phe-7 and Gly-10 for Thr-10, and with only the pentapeptide preceding it in precursor form(s) identical to the corresponding sequence of somatostatin-28. A dodecapeptide, urotensin II, has been isolated from the caudal neurosecretory system of the teleost *Gillichthys mirabilis* and found to have the sequence A G T A D C F W K Y C V. If urotensin II and somatostatin-14 are aligned from their N termini, it is seen that the amino acid residues are identical in positions 1–2 and 7–9 of the two peptides (Pearson *et al.*, 1980).

9. *Substance P*

In 1931, v. Euler and Gaddum found that extracts of various horse tissues, but particularly those of the intestine and the brain, contained a substance that caused contraction of the isolated rabbit jejunum *in vitro* and lowered the arterial blood pressure of the anesthetized rabbit

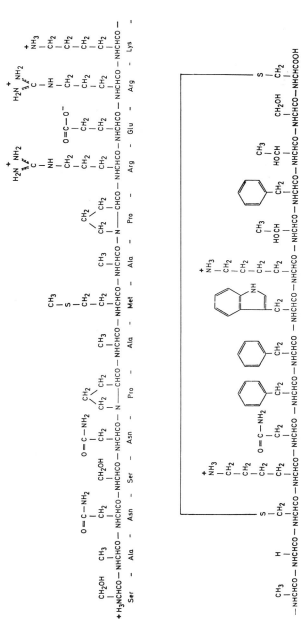

Fig. 8. Amino acid sequence of porcine somatostatin-28.

by way of peripheral vasodilatation. This substance was not acetylcholine since its effects were resistant to atropine and the muscular
contraction in response to it developed more slowly than it did in response to acetylcholine. It was first referred to as "powder P" or preparation "P" (v. Euler and Gaddum, 1931) and its peptide nature was
established by v. Euler (1936). Highly active preparations of substance
P were obtained by v. Euler and associates (v. Euler, 1942; Pernow,
1953) and others (Boissonnas et al., 1963; Zuber, 1963; Vogler et al.,
1963; Leeman and Hammerschlag, 1967; Zetler and Baldauf, 1967;
Lembeck and Starke, 1968). Substance P was isolated in a degree of
purity sufficient for structural work by Chang and Leeman, (1970a,b).
It was originally assumed that substance P had been isolated from
bovine hypothalamic tissue, but apparently the material used for the
amino acid sequence determination (Chang et al., 1971) had been isolated from bovine superior and inferior colliculi instead (Leeman and
Carraway, 1977; Carraway and Leeman, 1979). Only later was substance P isolated specifically from bovine hypothalamic tissue (Carraway and Leeman, 1979), but the peptides isolated from both tissues are
identical (Carraway and Leeman, 1979); they are also identical to substance P isolated from horse intestine (Studer et al., 1973). The amino
acid sequence of the undecapeptide amide substance P (Chang et al.,
1971) is

$$\text{Arg-Pro-Lys-Pro-Gln-Gln-Phe-Phe-Gly-Leu-Met-NH}_2$$

which is shown in formula form in Fig. 9.

10. Neurotensin

Neurotensin is a hypotensive peptide that was discovered in extracts
of bovine hypothalami by Carraway and Leeman (1971, 1973). In addition to being hypotensive, it stimulated in vitro the contraction of the
guinea pig ileum and rat uterus but relaxed the rat duodenum. The
sequence of its 13 amino acid residues was elucidated by Carraway and
Leeman (1975a). Immunoreactive neurotensin has been shown to be
present in organs other than the brain and in the rat; concentrations
are especially high in the jejunoileal part of the intestine (Carraway
and Leeman, 1976). In the dog, intestinal cells containing neurotensin
seem to be confined to the lower ileum (Orci et al., 1976) and in man to
the ileum (Polak et al., 1977a). Neurotensin was isolated from calf
intestinal tissue by Kitabgi et al. (1976) and shown to be identical to
hypothalamic neurotensin (Carraway et al., 1978). Hammer et al.
(1979) have isolated neurotensin from human intestinal mucosa and
presented strong evidence for its identity with bovine neurotensin.

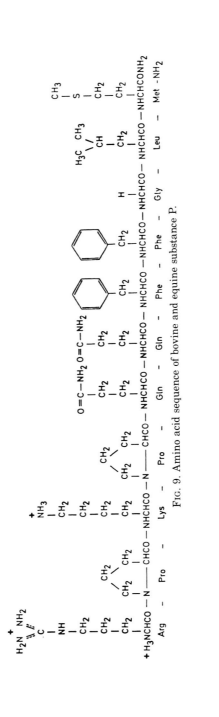

FIG. 9. Amino acid sequence of bovine and equine substance P.

The amino acid sequence of neurotensin (Carraway and Leeman, 1975a) is

Glp-Leu-Tyr-Glu-Asn-Lys-Pro-Arg-Arg-Pro-Tyr-Ile-Leu

shown in formula form in Fig. 10. Folkers *et al.* (1976) have discussed the possibility that in native neurotensin residue No. 4 might be one of glutamine rather than of glutamic acid.

11. *Glicentin*

Tager and Steiner (1973) isolated a contaminating peptide, possibly a fragment of proglucagon, from a preparation of crystalline bovine–porcine glucagon and found that it was composed of glucagon extended from its C terminus by the octapeptide K R N N K N I A. Sundby *et al.* (1976) isolated a peptide from porcine small intestinal tissue with glucagon-like immunoreactivity (GLI) that appeared to consist of 100 amino acid residues, incorporating pancreatic glucagon (Bromer *et al.*, 1957) in their 63–92 sequence (Jacobsen *et al.*, 1977). Its C-terminal octapeptide, extending the glucagon sequence, was found to have the sequence K R N K N N I A, which differs from the sequence that Tager and Steiner had found for the corresponding part of their C-terminally extended, pancreatic, glucagon-related peptide by a transposition of

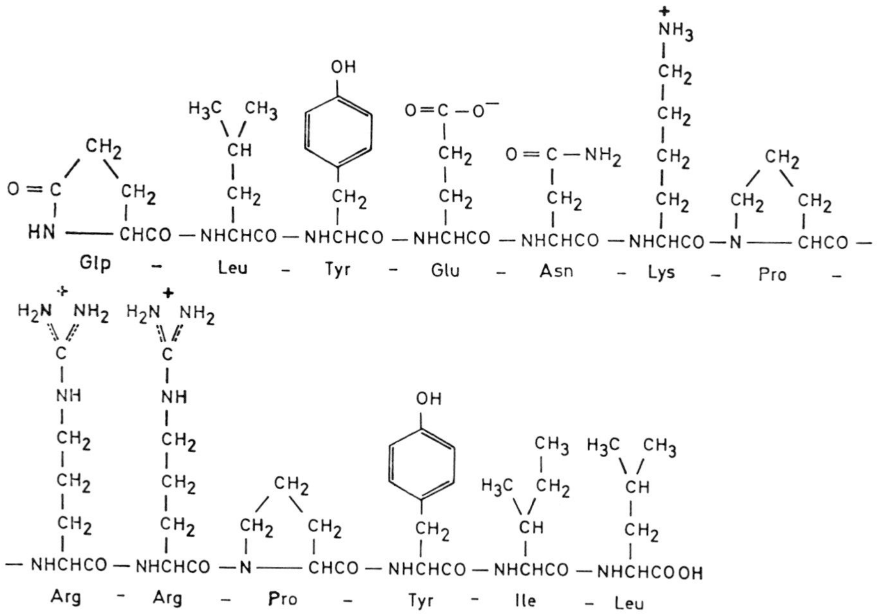

FIG. 10. Amino acid sequence of bovine and human neurotensin.

the amino acid residues in positions 4–5. Sundby *et al.* originally called the peptide they had isolated GLI-I, but subsequently they named it glicentin (Moody *et al.*, 1978). The N-terminal tridecapeptide sequence of glicentin was found to be R S L Q N T Z Z K A R S F (Sundby *et al.*, 1976). More recently, Thim and Moody (1981) have found that glicentin contains 69 instead of 100 amino acid residues in the sequence

R S L Q N T E E K S R S F P A P Q T D P L D D P D Q M T E D K R H S Q
G T F T S D Y S K Y L D S R R A Q D F V Q W L M N T K R N K N N I A

i.e., it is composed of glucagon extended N-terminally by a peptide of 30 amino acid residues and C-terminally by an octapeptide.

B. (GROUP 2) ISOLATED PEPTIDES WITH PARTIALLY DISCLOSED
SEQUENCE DATA

1. *Chymodenin PHI and PYY*

Adelson and Rothman (1974) described a peptide that appeared to effect a selective stimulation of chymotrypsinogen secretion from the pancreas of the anesthetized rabbit, and they named the active substance chymodenin. Chymodenin was isolated from a side fraction obtained during the isolation of secretin and cholecystokinin from a concentrate of porcine upper intestinal peptides (Adelson *et al.*, 1980; see also p. 286). It has hitherto been shown to have C-terminal isoleucine, the probable N-terminal sequence pyroglutamyl-cysteinyl-lysine, with the cysteine residue forming a disulfide bridge with another cysteine residue, and an internal B B R R A Z G T F P G K I sequence. *PHI* and *PYY* have been isolated from a side fraction obtained during the preparation of secretin from a concentrate of porcine upper intestinal peptides (Tatemoto and Mutt, 1980). The acronyms denote "peptide (P) with N-terminal histidine (H) and C-terminal isoleucine (amide) (I)" and "peptide with N-terminal tyrosine (Y) and C-terminal tyrosine (amide) (Y)," respectively. PHI is composed of 27 amino acid residues and PYY of 36. Partial sequences have been published, H A D G V F T – – – – – – – L I for PHI and Y P A K P E A P G – – – – – – – R Y for PYY. [Recently (porcine) PHI and PYY have moved into Group 1, i.e., their complete amino acid sequences have been published. See Note Added in Proof.]

2. *Oxyntomodulin*

Oxyntomodulin was so named because of its strong stimulatory activity on cAMP production in fundic, but not pyloric, gastric glands. It was isolated from pig distal small intestine and appears to be either identical with or very similar to the proglucagon fragment of Tager and Steiner (1973), except for the transposition, as in glicentin (Jacobson *et al.*, 1977), of an asparagine and a lysine in its C-terminal part (Bataille *et al.*, 1981).

C. (SUBGROUP 3a) KNOWN PEPTIDES NOT YET ISOLATED FROM GASTROINTESTINAL TISSUES BUT CLAIMED TO BE PRESENT THERE ON IMMUNOCHEMICAL EVIDENCE. VARIANT FORMS, NOT YET ISOLATED, OF PEPTIDES OF GROUPS 1 AND 2

There is convincing evidence that many, presumably all, of the hormones that have been hitherto isolated from gastrointestinal tissues occur in still other variant molecular forms that yet remain to be isolated and characterized.

D. HETEROGENEITY

1. *Types of Peptide Hormone Heterogeneity*

a. Variations in Amino Sequence and in Posttranslational Modifications. There are several ways, apart from aggregation or changes in conformation, in which a peptide hormone may exhibit heterogeneity. The most obvious is a difference in the amino acid sequence between two molecules of the hormone. This difference must be so located within the peptide chain that the general physiological characteristics of the hormone are not altered to such an extent that two functionally different, and therefore differently named, hormones are formed. For instance, the human and porcine calcitonins have different amino acid residues in 56% of the possible positions (Potts, 1970), but both are functionally calcitonins nevertheless, whereas oxytocin and vasopressin, which vary in only 22% of their positions (Dayhoff, 1972) are two different hormones. Differences often occur between peptide hormones isolated from different species, as first shown for insulin by Sanger (1949). The extent to which this occurs varies greatly from hormone to hormone. The difference between human and porcine calcitonin just mentioned is an extreme example. Glucagon is at the other extreme. The glucagons from the six mammalian species from which glucagon has been isolated are identical (Sundby *et al.*, 1974), and this mammalian glucagon differs from turkey and chicken glucagon (Markussen *et al.*, 1972; Pollock and Kimmel, 1975) in only one position and from duck glucagon (Sundby *et al.*, 1972) in only two.

As may be seen from the above presentation of the sequences of the gastrointestinal hormonal peptides of group 1, VIP seems to have been strongly conserved during evolution while gastrin shows moderate variability outside of its C-terminal functionally important sequence. There is evidence that this is so also for cholecystokinin (Straus and Yalow, 1978). Secretin would seem to be strongly conserved among mammalian species, but less so between mammals and birds; however, isolation from additional species will be necessary before it is known whether or not this is really so.

Another type of sequence variation, well known from other areas of protein chemistry, for instance the isozymes of enzymology, is due to sequence differences between different molecules of a peptide hormone in the same species. Examples are the two different rat and mouse insulins (Smith, 1966; Steiner *et al.*, 1969; Markussen, 1971; Bünzli *et al.*, 1972) and the variant form of human insulin in which phenylalanine is replaced by leucine in position 24 of the B chain (Tager *et al.*, 1980b). This type of heterogeneity has not yet been discovered among gastrointestinal hormones, but there is no reason to believe that it does not occur.

Another type of heterogeneity is found when the side chain of an amino acid residue is modified in some, but not other, molecules of a peptide hormone. One example is the esterification or nonesterification of the phenolic group of a tyrosine residue with sulfuric acid in gastrin. Cholecystokinin is, as yet, known in only the sulfated forms, but there is no evidence either for or against the existence in tissues or in the circulation of nonsulfated forms. Other factors that could give rise to this type of heterogeneity are, for example, partial deamidation of aspartyl or glutaminyl residues or oxidation of methionine residues to residues of methionine sulfoxide (Brewer *et al.*, 1968).

b. Size Heterogeneity. The most common reason for peptide hormone heterogeneity is nevertheless size heterogeneity, in which a hormone occurs in forms of different peptide chain lengths, the larger ones being extensions at either end, or at both ends, of the shorter forms.

c. Proteolytic Processing, Extra- and Intracellular, of Precursor Forms. It has long been known that peptide hormones may be formed by the proteolytic processing of large inactive precursor forms, and that such processing may take place over the formation of intermediate forms. The discovery of renin by Tigerstedt and Bergman (1898) led, by work in different laboratories, to the understanding that renin acts on a plasma protein angiotensinogen to release a weakly active decapeptide, angiotensin I, which is in turn enzymatically converted to the highly active octapeptide angiotensin II (Schwyzer, 1960). Similarly, the discovery of kallikrein (Kraut *et al.*, 1930) and of bradykinin (Rocha e Silva *et al.*, 1949) led to the unraveling of the kinin system, in which enzymes act on plasma proteins with the release of highly active kinin peptides (Schachter, 1969).

The formation of kinins and of angiotensin by enzymatic cleavage of precursor proteins takes place extracellularly. Intracellular cleavage of precursors into active hormones was suggested for vasopressin (Takabatake and Sachs, 1964), discussed for the β-lipotropin to γ-lipotropin to β-melanotropin conversions in sheep pituitaries by Chrétien and Li (1967), and unequivocally demonstrated for the proinsulin to insulin conversion in human islet cell adenoma tissue by Steiner and Oyer (1967).

The release of γ-lipotropin, which constitutes the Glu_1 . . . . Asp_{58} sequence, from β-lipotropin

$$Glu_1 . . . . . Lys_{39}\text{-}Lys_{40}\text{-}Asp_{41} . . . . . Asp_{58}\text{-}Lys_{59}\text{-}Arg_{60}\text{-}Tyr_{61} . . . . . Glu_{91}$$

necessitates cleavage of the $Asp_{58}\text{-}Lys_{59}$ bond. The further release of β-melanotropin from the γ-lipotropin necessitates the cleavage of the $Lys_{40}\text{-}Asp_{41}$ bond. Looking at the molecule of lipotropin, both cleavages seem to take place at "double basic" amino acid residue sequences, at the carboxyl side of the lysyllysyl residue, and at the amino side of the lysylarginyl residue. Work with other prohormone to hormone conversions has shown that cleavages at such double basic residues are catalyzed by enzymes with trypsin-like specificity and take place preferentially at the carboxyl side of both such residues, or between them, but never at the amino side of the first residue of the pair of basic residues. Cleavage of the bond involving the amino group of the latter residue is a secondary effect apparently catalyzed by another enzyme with carboxypeptidase B line activity (Tager *et al.*, 1980a). Consequently, in the β-lipotropin to γ-lipotropin conversion, the initial cleavage is of the $Arg_{60}\text{-}Tyr_{61}$ bond, and this is followed by secondary removal of the Arg_{60} and Lys_{59} from the γ-lipotropin intermediate. While then the presumable occurrence of this type of trypsin-like cleavage followed by carboxypeptidase B-like cleavage was implicit in the β-lipotropin to γ-lipotropin to β-melanotropin conversions (Chrétien and Li, 1967), it was first clearly suggested to occur in the proinsulin to insulin conversion after the isolation of proinsulin and the determination of its amino acid sequence (Chance *et al.*, 1968; Nolan *et al.*, 1971). Since then, cleavages at points containing two consecutive basic residues have been demonstrated to take place during the conversion of "pro" into shorter forms of many other hormones, such as glucagon (Tager and Steiner, 1973), parathyroid hormone (Hamilton *et al.*, 1974), gastrin (Gregory and Tracy, 1975), somatostatin (Pradayrol *et al.*, 1980; Schally *et al.*, 1980; Böhlen *et al.*, 1980), and γ-melanotropin (Nakanishi *et al.*, 1979; Håkanson *et al.*, 1980; Seidah *et al.*, 1980; Estivariz *et al.*, 1980), and also of other types of proteins, such as albumin (Russel and Geller, 1975). In the CCK-39 to CCK-33 conversion, however, cleavage takes place between the Arg-6 and Lys-7 residues of CCK-39 rather than between its Lys-7 and Ala-8 residues.

 d. *The Signal Hypothesis and Peptide Hormone Heterogeneity.* In the early 1970s it was shown (Milstein *et al.*, 1972; Devillers-Thiery *et al.*, 1975) that many such proteins secreted from cells are synthesized in "pre" forms with N-terminal extension of 15–30, mostly hydrophobic amino acid residues. This extension peptide seems to act as a signal (Milstein *et al.*, 1972; Blobel and Sabatini, 1971; Blobel and Dobberstein, 1975) for the attachment of the ribosomal translation complex to the endoplasmatic reticulum and to direct, concomitant with translation, the vectorial transport of the protein being synthesized (Redman *et al.*, 1966; Sabatini *et al.*, 1966) through the reticular membrane into the cisternal space. The signal peptide is usually removed as soon as it has directed the protein through the membrane. This type of mechanism for the synthesis of secreted proteins has been demonstrated for dozens of individual proteins (Austen, 1979) including several peptide hormones, such as insulin (Lernmark *et al.*, 1976; Permutt and Boime, 1975; Lomedico, 1975; Weber, 1975; Yip *et al.*, 1975; Chan *et al.*, 1976; Lomedico *et al.*, 1977), parathyroid hormone (Habener *et al.*, 1976, 1977, 1978), and somatostatin (Shields, 1980; Goodman *et al.*, 1980a; Hobart *et al.*, 1980). The complete amino acid sequence or sequences for angler fish preprosomatostatins have, as mentioned, been deduced by way of the nucleotide sequences of the genes coding for them by Goodman *et al.* (1980a) and by Hobart *et al.* (1980), who found two preprosomatostatins with variation also in the active tetradecapeptide moiety. The spatial and temporal aspects of the biosynthesis of the "pre" and the "pro" forms and the conversion of the "pre" to the "pro" form and further to the hormone have been described in considerable detail for parathyroid hormone (Habener *et al.*, 1977). The biosynthesis of hormones from "pre" and "pro" forms has also been the topic of a conference (Zimmerman *et al.*, 1980). An impetus for work on the precursor forms of peptide hormones is the repeatedly voiced expectation (Grube and Forssmann, 1979; Tager *et al.*, 1980a; Herbert *et al.*, 1980) of finding several different hormones as components of one and the same precursor, as was found to be the case for corticotropin and lipotropin (Lowry *et al.*, 1976; Mains *et al.*, 1977; Roberts and Herbert, 1977a,b; Herbert *et al.*, 1980; Mains and Eipper, 1980).

    e. Biosynthesis of C-Terminal α-Amide Structures. For certain peptide hormones, heterogeneity would seem to arise as a consequence of their C-terminal α-amide structures. Such hormones are, for example, vasopressin, oxytocin, α-melanotropin, gastrin, secretin, cholecystokinin, substance P, the vasoactive intestinal polypeptide (VIP), thyroliberin, gonadoliberin (Dayhoff, 1972), the bombesin-related gastrin-releasing peptide (McDonald *et al.*, 1979, 1980), PHI and PYY (Tatemoto and Mutt, 1980). There are indications (Gross, 1972; Smyth, 1975; Suchanek and Kreil, 1977) that such hormones may be formed by the cleavage of C-terminally extended precursor forms with retention of the amino group of the amino acid residue C-terminal to the point of cleavage as the —NH_2 component of the C-terminal α-amide group of the hormone.

2. *Heterogeneity of Gastrointestinal Peptides Reacting with Antibodies to Glucagon*

The gastrointestinal hormones are obviously not exempt from the various types of intracellular modifications of "pre" and "pro" forms and of extracellular proteolytic modifications. Concerning the latter, they fall into two main categories: (*a*) hormones, like secretin, where any fragmentation of the known form leads to a drastic decrease of activity and therefore may be considered as an inactivation rather than modification; (*b*) hormones like gastrin, cholecystokinin, substance P, the bombesin-related gastrin-releasing peptide, and somatostatin-28, where fragmentation of certain known forms leads to retention of activity in the C-terminal fragments but, at least in some cases, with qualitative differences in the action of these fragments as compared to the actions of the longer forms. For such hormones it will be an arduous task to determine whether various active forms that may be detected in, and eventually isolated from, the complex proteolytic environment of blood circulating through different vascular beds, represent meaningful physiological modifications of these hormones or merely random steps in their disintegration.

    a. Discovery of such Peptides and Preliminary Characterization as to Molecular Size and Electric Charge. The heterogeneity of gastrointestinal hormones seems first to have been described for glucagon, at a time (Samols *et al.*, 1966) when no form of glucagon had yet been isolated from gastrointestinal tissues. Work on glucagon and on gastrin has done much to clarify how peptide hormones become heterogeneous in blood and in their tissues of origin and is therefore discussed here in some detail. Sutherland and de Duve (1948) showed that a substance in pancreatic extracts from several mammalian species had glycogenolytic effects on rabbit liver slices *in vitro* and caused hyperglycemia when injected into rabbits, and that this "hyperglycemic glycogenolytic factor" was also present in extracts of the mucosa of the upper three-fourths of the dog stomach and of the rabbit stomach, but not in extracts of hog, beef, or sheep stomach. Small amounts of activity could be detected in extracts of dog duodenal and ileal mucosa. The presence of glucagon-like activity, assayed on the basis of its glycogenolytic action on liver slices, was found in extracts of human stomach, duodenum, jejunum, and ileum (Kenny and Say, 1962). Makman and Sutherland (1964) used stimulation of adenylate cyclase in particulate fractions of cat or dog liver as a basis for the assay of glucagon-like activity in various tissue extracts. They found such activity in extracts of both the mucosal and the muscular layers of human and of dog gastrointestinal tissues. In retrospect it is evident that the finding of glucagon-like bioactivity in a tissue extract does not prove that the extract contains glucagon since other peptides, such as VIP (Said and Mutt, 1970a) exhibit similar activities. However, other investigations definitely confirmed that gastrointestinal tissues do contain glucagon in various forms.

After the elaboration of a radioimmunochemical method for the assay of glucagon (Unger *et al.*, 1959, 1961a), material reacting with an antiserum to glucagon was shown to be present in extracts of dog stomach and duodenum, although in much lower concentrations than in corresponding extracts of pancreatic tissue. Calculated per unit weight of tissue, the stomach extracts were found to contain about one-tenth as much glucagon-like immunoreactive material as pancreatic extracts but about 20 times more than the duodenal extracts (Unger *et al.*, 1961b). Interest in gastrointestinal glucagon was greatly stimulated by the finding (Samols *et al.*, 1965b; Lawrence, 1966) that ingestion of glucose led, in man, to increased concentrations of plasma glucagon-like immunoreactive material, and the suggestion by Samols *et al.* (1965a,b) that this might be due to release, by the glucose, of glucagon-like material of intestinal origin, which possibly could lead to increased concentrations of plasma insulin and also directly affect the disposal of the absorbed glucose.

Unger *et al.* (1966) described the presence of glucagon-like immunoreactivity in extracts of human jejunum, dog stomach and duodenum, and rat stomach, duodenum, and jejunum. The patterns obtained on chromatography of the active material of such extracts on Sephadex gels as well as comparisons of immunoreactivities and bioactivities suggested that the glucagon-like substance in the dog stomach extracts was similar to pancreatic glucagon. Samols *et al.* (1966) found that beef and pork pancreatic glucagon showed identical crossreactivity with glucagon in extracts of human pancreas and colon whereas cross-reactivity between the pancreatic glucagon and the glucagon-like material in extracts of tissues from other parts of the gastrointestinal tract was less pronounced, suggesting that different types of molecules were reacting. Shortly thereafter, Unger *et al.* (1968) found that glucagon-like immunoreactive material extracted with acid ethanol from dog jejunal tissue behaved on chromatography on Sephadex G-25 as though it had about twice the molecular weight of glucagon. The jejunal material had no hyperglycemic activity when injected endoportally into dogs, was not glycogenolytic on the isolated perfused rat liver, and did not stimulate hepatic adenylate cyclase in the perfused rat liver. There was, however, some indication that it might stimulate insulin secretion. Further work by Unger and co-workers (Valverde *et al.*, 1968, 1970a) confirmed the presence in dog jejunal extracts of the large form of glucagon-like immunoreactive material, but also showed that in addition to this the extracts contained another type of material with glucagon-like immunoreactivity that appeared to be of approximately the same molecular size as glucagon. Like glucagon—but in contrast to the component of larger molecular size—it was glycogenolytic in the isolated perfused rat liver and hyperglycemic on injection into dogs, although there seemed to be some quantitative differences between it and glucagon (Valverde *et al.*, 1968, 1970a). Glucagon-like immunoreactivity was found to be exhibited by materials of two different molecular sizes also in extracts of human (Valverde *et al.*, 1973), pig, rabbit, and rat intestinal tissues and of pig intestinal mucosa. In the latter extracts, electrofocusing of material from either of the molecular-size fractions showed that more than one glucagon-like immunoreactive component was present in each fraction (Markussen and Sundby, 1973).

The possible physiological importance of gastrointestinal glucagon-like peptides was further stressed when several groups of workers showed that, whereas pancreatectomy in dogs led to a disappearance of insulin from the plasma, the plasma glucagon concentrations were not markedly lowered (Buchanan *et al.*, 1967; Unger *et al.*, 1968; Cherrington *et al.*, 1974; Vranic *et al.*, 1974; Matsuyama and Foà, 1974; Mashiter *et al.*, 1975), suggesting that a sizable part of plasma immunoreactive glucagon might normally be of gastrointestinal origin. Direct release in response to glucose of material with glucagon-like immunoreactivity from the rat jejunum *in vitro* was described by Luyckx and Lefebvre (1969) and Zandomeneghi and Buchanan (1972). In the cat, glucagon-like immunoreactive material, despite its presence in tissues from the stomach to the colon, was found to be released into the venous effluent by glucose only from the colon, and in quantities too small to affect plasma concentrations of glucagon-like immunoreactive material appreciably (Frame, 1977). There is less unanimity concerning the importance of the gastrointestinal tract for the plasma concentrations of immunoreactive glucagon in man than in the dog. Assan *et al.* (1967), Samols and Marks (1967), and Muller *et al.* (1974), and subsequently others (del Prato *et al.*, 1980, and others quoted by them) have found glucagon-like immunoreactive material to be present in the plasma of insulin-treated pancreatectomized patients, or patients with pancreatic atrophy, whereas Barnes and Bloom (1976) found no such immunoreactivity in the plasma of pancreatectomized patients. Morita *et al.* (1976) have commented on these discrepant findings and suggested that they may in part be explained by the use of different antisera, but also pointed out that canine plasma glucagon-like immunoreactivity is much more pronounced if the animals are in a state of insulin deficiency than when they are euinsulinemic.

b. *Types of Antisera.* Of great importance for work on gastrointestinal and pancreatic glucagon-related peptides has been the development of antisera that react differently with glucagon and with certain of the gastrointestinal peptides that show glucagon-like immunoreactivity (Eisentraut *et al.*, 1968; Heding, 1969, 1971; Buchanan *et al.*, 1974). It would appear (Senyk *et al.*, 1972; Assan and Slusher, 1972; Buchanan *et al.*, 1974; Holst, 1978; Conlon, 1980) that two main types of antisera are in use. One type, the so-called "crossreacting antisera" (Holst, 1978), are directed toward some sequence in the N-terminal or middle part of glucagon, or both, and react equally as well with glucagon as with various peptides in which glucagon is extended at one end or the other or at both ends, and also with N-terminal fragments of glucagon, either free or carrying N-terminal peptidal extensions (Holst, 1978; Conlon, 1980). Antisera of the other type, the so-called "specific" glucagon antisera (Holst, 1978; Conlon, 1980), are specific for the C-terminal structure of glucagon and will not react with peptides in which the glucagon sequence carries a C-terminal extension. They react, however, with peptides in which glucagon is N-terminally extended, and also with C-terminal fragments of glucagon. It also seems that only such glucagon-related peptides as contain the whole amino acid sequence of glucagon without any N-terminal extension exhibit the bioactivities of glucagon (Conlon, 1980).

c. *Attempts at Isolation from Tissue Extracts.* Much work has been carried out by various investigators to determine the chemical nature of the substances that exhibit glucagon-like immunoreactivity in the gastrointestinal tract. The work on glicentin and oxyntomodulin has been referred to above. One salient question has been whether or not glucagon itself, i.e., the 29 amino acid residue peptide (Bromer *et al.*, 1956, 1957), originally isolated from the pancreas of species not revealed (Staub *et al.*, 1953, 1955) but later disclosed as porcine (Bromer *et al.*, 1971), occurs as such in gastrointestinal tissues. Sasaki *et al.* (1975a) described the partial purification from porcine upper small intestine of a glucagon-like peptide, which on BioGel P-10 chromatography was indistinguishable from glucagon and on isoelectric focusing had the same p*I* value as the latter. It was also indistinguishable from glucagon in its reactivities with two antisera and in its ability to stimulate glycogenolysis in the perfused rat pancreas and adenylate cyclase in isolated liver cell membranes. Sasaki *et al.* (1975a) considered this peptide to be identical with glucagon. They also described another glucagon-immunoreactive intestinal peptide with, as estimated by gel chromatography, a lower molecular weight and a more basic electric charge than glucagon. This peptide reacted with only one of the two antisera and was considerably weaker than glucagon in its ability to activate adenylate cyclase and glycogenolysis in the systems mentioned above.

Holst (1977) carried out a careful study of the distribution of glucagon-like immunoreactive materials in different sections of the gastrointestinal tract of the pig. Gastric mucosal extracts of the esophageal, the fundic, and the pyloric gland area contained only traces of a glucagon-like peptide, but there was considerably more, 10–40 pmol eq per gram, in extracts of the mucosa of the cardiac gland region. On Sephadex gel chromatography, some 80% of the latter material migrated like glucagon and also reacted like glucagon in a radioreceptor assay, while the rest of the immunoreactive material appeared to have a higher molecular weight and did not react in the receptor assay. In extracts of the duodenal mucosa, the total amount of glucagon-like immunoreactive material was approximately the same as in extracts of the mucosa of the cardiac region, but only about 20% of it coeluted with glucagon on Sephadex. Four other components with different chromatographic properties were also present; two reacted with "specific" glucagon antisera, and the other two only with the nonspecific antisera. In extracts of the ileal mucosa, the total concentration of glucagon-like immunoreactive material was some 40 times higher than in extracts of the duodenal mucosa, and about 5% coeluted with glucagon on Sephadex G-50. Other chromatographic fractions contained two components reacting with "nonspecific" glucagon antisera and one component of apparently higher molecular weight than glucagon, which reacted with the "specific" sera. In extracts of colonic mucosa, the total amount of material showing glucagon-like immunoreactivity was roughly the same as in extracts of ileal mucosa and the same components seemed to be present. However, the concentration of what appeared to be glucagon was about twice as high in the colonic as in the ileal extracts.

Bataille *et al.* (1974) described the partial purification of a peptide material with glucagon-like immunoreactivity from porcine distal, small intestinal extracts that, in contrast to both secretin and VIP, seemed to bind to the same receptors in rat adipose tissue and liver cell membranes as glucagon. The action of this peptide was relatively weak on the liver cell membranes. On the basis of glucagon-like immunoreactivity, about 10 times more of it than of glucagon was necessary for half-maximal stimulation of cAMP production, whereas in the adipose tissue cell membranes, on the contrary, about one-thirtieth of the amount of glucagon was needed for half-maximal stimulation of cAMP production. In part, this latter activity appeared to be due to contamination of the intestinal peptide material with VIP or some VIP-like substance. Continuation of this work by Bataille and co-workers led to the isolation of oxyntomodulin (p. 261).

Buchanan and co-workers have used Sepharose-4B-coupled rabbit antibodies to porcine glucagon for the purification of peptides, showing crossreactivity with such antibodies from porcine ileal (Murphy *et al.*, 1971, 1973) and colonic (Conlon *et al.*, 1979) tissues. The ileal material, eluted from the immunoadsorbent columns, could be subfractionated by chromatography on Sephadex G-50 into material with an apparent molecular weight of about 12,000. This constituted about 95% of the total immunoreactive material and the remainder, with a molecular weight of about 3500, i.e., approximately that of glucagon. Only the latter fraction showed the biological activities of glucagon on testing in several different assay systems. The material of approximately 12,000 molecular weight showed three N-terminal amino acids, glycine, alanine, and methionine. The N-terminal arginine of glicentin (Sundby *et al.*, 1976) was not observed. Electrophoresis on polyacrylamide gels resolved it into three components. Which of the N-terminal amino acids were in these components was, however, not mentioned. Immunoaffinity chromatography of extracts of colonic tissue resulted in material that, after pretreatment with sodium dodecyl sulfate, could be further fractionated by chromatography in 0.2 *M* acetic acid on Sephadex G-50 into components with apparent molecular weights of 12,000, 8000, 5000, and 3000. All of these reacted much more strongly with antisera directed toward the N-terminal part of the glucagon molecule than with antisera directed toward its C-terminal part. The 8000 and 3000 molecular weight fractions were homogeneous on isoelectric focusing with pI values of 6.2 and 10, respectively, and the other two fractions each showed several components with different pI values.

Apart from work on porcine extracts, most work on gastrointestinal peptides showing glucagon-like immunoreactivity has been carried out on such peptides extracted from dog stomach and intestinal tissues, i.e., tissues where gastrointestinal glucagon-like bioactivity was originally discovered by Sutherland and de Duve (1948). Morita et al. (1976) found that the fundus and corpus of the dog stomach contained large quantities of peptide material that reacted with antisera specific for glucagon. On BioGel P-30 chromatography, a substantial part of this material eluted like glucagon, but on polyacrylamide electrophoresis this fraction resolved into three components, only one of which migrated indistinguishably from glucagon. Material reacting with the specific antibodies was present also, although in lower concentrations, throughout the rest of the gastrointestinal tract and also in the salivary glands. Morita et al. (1976) also observed glucagon-like immunoreactivity associated with an apparently smaller molecule, as had been noted by Sasaki et al. (1975a) for material from porcine upper intestine, but only under conditions where enzymatic degradation had not been minimized. Srikant et al. (1977) found that the glucagon-like immunoreactivity in extracts of dog gastric mucosa was exhibited by substances with molecular weights (M_r); as estimated from chromatography on BioGel gels, of 2000, 3500, 9000, and 65,000. The M_r 3500 material was similar to glucagon not only in molecular weight but also in its glycogenolytic activity in the isolated rat liver. However, it differed from glucagon by having a relatively stronger activating effect on rat liver cell membrane adenylate cyclase. It also seemed to be slightly more acidic than glucagon, its pI being 6.15 rather than the 6.25 of glucagon.

Partial purification by affinity chromatography of peptides with glucagon-like immunoreactivity extract from dog jejunoileal mucosa has been described by Ohneda et al. (1976). Doi et al. (1979) extracted dog gastric fundic mucosa with aqueous ethanol acidified with hydrochloric acid and purified a glucagon immunoreactive component from this extract by two consecutive chromatographies, in different buffers, on a polyacrylamide gel followed by anion-exchange and then cation-exchange chromatography. The material obtained showed a single band on polyacrylamide electrophoresis and migrated with the same velocity as pancreatic glucagon. The effects of the purified material on glycogenolysis, gluconeogenesis, production of urea, lactate, and pyruvate in isolated rat hepatocytes were compared with the effects of pancreatic glucagon on these processes, and no differences, qualitative or quantitative, were noted. These results strongly suggest that this component of dog gastric glucagon-like immunoreactivity may be identical to pancreatic glucagon. No structural studies to prove this, however, have been described. Doi *et al.* (1979) also reported on the occurrence in extracts of dog fundic mucosa of another peptide with glucagon-like immunoreactivity that also was approximately the same size as pancreatic glucagon but differed from it by being much more basic.

Gutman *et al.* (1973) showed that rat small intestinal tissue contained peptides with glucagon-like immunoreactivities, which like the corresponding porcine and canine peptides could be separated by gel chromatography into two fractions, one containing peptide(s) the size of glucagon and the other peptides about twice this size. Frame (1976) found that in rat intestine, glucagon-like immunoreactivity was present from the duodenum to the colon, the concentration being highest in the ileum, somewhat lower in the colon, considerably lower in the jejunum, and lowest in the duodenum. Intestinal administration of glucose resulted in approximately equal elevations of plasma glucagon-like immunoreactivity levels from the proximal and the distal half of the gut, despite the much higher total levels of glucagon-like immunoreactivity in the latter.

O'Connor *et al.* (1979) described a model in which the isolated perfused rat intestine was shown to release glucagon-like immunoreactive peptides into its serosal secretions. The peptides consisted of several molecular species, one of about M_r 12,000, several smaller, and possibly one larger. The authors suggested that this type of perfused intestine could be used to study the release of other intestinal peptides.

An important and obvious problem is the relation of glucagon to all the various other peptides showing glucagon-like immunoreactivity. Rigopoulou *et al.* (1970) showed that although about 90% of the glucagon-like immunoreactivity in extracts of dog pancreas seemed to be exerted by glucagon itself, the remainder was associated with peptide material having approximately twice the molecular weight of glucagon. A similar pattern of immunoreactivity was found in pancreatic extracts of man, duck, beef, and rat.

Valverde *et al.* (1970b) found that the plasma of fasting dogs contained peptides with glucagon-like immunoreactivity that could be fractionated by gel chromatography into two fractions, one containing peptide(s) the size of glucagon, and the other containing larger peptides. They also found that mesenteric vein plasma contained the large and small peptides in about equal amounts in contrast to the pancreaticoduodenal vein plasma, in which the predominant part of the glucagon-like immunoreactivity was associated with glucagon-sized peptide(s) while smaller quantities consisted of the large peptides. As mentioned above, Tager and Steiner (1973) isolated from a highly purified preparation of bovine and porcine glucagon extracted from the pancreas a peptide with the amino acid sequence of glucagon extended from its C terminus by an octapeptide. They considered the possibility that this peptide was a fragment of proglucagon, a precursor of glucagon first observed during the biosynthesis of glucagon in angler fish islets by Noe and Bauer (1971), in pigeon islets by Tung and Zerega (1971), guinea pig islets by Hellerström et al. (1972), and in the perfused rat pancreas by O'Connor et al. (1973). Jacobsen et al. (1977) discussed the possibility that the biosynthesis of GLI-I (glicentin) and of glucagon starts with an identical precursor that, in the pancreas, is shortened to glucagon and in the intestine to glicentin and perhaps smaller peptides. This possibility has become increasingly probable in view of more recent work.

Tager and Markese (1979) extracted peptides reacting with a "nonspecific" glucagon antiserum from rabbit pancreas and small intestine and analyzed their gel chromatographic and polyacrylamide electrophoretic properties and the effects that treating the peptides with trypsin and carboxypeptidases A and B had on these properties and the reactivities of the peptides with a specific glucagon antiserum. The results indicated that identical peptides, with approximate molecular weights of 12,000 and 8000, were present in both pancreas and intestine. Glucagon itself also appeared to be present in both locations, but in much higher concentrations in the pancreas than in the intestine. In addition, the pancreas, but not the intestine, contained a peptide with a molecular weight of 9000. Immunochemical evidence suggested that this peptide consisted of glucagon extended from its N terminus only, while the 12,000 and 8000 M_r peptides consisted of glucagon extended from its C terminus with an identical peptide, but with N-terminal extensions of different length. Tager et al. (1980a) concluded that in all probability the biosynthesis of glucagon and related peptides starts by the synthesis of the same primary product in the pancreas and the intestine and that the same partially proteolysed fragments of this primary product are also found in both locations, but in different proportions. If, as seems probable, this is so, then the elucidation of the amino acid sequences of the precursor forms of glucagon in the pancreas will help to clarify also the chemistry of the intestinal peptides with glucagon-like immunoreactivities, and vice versa.

Patzelt et al. (1979) obtained evidence that a precursor form of glucagon in rat pancreatic islets has a molecular weight of 18,000 and that the release of glucagon from the precursor is accompanied by the formation of a 10,000 M_r protein of unknown function. A report has ap-

peared on the isolation of a 78-amino acid residue precursor to glucagon from angler fish islets, but no sequence data have yet been given,
apart from the statement that the peptide was found to have
N-terminal histidine (Trakatellis *et al.*, 1975).

d. Translation of Messenger RNA for Glucagon Precursors. Lund *et
al.* (1980) found that translation in a heterologous system of messenger
RNA extracted from angler fish pancreatic islets resulted in the formation of two proteins that could be precipitated by antibodies to glucagon with a double antibody technique. The molecular weights of these
proteins, as estimated from polyacrylamide electrophoresis in the presence of SDS, appeared to be 14,500 and 12,500. If dog pancreatic microsomal membranes were added to the translation mixture, the
amount of the 14,500 M_r protein decreased and that of the 12,500 M_r
protein increased. Somewhat surprisingly the 12,500 M_r protein was
not degraded further by either trypsin or chymotrypsin. The authors
suggested the possibility that it might have been segregated within
microsomal membranes, and that the 14,500 M_r peptide might be pre-
proglucagon and the 12,500 M_r peptide a proglucagon. In conformity
with this are observations suggesting that the much larger peptides
reacting with antisera to glucagon, occasionally observed by various
workers, probably do not contain glucagon but do contain some short
sequence(s) that will react with glucagon antisera (Rehfeld, 1979).

e. Terminology. The existence in the pancreas, and presumably in
the intestine, of glucagon itself and of various other peptides reacting
with antisera to glucagon has inevitably led to discussions concerning
the terminology for these substances. At a glucagon symposium in
Dallas, Texas it was suggested (Unger, 1976) that the word glucagon be
used only for the nonacosapeptide (Staub *et al.*, 1953; Bromer *et al.*,
1957) and that, in referring to immunochemical measurements on
plasma or tissue extracts, the term IRG (immunoreactive glucagon) be
used for peptides reacting with "specific" antisera (i.e., antisera directed toward the C-terminal sequence of glucagon). A superscript
should then be added when the (approximate) molecular weight of the
reacting peptide has been determined—for instance, IRG[3500] for glucagon itself, if determined immunochemically. Peptides reacting with
"nonspecific" sera, directed toward the N-terminal or middle sequences
of glucagon but not with the C-terminal antisera should, according to
this suggestion, be referred to as GLI (glucagon-like immunoreactivity), and again a superscript should be added when the molecular
weight is known. Glicentin would thus be GLI[8100]. The term GLI
should, consequently *not* be used for the total quantity of material reacting with glucagon antisera, if this material should be composed of
both GLI and IRG. It was also suggested that the term enteroglucagon

should not be used for GLI on the grounds that GLI is not glucagon. Another reason, the opposite, for not using the term enteroglucagon has been given by Murphy (1979). If glucagon and various glucagon-related peptides should be the same in the intestine and the pancreas, then "enteroglucagon" could cause confusion by suggesting that they were in fact different. Likewise, IRG could be ambiguous if taken to imply that there was another glucagon that did not react with antisera to the known glucagon. It is true that enteroglucagon would make better sense if it could be shown that there is in intestinal tissue some glucagon-related peptide that does not occur in the pancreas. On the other hand, if there is no such peptide it may nevertheless by useful to speak of intestinal, i.e., enteroglucagon, as a physiological entity.

Conlon (1980), in a review of the various glucagon-like peptides known by now, suggested that the IRG-GLI terminology, with superscripts when appropriate, as recommended at the Dallas conference, be followed. This seems most reasonable, at any rate for immunochemical purposes at present. However, when the amino acid sequences of the various IRG and GLI components have been established, some other terminology might prove to be more descriptive, at least in chemistry. For instance, if, as seems probable, the various IRG and GLI peptides are found to be composed of the glucagon sequence carrying C- or/and N-terminal extensions, it might be reasonable to use the glucagon sequence as the reference point and indicate the number of amino acid residues in the extensions. The "proglucagon fragment" of Tager and Steiner (1973) could be written as glucagon-8 and glicentin (Thim and Moody, 1981) as 32-glucagon-8. Alternatively it may be reasonable to let the number to the left of "glucagon" indicate *all* the amino acids from the C terminus of glucagon, the proglucagon fragment then becoming 29-glucagon-8, and glicentin 61-glucagon-8. This would simplify the description of C-terminal *fragments* of glucagon. Similar considerations of terminology apply to the other gastrointestinal hormones and their precursor "pre" and "pro" forms.

3. Heterogeneity of Gastrin

a. Discovery of Gastrin Heterogeneity. Although the heterogeneity of gastrointestinal hormonal peptides was first described for glucagon-related peptides, it is in connection with gastrin that heterogeneity has been studied most thoroughly. Yalow and Berson (1970) found that only a small fraction of the peptides in human peripheral plasma that reacted with antibodies to gastrin had the characteristics of the then known heptadecapeptide gastrins, whereas a major portion of gastrin-like immunoreactivity appeared to consist of peptides that, judging from their Sephadex chromatographic properties, were of a larger molecular size than the heptadecapeptides and also differed from them by migrating as less acidic peptides on starch gel and paper electrophoresis. Soon thereafter, Yalow and Berson (1971a) showed that the "big gastrin" could be converted by trypsin into gastrin-immunoreactive material with certain chromatographic and electrophoretic properties similar to those of the heptadecapeptide gastrins. Berson and Yalow (1971) then showed that the "big gastrin," apparently of the same type as found in plasma, was also present in extracts of human antrum, duodenum, and proximal jejunum. The ratio of the concentrations of "big" to "little" gastrin increased from proximal to distal gut with the total concentrations of both forms decreasing distally.

The finding by Berson and Yalow of the size heterogeneity of plasma and gut tissue gastrin undoubtedly drew attention to this facet of the gastrin problem and presumably accelerated the isolation of the tetratriaconta- and tetradecapeptide gastrins by Gregory and Tracy (p. 240). It did not quite, however, come as a revelation. Gregory had repeatedly pointed out that the relation of the heptadecapeptide gastrin(s), which he and Tracy had isolated from antral mucosa, to the circulating form of gastrin, and indeed to the storage form of it in the mucosa, remained to be established (Gregory and Tracy, 1964; Gregory, 1968). Besides, the Liverpool workers had in 1968 made unpublished observations suggesting the occurrence of a larger form of gastrin than the heptadecapeptides, in addition to the latter, in extracts of pig antral mucosa and of Zollinger–Ellison tumor tissue (Gregory and Tracy, 1975). There were also a few reports from other laboratories that seemed to suggest that gastrin could occur in a form larger than the heptadecapeptide. Subsequently, Yalow and Berson (1972) found that a minor component of the material that reacted with antibodies to gastrin in the plasma of patients with the Zollinger–Ellison syndrome, and in extracts of jejunal tissue of these (?) patients, appeared in the void volume on Sephadex G-50 chromatography, thereby behaving as though it had a molecular size much larger than that of even "big" (i.e., tetratriacontapeptide) gastrin. Among the split products obtained on treating plasma fractions containing such "big-big" gastrin with trypsin was a gastrin-immunoreactive component of the size of the heptadecapeptides.

In further work on "big-big" gastrin, Yalow and Wu (1973) found that it appeared to constitute a major fraction of the total gastrin immunoreactivity in the normal nonstimulated state of human, canine, and porcine plasma. Later work, however, seems to suggest that plasma "big-big" gastrin is an artifact in part due to adsorption of other forms of gastrin to some plasma protein(s) of large molecular size (Rehfeld et al., 1975) and in part due to nonspecific interference in the radioimmunoassay by nongastrin protein (Rehfeld, 1979). A real "big-big" gastrin may, nevertheless, be present in extracts of gastrinoma tumors and of normal antral tissue (Rehfeld et al., 1974). However, other structurally as yet uncharacterized peptides contribute to true gastrin heterogeneity. By Sephadex G-50 chromatography of sera from patients with either pernicious anemia, or the Zollinger–Ellison syndrome, followed by further resolution of the fractions obtained on aminoethyl cellulose, Rehfeld et al. (1974) found evidence for the occurrence in these sera of the pairs of the tetradecapeptide gastrins (component IV of the chromatography on Sephadex G-50 superfine), the heptadecapeptide gastrins (component III), the tetratriacontapeptide gastrins (component II), and of a monophasic gastrin-immunoreactive component that on gel chromatography eluted before the tetratriacontapeptide gastrins, in approximately the same fractions as proinsulin would have eluted. On degradation with trypsin this component I gastrin, which was not identical with "big-big" gastrin, released a component with the chromatographic properties of heptadecapeptide gastrin I. Earlier, Rehfeld (1972) had obtained evidence for the existence of component I in normal human serum, and a partial purification of this form of gastrin has been achieved (Gregory, 1979a).

There is evidence that the heterogeneity of gastrin, both when circulating in the plasma (Rehfeld et al., 1975) and in the tissues of its biosynthesis (Gregory, 1979a), may be still much greater than what would appear from the description above. On analyzing plasma gastrin from a patient with the Zollinger–Ellison syndrome by combinations of high-resolution gel chromatography, ion-exchange chromatography, and disc-gel electrophoresis, Rehfeld et al. (1975) found that components I and II could be resolved into six components each, instead of only two, as would have been expected, and to the presence of nonsulfated and sulfated forms in each component. Later work (Rehfeld, 1979) showed that components III and IV could each be resolved into four subcomponents, instead of only two.

b. Terminology. Rehfeld (1979) uses the term macroheterogeneity to describe the various forms of a peptide hormone that may be formed from a common precursor by enzymically catalyzed cleavages, and the term microheterogeneity to describe posttranslational covalent modifications of single amino acid residues, such as the esterification of a tyrosine residue with sulfuric acid. These terms are descriptive. However, microheterogeneity has been used in protein chemistry to describe also genetically determined replacements of amino acid residues in a peptide chain (Colvin et al., 1954) and therefore the o and m ("original" and "modified") terminology of enzymology (IUPAC–IUB

Commission on Biochemical Nomenclature (CBN), 1977) may be preferable for describing posttranslational modifications of single residues. Instead of macroheterogeneity, the term size heterogeneity is also used (Yalow and Berson, 1971b). This is a suggestive term, but strictly speaking not very revealing, since a hormone may exhibit size heterogeneity by occurring in forms of different chain length, but any modification of an amino acid residue will also almost always lead to differences in size between the o and the m form of the hormone. "Chain-length heterogeneity" or "number of residues heterogeneity" might be more accurate. The latter expression is somewhat cumbersome in English, but not in some other languages, which have separate words for "number" and "number of." Considerable interest centers at present on the question of whether, or rather to what extent, the common C-terminal tetrapeptide amide of gastrin and of cholecystokinin "G/CCK-4" occurs in the circulating blood and/or in tissues (Rehfeld and Larsson, 1979; Rehfeld *et al.*, 1980; Dockray and Gregory, 1980). Similar to other naturally occurring peptides with C-terminal α-amide structures, gastrin may be expected to have precursor forms extended C-terminally past the C-terminal phenylalanine amide of the forms with known structures, and there are reports by Gregory (1979b) and more definitely by Rehfeld (1980) that such forms have been sighted.

  c. Evidence for Existence of Forms Not Yet Isolated. During the isolation of porcine heptadecapeptide gastrins from hog antral mucosa, Gregory and Tracy observed the presence in the partially purified preparations of two peptides corresponding to the 1–13 sequences of, respectively, the sulfated and nonsulfated heptadecapeptides (Gregory, 1974). Dockray and Walsh (1975) subsequently provided strong immunochemical evidence for the occurrence of the 1–13 fragment of G-17 in the sera of patients with the Zollinger–Ellison syndrome. Whether this gastrin fragment from the serum was sulfated or not, or a mixture of sulfated and nonsulfated forms, was not mentioned. This 1–13 fragment is of particular importance, since its removal from the heptadecapeptides should result in the release of the C-terminal tetrapeptide amide of the gastrins—and of the cholecystokinins (Gregory, 1974, 1979a; Dockray and Walsh, 1975). Gregory has reported on a peptide that might be the 1–30 sequence of the tetratriacontapeptide gastrin (Gregory, 1979a). The heterogeneity of gastrin has been discussed in many earlier reviews, in this series (McGuigan, 1974) and elsewhere (Gregory, 1974; Walsh, 1975; Gregory, 1979a,b; and Rehfeld, 1979).

  d. Determination of Amino Acid Sequences of Naturally Occurring Peptides via Sequencing of Their Corresponding Nucleic Acids. Use of

Such Techniques for the Determination of the Amino Acid Sequences of Preprogastrin, Preprosomatostatin, and Other Peptides. An important development in biochemistry has been the demonstration of the feasibility, although there may be pitfalls, of determining amino acid sequences of naturally occurring polypeptides by way of the nucleotide sequences of their corresponding messenger RNAs or of the genes coding for these mRNAs (Schulz and Schirmer, 1979). This became practical owing to the development of swift and reliable methods for the determination of nucleotide sequences in DNA (Sanger *et al.,* 1977; Maxam and Gilbert, 1977). The remaining difficulty is not the sequencing, which seems to be easy compared to that of polypeptides, but the isolation of the correct DNA for sequencing. For this, many methods have been described, most of which start not directly with DNA, but with the isolation of the corresponding messenger RNA followed by reverse transcriptase-catalyzed synthesis of its complementary DNA (Ross *et al.,* 1972; Verma *et al.,* 1972; Kacian *et al.,* 1972). Riccardi *et al.* (1979) do, however, describe a method in which *fragments* of DNA, obtained by cleavage of DNA with restriction enzymes, are separated and used to isolate, from total cellular RNA, mRNAs with sequences complementary to those of the DNA fragments; the mRNA nature of the hybridized RNA being established, after elution from the DNA fragments, by its ability to stimulate polypeptide synthesis in a cell-free system. A somewhat similar technique for obtaining specific fragments of DNA by cleaving DNA complementary to human placental and rat pituitary mRNAs has been described by Goodman and co-workers (see later). Apart from the preparation of cDNA, mRNA has been used as such, in heterologous translation systems, for investigations of polypeptide or protein biosynthesis, as shown for hemoglobin by Laycock and Hunt (1969) and by Lockard and Lingrel (1969). This type of work has been particularly useful for the identification of biosynthetic precursor forms, for immunoglobulins (Milstein *et al.,* 1972), several pancreatic secretory proteins (Devillers-Thiery *et al.,* 1975), proinsulins from various species (Permutt and Boime, 1975; Weber, 1975; Lomedico, 1975; Yip *et al.,* 1975; Lomedico *et al.,* 1977; Shields and Blobel, 1977), parathyroid hormone (Kemper *et al.,* 1974), glucagon (Lund *et al.,* 1980), somatostatin (Shields, 1980; Goodman *et al.,* 1980a), and many others.

The isolation of mRNA is consequently important. In principle, published isolation methods fall into two categories. In one, the whole complex mRNA fraction of a tissue that synthesizes a certain polypeptide is isolated and used as such for DNA or polypeptide synthesis. This is reasonable when the cells synthesizing the polypeptide occur in high concentration in a tissue and also synthesize the polypeptide in question in a high concentration compared with other polypeptides. Obviously this is so for the synthesis of globin by reticulocyte mRNA (Ross *et al.*, 1972), but also in several other less obvious, cases partially purified mRNA has been successfully used. For instance, Shields and Blobel used the complex mRNA fraction from the islets of Langerhans of the angler fish to study the biosynthesis of both preproinsulin (Shields and Blobel, 1977) and of preprosomatostatin (Shields, 1980) in a wheat germ cell-free system, this being possible because these two peptides were prominent among the translation products and apparently were easily separable from each other and other peptides by electrophoresis in polyacrylamide gels. Chan *et al.* (1976) did not even find it necessary to separate the mRNA complex of rat Langerhans islets from other types of nucleic acids before using it for stimulating preproinsulin synthesis in a cell-free system. Ullrich *et al.* (1977) used DNA obtained by reverse transcription of the complex mRNA fraction of rat islets of Langerhans for the preparation of recombinant DNA bacterial plasmids that were then found to contain DNA sequences coding for various fragments of the two preproinsulins of the rat. Kronenberg *et al.* (1977) used a bovine parathyroid mRNA fraction to synthesize cDNA, which in a linked transcription–translation system directed the synthesis of preproparathyroid hormone. Later, Kronenberg *et al.* (1979) used such cDNA for the construction of bacterial plasmids and found that one of the 49 colonies that were investigated produced DNA with the whole coding region for preproparathyroid hormone, with noncoding polynucleotide extensions at both the 5′ and 3′ ends of this sequence. Determination of the nucleotide sequence of this DNA served to clarify an obscure point in the earlier known amino acid sequence of preproparathyroid hormone. Likewise, Hobart and co-workers and Goodman and co-workers used DNA complementary to complex angler fish Brockman body mRNA for preparing clones of bacterial recombinant DNA plasmids and could select clones coding for the entire sequence of preprosomatostatin (Goodman *et al.*, 1980a,b) or, unexpectedly, for two different preprosomatostatins (Hobart *et al.*, 1980).

Where complex tissue mRNA has been used for the preparation of cDNA, the mRNA complex has in most cases been separated from other types of RNA. This has proved to be possible by taking advantage of the finding (Lim and Canellakis, 1970; Darnell *et al.*, 1971; Lee *et al.*, 1971; Edmonds *et al.*, 1971; Burr and Lingrel, 1971) that mammalian mRNAs characteristically have polyadenylate sequences at their 3′ termini. This chemical characteristic makes it possible to hybridize them reversibly (Nakazato and Edmonds, 1972; Aviv and Leder, 1972) to immobilized polythymidylate (Gilham, 1964), but also imparts to them other solubility and adsorptive properties useful for purification purposes (Brawerman *et al.*, 1972).

The other category of mRNA isolation methods aims at a high purity of a specific mRNA before it is used for reverse transcription or polypeptide synthesis. Several different methods have been devised for such isolations. Immunoadsorbent or immunoprecipitation techniques directed toward the specific peptide translated by the mRNA have been used to isolate the corresponding polysomal mRNA–protein complex, with subsequent separation of the nucleic acid from the protein (Palacios *et al.*, 1973; Schechter, 1973). Isolation of mRNAs has, however, also been accomplished by the application of ordinary biochemical chromatographic and electrophoretic fractionation methods to the mRNA fraction of a tissue. After purification by translating aliquots of the various fractions obtained in a cell-free system, the purification is continued until a fraction is obtained that translates only the protein corresponding to the mRNA sought. This type of approach was used for the isolation of ovalbumin mRNA from hen oviducts (Woo *et al.*, 1975) and more recently for the isolation of the mRNA for the bovine corticotropin–lipotropin precursor (Kita *et al.*, 1979). The cDNA to this mRNA was then used for the construction of bacterial plasmids that were found to synthesize the DNA coding for the complete sequence of the protein. The nucleotide sequence of the DNA was determined, and the amino acid residue sequence of the protein was deduced from this (Nakanishi *et al.*, 1979).

For preparing DNA coding for human chorionic somatomammotropin, Seeburg *et al.* (1977a) started with the complex mixture of mRNAs from human placental tissue and prepared the corresponding cDNA. This was subsequently cleaved with restriction endonucleases, and the fragments obtained were separated by electrophoresis in polyacrylamide gels. Fragments complementary to the mRNA for somatomammotropin were identified and used for sequencing and in subsequent work for the construction of recombinant bacterial plasmids. DNA, from a clone of the latter, was used for sequencing and the previously known amino acid sequence of the hormone (Niall *et al.*, 1971) was confirmed (Shine *et al.*, 1977). Work along similar lines led to the establishment of the nucleotide sequence of the DNA directing the synthesis of rat somatotropin and its precursor form and thereby of the amino acid sequences of these proteins (Seeburg *et al.*, 1977b). Only a partial sequence of rat somatotropin had at that time been determined by amino acid residue sequence analysis (Wallis and Davies, 1976).

A rather different approach to mRNA purification has been described by Agarwal and co-workers (Noyes *et al.*, 1979; Mevarech *et al.*, 1979).

They synthesized oligodeoxynucleotides with sequences complementary to a hypothetical mRNA for gastrin, the nucleotide sequence of which was constructed from the known amino acid sequence of the peptide. These oligonucleotides were then used as hybridization probes for the identification of the true mRNA for gastrin in antral extracts and for the priming of the synthesis of cDNA to this mRNA. The deduction of mRNA sequences from amino acid sequences is known to be very difficult (Fitch, 1976). In working with gastrin, Agarwal and coworkers could make good use of the methionyltryptophanyl sequence, since methionine and tryptophan are exceptional by having unique codons. It will be interesting to see whether their elegant oligodeoxynucleotide method can be applied to peptides not containing residues of these two amino acids. The work of Noyes et al. (1979) on the nucleotide sequence of the DNA complementary to the mRNA of porcine gastrin confirmed the amino acid sequence that had been deduced for it and showed, in addition, that the pyroglutamyl residue of pG-34 was in the precursor a residue of glutamine, which in turn was preceded by a histidyl-arginyl-arginyl sequence, and that preprogastrin was a peptide of between 110 and 140 amino acid residues incorporating G-34 extended from both ends.

  e. *Evidence for Heterogeneity of VIP, Secretin, and GIP and for the Existence of Still Uncharacterized Forms of Cholecystokinin.* Compared to the extensive studies on the heterogeneity of glucagon and gastrin, only little work has yet been carried out on other gastrointestinal hormonal peptides. Dimaline and Dockray (1978) have found that in extracts of human colonic mucosa reactivity with antibodies to VIP is associated with four different types of peptides: one with the gel filtration and cation-exchange chromatographic properties of the known octacosapeptide, one of apparently smaller size, and two of the same size as VIP, but less basic. Yamaguchi et al. (1980) detected in extracts of certain pancreatic tumors large amounts of a peptide that reacted with antibodies to VIP but appeared to be some 4–5 times larger than VIP, possibly a precursor form. Mason et al. (1979) conjugated antibodies with specificity to the C-terminal part of porcine secretin to Sephadex and used these conjugates to purify *plasma immunoreactive secretin.* They found that during starvation plasma concentration of secretin-like immunoreactivity increased and seemed to be due to three types of peptides, secretin itself, peptide(s) smaller than secretin, and peptides about four times larger than secretin, presumably precursor form(s). Tatemoto (1980) has isolated a variant form of porcine secretin and localized the difference to the N-terminal part of the molecule, but the exact nature of this difference has not yet been clarified.

  In addition to the three forms of CCK that have been isolated from porcine and ovine tissues, Rehfeld (1978b) has, with sequence-specific radioimmunnoassays, found evidence for the occurrence in extracts of human and porcine upper intestinal tissues of several additional forms of CCK. Tatemoto (1980) has obtained evidence for the occurrence in porcine intestinal tissues of a CCK-bioactive peptide, which is more basic than either CCK-33 or CCK-39 and has N-terminal arginine, instead of the N-terminal lysine and tyrosine, respectively, of the latter two peptides. Ryder *et al.* (1981) has presented immunochemical evidence for the occurrence in pig and rat brain of C-terminally extended forms of cholecystokinin. Brown and co-workers (1980) have found evidence for the occurrence in porcine intestinal extracts of a larger form of GIP than the known dotetracontapeptide.

   f. Evidence for the Presence in Gastrointestinal Tissues of Materials with Corticotropin-like, Urogastrone-like, Enkephalin-like, and Physalaemin-like Immunoreactivities. The presence of peptides with corticotropin-like immunoreactivity in certain pancreatic islet cell tumors was described by Orth and Nicholson (1977). Larsson (1977) first described immunocytochemical studies suggesting the presence of peptide(s) reacting with antisera to the C-terminal part of corticotropin in certain cells of the dog, cat, and rat antropyloric mucosa and pancreas. Such cells also occurred in human and monkey antropyloric mucosa but were very rare. Later, Larsson described the simultaneous presence of corticotropin- and gastrin-like immunoreactivity in cells of rat antropyloric mucosa, both in the G cells earlier known to produce gastrin and in another type of cell that he classified as G_a (Larsson, 1978). Feurle *et al.* (1980) found that acid extracts of human antrum and pancreas contained peptides reacting with antisera to corticotropin and that the gel chromatographic properties of these peptides suggested the presence in the extracts of both corticotropin itself and two apparently glycoprotein precursor forms. The presence in extracts of rat gastrointestinal tissues of material reacting with antisera to thyroliberin and showing gel and cation chromatographic properties indistinguishable from the latter, has been demonstrated by Leppäluoto *et al.* (1977, 1978) and by Morley and co-workers (Morley *et al.*, 1977; Morley, 1979).

   A factor in urine that inhibits gastric secretion (Gray *et al.*, 1939; Friedman *et al.*, 1939) was named *urogastrone* by Gray *et al.* (1940), because of its similarity in action to the hypothetical enterogastrone (Kosaka and Lim, 1930). Many methods were described for the isolation of urogastrone (Gregory, 1955), but it was not until 1975 that urogastrone was isolated, from normal male urine, by means of a 12-stage purification process and found to be a mixture of two peptides, one named β-urogastrone composed of 53 amino acid residues, and the other, named γ-urogastrone, with 52 residues. γ-Urogastrone differed from β-urogastrone only by lacking the C-terminal arginine residue of the latter. The amino acid residue sequence of β-urogastrone (Gregory, 1975; Gregory and Preston, 1977) is N S D S E C P L S H D G Y C L H D G V C M Y I E A L D K Y A C N C V V G Y I G E R C Q Y R D L K W W E L R.

The disulfide bridges join cysteine residues 6–20, 14–31, and 33–42. Urogastrone was, unexpectedly, found to be markedly similar in sequence with the mouse epidermal growth factor, a substance originally discovered by Cohen (1962) in the submaxillary glands of male mice that, on administration to newborn mice, induced premature eye opening and eruption of incisors. Perhaps it should not have been such a surprise since Sandweiss (1943) had claimed that urine contained a substance, which he called anthelone, that produced fibroblastic proliferation and epithelization of the mucosa. However, he considered urogastrone and anthelone to be two separate substances. The sequence of the 53 amino acid residues of mouse epidermal growth factor was worked out by Savage et al. (1972). Human epidermal growth factor was isolated from pregnancy urine by Cohen and Carpenter (1975). Small differences in its amino acid composition and that of the urogastrone isolated by Gregory (1975) were observed, but apparently it could not be excluded that these could be attributed to technical inadequacies in the analytical methods used (Carpenter, 1978). Although epidermal growth factor–urogastrone, EGF–URO as it has been called (Hollenberg and Gregory, 1980), has not been isolated from gastrointestinal tissues, Heitz et al. (1978) and Elder et al. (1978) have presented immunocytochemical evidence for its presence in man, in special cells of the submandibular salivary glands and in the glands of Brunner of the duodenum. EGF–URO has been reviewed in this series (Hollenberg, 1979).

Elde et al. (1976) found leu-enkephalin-like immunoreactive material to be present in the myenteric plexus of the rat gastrointestinal tract, and Polak et al. (1977b) found met-enkephalin-like immunoreactive material in extracts of human antral and upper small intestinal tissues, and also that, in the pyloric antrum, met-enkephalin-like immunoreactivity was present in gastrin-containing cells. Alumets et al. (1978) could not confirm these results concerning the gastrin cells, but did find enkephalin-like immunoreactivity in gastrointestinal tissues. Ito et al. (1979), however, came to the same conclusions as Polak and co-workers and found in addition that also in the antropyloric mucosa of the dog, gastrin- and met-enkephalin-like immunoreactivities were seen in the same cells. The amino acid sequences of the two enkepha-lins (Hughes *et al.*, 1975) are Tyr-Gly-Gly-Phe-Met and Tyr-Gly-Gly-Phe-Leu, respectively.

Lazarus *et al.* (1980) have presented immunochemical and chromatographic evidence for the occurrence in extracts of rabbit, guinea pig, rat, and mouse stomach tissues, of guinea pig duodenum, and, in lower concentration, of other guinea pig tissues, of a peptide similar to, or identical with physalaemin, the undecapeptide with the sequence Glp-Ala-Asp-Pro-Asn-Lys-Phe-Tyr-Gly-Leu-Met-NH$_2$ (Anas-tasi *et al.*, 1964) from the skin of the South American amphibian *Physalaemus fuscumaculatus*.

III. Isolation of Gastrointestinal Hormones

In a review of what was then known about gastrointestinal hor-mones, Greengard wrote: "So numerous have been the attempts to obtain secretin in a chemically pure form that it is not expedient to enumerate them all" (Greengard, 1948). This is true not only for secre-tin, but also for gastrin, cholecystokinin, and substance P. It may, however, be remembered that in many cases pieces of information ac-quired by the early workers have been used to develop the methods that finally, in another technological age, led to the isolation of the hormones.

The way a peptide is extracted from a tissue is important for any isolation procedure. In the field of gastrointestinal hormones, three main types of extraction techniques have proved to be particularly useful. All three aim at preventing proteolytic degradation of the pep-tides during the extraction. The method used for gastrin by Gregory and Tracy (1964) is the simplest: the peptide is extracted by boiling water. That this would be possible had already been demonstrated by Edkins (1906) and by Blair *et al.* (1961). This technique has also been used for the isolation of 8-CCK from sheep brain (Dockray *et al.*, 1978a). The second method entails boiling of the tissue, briefly, in water, followed by extraction of the peptides by cold dilute aqueous acid. This technique seems to have been first used by Jorpes and Mutt (1961c) for the purification of secretin and cholecystokinin, although it was implicit already in the work of Bayliss and Starling (1902a,b). Subsequently it has been used for the extraction of GIP (Brown *et al.*, 1970), motilin (Brown *et al.*, 1971), VIP (Said and Mutt, 1972), chymodenin (Adelson *et al.*, 1980), the bombesin-related gastrin-releasing peptide (McDonald *et al.*, 1979), somatostatin-28 (Pradayrol *et al.*, 1980), PHI, and PYY (Tatemoto and Mutt, 1980). In contrast to this, extraction by boiling dilute acid has frequently been used. It would, however, seem that heating at a low pH might disrupt acid-labile peptide bonds (Piszkiewicz et al., 1970; Jauregui-Adell and Marti, 1975). It has indeed been asked what effect "cooking" in even neutral solution might have on peptides (Blundell et al., 1976). This has not been investigated quite as systematically as it, perhaps, should have been. Nevertheless, Gregory and Tracy (1973) found no difference in G-34 if it was extracted from hog antral mucosa with a cold phosphate buffer or with boiling water, although the yield was lower in the former case. Likewise Holst (1977) found no difference in the immunochemical properties of peptides reacting with antisera to glucagon whether they had been extracted with dilute acetic acid from briefly boiled, or with acid ethanol from unheated, porcine gastrointestinal tissues.

It is not quite clear why the acidic peptides gastrin and 8-CCK are easily extracted from tissues by boiling water whereas basic peptides like secretin and the larger forms of CCK need acid to be extracted. One suggestion (Jorpes, 1968) is that, since the bulk of the insoluble structural tissue proteins are negatively charged at neutral pH values, they may electrostatically bind positively charged, basic, but not negatively charged, acidic, peptides whereas at low pH values both protein and peptide will be negatively charged and will not interact. It may be mentioned that, in the method for extracting substance P from horse intestine that v. Euler and his co-workers had devised (Pernow, 1953), extraction was admittedly carried out by boiling in dilute acid, but very dilute indeed.

In the third type of procedure, extraction is with mixtures of water with some organic solvent, usually ethanol or acetone. Some acid is also usually added to facilitate extraction. This type of procedure was used for the extraction of insulin from beef pancreas by Banting et al. (1922) and has ever since, in various modifications, been used for the preparation of insulin, glucagon, and the pancreatic polypeptide (Kimmel et al., 1975). Instead of acid alcohol, Lyons (1937) used acid acetone for the extraction of corticotropin and prolactin from sheep pituitaries, and this extractant has found extensive use in work on anterior pituitary hormones (Li, 1952; Li et al., 1978). It has also been used during the isolation of substance P (Chang and Leeman, 1970b) and of neurotensin (Carraway and Leeman, 1973) from bovine hypothalamic extracts. That peptides may form condensation products with acetone was demonstrated by Yamashiro et al. (1965). It has been pointed out (Murphy, 1979) that the extraction methods commonly used may have discriminated against large precursor forms. This may well be true, and not only concerning precursor molecules. It is quite possible that there are yet unknown gastrointestinal hormones that have been either destroyed or left unextracted by the various types of extraction procedures.

Three fairly distinct stages are discernible in the types of methods that have been used for the isolation, or attempted isolation, of individual gastrointestinal hormones from these various types of extracts. Until the mid-1950s the methods were such as had been developed already by the protein chemists of the nineteenth century and the early twentieth century. These fractionations of aqueous solutions at various acidities with neutral salts and/or organic solvents, and isoelectric precipitations, led to important results especially outside the field of gastrointestinal hormones. Both insulin (Abel, 1926) and glucagon (Staub *et al.,* 1955) were isolated in crystalline form by the use of such methods exclusively. No gastrointestinal hormone was, however, isolated at this stage, although pharmacologically acceptable preparations of secretin were obtained. It was not until these early methods were supplemented by a newer set of methods that had been developed in various other areas of biochemistry, methods like chromatography on ion-exchange resins (Paleus and Neilands, 1950), cellulose-based ion exchangers (Sober and Peterson, 1954), gels of crosslinked dextran (Porath and Flodin, 1959), and countercurrent distribution (Craig, 1962) that first gastrin and secretin and thereafter other peptides could be isolated from gastrointestinal tissues in degrees of purity sufficient for determination of their amino acid seqeunces.

During the 1970s there has again been an accelerated influx of newer techniques into the area, and important results have been obtained by the use of immunoaffinity chromatography and high-performance liquid chromatography. The value of the latter technique was first clearly demonstrated, outside of the gastrointestinal field, by its use for the isolation of the enkephalins (Hughes *et al.,* 1975). The available techniques are now so efficient that it seems possible to isolate any peptide from an extract fairly quickly, and the problem is increasingly turning from how to isolate to what to isolate. One approach would obviously be to isolate every peptide from an extract. This would, owing to the often great complexity of the peptide patterns in tissue extracts, certainly demand much work but could presumably be done. Until recently it would have been a rather pointless undertaking, since the small amounts of pure peptides that would have been obtained would not have sufficed for sequence determinations or analyses of biological effects. Advances in automatization of sequence work, especially if combined with deduction of amino acid sequences from polynucleotide sequences, and the possibility of thereafter obtaining replicates of the natural peptide through synthesis by organic chemical methods, or by recombinant DNA technology, tend to make it more reasonable. Nevertheless, the work that would have to follow of establishing which of the isolated peptides have hormonal properties, and which are fragments of structural proteins, enzymes, respiratory proteins, etc. or inactive precursors that must be cleaved in unknown ways, does not make it very tempting, and it would seem advisable to continue to have some form of selection. The classic way of finding a hormonally active peptide is by the discovery of a certain type of hormonal activity in an extract and purification of the agent exerting this activity, whereby the purification is monitored by determining the distribution of the activity into the various fractions obtained. This procedure resulted in the isolation of gastrin and of secretin. In the case of cholecystokinin and pancreozymin there was a surprise—following either of these activities resulted in one peptide, exhibiting both activities (Jorpes and Mutt, 1966). There is no doubt that this type of approach will continue to be used in hormone chemistry. There are, however, a few alternatives.

Immunological crossreactivity can obviously be used for the isolation of unknown peptides. In other cases radioimmunoassay can be used indirectly for following the purification of a liberin or statin by measuring the effects of material from various fractions on the plasma levels of the known substance—the release of which is either stimulated or inhibited. A peptide may be isolated purely by chance and turn out to have hormonal activity, as happened in the case of lipotropin (Li, 1968) and the pancreatic polypeptide (Kimmel et al., 1968). It may, however, also turn out to be a fragment of some known protein and very probably without any hormonal activity (Chang et al., 1980). It may therefore be worthwhile to attempt to increase the probability that the peptides isolated are hormonally active by isolating such peptides as have some chemical feature known to occur often in hormonally active peptides. The C-terminal α-amide would appear to be one such structure, and the isolation from extracts of porcine intestinal tissue of two previously unknown peptides, which were identified on the basis of such a structure (Tatemoto and Mutt, 1980), resulted in the finding that both these peptides did indeed exhibit hormone-like activities, at any rate pharmacologically.

IV. WORK ON STRUCTURES OF GASTROINTESTINAL HORMONES

Compared to the extensive investigations of the secondary and tertiary structures of polypeptide hormones like insulin (Blundell et al., 1971), oxytocin and vasopressin (Walter, 1971; Smith and Walter,

1978), glucagon (King, 1959; Blanchard and King, 1966; Gratzer *et al.*, 1968, 1972; Gratzer and Beaven, 1969; Swann and Hammes, 1969; Schiffer and Edmundson, 1970; Bornet and Edelhoch, 1971; Low *et al.*, 1971; McBride-Warren and Epand, 1972; Epand and Grey, 1973; Contaxis and Epand, 1974; Panijpan and Gratzer, 1974; Chou and Fasman, 1975; Sasaki *et al.*, 1975b; Blundell *et al.*, 1976; Moran *et al.*, 1977; Ross *et al.*, 1977; Deranleau *et al.*, 1978; Johnson *et al.*, 1979), and, more recently, the "pancreatic polypeptide" (Pitts *et al.*, 1979), work on the structures of gastrointestinal hormones has as yet mainly been concerned with amino acid sequence determination. This is due in part to the fact that none of these hormones has yet been obtained in the form of crystals suitable for X-ray crystallographic studies. Nevertheless, some attempts to gain insight into their secondary and three-dimensional structures have been described. Bodanszky *et al.* (1969) concluded from investigations of rotatory dispersion and circular dichroism spectra of porcine secretin that secretin in aqueous solution existed as a peptide of low, but definite, helix content. The spectra of various fragments of secretin seemed to suggest that there were two helical turns, most probably in the sequence 6–13, and that this helical structure, containing hydrophobic amino acids in positions 6, 10, and 13, might be stabilized by hydrophobic acid residues in positions 22, 23, 26, and 27 in the C-terminal part of secretin brought into proximity of the helical region by a reverse turn of the peptide chain. Stabilization of helical structures by interaction of sequence structures that would be distant from each other in the extended peptide chains had been described for other polypeptides (Epand and Scheraga, 1968). Further work by Bodanszky and co-workers, also by the analysis of nuclear magnetic resonance (NMR) spectra (Patel *et al.*, 1970), provided additional evidence for the stabilization of a helical section in secretin through the interaction of hydrophobic amino acid residues in these two parts of the chain, but also suggested that the helical stretch occurred in the C-terminal part instead and was stabilized by the hydrophobic residues Phe-6, Leu-10, and Leu-13, which themselves were in a nonhelical region (Bodanszky and Fink, 1976; Bodanszky *et al.*, 1976). Such a structure, with the bend of the chain localized to the region of Leu-13 and Arg-14, could be further stabilized by ion-pair formation between Glu-9 and Arg-18 and between Asp-15 and Arg-12 (Makhlouf *et al.*, 1978). Bodanszky *et al.* (1974a) found that VIP in aqueous solution showed optical rotatory spectra suggesting a helix content of about 20%. The helical nature became more pronounced on addition of organic solvents, and especially 2-trifluoroethanol added to the solution markedly enhanced the helical nature of the spectra.

It has been suggested by other workers that the circular dichroism

(CD) spectra of cell membrane proteins in water-trifluoroethanol mixtures may be more like the spectra of these proteins in their natural, partly hydrophobic, environment than those they exhibit in purely aqueous solution (Urry, 1972; Long et al., 1977). Wünsch and co-workers synthesized three analogs of porcine secretin in which the N-terminal pentapeptide of secretin was converted to the corresponding sequence of glucagon (glucagon-secretin; Gln^3-secretin), VIP (VIP-secretin; Ala^4, Val^5-secretin) and GIP (GIP-secretin; Tyr^1, Ala^2, Glu^3-secretin), respectively, and a fourth analog in which the N-terminal tetrapeptide was replaced by the 6–9 sequence of somatostatin-14 (somatostatin-secretin; Phe^1, Phe^2, Trp^3, Lys^4-secretin) and compared the CD spectra of these analogs with the spectra of secretin (Jaeger et al., 1979). In water solution, all the spectra in the far ultraviolet were quite similar in accordance with the suggestion of Blundell et al. (1976) that the N-terminal pentapeptide of secretin is not involved in the stabilization of the preferred conformation of the peptide backbone of secretin. The CD spectra in the near ultraviolet indicated, however, that amino acid residues in the N-terminal pentapeptide sequence could exert effects on the conformation of the side chain of Phe-6. In trifluoroethanol solution, the helicity of all peptides increased and VIP-secretin differed from the others by having an additional extension of helical structure toward the N-terminus. These authors further found that the CD spectra of secretin were dependent on the pH of the secretin solution. Such pH dependence had been shown for human gastrin-17 ns by Piszkiewicz (1974), whose findings suggested that this gastrin was helical in aqueous solution at acid but of "random coil" conformation at neutral pH values.

Studies that involved NMR spectroscopy of the conformational properties of the N-butyloxycarbonyl-β-alanyl derivate of the C-terminal tetrapeptide amide of gastrin ("pentagastrin") and of some of its component peptides have been described by Feeney et al. (1972). Bleich et al. (1976) attempted to gain insight into the intramolecular micro-dynamical and conformational properties of the tetrapeptide amide by studying ^1H and ^{13}C NMR spin lattice relaxation properties of its dimethyl sulfoxide solutions. They concluded, inter alia, that the motional characteristics of the side chains of tetragastrin vary considerably and that the most rigid side chain is that of tryptophan while the β-carbon of the aspartic acid residue exhibits considerable motional freedom relative to the main chain, that in the methionine side chain there is increasing motional freedom from $C\alpha$ to the methyl carbon, and that internal reorientation takes place in the ring of the phenylalanine residue.

Pham Van Chuong et al. (1979) found that the CD spectra of human

G-17 ns in water and in 2-trifluoroethanol were rather similar in the near ultraviolet but differed markedly in the far ultraviolet. In trifluoro-ethanol, the peptide exhibited a spectrum suggesting some 47% helical structure, presumably localized to the sequence 4–11, whereas in water the conformation was predominantly random coil. Investigation of spectra of the C-terminal peptide amides of different chain length in trifluoroethanol–water mixtures showed that in the di- and tripeptide signals from the phenylalanine residue could be registered, but that there was no evidence for a rigid conformation of the peptide chain. In the tetrapeptide and various acylated derivatives of it, the spectra suggested that some interaction between the phenylalanine and the tryptophan rings was taking place. There was no evidence for a helical structure in the tetrapeptide, but some kind of folded structure permitting this interaction between the aromatic rings seemed probable. The spectrum of cerulein was similar to that of tetragastrin, indicating that extension of tetragastrin from its N terminus by the peptide Glp-Glu-Asp-Tyr(SO_3)-Thr-Gly did not result in a helical peptide. However, when the tetrapeptide was instead extended to (human) gastrin-17, in particular upon the addition of the pentaglutamyl sequence, spectral evidence for a helical structure appeared. The authors suggested that the folded structure in the C-terminal part of the gastrin chain, which allowed interaction between the phenylalanine and tryptophan rings, might be further stabilized by the side chains of the hydrophobic amino acid residues in the helical part of G-17 ns, i.e., the side chains of Trp-4, Leu-5, and Ala-11.

Already earlier, Schiller *et al.* (1978) had, by measurement of fluorescence enhancement, evaluated the intramolecular resonance energy transfer between tryptophan and tyrosine residues in the *N-tert*-butyloxycarbonyl (Boc) derivative of the unsulfated analog of 7-CCK, Boc-Tyr-Met-Gly-Trp-Met-Asp-Phe-NH_2, and concluded that there must be some kind of folded conformation in the peptides bringing the tyrosine and tryptophan residues closer together than they would have been in the fully extended peptide chain. Analysis of optical rotatory and circular dichroism spectra of 33-CCK in aqueous solution did not provide evidence for any helicity in 33-CCK (Bodanszky *et al.*, 1970).

Mehlis *et al.* (1975) studied circular dichroism and infrared spectra of aqueous solutions of substance P and some of its C-terminal component peptides and concluded that there was evidence for intramolecular hydrogen bonding in substance P, whereas, in its C-terminal octapeptide, intermolecular association was prominent. These conclusions were supported by the results of hydrogen–deuterium interchange studies of films of these substances in contact with gaseous D_2O. Mutter *et al.* (1976) investigated the CD spectra of various C-terminal component peptides of substance P, linked at their C termini to polyethylene glycol during the synthesis of substance P by a stepwise chain elongation method. Evidence for the appearance of secondary structure during chain-elongation was obtained. Holladay and Puett (1976) concluded from investigations of CD spectra, diffusion, and sedimentation equilibria that somatostatin was not helical in aqueous solution but did have some other type of ordered structure, possibly a hairpin bend leading to several amino acid residues forming an antiparallel β-pleated sheet. Hallenga *et al.* (1979) used high-resolution NMR to study the conformational properties of the tetrapeptide corresponding to the somatostatin sequence Thr[10]-Phe[11]-Thr[12]-Ser[13] and some of its component peptides in water or dimethylsulfoxide solution and found evidence for inequivalence of the two threonine residues in the tetrapeptide suggesting a folded structure with shielding of Thr[10] by Phe[11]. It may be remembered that this tetrapeptide sequence is also present in secretin and in glucagon, where it constitutes the 5–8 sequences.

For the determination of the amino acid sequences of the gastrointestinal hormonal polypeptides, the phenylisothiocyanate method of Edman (1950) and the subtractive "dansyl-Edman" (Gray and Hartley, 1963) have been important, although in some cases these methods have had to be supplemented by other techniques and, in a few other cases, other methods have been used throughout. Obviously, in those forms of gastrin and in neurotensin, where no free N-terminal amino group is present, direct application of the Edman method was impossible. In these cases the use of pyrrolidonecarboxylyl peptidase (Doolittle, 1972) for enzymatic removal of the N-terminal pyroglutamyl residue in these peptides proved to be useful (Gregory, 1979a; Carraway and Leeman, 1975a). In many cases, peptide synthesis has played an important role for peptide sequence determination, since the natural peptides and their synthetic replicates must be identical in all comparisons they are exposed to, and any difference must lead to a revision of the sequence of the natural substance, provided that the synthetic product has the given structure. In our determination of the amino acid sequence of porcine secretin, we were at one stage aided by the synthesis by Levine and Bodanszky (1966) of two hexapeptides with identical amino acid compositions but with reversed sequences in a component dipeptide.

The amino acid sequence of human G-17 ns was determined by Bentley *et al.* (1966). The amount of peptide material available was too small to permit direct determination of the amino acid residue in each of the 17 positions. Instead, the total amino acid composition of the peptide was determined and then parallel degradations by papain of the human and porcine gastrins were carried out. The fragment peptides were separated by paper electrophoresis and thin-layer chromatography, and their amino acid compositions were determined. It was found that most of the peptides, comprising the N-terminal sequences 1–5 and 1–6, were different owing to the presence of a leucine residue in the human and a methionine residue in the porcine peptides (in position 5) according to the proposed sequence. The synthesis of hG-17 ns was described by Beacham et al. (1966), and comparisons by electrophoresis and thin-layer chromatography of papain degradation products of the natural hormone and of its synthetic replicate did not reveal any differences between the natural and synthetic peptides.

A peptide for which structure determination relied unusually heavily on synthesis is canine G-17 ns. The amount of peptide available for structural work was again very small, and ambiguity arose concerning the sequence 6–10 found to be composed of four residues of glutamic acid and one residue of alanine. The problem was solved by the synthesis of all five possible isomers, i.e., with alanine in each of the positions 6 to 10, and comparison of the products obtained on fragmentation of the synthetic heptadecapeptides with those obtained on exposure of the natural peptide to identical conditions of fragmentation. The results unequivocally showed that the alanine residue was in position 8 of canine gastrin (Agarwal et al., 1969a). The sequence of feline gastrin was determined mainly with the use of mass spectrometry (Agarwal et al., 1969b). A most unusual situation developed concerning the sequences of porcine and human tetratriacontapeptide gastrins. Here, the synthetic (Choudhury et al., 1976, 1979; Wünsch et al., 1977a) and natural substances were identical in a variety of chemical and pharmacological comparisons. However, Dockray et al. (1978b), with sequence (or region) specific antisera (Agarwal et al., 1971), found that the synthetic replicates of porcine and human G-34 reacted identically to the corresponding natural peptides with an antiserum specific for the C-terminal part of natural porcine G-34 s, but that each natural peptide reacted more than a thousand times more strongly than its synthetic counterpart with an antiserum directed toward the N-terminal sequence of natural G-34. The following up of these observations led to the already mentioned revision of the N-terminal sequences of both porcine (Dockray et al., 1979a) and human (Choudhury et al., 1980) G-34.

An elegant example of the application of synthetic organic chemistry in combination with physiology to the elucidation of a peptide sequence is given by the work of Gregory and co-workers on "minigastrin." Originally, minigastrin was believed to be the C-terminal tridecapeptide amide of the gastrins, and its replicate was synthesized on this assumption (Gregory, 1979a). On comparing the stimulatory effects of natural minigastrin and natural G-17 on gastric acid secretion in dogs, Debas *et al.* (1974a) found that minigastrin was on a molar basis only half as effective as G-17. This was somewhat unexpected in view of earlier findings that up to five amino acid residues could be removed from the N terminus of G-17 without loss of activity (Grossman, 1970b). When synthetic G-13 became available it was found, however, to be essentially as potent as G-17. This led to a reinvestigation of the sequence of minigastrin, and it was found that instead of being G-13 it was G-14, the N-terminal tryptophan having been overlooked in the earlier work. For the original comparative bioassays, minigastrin and G-17 had been made up to what were believed to be equimolar injection solutions on the basis of their spectroscopically determined contents of tryptophan (the main contributor to the light absorbance at the wavelength chosen) and tyrosine. Consequently, the assumption that minigastrin had only one residue of tryptophan, in contrast to the two residues in G-17, had led to undue dilution of the minigastrin solution. Synthetic G-14 was found to be roughly as potent as G-17, possibly slightly weaker (Carter *et al.*, 1979).

In our work on the amino acid sequences of porcine secretin and 33-CCK, we found thrombin useful, since in both these peptides it cleaved only one of the four bonds susceptible to cleavage with trypsin and this assisted the alignment of the tryptic peptides. For the determination of the sequence of the N-terminal hexapeptide, which in 39-CCK extends N-terminally, the sequence of 33-CCK degradation with dipeptidyl aminopeptidase I (McDonald *et al.*, 1969) was interesting since the cleavage proceeded with removal, in turn, of the dipeptides Tyr-Ile, Gln-Gln, and Ala-Arg, whereupon, as could have been expected from the known specificity of the enzyme, it stopped, leaving 33-CCK intact (unpublished). Removal of N-terminal dipeptides from promelittin by dipeptidylpeptidase IV has been suggested to be a possible mechanism for the biosynthesis of melittin from promelittin (Kreil *et al.*, 1980). In the sequence of VIP, both porcine and chicken, kallikrein was found to cleave only one of the five bonds that may be cleaved by trypsin. Incidentally, the sequence of porcine VIP was deduced exclusively by a series of selective enzymic degradations and determination of the amino acid compositions and N-terminal amino acid residues of the subpeptides formed. In the future, the use of such enzymic cleavages in sequence work on relatively short polypeptides is going to become less common as automatic stepwise degradation methods (Edman and Begg, 1967) will increasingly be used. We have, in collaboration with H. Jörnvall at the Department of Chemistry at this Institute, used such methodology for the sequence determination of several peptides, such as porcine GRP (McDonald *et al.,* 1979), somatostatin-28 (Pradayrol *et al.* 1980), chicken secretin (Nilsson *et al.,* 1980), chicken GRP (McDonald *et al.,* 1980), bovine VIP (Carlquist *et al.,* 1979), bovine secretin (Carlquist *et al.,* 1981a), and also for a revision of the sequence of porcine GIP (Jörnvall *et al.,* 1981a).

The continuing improvement of automatic degradation techniques and their adaptation to increasingly small quantities of peptide (Wittmann-Liebold, 1980; Hunkapiller and Hood, 1978) will presumably make the isolation of gastrointestinal hormones from distant species for studies of evolutionary relationships (Dockray, 1979a,b) a reasonable undertaking. In view of the exorbitant price of commercial instruments for automatic peptide degradation, manual methods will nevertheless be used in many laboratories. Perhaps this is as well, since interesting properties of peptides may at times be overlooked when automatic techniques are used. Two promising developments are the introduction of a highly colored isothiocyanate for the Edman procedure (Chang *et al.,* 1978) and the application of the angiotensin converting enzyme to the removal of dipeptides from the C termini of polypeptides (Krutzsch, 1980). The determination of amino acid sequences of peptides via the nucleotide sequences of their corresponding nucleic acids has been mentioned above (p. 279).

V. General Sequence Characteristics of Gastrointestinal Hormonal Peptides That Have Been Isolated

Unlike the glycopeptide hormones of the anterior pituitary, which are composed of two different noncovalently bound peptide chains, and unlike insulin and relaxin, which are composed of two different covalently linked peptide chains, all gastrointestinal hormones with known sequences are single-chain peptides. None of them contain carbohydrate,* and the only nonpeptide constituent known to occur in them is the sulfuric acid that esterifies the phenolic group of the tyrosine residue in cholecystokinin and may or may not do so in gastrin. With

---

* Seppälä and Wahlström (1980) have, however, presented immunochemical evidence for the presence of the α-subunit of the glycoprotein hormones in human pancreatic islets, and Carrea and co-workers (1976) have described a porcine duodenal glycoprotein with gastric antisecretory properties (p. 310).

three exceptions, all these peptides are of the straight-chain type. The exceptions are somatostatin-28, which has a disulfide loop in its somatostatin-14 part; urogastrone, which has three such loops; and chymodenin, which is stated to have two loops. The largest of these hormonal or prohormonal peptides isolated to date from gastrointestinal tissues is glicentin with 69 amino acid residues; the smallest is 8-CCK, although there is some evidence that 4-G/CCK also might occur free in tissues (Rehfeld and Larsson, 1979). None of these hormones and prohormones contain a complete set of the amino acid residues commonly found in proteins. For instance, porcine glicentin lacks cysteine (Sundby *et al.*, 1976); porcine G-34 lacks arginine, asparagine, cysteine, isoleucine, serine, and threonine; porcine secretin lacks asparagine, cysteine, isoleucine, lysine, methionine, proline, tryptophan, and tyrosine (Mutt *et al.*, 1970); and porcine VIP lacks cysteine, glutamic acid, glycine proline, and tryptophan (Mutt and Said, 1974). In itself probably only a reflection of the relatively small size of these peptides, the absence of certain types of amino acid residues is quite useful as a criterion of purity during their isolation from tissues. All the gastrins and 8-CCK are acidic peptides, glicentin is neutral (Sundby *et al.*, 1976), all others are basic from weakly (motilin) to strongly (VIP). There is no category of chemical structures that has been found to occur exclusively in gastrointestinal hormones, although the sulfuric acid of the tyrosine ester residue as in the sulfated forms of gastrins and in CCK, the N-terminal pyroglutamyl structure as in many of the gastrins and in neurotensin, and the C-terminal amide structures as in gastrin, secretin, CCK, VIP, and substance P, are by no means common among other types of peptides and proteins.

SOME SEQUENCE COMPARISONS

Even the most casual observer will note that the gastrointestinal hormones do not comprise many unrelated peptides, but that some of them quite obviously belong to certain groups on the basis of their sequence similarities (Dayhoff, 1972; Mutt, 1972; Mutt and Said, 1974). A closer examination also shows possible intergroup relationships (Jörnvall *et al.*, 1982) and, for some of the peptides, ambiguities as to group distribution.

It was first found that porcine secretin had the same N-terminal dipeptide sequence as glucagon (Jorpes *et al.*, 1962), and further work showed that, in no fewer than 14 of the 27 possible positions, the amino acid residues were identical in the two hormones (Mutt *et al.*, 1970). Subsequently it was found that the His_1 . . . . . -Phe_6-Thr_7- sequence is present also in VIP (both porcine and chicken) and in porcine PHI. In GIP there is Tyr_1 . . . . -Phe_6. All these peptides show additional similarities in sequence. It has been noted (Jörnvall *et al.*, 1981b) that the His_1 . . . . -Phe_6-Thr_7- structure has a counterpart in the His_{90} . . . . -Phe_{95}-Thr_{96}- sequence of human prealbumin (Kanda *et al.*, 1974) and also resembles the His_3 . . . . Phe_8- structure in the heavy chain of the human histocompatibility antigen HLA-B7 described by Terhorst *et al.* (1977).

Gastrin (Gregory *et al.*, 1964) at first did not seem to have any obvious relations to other peptides, but was later found to be similar to CCK (Mutt and Jorpes, 1967a) and to cerulein, a decapeptide from the skin of the frog *Hyla caerulea* (Anastasi *et al.*, 1967). The similarities in this group of peptides are, if anything, still more striking than those in the glucagon–secretin–VIP–PHI–GIP group. Gastrin, CCK, and cerulein all have identical C-terminal pentapeptide amide structures, -Gly-Trp-Met-Asp-Phe-NH_2, and CCK and cerulein both contain a residue of tyrosine-O-sulfate, which is separated from this pentapeptide amide by one amino acid residue, a residue of methionine in CCK, and one of threonine in cerulein. In gastrin s there is also a residue of tyrosine-O-sulfate, but this is attached directly to the pentapeptide amide. Gastrin ns has the same C-terminal hexapeptide amide sequence as gastrin s, but the phenolic group of the tyrosine residue is not esterified but is free. A gastrointestinal peptide, obviously not belonging to either of the two groups just mentioned but rather to a third, earlier known (Erspamer, 1971; Dayhoff, 1972) group containing certain amphibian peptides has been isolated. This is the "gastrin-releasing peptide" (GRP), obviously the mammalian (McDonald *et al.*, 1979) and the avian (McDonald *et al.*, 1980) analog of the amphibian peptides bombesin and alytesin (Anastasi *et al.*, 1971). Chicken GRP, porcine GRP, alytesin, and bombesin all have identical C-terminal heptapeptide amide structures, -Trp-Ala-Val-Gly-His-Leu-Met-NH_2. The amino acid residue preceding this heptapeptide amide is histidine in the mammalian and avian peptides, but glutamine in the amphibian ones. This histidine residue is in turn preceded by a glycylasparaginyl sequence in bombesin and porcine GRP, a glycylseryl sequence in chicken GRP, and a glycylthreonyl sequence in alytesin. There is some ambiguity concerning the group relationship of motilin, since sequence similarities to both secretin and gastrin have been pointed out (Track, 1976; Mutt, 1978). A comparison of various gastrointestinal hormone sequences has suggested a similarity between motilin and somatostatin-28, and between GRP and VIP (Jörnvall *et al.*, 1982).

In addition to the intragroup similarities that, in the secretin group, are concentrated to the N-terminal parts of the peptide chains, there are intergroup similarities. The latter seem to be concentrated to the C-terminal parts of the peptide chains, possibly indicating more distant evolutionary relationships and/or structural requirements for interactions with receptors for these parts of the molecules (Jörnvall *et al.*, 1982). Already earlier, a slight similarity in the C-terminal sequences of CCK, VIP, and glucagon had been noticed (Mutt, 1974). Other comparisons (Mutt, 1972) showed similarities between the 16–23 sequences of porcine CCK, *leu*$_{16}$-Asp-Pro-Ser-*His-Arg*-Ile-*Ser*$_{23}$-, and of porcine calcitonin *Leu*$_{16}$-Asn-Asn-Phe-*His-Arg*-Phe-*Ser*$_{23}$- (Potts *et al.*, 1968). Some similarities between neurotensin and PYY and between PYY and the "pancreatic polypeptide" have been pointed out (Tatemoto and Mutt, 1980). Another similarity is between bradykinin *Arg-Pro*-Pro-Gly-Phe-Ser-Pro-*Phe*-Arg (Boissonas *et al.*, 1960; Elliott *et al.*, 1960) and substance P (Chang *et al.*, 1971) *Arg-Pro*-Lys-Pro-Gln-Gln-Phe-*Phe*-Gly-Leu-Met-NH$_2$. A certain degree of sequence similarity has been noted between the N-terminal octadecapeptide of porcine CCK and the N-terminal hexadecapeptide of porcine GRP, particularly if a deletion of one amino acid residue is assumed to have occurred in the GRP sequence (McDonald *et al.*, 1979).

In sequence comparisons it is tempting to simplify matters to a registration of amino acid residue identities. This can, however, lead to misleading conclusions. As mentioned earlier (Mutt, 1978), it was found (Christophe *et al.*, 1976a) that a peptide with the porcine secretin sequence 14–27 was more effective in inhibiting the binding of ^{125}I-labeled VIP to dispersed guinea pig pancreatic cells than was a peptide comprising the 1–14 secretin sequence, despite the fact that the sequence of the latter shows eight positional identities with the corresponding part of the VIP sequence as against only two such identities in the former. As pointed out by Christophe *et al.* (1976a), the explanation most probably is that although X$_{14-27}$ has only two identities with VIP$_{14-27}$, there are several positions in which chemically similar, although not identical, amino acids occur in these two peptide sequences, as may be seen from Figs. 3 and 4.

VI. A Brief Look at Synthesis

Peptide synthesis by organic chemical methodology has several objectives. One, where recombinant DNA techniques (Itakura *et al.*, 1977) also will be increasingly used, is to prepare replicates of the natural substances in large quantities for scientific and clinical use.

This is a technical problem and will at times raise the question of what should be done with the natural substances as long as the tissues for their extraction are freely available owing to the use of animals for food. Should they be allowed to go to waste? This question is particularily relevant in the case of hormones like glucagon and presumably VIP, which are identical in man and common domestic animals, or when the difference is very small as in insulin where the porcine and human forms differ in one residue of a total of 51. For hormonal peptides like calcitonin (Potts, 1970) and presumably relaxin (John et al., 1981), where the differences between the human and the animal forms are large, it is obvious that it will be useful to have synthetic replicates of the human peptides freely available.

As already mentioned, synthetic chemistry has made important contributions to the validity of the work on peptide sequences. Perhaps its most important contribution has nevertheless been, and will continue to be, in the understanding of the structural requirements for hormone action and for the construction of peptide hormone analogs that in some respect are better than the natural hormones. In leaving the time-honored natural substances, the possibility of unexpected pharmacological side reactions may turn out to make such hormone analogs not better at all, although they may seem to be so in some restricted assay system. Nevertheless, the construction—starting from conformational considerations—by Smith and Walter (1978) of a vasopressin analog with much higher diuretic activity and much lower pressor activity than vasopressin itself does make this line of approach interesting. In the field of gastrointestinal hormones, no such dramatic separations of the various activities of the natural hormones have hitherto been achieved, but, as will be briefly mentioned in Section VIII on structure—activity relationships, there are some indications that this may not be impossible to achieve in at least some cases.

An important objective for synthetic chemistry is the attempted construction of selective antagonists for peptide hormone action (Kenner, 1972). Porcine G-17 ns was synthesized by Anderson et al. (1964). The N-terminal nonadecapeptide corresponding to human G-34 ns has been synthesized by Choudhury et al. (1980), and the complete replicate of G-34 ns by Wünsch et al. (1981b). The replicate of human minigastrin, G-14, was synthesized by Gregory et al. (1979). The replicate of porcine secretin was first synthesized by Bodanszky et al. (1966, 1967). It was subsequently synthesized by Wünsch and co-workers (Wünsch, 1972) with methodology that they had developed during their synthesis of glucagon (Wünsch et al., 1968). Thereafter, other syntheses, with again other methods, have been described by van Zon and Beyerman

(1976), Hemmasi and Bayer (1977), and others. The C-terminal octapeptide amide of CCK, 8-CCK, and the corresponding 12-CCK were first synthesized by Ondetti *et al.* (1970a). The N-terminal hexapeptide and a protected N-terminal octapeptide of 33-CCK were synthesized by Bodanszky *et al.* (1972). The synthesis of a protected peptide corresponding to the 17-23 sequence of 33-CCK was described by Klausner and Bodanszky (1977). A synthesis of the C-terminal decapeptide amide of CCK, with a new method for the introduction into the peptide chain of tyrosine-*O*-sulfate residues (Moroder *et al.*, 1979), has been described by Wünsch *et al.* (1981a). The synthesis of the complete tritriacontapeptide corresponding to a desulfated 33-CCK has been described by Yajima *et al.* (1976), the synthesis of porcine motilin by Yajima *et al.* (1975a) and by Izeboud and Beyerman (1980), the synthesis of 13-leucine motilin and of 13-norleucine motilin by Wünsch *et al.* (1976), the synthesis of substance P by Tregear *et al.* (1971), and the synthesis of neurotensin by Carraway and Leeman (1975b). Syntheses of somatostatin-28 have been described by Ling *et al.* (1980) and Wünsch *et al.* (1980), a synthesis of porcine VIP by Bodanszky *et al.* (1974b), and synthesis of chicken VIP by Bodanszky *et al.* (1978a) and Yajima *et al.* (1980). Synthesis of partial sequences of glicentin have been described by Kaneko *et al.* (1979).

A peptide with the tritetracontapeptide sequence proposed for porcine GIP by Brown and Dryburgh (1971) has been synthesized by Yajima *et al.* (1975b), but the synthesis of a peptide corresponding to the revised sequence of GIP (Jörnvall *et al.*, 1981a) has not been reported yet.

VII. Some Physiological Aspects

Physiological experimentation with gastrointestinal hormones antedates by far the availability of pure, or rather essentially pure, preparations of such hormones. Important observations were made with the use of crude preparations or no preparations at all, but by observing the physiological effects of the release or inhibition of release of the endogenous hormones. The classical endocrinological method where the function of a hormone is investigated by observing the physiological changes after the removal of the gland(s) producing it could as a rule not be applied to the gastrointestinal hormones, which are not found in cells concentrated to special glands but are widely dispersed throughout the tissues of the gut. Nevertheless, several important observations, particularly in the case of gastrin, of the effects of removal of the portion of the gastrointestinal tract where the major portion of a hormone is normally biosynthesized and/or stored, have been made. Obviously, however, when essentially pure preparations of these hormones and their synthetic replicates became available, the pace of physiological, pharmacological, and clinical experimentation in the field increased tremendously. Fortunately this took place at approximately the time when the then new methodology of radioimmunoassay made it possible for the first time to measure peptide hormones in concentrations as low as those occurring in the circulating blood. In many cases the observations that had been made by workers with crude hormone preparations were confirmed; in others, revisions became necessary. In addition much new knowledge has been acquired.

Here only a very brief outline of the physiology of the gastrointestinal hormones in relation to their chemistry is given. The early work in the field has been reviewed by, among others, Ivy (1930), Greengard (1948), Babkin (1950), and Grossman (1950). A book by Gregory (1962b) and a review article by Jorpes and Mutt (1961b) are from immediately before the time when the first of the gastrointestinal hormones became known by their structural characteristics instead of by their physiological properties only. The more recent work has been repeatedly reviewed e.g., by Gregory (1974), Rayford et al. (1976a,b), Varró (1976), Bloom (1977), Chey and Gutierrez (1978), Lamers (1978), McGuigan (1978), Straus (1978), Vigouroux and Thomas (1978), Debas (1979), Jaffe (1979), and Klapdor (1979).

There have been several International Conferences devoted entirely to gastrointestinal hormones, and the published proceedings of the conferences contain a wealth of information on the physiological and pharmacological properties of these substances, on their clinical applications, their cellular origins, and methods for their bioassay and immunoassay. Such proceedings of conferences covering the whole field have been edited by Demling (1972), Andersson (1973), Chey and Brooks (1974), Thompson (1975), Grossman et al. (1978), Myren et al. (1978), Miyoshi (1979), and Bloom and Polak (1980a,b). Two conferences have been devoted specifically to gastrin, one exclusively (Grossman, 1966), the other to gastrin and cholecystokinin (Rehfeld and Amdrup, 1979), and two conferences to peptides common to the brain and the gastrointestinal tract (Zimmermann, 1979; and Basso et al., 1981). The gastrointestinal hormones also played a prominent part at the Symposia on Stimulus-Secretion Coupling (Case and Goebell, 1976) and on Hormonal Receptors in Digestive Tract Physiology (Bonfils et al., 1977; Rosselin et al., 1979).

In addition, multiauthored compilations on gastrointestinal hormones have been edited by Berson and Yalow (1973), Holton (1973), Jorpes and Mutt (1973), Bloom (1978), Glass (1980), and Bloom and Polak (1981). In this series, gastrin (McGuigan, 1974), substance P (Mroz and Leeman, 1977), and urogastrone (Hollenberg, 1979) specifically, have been reviewed.

Not only the hormones may show species specificity, which has been demonstrated time and again, but almost certainly their receptors will be found to do so too. Anyhow, the responses of different experimental animals to the same hormone may be very different. The difference may be quantitative as when Dockray (1973) found that compared to porcine secretin, porcine VIP was a weak stimulant of pancreatic secretion in the rat but about 30 times stronger than secretin in the turkey. It may, however, also be qualitative: in the dog, secretin is known to inhibit strongly the secretion of gastric acid, but in the chicken it stimulates (Burhol, 1974). In all of several mammalian species where it has been tested, somatostatin has been found to inhibit the release of glucagon. In the duck, however, it stimulates glucagon release (Strosser et al., 1980).

A. Effects on Motility and Secretion

It would appear that almost, although perhaps not strictly, all types of gastrointestinal secretory and motor activity may be influenced in a stimulatory or inhibitory fashion by some gastrointestinal hormone(s).

1. Salivary Secretion

Salivary secretion was long considered not to be influenced by peptide hormones (Greengard, 1948), but this may not be so. Substance P was shown to be a sialogogue (Chang and Leeman, 1970a,b), and Denniss and Young (1978) have found that in the main excretory duct of the mandibular gland of the rabbit, VIP and GIP at concentrations within the range of their normal plasma concentrations reduced net Na^+ movement from lumen to interstitium and VIP also reduced the transepithelial potential difference. The effects of VIP and GIP were found to be counteracted by physalaemin, known to have a substance P-like action on the salivary secretion. Secretin and gastrin both had GIP- and VIP-like actions, but only at concentrations much higher than those in which they normally occur in plasma. The latter observation is in accordance with the finding by Clendinnen et al. (1970) that in dogs neither exogenous gastrin or CCK nor secretin had any noticeable effect on salivary volume or protein output. In man, however, Mulcahy et al. (1972) found that both secretin and CCK increased the amylase concentration in human parotid saliva. The results were confirmed by Malfertheiner *et al.* (1980), who further showed that pentagastrin had a similar effect.

There was, however, a considerable variation in the responses of different subjects to the hormones. Bloom *et al.* (1979) found VIP-like immunoreactivity, apparently located in nerves, to be present in the salivary glands in several mammalian species. Stimulation of the chorda tympani in cats (Bloom and Edwards, 1979) produced an abrupt rise of immunoreactive VIP concentration in the submaxillary venous effluent plasma that was accompanied by an increase in submaxillary blood flow. The salivary vasculature was some 20 times more sensitive to VIP than to acetylcholine. Lundberg *et al.* (1979) described experiments indicating that VIP occurred in cholinergic neurons in several exocrine glands and suggested that such nerves released both acetylcholine and VIP, causing secretion and vasodilatation, respectively. These studies were extended by Lundberg *et al.* (1980a), who obtained evidence for the occurrence of VIP and acetylcholine in nerves of the submandibular gland of the cat. Preganglionic stimulation of the chorda lingual nerve resulted in the release of immunoreactive VIP into the venous effluent from the submandibular gland and also in increased blood flow. This was accompanied by an increase in salivary secretion, which, in contrast to the release of VIP and to the increase in blood flow, could be blocked by atropine. More recently, Lundberg *et al.* (1980b) have found that the atropine-resistant vasodilation can be inhibited by the avian pancreatic polypeptide. A stimulating effect of human calcitonin on the secretion of salivary amylase in man has been described by Koelz *et al.* (1976), who further found that calcitonin also stimulated amylase secretion *in vitro* from isolated rat salivary gland cells.

2. *Lower Esophageal Sphincter Pressure*

The correct tone of the lower esophageal sphincter (LES) is of importance to prevent reflux as well as achalasia. During the past decade many investigations have been concerned with the effects of different gastrointestinal hormones on the LES tone, but no clear picture has yet emerged of either the physiological or pathological importance (or unimportance?) of these hormones for the regulation of this tone. Some observations are mutually contradictory and may partly be explained by species differences. Giles *et al.* (1969) demonstrated that gastrin increases LES pressure in man. They administered either pG-17 s, pG-17 ns, or "pentagastrin" intravenously to volunteers and found that each of the peptides led to an increase in LES pressure. This effect was not secondary to the acid secreted in response to the peptides, since it occurred also when the acid was neutralized by intragastric administration of sodium bicarbonate. The effect was, however, prevented by atropine. Independently of Giles *et al.* (1969), the stimulating effect of pentagastrin on LES pressure in man was observed by Castell and Harris (1970). Since then it has been abundantly confirmed by many workers that gastrin has a stimulating effect on LES pressure in man and in experimental animals.

The importance of this stimulating effect in physiology and pathology is, however, a matter of considerable controversy, or rather uncertainty. Goyal and McGuigan (1976) found in the anesthetized opossum that the intravenous administration of an antiserum to gastrin had no influence on basal LES pressures, whereas the stimulatory effect of the administration of hG-17 s on the acid secretion and sphincter pressure was completely abolished. This was taken to indicate that endogenous gastrin is of little or no importance for the maintenance of LES tone under physiological circumstances. Apart from these discussions, Siewert *et al.* (1974a) found a pentagastrin test of lower esophageal pressure useful in grouping patients with hiatus hernia as regards difference in disease severity. Resin *et al.* (1973) and Fisher *et al.* (1975) found that LES pressure was decreased in man by the administration of 8-CCK and suggested that this effect was due to a competitive inhibition of the effect of the structurally related endogenous gastrin on the sphincter. The latter authors described a similar effect of 8-CCK on the LES of the anesthetized opossum, but another group of workers have found that in this species 8-CCK causes contraction of the LES (Dent *et al.*, 1980). From a study in cats, Behar and Biancani (1977) concluded that the effect of CCK on the LES is a dual one, an activation of putative inhibitory nerves to the sphincter causing relaxation after swallowing and another direct contractile effect on the muscle. A paradoxical effect of CCK on the LES in patients with achalasia has been described by Dodds *et al.* (1981).

Secretin was found to inhibit the stimulatory action of gastrin on the LES in man (Cohen and Lipshutz, 1971), and the inhibition appeared to be of competitive character, which is somewhat surprising in view of the great structural difference between the two hormones. Hoke *et al.* (1972), Waldeck *et al.* (1973), and Hogan *et al.* (1975) showed that in man glucagon inhibited LES pressure, both basal and when stimulated with pentagastrin. Waldeck *et al.* (1973) further found that calcitonin, too, inhibited the pentagastrin-stimulated increase in LES pressure but, contrary to glucagon, had no effect on basal pressure. Christiansen and Borgeskow (1974) found that in man both glucagon and secretin decreased resting and pentagastrin stimulated LES pressure, but that there seemed to be no interaction between secretin and glucagon in this action.

Gastric inhibitory peptide, like secretin and like glucagon, has been found to inhibit both basal and pentagastrin-stimulated LES pressure in cats (Sinar *et al.*, 1978). Vasoactive intestinal polypeptide was shown to lower basal LES pressure in anesthetized opossums (Rattan *et al.*, 1977). The effect of VIP may be of particular interest in view of the demonstration by Alumets *et al.* (1979) of a rich supply of VIP-immunoreactive nerves in the smooth muscle of all recognized sphincters in the cat. Substance P has been found to increase LES pressure in the opossum (Mukhopadhyay, 1978), and (Gln[4]) neurotensin to decrease it in man (Rosell *et al.*, 1980).

The effects of gastrointestinal hormones on the LES have been repeatedly reviewed, e.g., by Cohen and Harris (1972), Cohen (1972), Rösch (1974), Siewert *et al.* (1974b), Christensen (1975), Snape and Cohen (1976), and Rozé (1980).

3. *Gastric Acid, Pepsin, and Mucous Secretion, Gastric Emptying and Motility; Enterogastrone*

All the various chemically defined forms of gastrins that terminate C-terminally with the tetrapeptide amide -Trp-Met-Asp-Phe-NH$_2$ have been found, in every species studied, to stimulate gastric acid secretion. Assayed in dogs, the heptadecapeptides were found to differ from the tetratriacontapeptides in potency, time interval between injections and onset of response, and duration of the latter (Gregory and Tracy, 1973). A careful analysis of the dose-response relationships showed that the stimulation of acid secretion at a certain molar concentration of gastrin in the plasma was weaker for G-34 than for G-17, but, since the action of G-34 was more prolonged, the total amounts of acid secreted to equal molar doses of G-34 and G-17 were roughly identical (Walsh and Grossman, 1973). In the dog, high doses of gastrin injected intravenously will *inhibit* gastric acid secretion (Gillespie and Grossman, 1963; Gregory and Tracy, 1964). This does not, however, seem to be an effect on the acid secretory mechanism of the parietal cells as such but to be caused, in some way, by obstruction of flow (Adkins *et al.*, 1967). Such an inhibitory effect is not seen in the stimulatory action of porcine gastrin on the isolated gastric mucosa of the bullfrog (Davdison *et al.*, 1966). The latter study, incidentally, shows that gastrin stimulates acid secretion by acting on the gastric mucosa, not, as could have seemed possible, although improbable, from the results of experiments in intact animals, by way of the release of some other hormone.

An analysis of the effects of specifically hG-17s on acid secretion in man was carried out by Makhlouf *et al.* (1964). On a molar basis, the gastrin was found to be some 500 times more effective than histamine. The maximal responses obtained were slightly higher for gastrin than for histamine, but essentially the same. A multicenter study (1967) compared the effects of the *N-tert-*butyloxycarbonyl β-alanyl derivative of G-4 "pentagastrin" with those of histamine. It was found that "pentagastrin" gave essentially the same maximal responses as histamine, but that side reactions were less frequent and less severe.

The relative importance for the secretion of gastric acid of the gastrin mechanism and direct vagal stimulation of the parietal cells has proved to be complicated to evaluate. Lanciault *et al.* (1972) investigated whether any correlation could be established between plasma gastrin levels and acid secretion in the fasting state in conscious miniature pigs or monkeys and found that there did not seem to be any correlation. However, in the vagotomized and anesthetized dog there was a positive correlation between acid secretion and immunoreactive plasma gastrin concentrations. Other factors besides gastrin and vagal stimulation may influence acid secretion. CCK can stimulate acid secretion in man (Celestin, 1967), in dogs (Preshaw and Grossman, 1965; Murat and White, 1966; Magee and Nakamura, 1966), and in other species. It also stimulates acid secretion in the isolated gastric mucosa of the bullfrog (Davidson *et al.*, 1969a). The situation is simple in the cat, where CCK is a full agonist (Way, 1971). It is somewhat more complicated in other species, like man and the dog, where CCK is only a partial agonist. When given alone it stimulates acid secretion, but, given together with gastrin, it, being the weaker agonist, inhibits competitively the action of gastrin. The inhibitory properties of CCK on acid secretion will be referred to again below under the heading Enterogastrone. Exogenous gastrin was shown to release pepsin in conscious dogs (Gregory and Tracy, 1964). Nakajima and Magee (1968) carried out experiments suggesting that endogenous gastrin also released pepsin in this species, but that "pentagastrin" had only a weak activity. Secretin too, despite its structural dissimilarity to gastrin, has been shown to release pepsin in anesthetized cats (Pratt, 1940), conscious dogs (Magee and Nakajima, 1968a,b; Stening *et al.*, 1969a), conscious cats (Stening *et al.*, 1969a), and man (Wormsley, 1968b; Berstad, 1969). Ruppin *et al.* (1975) showed that 13 Nle-motilin stimulated pepsin secretion in man. Sjödin and Miura (1974) found that there was no difference in the stimulatory effect of secretin on pepsin secretion in vagally innervated or denervated fundic pouches in dogs. They pointed out that the effect of secretin was, however, quite weak as compared to that of cholinergic stimulation.

Pentagastrin has been found to stimulate the secretion of gastric mucus in cats. Both mucopolysaccharide and glycoprotein secretion was stimulated (Vagne and Fargier, 1973). Secretin was found to stimulate gastric mucous secretion in man (André *et al.*, 1972) and in the isolated, perfused dog stomach (Kowalewski *et al.*, 1978). Kaura *et al.* (1980) found that administration of secretin to conscious cats resulted in what appeared to be a real stimulation of mucous secretion, while the effect of "pentagastrin" appeared to be a washing out of preformed mucus.

Porcine gastrin 17 s was shown to inhibit gastric emptying in man (Hunt and Ramsbottom, 1967) although Gregory and Tracy (1964) had shown in dogs, and Smith and Hogg (1966) in man, that it stimulated gastric motility. Hunt and Ramsbottom hypothesized that the decrease in emptying might be explained by a general increase in the tone of the gut, which would give the upper intestine with its smaller diameter a mechanical advantage over the stomach. Chey *et al.* (1970) found that in man both exogenous secretin and CCK could inhibit gastric emptying, and to the same extent. From experiments in dogs, Debas *et al.* (1975) concluded that the plasma concentrations of CCK necessary for inhibition of gastric emptying were such that CCK probably could have this function physiologically. In healthy volunteers, Meves *et al.* (1975) found that gastric emptying was impeded by pG-17 ns, pentagastrin, secretin, and glucagon. The authors suggested that the first two probably acted by increasing intraduodenal pressure, which overcomes their stimulatory effect on antral motor activity, and the latter two by inhibiting antral motor activity.

Motilin has been suggested to regulate *interdigestive* motor activity of the stomach and the upper intestine (Itoh *et al.*, 1976; Wingate *et al.*, 1975). Valenzuela (1976) found in dogs that intergastric pressure was decreased by the administration of either secretin, CCK, VIP, glucagon, or GIP, less so by the latter two than by the former three. Motilin caused an increase, of short duration, of intragastric pressure. The doses necessary for the effects suggested that both secretin and CCK might be involved in the physiological regulation of gastric pressure. Glucagon, like secretin, has been shown to reduce gastric motility (Robinson *et al.*, 1957; Paul, 1974) and duodenal motility (Paul, 1974), but, unlike secretin, it inhibited also colonic motility (Paul, 1974) and the secretion of pepsin (Cohen *et al.*, 1959).

Enterogastrone. Inhibition of gastric motility is part of the complex enterogastrone problem. The early history of enterogastrone has been reviewed by Greengard (1948). The name was created by Kosaka and Lim (1930) to describe a "humoral agent" that they found could be extracted from the intestinal mucosa of dogs if the intestines had immediately previously been exposed to fat. On subcutaneous or in-travenous injection, enterogastrone inhibited, in dogs with Heidenhain pouches, the stimulation of acid secretion that followed upon feeding. Enterogastrone attracted much attention and many efforts were made to isolate it, but with indecisive results. In addition to inhibition of acid secretion it was also believed to inhibit gastric motility (Gray et al., 1937).

An unexpected development started with the observation by Green-lee et al. (1957) that, in dogs with Heidenhain-type (vagally dener-vated) pouches, the intravenous administration of a secretin prepara-tion profoundly inhibited pouch gastric acid secretion in response to feeding. Little or no inhibition was noticed in dogs with the Pavlov (vagally innervated) type of pouches. Jordan and Peterson (1962) con-firmed these observations with a purer preparation of secretin and also cursorily noted that a preparation of CCK had an inhibitory effect similar to that of secretin. Investigation of the inhibition of gastric acid secretion by known peptides, first by secretin and CCK, subsequently by many others, started in earnest in 1964. Gillespie and Grossman (1964b) showed that in dogs with Heidenhain pouches essentially pure porcine secretin inhibited gastric acid secretion if stimulated by gastrin, but not by histamine, and that a preparation of CCK was a stronger inhibitor of acid secretion than was secretin. The CCK prepa-ration also inhibited histamine-stimulated secretion. Stening et al. (1969b) found that CCK inhibited acid secretion in Heidenhain pouch dogs if it was induced by gastrin or by low doses of histamine, but in-creased secretion in response to intermediate doses of histamine. In retrospect it is not clear to what extent this action of CCK was due to CCK itself or to contamination of the preparation by GIP (Brown, 1974). Wormsley and Grossman (1964) found that in dogs with Pavlov pouches secretin to a certain extent inhibited also histamine-stimu-lated acid secretion. Kamionkowski et al. (1964) showed that exo-genous secretin inhibited gastric acid secretion in response to a meal in man. Inhibition of mecholyl-stimulated pepsin secretion by CCK was demonstrated by Nakajima and Magee (1970a) in dogs with Heidenhain pouches.

Many other investigators entered the field, and inhibition of gastric acid secretion has been shown, in some species under certain condi-tions, to be elicited not only by secretin and CCK, but also by GIP (Maxwell et al., 1980), VIP (Konturek et al., 1975, 1976b), somatostatin (Albinus et al., 1975), neurotensin (Andersson et al., 1976b), urogas-trone (Elder et al., 1975), and calcitonin (Barlet, 1974). (The references given are not necessarily to the first publications describing the gastric antisecretory effects of the particular hormone, but may have been chosen from among many as being illustrative and also referring to the earlier work.) Enteroglucagon has been suggested as yet a candidate for inhibition of gastric secretion in man (Christiansen *et al.*, 1979). A glycoprotein was isolated from human urine and found to have gastric antisecretory activity in rats and dogs (Niada *et al.*, 1979), but it has been suggested that its activity might be due to a contaminant (Impicciatore *et al.*, 1980). This glycoprotein may biosynthetically be of duodenal origin since its C-terminal amino acid sequence was found to be Phe-Tyr-Leu-Val (Lugaro *et al.*, 1976), and the C-terminal sequence of a glycoprotein with gastric antisecretory activity isolated from porcine duodenal tissue was found to be Phe-Tyr-Leu (Carrea *et al.*, 1976).

Work on the gastric antisecretory properties of these various peptides has given much information concerning the possible role of at least some of them as endogenous physiological regulators of gastric acid secretion. This physiological problem complex, however, will not be discussed here. There are discussions of it based on the earlier work by Johnson and Grossman (1971) and Brown (1974). The finding that so many peptides can inhibit gastric acid secretion has necessitated a revision of what is meant by enterogastrone, originally a name for a hypothetical substance (Kosaka and Lim, 1930). Gregory (1967) suggested that the term could describe any hormone of the upper intestinal mucosa that was liberated by fat or its digestion products, by hypertonic solutions, or by acid and which inhibited gastric secretion or motility. A still broader definition was used by Johnson and Grossman (1971), who considered any hormone that was released from the upper intestine to be an enterogastrone if it inhibited gastric acid secretion. That is probably the limit for extension of the concept in view of the name, although inhibition of acid secretion by calcitonin does raise a question of nomenclature.

It may be mentioned, concerning the physiological importance of enterogastrone, that Sjödin (1972) found, in dogs with Heidenhain pouches, that while exogenous secretin and CCK inhibited gastric secretion if it was stimulated by gastrin, the secretion stimulated by food was inhibited only weakly by these two hormones. Other enterogastrones may be more important. Klein and Winawer (1974) described a patient with gastric hypersecretion after small bowel resection, and Moossa *et al.* (1976) found in rhesus monkeys that 50% distal small bowel resection resulted in persistent gastric hypersecretion. The surprising finding (Barlet, 1974; Hotz *et al.*, 1980) that intragastric calcitonin inhibits acid secretion brings to mind the casual mention by Gray *et al.* (1937) that their crude enterogastrone preparations seemed to have some activity on oral administration to dogs, something that probably has been dismissed by later workers as impossible because of the lability of peptide hormones to proteolytic degradation.

Two other groups of substances have impinged on the enterogastrone field. They are the histamine H_2 receptor inhibitors (Black et al., 1972)—a review of recent developments in this area is given by Bertaccini and Dobrilla (1980)—and certain types of prostaglandins (Ippoliti et al., 1981).

4. Pyloric Sphincter

Fisher et al. (1973) studied the effects of gastrin, CCK, and secretin on the human pyloric sphincter in vivo and on the circular muscle of the opossum sphincter in vitro. In both cases, secretin and CCK contracted this sphincter whereas gastrin had no apparent effect of its own but counteracted the effect of CCK, possibly also the effect of secretin. Eklund et al. (1979) have shown that VIP causes prolonged relaxation of the cat stomach, and Edin et al. (1979) found a high concentration of immunoreactive VIP in the cat pyloric sphincter.

5. Pancreatic Secretion

Pavlov and his co-workers stressed the importance of nerves for the regulation of pancreatic function (Kudrewetzky, 1894). After the discovery of secretin, Mellanby (1925) proposed that the vagus nerves stimulated the secretion of enzymes from the pancreas, and secretin stimulated the secretion of water and bicarbonate. After the discovery of pancreozymin (Harper and Raper, 1943), it might have appeared that nerves were unnecessary for the regulation of pancreatic secretion, since this could be achieved by the combined work of the two hormones secretin and pancreozymin. Today it is known that the regulation of pancreatic secretion is probably far more complex. It will not be discussed here except for some illustrative details.

Hickson (1970) found that in the pig, in contrast to the dog, stimulation of the vagus nerves resulted in a copious flow of pancreatic juice and that was not prevented by atropine. The possible importance of vagal release of VIP for this type of stimulation of secretion has been discussed by Fahrenkrug et al. (1979). Blood-borne VIP is known to stimulate pancreatic secretion in a secretin-like fashion, but is much weaker than secretin (Domschke et al., 1977). Suggestions that gastrin may play a role in a gastric phase of pancreatic secretion (Preshaw and Grossman, 1965; Blair et al., 1966) have received support from findings that, in the isolated perfused pig pancreas, different forms of gastrin, in concentrations in which they are known to occur in the plasma, stimulated exocrine pancreatic secretion of both bicarbonate and enzymes (Jensen et al. 1980). The physiological importance of the stimulatory effect of GRP on pancreatic secretion, both indirectly by the release of gastrin and CCK and by reacting directly with receptors on the acinar cells (Jensen *et al.*, 1978), is yet quite unclear.

Several hormonal peptides are known pharmacologically to inhibit exocrine pancreatic secretion with certain differences in degree of inhibition of enzyme compared to bicarbonate secretion and also with considerable species differences. Among such peptides are somatostatin (Miller *et al.*, 1979), vasopressin (Schapiro, 1975), and calcitonin (Petrin, 1974). Neurotensin was found to depress basal pancreatic secretion in rats but to have no effect on secretion stimulated by secretin or CCK. It was suggested that neurotensin might be acting by suppressing the normal release of intestinal hormones (Demol *et al.*, 1979). A question of long standing is whether secretin stimulates the pancreas to secrete water and inorganic electrolytes only, or to some extent of enzymes too (Lagerlöf, 1942; Wang *et al.*, 1948). The correlate to this question is whether CCK stimulates the pancreas to secrete enzymes only, or also water and bicarbonate (Wang *et al.*, 1948).

It may be that there is no unambiguous answer to these questions since there seem to be considerable differences in detail in the way in which pancreatic secretion is regulated in different species. Wormsley (1968a) found that in man, low doses of secretin stimulated but high doses inhibited the secretion of trypsin; and Henriksen and Möller (1971) found that in dogs secretin did have a weak stimulating effect on the secretion of protein. No such effect was seen, however, by Douglas and Duthie (1971). Debas and Grossman (1973) found that porcine 39-CCK and 33-CCK did stimulate, although weakly, the secretion of bicarbonate and water in dogs. However, there is reason to believe that the main actions of secretin and of CCK are on different cell types. It was first suggested by Grossman and Ivy (1946) that secretin acted on the duct cells of the exocrine pancreas and CCK on the acinar cells. This assumption has received strong support from analysis of the effects of secretin and CCK on the composition of the pancreatic juice obtained by micropuncture from the acinar and the ductal system (Schulz *et al.*, 1969). In accordance with this, Dean and Matthews (1972) found that *in vitro* CCK depolarized the exocrine acinar cells of the mouse pancreas but secretin had no such effect. Greenwell (1975) found that *in vitro* CCK depolarized the cell membranes of mouse acinar cells whereas secretin hyperpolarized those of the duct cells.

Henriksen (1969) found that in dogs atropine increased the secretion of bicarbonate and water in response to CCK but had no effect on secretion in response to secretin. This suggested that secretin and CCK were stimulating water and bicarbonate secretion by different mechanisms. Petersen and Ueda (1975), with microelectrodes, investigated the effects of gastrin, secretin, and CCK on the acinar cells of the rat pancreas and found that, in contrast to both gastrin and CCK, secretin had no effect on the bioelectric properties of these cells. This suggested that there were no physiologically important secretin receptors in rat acinar cells. The picture is complicated by the finding that, nevertheless, there are receptors on guinea pig acinar cells that are capable of reacting with secretin (Christophe *et al.,* 1976a) and also raises the question of the mechanism by which the well known potentiation of the secretin effect by CCK (Brown *et al.,* 1967; Henriksen and Worning, 1967; Meyer *et al.,* 1971) takes place. Such potentiation may be of considerable physiological importance (Grossman, 1979a) in view of the finding by several groups of workers that the increases in plasma secretin concentrations, in association with meals, are remarkably small (Häcki *et al.,* 1978; Rhodes *et al.,* 1974).

A problem of considerable interest and controversy is whether the secretion of pancreatic enzymes always takes place in a parallel fashion or if different methods of stimulation may lead to changes in relative amounts of the different enzymes secreted (Glazer *et al.,* 1976; Rothman, 1977). This problem must be kept clearly apart from another: the adaptation of pancreatic enzyme synthesis to different diets. Both Pavlov (1900) and Bayliss and Starling (1904) described work carried out in their respective laboratories suggesting that such an adaptation did in fact take place. More recent investigations seem to confirm this early work (Morisset and Dunnigan, 1967).

6. *Sphincter of Oddi and Putative Pancreatic Duct Sphincter*

Secretin was shown to dilate the opening of the pancreatic duct and to decrease the resistance to the flow of pancreatic juice into the duodenum in dogs. This suggested the existence of a pancreatic ductal sphincter mechanism (DiMagno *et al.,* 1981).

Soon after the discovery of CCK (Ivy and Oldberg, 1928), Sandblom *et al.* (1935) showed that, although CCK contracted the musculature of the gallbladder, it, a short distance away, relaxed the muscle of the sphincter of Oddi. It is, however, not accepted by all workers that expulsion of gallbladder bile takes place by the simple mechanism that this contraction and relaxation brings to mind (Stasiewicz and Wormsley, 1974).

Toouli and Watts (1972) carried out experiments suggesting that rhythmic contraction and relaxation of the sphincter may be involved in gallbladder evacuation both in man and in dogs. Behar and Biancani (1980) found that CCK caused a relaxation of the sphincter in anesthetized cats but that pharmacologically it could be shown that there were two CCK receptors in the sphincter, one inhibitory and the other excitatory. Jansson *et al.* (1978) found that, in the cat, VIP stimulated fluid secretion from the wall into the lumen of the gallbladder. Vasoactive intestinal polypeptide has been shown to decrease opossum gallbladder pressure *in vivo* and to counteract the stimulatory effect of CCK on it (Ryan and Cohen, 1977). Calcitonin has been found to inhibit gallbladder contraction in man (Winckler *et al.*, 1973).

7. *Hepatic Bile*

Already Bayliss and Starling (1902b) stated that, in addition to stimulating the secretion of pancreatic juice, secretin also stimulated the secretion of hepatic bile, and when secretin was isolated it was shown that it did have choleretic properties. This was originally demonstrated in the dog (Jorpes *et al.*, 1965) and the cat (Scratcherd, 1965) and subsequently in many other species. The extent to which secretin stimulates bile secretion varies widely between species. In sheep (Caple and Heath, 1972) the volume of bile secreted in response to it is larger than the volume of pancreatic juice, but in the rabbit the response has been variously described as nonexistent (Scratcherd, 1965) or weak (Esteller *et al.*, 1977). Cholecystokinin, too, stimulates hepatic bile secretion. In the dog, the bile secreted in response to CCK was found to have the same type of electrolyte composition as that secreted in response to secretin (Jones and Grossman, 1970). Porcine G-17 s was also found to be a choleretic in the dog (Jones and Grossman, 1970; Kaminski and Deshpande, 1979). Russell *et al.* (1975) found that, in dogs, the principal choleretic action of secretin was exerted on the ducts but that of taurocholate was on the canaliculi; and Shaw and Jones (1978) found, also in dogs, that the principal choleretic action of CCK, too, was on the ducts. More detailed discussions of the choleretic effects of gastrointestinal hormones, the physiological importance of hormonal stimulation of bile flow in relation to bile flow dependent on the synthesis and excretion of bile salts by the liver, and the enterohepatic circulation of these salts may be found in two reviews (Kaminski and Nahrwold, 1979; Jones and Meyers, 1979).

8. *Intestinal Secretion of Fluid and Enzymes, Intestinal Motility*

Nasset (1938) described experiments suggesting that the tissue of both the small and the large intestine in man and in several animal species contained a specific hormone, enterocrinin, that stimulates the glands of the small intestine to secrete fluid and enzymes. Like enterogastrone, enterocrinin seems to have turned into a concept. Several workers have shown that different peptide hormones may stimulate intestinal secretion of fluid and in some cases stimulation of enzyme secretion has been stated to occur also. Secretin was found to stimulate the secretion of the glands of Brunner in dogs (Love *et al.,* 1968; Stening and Grossman, 1969b) and in cats (Stening and Grossman, 1969b). Glucagon was shown to have a similar effect (Jones and Hall, 1969). Warnes *et al.* (1969) found that in patients with complete biliary and pancreatic obstruction both secretin and CCK increased the amount of alkaline phosphatase in the duodenal contents, suggesting that the hormones were stimulating secretion of this intestinal brush border enzyme into the lumen.

Goldman *et al.* (1971) found that in dogs glucagon stimulated the secretion of enterokinase in Brunner gland area pouches. Nasset (1972) found that in rats and in dogs administration of CCK and 8-CCK induced a marked increase in the intraluminal content of several intestinal enzymes in the jejunum without increasing the DNA content, suggesting that the increase in enzyme content was not due to desquamation of cells.

In rats, Götze *et al.* (1972) found that CCK-PZ strongly increased the release of the intestinal hormones enterokinase, alkaline phosphatase, and sucrase into the intestinal lumen. The action of the hormone was strongly augmented, but not dependent, on the presence of bile in the intestine. Secretin also had a weak effect on enzyme release, but this was observed only in the presence of bile in the intestine. Nordström (1972), however, found in rats that, although secretin and CCK did release enterokinase, alkaline phosphatase, and disaccharidases into the intestinal lumen, the effects were weak and possibly dependent on the stimulation of motility and fluid secretion by the hormones.

Dyck *et al.* (1974) investigated in anesthetized dogs the effect of intravenous injections of secretin and CCK on the secretion of sucrase, maltase, and lactase in perfused jejunal loops from which pancreatic juice and bile had been excluded. Secretin had a weak, but CCK a pronounced, effect on the secretion of all three enzymes. In no case did the conent of the enzymes in the mucosa vary noticeably. The authors concluded that the response to CCK was a true hormone-mediated stimulation of the secretory process.

Eloy *et al.* (1978) demonstrated in the rat that low doses of either "pentagastrin," cerulein, or glucagon resulted in an increased secretion of several intestinal enzymes into the lumen. Because of difficulties in the establishment of dose-effect relationships they left open the question as to the nature of the hormone-stimulated secretion of enzymes. Working with sacs of hamster everted small intestine, Gardner *et al.*

(1967) found that porcine secretin, as well as partially purified CCK and gastrin, all induced significant decreases in the net mucosal to serosal transfer of fluid, sodium, and chloride, but not of potassium, in sacs from the distal third of the small intestine. In sacs from the middle and proximal thirds of the small intestine none of the hormones had any effect on net transfer in these segments. Analyzing the effects of the hormones on unidirectional movements of sodium, it was found that in sacs from the distal third of the small intestine all three hormones decreased the mucosal to serosal sodium movement; gastrin, but not secretin or CCK, decreased the serosal to mucosal movement also.

In man, Matuchansky *et al.* (1972) found that CCK increased the secretion of water, sodium, and chloride into the lumen of the jejunum, but pointed out that this effect could be secondary to the decrease in intestinal transit time also effected by CCK.

Moritz *et al.* (1973), however, found that both secretin and CCK significantly inhibited the absorption of water, sodium, potassium, and chloride in the jejunum, despite that they had opposite effects on motor activity, and suggested that at any rate the effect of secretin on absorption was probably not related to its action on motor activity. CCK does speed up intestinal transit. This has been found to be useful clinically (Monod, 1964; Dahlgren, 1966; Morin *et al.*, 1966; Parker and Beneventano, 1970). Gutiérrez *et al.* (1974) demonstrated that in man the motor activity of the duodenum and jejunum was stimulated by CCK and inhibited by secretin. Dinoso *et al.* (1973) found effects of CCK and secretin on the sigmoid colon, but neither of the hormones influenced the motor activity of the rectum. Waller *et al.* (1973) also found that CCK had no effect on the rectum, but they did not find it to cause any meaningful changes in colonic motility either.

Chijikwa and Davison (1974) showed in the guinea pig that CCK in doses that were only threshold for contraction of the guinea pig small intestine strongly stimulated its peristaltic reflex. Frigo *et al.* (1971) had made similar observations with cerulein.

Barbezat and Grossman (1971) observed that both GIP and VIP had a stimulating action on small intestinal secretion in dogs. Considerable interest has been shown in the stimulatory effect of VIP on secretion in various segments of the intestine (Krejs *et al.*, 1980). High-affinity receptors to VIP have been found on rat (Laburthe *et al.*, 1979) and guinea pig (Binder *et al.*, 1980) small intestinal cells. It is also of interest that immunoreactive VIP has been found throughout the length of the wall of the gastrointestinal tract (Bloom and Polak, 1978).

Du Pont *et al.* (1980) have found remarkable species differences in the ability of VIP and secretin to stimulate the production of cAMP in the fundic and the antral gastric epithelium. In man, VIP was by far the more efficient stimulator, and also active at very low concentrations, whereas in the dog and in the rat secretin was 200 times stronger than VIP. Distinct receptor sites for VIP and for certain prostaglandins in human colonic mucosa have been described by Simon and Kather (1980).

In the rat colon, *in vivo* (Wu *et al.*, 1979) and *in vitro* (Racusen and Binder, 1977), VIP was found to reverse net absorption of electrolytes and water to net secretion. Small intestinal motility has been found to be retarded by VIP in dogs (Kachelhoffer *et al.*, 1976) and in rats (Gustavsson *et al.*, 1977).

Somatostatin has been shown to inhibit motilin-induced interdigestive contractile activity in dogs (Ormsbee *et al.*, 1978).

Neurotensin was found to relax the rat ileum but to contract the guinea pig ileum and to have a biphasic response, relaxation followed by contraction, on guinea pig ileum that had contracted in response to histamine (Kitabgi and Freychet, 1978).

Calcitonin has been found to cause secretion of fluid and electrolytes in the human jejunum (Gray *et al.*, 1976).

Angiotensin has been found to have a dose-depressant biphasic action on fluid absorption in the rat jejunum. Low doses stimulate absorption, but high doses inhibit it (Bolton *et al.*, 1974).

A contractile action of VIP on guinea pig ileum and rabbit jejunum *in vitro* has been described by Cohen and Landry (1980). Inhibition by opiate agonists of fluid secretion stimulated in rat small and large intestines by VIP, as well as some other substances, has been described by Beubler and Lembeck (1979). Naloxone was found to enhance the effect of VIP and of the prostaglandin PGE on fluid secretion.

B. Effects on Blood Flow through Gastrointestinal Organs

Gayet and Guillaumie (1930) found that stimulation of pancreatic secretion by secretin led to an increase in blood flow through the gland in dogs. It is tempting to assume that there must be a simple relationship between the activity of a gland and the amount of blood flowing through it. Such relationships apparently exist but may not always be revealed by simply measuring the flow from the gland at rest and at work.

It has been pointed out (Harper, 1972) that most of the published evidence suggests that when the resting pancreas is stimulated to secrete by an injection of secretin there is an increase in blood flow through the gland, but that this subsides before the pancreatic secretion does and that subsequent injections of secretin will have little effect on blood flow despite continued stimulation of secretion.

Fasth and Hultén (1971) found in anesthetized cats that glucagon increased intestinal blood flow but inhibited motility. The inhibition, but not the increase in blood flow, was evidently mediated by a release of catecholamines from the adrenals.

Kachelhoffer et al. (1974) found that VIP dilated the vascular bed in a dose-dependent fashion in perfused isolated canine jejunal loops. This effect was not inhibited by either propranolol or atropine. However, the large doses necessary and the occurrence of an "escape" phenomenon seemed to indicate that the vasodilatory effect of VIP was of doubtful physiological significance.

Jacobson et al. (1967) stressed the importance, when studying relationships between secretory activity and blood flow in glandular organs, of recording not only total blood flow through the organ but also flow through that part of it that was directly involved in secretory activity. Thus, in dogs with Heidenhain pouches, it was possible with graded doses of histamine to obtain a sixfold increase in acid secretion accompanied by a fourfold increase in mucosal blood flow without any significant change in total pouch inflow, suggesting that a redistribution of blood flow within the wall of the stomach had occurred.

Fara and Madden (1975) found in anesthetized cats that secretin caused a redistribution of blood away from the jejunal mucosa to the submucosa while CCK had an opposite effect, and Beijer et al. (1979) found in anesthetized dogs that the blood flow increase after administration of secretin was highest in the pancreatico-duodenal artery out of 18 arteries investigated.

Goodhead et al. (1970), nevertheless, found in anesthetized dogs that secretin caused a marked increase in duodenal and pancreatic blood flow, and Vaysse et al. (1973) found that in the isolated perfused dog pancreas, CCK in the range of 2.5 to 25 Ivy dog units caused a dose-related increase in blood flow.

Richardson and Withrington (1977) found that both secretin and CCK caused hepatic arterial vasodilation in anesthetized dogs. Chou et al. (1977) concluded from experiments in dogs that CCK, but not secretin, may contribute to the postprandial intestinal hyperemia.

Thulin and Samnegård (1978) have pointed to qualitative differences in the patterns of the effects of different gastrointestinal hormones on different vascular beds in the splanchnic area.

C. Trophic Effects

Among the various actions that Gregory and Tracy (1964) described for the gastrin that they had isolated they did not include one, unknown at the time, that according to some investigators (Johnson *et al.*, 1975b) may turn out to be the most important of all its many actions. In retrospect, it is evident that there were at the time stray pieces of information in the literature that may have been taken to suggest that gastrin and other gastrointestinal hormones could have trophic effects on their target organs. Daly *et al.* (1952) had found that more nitrogen from ^{15}N-labeled glycine was incorporated into the pancreas of fed than of starving mice. Hunt (1957) found that refeeding of fasted rats led to a marked increase in the mitotic activity of their gastric glands, and Polacek and Ellison (1963) had found that the parietal cell mass in a patient with the Zollinger–Ellison syndrome was some eight times greater than in control subjects. Subsequently, Pearl *et al.* (1966) showed that electrical stimulation of the anterior hypothalamic area in cats resulted in marked hyperplasia of all types of gastric fundic mucosal cells, provided that the vagi were intact—and presumably stimulating the release of gastrin (Uvnäs, 1942). No such effect was seen if the vagi were severed. Martin *et al.* (1970) showed that antrectomy in rats led to a marked reduction in the number of parietal cells, but also of the peptic cells in the fundic mucosa. Salganik *et al.* (1971) found that administration of pentagastrin to anesthetized rats stimulated RNA synthesis in their gastric mucosa, whereas histamine had no such effect. These authors considered the effect on RNA synthesis to be involved in the mechanism of the stimulation of acid secretion by gastrin, since prevention of RNA synthesis by an actinomycin-related antibiotic also prevented the stimulation of acid secretion.

Gillespie *et al.* (1960) showed that the maximal gastric acid response to histamine was strongly suppressed in patients who had undergone antrectomy and considered this to be in line with the suggestion of Uvnäs (1942) that the full functioning of the antral and nervous phases of acid secretion were dependent on one another. Subsequently, Passaro *et al.* (1963) did demonstrate a potentiating effect of histamine on acid secretion elicited by exogenous gastrin in dogs with Heidenhain pouches. Broomé and Olbe (1969) were, however, unable to demonstrate such a potentiating effect of pentagastrin on histamine-stimulated acid secretion in man and suggested that the effect of antrectomy might instead be explained by it causing an atrophy of the parietal cell area of the gastric mucosa. This, in view of the work of

Crean and co-workers, who, starting from the assumption that the gastric hypersecretion known to occur in duodenal obstruction might be an effect of continuous gastrin release due to antral distension (Crean *et al.*, 1969a), injected rats with large doses of pentagastrin for a period of 3 weeks and found that the weights of their stomachs had increased markedly and that there was hyperplasia of the parietal cells. The apparent increase in number of peptic cells was not statistically significant. There was no significant change in the mass of the antral mucosa. The authors ascribed the hyperplasia to either a trophic effect of pentagastrin or to an effect secondary to the stimulation of acid secretion. The latter seemed, however, to be unlikely, since stimulation of acid secretion with histamine did not lead to any hyperplasia (Crean *et al.*, 1968, 1969b). Johnson *et al.* (1969b) showed that if rats were pretreated with pentagastrin, then homogenates of their gastric oxyntic gland area and duodenal mucosa showed an increased incorporation of L-[^{14}C]leucine into proteins, whereas, homogenates of liver or skeletal muscle were not influenced in this way by pretreatment with pentagastrin, and pretreatment with histamine had no effect on leucine incorporation in any of these tissues. The authors concluded that gastrin might be a trophic hormone for the gastric and duodenal mucosa. This conclusion was supported by results from *in vivo* experiments in rats where either pentagastrin or "synthetic human gastrin" (presumably G-17 ns) stimulated leucine incorporation into duodenal and oxyntic gland mucosa, whereas there was no effect on incorporation into liver proteins and incorporation into skeletal muscle was actually depressed.

Miller *et al.* (1973) found that pentagastrin inhibited outgrowth of fibroblasts and stimulated proliferation of epithelial cells in cultures of rat and human gastric mucosa from the oxyntic gland region. Similarly, Lichtenberger *et al.* (1973) found that in cultures of rat duodenal cells, pentagastrin preferentially supported the growth of epithelial cells. Johnson and Chandler (1973) found that, in rats, antrectomy decreased the oxyntic glandular and duodenal content of DNA and RNA. Treatment of the animals with pentagastrin partially restored the gastric mucosal content of RNA but not of DNA. In the duodenal cells, the content of RNA was fully restored and that of DNA partially. Subsequently, however, Johnson and Guthrie (1974a) found that the DNA-synthesizing activity of rat gastric mucosa was enhanced by treatment with pentagastrin. They devised a method for assessing the growth-promoting action of gastrointestinal hormones on gastrointestinal tract tissues; rats were pretreated with the hormone(s) in question, whereupon pieces of tissue were removed and incubated *in vitro* with [³H]thymidine and the incorporation of radioactivity into DNA was measured. With this method they found that, in rats, pentagastrin stimulated DNA synthesis in the tissues of the oxyntic gland area, the duodenum, and especially strongly, the ileum, whereas no stimulation took place in the liver.

The effect on DNA synthesis was not confined to the rat. Willems *et al.* (1972), with a method similar to that of Johnson and Guthrie, found in dogs that, 12 hours after treatment with porcine G-17, fundic mucosal biopsies showed an intense DNA-synthesizing activity and, at 20 hours, mitotic activity. Histamine in doses giving the same acid secretory response had no effect on cell proliferation. No effect of gastrin on DNA synthesis in dog antral mucosa could be demonstrated (Willems and Vansteenkiste, 1974). An apparent discrepancy with the latter finding is the observation of Lehy *et al.* (1975) that hyerplasia of, also, the gastrin-producing cells of the antrum develops in rats with the antrum surgically transpositioned into the colon. Such animals are known to have increased plasma gastrin levels due to elimination of acid feedback inhibition of gastrin release. Johnson (1976) has suggested that this type of hyperplasia is not due to a trophic effect of gastrin but is secondary to the removal of the acid inhibition of gastrin release from these cells.

Sutton and Donaldson (1974) showed that pentagastrin stimulated incorporation of [¹⁴C]leucine into protein in rabbit gastric mucosa in organ culture, and Enochs and Johnson (1974) similarly showed increased *in vitro* incorporation of ¹⁴C amino acids into protein in pieces of rat oxyntic gland and duodenal tissues. In rats, Pansu *et al.* (1974) observed a stimulatory effect by pentagastrin on renewal of jejunal mucosal cells, and Johnson (1977) on DNA synthesis in the colon mucosal cells. Enochs and Johnson (1977) considered gastrin to stimulate protein synthesis in the mucosa along the entire length of the gut with the exception of the esophagus and antrum. There is substantial evidence indicating that such stimulation is not a pharmacological curiosity but has profound physiological relevance. Zelenková and Gregor (1971) found (by bioassay) that the antral content of gastrin in rats was very low during the newborn period and increased dramatically during weaning. This was confirmed by Lichtenberger and Johnson (1974), who further presented evidence that this rise in gastrin concentration, also demonstrated by radioimmunoassay, in plasma went in parallel with a rapid development of the intestine toward its adult form.

Lichtenberger *et al.* (1976) found that during starvation the DNA, RNA, and protein content of the intestinal tissue was decreased to a proportionally greater extent than the body weight. In confirmation of some (but not other) earlier findings, the intestinal lactase and maltase activities *increased* with starvation while antral gastrin concentrations fell. Administration of "pentagastrin" reversed all these effects of starvation, but only partially. Instead of investigating starved animals, Johnson and co-workers (1975a) studied parenterally fed rats and found, as compared to orally fed control animals, tissue weight: total body weight ratios to be significantly decreased for the oxyntic gland area, the small intestine, and the pancreas, but not for the antral area, the spleen, or the kidneys. The RNA:DNA ratio in the small intestine almost doubled. The antral gastrin concentrations of parenterally fed animals fell to about one-thirtieth of those of the controls, but, contrary to the findings in the starved animals, the intestinal disaccharidase concentrations also fell. "Pentagastrin," but not histamine, reversed completely the effect of parenteral feeding both on the tissue weight:body weight ratios and on the enzyme activities (Johnson *et al.*, 1975b).

Granting that gastrin is important for the preservation of the normal functional state of a large section of the gastrointestinal canal and of the pancreas, the question arises whether there is any physiological mechanism that balances its activity. Stanley *et al.* (1972) showed that the trophic action of chronically administered pentagastrin on the fundic mucosa of the rat stomach, including the resultant increase in acid secretory capacity, could be blocked or reversed by the administration of (large doses of) secretin. Johnson and Guthrie (1974b) investigated the effect of secretin further and showed that secretin prevented the DNA synthesis-stimulating action of pentagastrin not only on the rat fundic mucosa, but also on the duodenal and ileal mucosa. The effect was not secondary to inhibition by secretin of acid secretion (Tumpson and Johnson, 1969), since inhibition of acid secretion by the histamine H_2 receptor blocker, metiamide, did not prevent the trophic effect of gastrin. Secretin by itself did not influence DNA synthesis in any of the gastrin-responsive tissues. Pansu *et al.* (1974) observed an inhibitory effect of secretin on jejunal cell renewal in rats, but since the experiments were carried out *in vivo* it is possible that the exogenous secretin was counteracting the stimulating effect of endogenous gastrin. Rommel and Böhmer (1974) found that administration of secretin to rats increased the activities of maltase and sucrase in their jejunal mucosa. Lactase was not stimulated and neither enzyme was stimulated by CCK. Here again it is possible that secretin was acting by counteracting endogenous gastrin. In man, Mitznegg *et al.* (1975) found that pentagastrin treatment increased the subsequent incorporation of

[^{14}C]leucine into the proteins of gastric fundic mucosal biopsy samples and that this effect of pentagastrin could be abolished by pretreatment with secretin but also by motilin (the 13-norleucine analog of porcine motilin was used). Rudo et al. (1976) found that, in rats, prolonged administration of glucagon (chemically related to secretin) or semi-starvation, presumably resulting in hyperglucagonemia, resulted in a decrease of jejunal villous height. Johnson and Guthrie (1978) found that secretin and VIP inhibited the DNA synthesis-stimulating effect of pentagastrin on rat colonic mucosa and had no effect on this synthesis by themselves. Glucagon, on the other hand, did not inhibit the effect of pentagastrin and stimulated DNA synthesis when given alone. The authors drew attention to the finding of Williamson et al. (1978) that resection of the proximal small intestine, which contains the major part of secretin, results in hyperplasia of gastrointestinal mucosa, including the colonic. Evans and Lin (1971) reported differences in the effect of pentagastrin on the rates of incorporation into rat stomach proteins of histidine and phenylalanine. Majumdar and Goltermann found that pretreatment of rats or rabbits with gastrin enhances the subsequent ability of their gastric, colonic mucosal, and pancreatic ribosomes to synthesize protein in cell-free systems (Majumdar, 1979).

If, as seems probable, gastrin does not have a trophic effect on the cells synthesizing it, the question as to the possible existence of some other factor(s) with such an effect arises. There are some indications that such factors do exist. In one study (Creutzfeldt et al., 1971) it was found that patients with primary hyperparathyroidism and acromegaly had hyperplasia of antral gastrin cells and increased amounts of gastrin in the antrum. This was, however, not confirmed on additional investigations by the same group of workers (Creutzfeldt et al., 1974). In hypophysectomized rats, both serum gastrin and antral gastrin concentrations were markedly lower than in normal controls, and treatment of the hypophysectomized animals with growth hormone or with cortisol elevated both concentrations to normal levels (Enochs and Johnson, 1977). Friesen (1968) described a patient with the Zollinger–Ellison syndrome in whom regression of metastatic tumors in the liver and lung followed on total gastrectomy and postulated the existence of a "gastric factor" supporting the growth of these tumors. He further drew attention to the high levels of somatotropin in the plasma of many patients with this syndrome and speculated on the possibility that the "gastric factor" might in turn be under hypothalamic and/or pituitary influence. Johnson (1976) has drawn attention to the paradoxical situation in pernicious anemia, where high levels of circulating gastrin are accompanied by atrophy of the oxyntic gland area of the stomach and suggested as a possible explanation that the circulating gastrin in this condition might for some reason be biologically inactive, as indeed could be inferred from the work of Hansky *et al.* (1973b).

Next to the mucosa of the gastrointestinal tract, most investigations on the trophic effects of the gastrointestinal hormones have been carried out on the pancreas. Work with slices of pigeon pancreas *in vitro* seemed to indicate that pancreozymin stimulated the expulsion of enzymes from the pancreas, but not the synthesis of new enzyme (Hokin and Hokin, 1956). However, it was subsequently found that, if pancreozymin was administered to the pigeons *in vivo,* pancreatic slices from the birds showed an increased uptake of L-[^{14}C]phenylalanine compared with pancreatic slices from birds that had not been treated (Webster and Tyor, 1966).

Rothman and Wells (1967) found that prolonged administration of exogenous pancreozymin to rats resulted in an increase in the wet weight of the pancreas, whereas the administration of metacholine had no such effect and the administration of secretin had only a very weak effect that was attributed to contamination of the secretin preparation with pancreozymin. In view of later findings (see later), the latter assumption was unwarranted. The amylase, chymotrypsinogen, and trypsinogen content of the enlarged pancreas was found to be increased, but in an unparallel fashion, since the content of trypsinogen had increased far less than that of amylase and chymotrypsinogen. Microscopic examination showed moderate enlargement of the acinar cells without observable increase in number of mitotic figures.

Barrowman and Mayston (1971) found that chronic administration of pentagastrin to rats resulted in a hypertrophy of the acinar cells of the pancreas, while islet cells, blood vessels, etc. did not seem to be influenced. A segment of the duodenum also showed signs of hypertrophy. The authors concurred with Johnson *et al.* (1969a) that the C-terminal tetrapeptide sequence of gastrin and cholecystokinin might exert trophic influences on a number of tissues of the gastrointestinal tract. A dose-related stimulation of amylase synthesis in rat pancreas *in vivo* was described by Leroy *et al.* (1971). Continuing with a study of the effects of CCK on the rat pancreas, Barrowman and Mayston (1974) found that prolonged treatment with the hormone increased the content of DNA, amylase, and proteolytic enzymes, but not lipase, in the gland.

Mainz *et al.* (1973) found that chronic administration of CCK to rats was associated with an increased RNA, protein, and DNA content of the pancreas and with stimulation of [^{14}C]thymidine incorporation into DNA. Bethanecol, likewise, increased RNA and protein content, but not that of DNA. The authors concluded that both stimulants led to hyperplasia of the pancreatic cells.

Petersen *et al.* (1973) found that the maximal bicarbonate secretory capacity of the pancreas was greater in patients with hypersecretion of gastric acid than in patients with hyposecretion of acid and suggested that a conditioning of the pancreas to a higher secretory activity might have taken place by the secretin released by the acid. Ihse *et al.* (1976) found that in rats both 8-CCK and a "10% pure" preparation of CCK caused an increase in the pancreatic weight and the pancreatic content of amylase, lipase, and trypsinogen, in a parallel fashion. Johnson and Guthrie (1976) also found that 8-CCK could exert a trophic effect on the rat pancreas and at plasma concentrations of the hormone that had no noticeable such influence on the duodenum or the oxyntic gland area of the stomach. At higher 8-CCK concentrations, stimulation of DNA synthesis in the duodenum did take place, but not in the oxyntic area; and at still higher concentrations of 8-CCK, stimulating action of pentagastrin on these tissues could be prevented.

Fölsch *et al.* (1978) found that treatment of rats with secretin and CCK in large doses resulted in increased pancreatic content of amylase and trypsinogen, but not of lipase, and the same pattern was found in the pancratic juice secreted by these animals. This observation is consistent with the earlier finding of Barrowman and Mayston (1974). Petersen *et al.* (1978) investigated the effects of pentagastrin, secretin, and a partially purified preparation of CCK in a subcutaneous depot carrier over a period of 15 days by recording the pancreatic weights and secretory properties in rats. All three agents resulted in increases in weight, but CCK was by far the strongest agent in this respect. In the CCK-treated animals, the maximal protein and bicarbonate outputs in response to CCK increased proportionally to the increase in pancreatic weight, but the maximal bicarbonate and protein outputs in response to secretin stimulation remained unchanged. The secretin-treated animals, unexpectedly, showed a lower sensitivity to stimulation with secretin, but the maximal responses obtainable remained unchanged.

In continuation of these experiments, Petersen *et al.* (1979) treated rats with a combination of secretin and CCK (the CCK analog cerulein was used). The results were surprisingly different from those of treatment with either agent separately. In addition to the trophic effect on the acinar cells, seen by treatment with CCK only, a trophic effect on the ductule cells also was now evident, since the maximal response to secretin was almost doubled.

An attempt to investigate the effect of chronic endogenous hypergastrinemia on the pancreas of the rat was made by Chariot *et al.* (1974), who investigated the effects on the pancreas of transplantation of the antrum into the colon. The DNA content of the pancreas increased, but there was no increase in the weight of the gland or in its enzyme content. Dembinski and Johnson (1979) found that in rats antrectomy, i.e., removal of the main source of endogenous gastrin, led to decreased DNA synthesis and DNA content in the pancreas, the oxyntic gland area, the duodenum, and the colon and that these effects were reversed by treatment with pentagastrin. More recently, Dembinski and Johnson (1980) found that secretin alone and cerulein alone increased DNA synthesis and the DNA content of the rat pancreas *in vivo* and that, given together, the hormones potentiated each other's actions. Analysis of RNA:DNA ratios suggested that both hypertrophy and hyperplasia of the pancreatic cells were taking place. Unexpectedly, secretin not only did not potentiate the stimulating action of pentagastrin on pancreatic DNA synthesis, but actually inhibited it.

Creutzfeldt *et al.* (1975) pointed out that in patients with the Zollinger–Ellison syndrome, hyperplasia of the pancreatic islets is a common finding, suggesting that gastrin exerts a trophic influence on the islet tissue, also. However, as mentioned (p. 324), Barrowman and Mayston (1971) did not see any effect on islet cells of treatment of rats with large doses of pentagastrin, and Petersen *et al.* (1978) did not find any histological evidence of a trophic effect on the rat endocrine pancreas of treatment with secretin or CCK. It cannot be excluded that the tumors of the Zollinger–Ellison type are secreting some other factor, in addition to gastrin, that may be exerting a trophic influence on the endocrine pancreas.

A trophic effect of CCK (cerulein) on mouse gallbladder epithelium has been reported (Putz *et al.*, 1980).

D. RELEASE OF GASTROINTESTINAL HORMONES

To act, the gastrointestinal hormones must be released from their cells of biosynthesis. Much information exists concerning one type of release, that into the blood stream. Some information exists about another type of release, secretion into the lumen of the gastrointestinal tract (Jordan and Yip, 1972; Andersson and Nilsson, 1974; Uvnäs-Wallensten and Rehfeld, 1976; Uvnäs-Wallensten, 1977; Lund *et al.,* 1979). No methodology has yet been worked out for quantitating the presumably important paracrine release of certain hormones to influence other cells in the neighborhood of their cells of origin (Grossman, 1979a).

There are several mechanisms known for the release of gastrin, but two of them, release after stimulation of the vagus and release after contact of the antral mucosa with low molecular weight peptides or amino acids appear to be of predominant physiological importance. The release of gastrin by vagal stimulation and its subsequent interaction with the vagal impulses to the parietal cells is probably the best known example of the coordination of the physiological activities of a peptide hormone and the nervous system. The first to note this interplay seems to have been Straaten (1933), who showed in dogs that the vagally mediated first or "psychic" phase of gastric secretion was strongly dependent on the presence of the pyloric glands. If these were surgically removed, sham feeding did not elicit any pronounced acid secretory response.

Uvnäs (1942) found in anesthetized cats and dogs that electrical stimulation of the vagus nerves failed to stimulate gastric secretion if the antral mucosa had been excised or if it was cocainized. He also found that acid secretion after vagal stimulation was strongly enhanced by the intravenous administration of small doses of a crude preparation of gastrin. This suggested that stimulation of the vagi might cause release of gastrin, but also that gastrin and vagal impulses might be potentiating each other's effects at the parietal cell level. Many workers have contributed to show that this is indeed so. However, for many years experimental findings remained inconclusive. The main reason for this seems to have been the feedback inhibition of gastric acid secretion due to acidification of the pyloric region. Indeed, it had been shown already by Szokolow (1904) that acid secretion from Pavlov pouches was depressed if the content of the main stomach became strongly acidic.

Wilhelmj et al. (1937) suggested that acid inhibition of gastrin activity might be an important physiological regulatory mechanism. Woodward et al. (1954) showed that application of foods to the mucosa of the antrum elicited acid secretion from the fundus and body of the stomach, but only if the reaction at the mucosal surface was neutral or faintly acidic. Spontaneous secretion of acid was inhibited by acidification of the mucosa. Acidification of the mucosa, however, did not have any effect on histamine-stimulated acid secretion. The authors therefore concluded that acidification acted by preventing release of gastrin, not by the release of an inhibitory hormone. They further found that cocainization or atropinization of the antral mucosa prevented topical application of foods from stimulating acid secretion. Andersson et al. (1958) found that exclusion of the antrum in dogs resulted in acid hypersecretion in Pavlov pouch dogs and that this hypersecretion was abolished on resection of the antrum.

Pe Thein and Schofield (1959) showed, in dogs with pouches of the pyloric antrum and either Heidenhain-type or transplanted fundic pouches, that sham feeding produced marked acid responses provided that the antral pouches were not exposed to acid. Denervation of the antral pouch or acidification of its mucosa abolished the acid response to sham feeding. Already earlier, Robertson et al. (1950) had shown that, in dogs, irrigation of the pyloric area of the stomach with acetylcholine resulted in acid secretion. They attributed this effect of acetylcholine to gastrin release. Gillespie and Grossman (1962) showed in Heidenhain pouch dogs that although acidification of isolated pyloric pouches prevented acetylcholine perfusion of the latter from stimulating acid secretion via liberation of endogenous gastrin, it did not prevent the effect of exogenously administered gastrin, thus indicating that the acidification did not inhibit acid secretion via the release of an inhibitory hormone.

Gillespie and Grossman (1964a) studied the effects of urecholine and gastrin on acid secretion in Heidenhain pouch dogs and found that there was true potentiation between the effects of the two agents, since the combined effects were greater than the sum of the actions of either agent acting by itself would have been.

In all the early work, acid secretory responses to, for instance, irrigation of pyloric mucosa with acetylcholine or to vagal stimulation were taken to indicate gastrin release and used to estimate its magnitude. Later, when it became possible to measure gastrin by radioimmunoassay, it was fortunately found that, in dogs, treatment of the pyloric mucosa with acetylcholine (Jackson et al., 1972) and direct electrical stimulation of the vagus nerves (Lanciault et al., 1973) do in fact release gastrin, or at any rate material reacting with antibodies to gastrin. Interestingly, atropine does not block vagally stimulated gastrin release, at least in dogs (Smith et al., 1975). The finding that the vagus nerve itself contains gastrin-like immunoreactive material is interesting, although its physiological importance is not yet known (Uvnäs-Wallensten et al., 1977). The vagal release of gastrin and the various interactions between gastrin and the vagus were reviewed by Olbe (1966) and have been the topic of a special conference (Rehfeld and Amdrup, 1979).

Debas et al. (1974b) found that, in dogs, application of large polypeptides, but not of whole protein, to the mucosa of vagally denervated antral pouches resulted in secretion of gastric acid, presumably via release of gastrin. The effect of the polypeptides and of several other stimulants of gastrin release was increased by distension of the antral pouches.

Elwin (1974) investigated the effect on acid secretion and presumably gastrin release of irrigating the antrum in dogs with Heidenhain and Pavlov pouches with protein hydrolyzates fractionated on the basis of molecular weight. The low molecular weight fractions, containing free amino acids and small peptides, were the strongest stimulators of acid secretion. Among amino acids there were distinct differences in activity.

Feldman and Grossman (1980) found that a liver extract and its free amino acid component were, on application, equipotent in stimulating gastric acid secretion in dogs. Grossman et al. (1948) showed in dogs that distension of the antral part of the stomach caused acid secretion in a subcutaneously transplanted fundic pouch and conversely distension of a transplanted pouch of the antral area acid secretion in the remainder of the stomach. Trudeau and McGuigan (1969) found that, in a patient with the Zollinger–Ellison syndrome, infusion of calcium gluconate resulted in marked increases in plasma immunoreactive gastrin. Subsequently, it was shown that calcium infusion or the use of calcium carbonate as an oral antacid raises serum gastrin concentrations in normal control subjects also (Reeder et al., 1971; Levant et al., 1973). Barreras (1973) drew attention to marked differences between various species in their gastric secretory responses to calcium. In the dog and the rat, for instance, hypercalcemia inhibits gastric secretion, whereas in the ferret, the cat, and the monkey, as in man, it stimulates secretion.

Hayes et al. (1972) found increased plasma gastrin levels in patients with pheochromocytoma and, after showing that in dogs adrenaline produced a rise in plasma gastrin concentrations, concluded that catecholamines stimulate gastrin release. This has been confirmed by different workers. Seino et al. (1980) found that increases in plasma gastrin in man after arginine injection were blocked by the β-adrenergic blocking agent propranolol.

Thomas and Crider (1940) found that the threshold value for acidification of the duodenum to stimulate pancreatic secretion was at about pH 5 in dogs. Thomas and Crider (1941) found that infusion of peptone solutions into the upper intestine of dogs stimulated pancreatic secretion and that, compared with the secretion in response to acidification of the duodenum, the volume of the juice secreted was small, but had a high concentration of enzymes. They assumed, however, that the peptones acted through a nervous mechanism.

After the discovery of pancreozymin by Harper and Raper (1943), Wang and Grossman (1951) carried out an extensive study of the effects of the introduction of various types of substances into the upper intestine on the release of secretin and of pancreozymin in dogs. As a criterion of secretin release, they took the secretion of bicarbonate and water from pancreatic autotransplants; and for pancreozymin release, the enzyme content of the juice secreted. They found that the introduction of dilute HCl into the upper intestine led to a strong release of secretin, but also to a weak release of pancreozymin. Protein hydrolyzates, as well as the amino acids leucine, tryptophan, and phenylalanine, were potent pancreozymin releasers, but also rather strong secretin releasers. Fats and, especially, soap also released pancreozymin and, to a lesser extent, secretin. Carbohydrates, on the other hand, showed no release properties. In passing, Wang and Grossman mentioned that the substances that released pancreozymin were the same as those that released cholecystokinin, an observation that was confirmed in an unexpected manner (Jorpes and Mutt, 1966). The assumption that acid releases not only secretin but also CCK found strong support in the work of Barbezat and Grossman (1975), who stimulated pancreatic secretion in dogs maximally by exogenous secretin and during this stimulation introduced acid into their duodeni. This resulted in increased secretion of protein in the pancreatic juice. The amount of protein secreted in response to acidification was compared with the amount secreted by giving different doses of CCK. In this way it could be estimated that acid was some five times more effective as a releaser of secretin than of CCK.

Nakajima and Magee (1970b) found that duodenal acidification in the pH range 5.0–3.0 in conscious dogs with Heidenhain pouches increased pouch pepsin secretion in response to either "pentagastrin," histamine, or metacholine. Lowering the pH further led to a fall in pepsin concentrations. Since secretin had been found to stimulate pepsin secretion and CCK to inhibit it, these findings were interpreted to suggest that mainly secretin was being released in the pH 5.0–3.0 range and both CCK and secretin at lower pH values. Since the acidity of the duodenal contents must increase to pH 5 or below (Thomas and Crider, 1940), and since the chyme from the stomach is quickly partly neutralized by the pancreatic and small intestinal secretions, it had been questioned whether the pH of the intestinal contents physiologically ever falls low enough for substantial quantities of secretin to be released (Thomas, 1950). The problem was investigated in dogs by Grossman and Konturek (1974), who reached the conclusion that gastric acid does indeed drive pancreatic bicarbonate secetion. Nevertheless, they pointed out that the amounts of secretin released might be rather small, but were physiologically important because of the potentiation of secretin activity by the CCK released by other constituents of the meal.

Chey et al. (1974) found by the use of radioimmunoassay that intraduodenal infusion of acid in man raised serum immunoreactive secretin levels. Glucose had no such effect. Also with radioimmunoassay, Boden et al. (1974) found that introduction of dilute HCl into the duodenum in dogs resulted in an increase of plasma concentrations of secretin-like immunoreactivity. Introduction of an amino acid mixture, solutions of fructose, sucrose, hyperosmotic sodium chloride, sodium oleate, or a mixture of sodium oleate and bile did not result in any such increase (Boden et al., 1975). The effect of bile is somewhat of a mystery. Originally it was found by Mellanby (1926) to stimulate pancreatic secretion in anesthetized cats. Other workers found no such effect, either in cats (Mutt and Söderberg, 1959) or in dogs (Thomas and Crider, 1941). Others again have confirmed stimulation of pancreatic secretion by intraduodenal bile. Osnes et al. (1980) have described rises in plasma immunoreactive secretin concentrations in man after intraduodenal infusion of cattle bile. Earlier, Forell and co-workers had described a stimulatory effect of intraduodenal bile on pancreatic enzyme secretion in man, but not on secretion of bicarbonate (Forell et al. 1965; Forell, 1973). Malagelada et al. (1972) found that, in man, intraduodenal bile acids at high concentrations inhibited gallbladder contraction and pancreatic enzyme secretion in response to intraduodenal fat or amino acids, presumably by inhibiting release of CCK. Malagelada et al. (1973) thereupon found that the threshold dose of CCK necessary for stimulation of pancreatic secretion in man was about 8 times lower than the threshold dose for stimulation of gallbladder contraction. This suggested the existence of a physiological control mechanism: Low doses of CCK lead to the secretion of pancreatic enzymes that act on fats and proteins to release fatty acids and amino acids that are efficient releasers of more CCK. After gallbladder contraction, the high concentrations of duodenal bile acids inhibit the release of additional CCK, giving the gallbladder an opportunity to refill.

A most interesting observation is that, while intraduodenal infusion of L-phenylalanine stimulates pancreatic secretion, presumably via release of CCK, infusion of D-phenylalanine is ineffective (Meyer and Grossman, 1972a). Incidentally, D and L isomers of serine and alanine were found to be equally effective, on application to the pyloric mucosa, in stimulating acid secretion in Pavlov pouch dogs, presumably via release of gastrin (Csendes and Grossman, 1972). However, in another mechanism for stimulation of acid secretion, application of amino acids directly to the acid-producing oxyntic gland area, L amino acids were found to be effective, and D amino acids completely ineffective (Konturek et al., 1976a).

Holtermüller et al. (1976) showed that intraduodenal perfusion with

$CaCl_2$ solutions in man results in secretion of pancreatic enzymes and gallbladder contraction, presumably via release of CCK by the calcium ions. Also, intraduodenal magnesium has such effects (Holtermüller, 1976). A calcium-dependent release in response to depolarizing stimuli of immunoreactive 8-CCK from rat brain synaptosomes has been described (Klaff et al., 1981). It is not known whether the agents that release secretin or CCK, or other gastrointestinal hormonal peptides, act directly on the cells storing these hormones or activate other release mechanisms, neural or hormonal (Meyer and Grossman, 1972b).

Schapiro and Woodward (1965) found that if several different types of local anesthetics were applied to the duodenal mucosa of dogs, then subsequent application of dilute hydrochloric acid to the anesthetized mucosa resulted in a much weaker secretion of pancreatic juice compared to the response of the unanesthetized mucosa to the acid. This suggested that the anesthetics interfered in some way with the release of secretin. Support for the latter assumption was provided by Slayback et al. (1967), who found that, in dogs, the response of the pancreas to exogenous secretin had not been diminished by application of local anesthetics to the mucosa. These workers further showed that the pancreatic secretion of enzymes in response to the application of a solution of peptides to the mucosa was inhibited if the mucosa had been pretreated with local anesthetics. The response to exogenous CCK was unaffected by anesthetization of the mucosa. These findings seemed to suggest that local neural mechanisms might be involved in the release of secretin and CCK from the intestine.

Some doubt seems to have been cast on the existence of neural mechanisms for CCK release. Not only has topical application of local anesthetics to the intestinal mucosa been claimed to interfere with this hypothetical mechanism, but also atropinization of the experimental animal as such (Konturek et al., 1972). Solomon and Grossman (1979) have found, however, that while atropinization does decrease the stimulating effect of intraduodenal sodium oleate (assumed to be acting by release of CCK) on the pancreas in dogs, it has no such effect on pancreatic autotransplants in these animals. The authors concluded that atropinization may, instead of impeding CCK-release, block an enteropancreatic reflex. As repeatedly referred to above, the interactions between the peptide hormones secretin and CCK are most probably of physiological importance; likewise, the interactions between the vagus and the gastrins. These are examples of what is presumably a very intricate fabric of interactions between different peptide hormones and of hormones with nerve impulses. One special type of interaction between hormones is their ability *to release each other* into the blood stream or prevent such release. A vast amount of information exists about such release phenomena, and only a few examples will be given here and in the following section. Very little is yet known about the mechanism(s) involved in these effects on hormone release. Or, rather, nothing is definitely known, but there are suggestions as to the involvement of cyclic nucleotides, prostaglandins, and calcium ions. These aspects of hormone release will not be discussed here.

Bombesin was shown to release gastrin from the antrum of dogs, and this release was found to be largely refractory to the usual acid inhibition of gastrin release (Impiccatore et al., 1974). Like bombesin, GRP released gastrin in dogs (McDonald et al., 1979).

Exogenous secretin was found to diminish basal immunoreactive plasma gastrin concentrations in man in one study (Hansky et al., 1971), whereas in another it was found not to affect basal concentrations but to suppress the expected postprandial rises (Thompson et al., 1972). A paradoxical effect of secretin has been found in many, although not all, cases with the Zollinger–Ellison syndrome. Instead of depressing plasma gastrin concentrations, these were increased (Isenberg et al., 1972; Thompson et al., 1972). Glucagon, too, has been found to decrease plasma gastrin concentrations in man (Hansky et al., 1973a; Becker et al., 1973). In dogs, food-stimulated release of gastrin was found to be suppressed by both VIP and GIP (Villar et al., 1976).

Release of immunoreactive VIP has been described after intraduodenal infusion of calcium (Ebeid et al., 1977b), hypertonic saline (Ebeid et al., 1977a), cattle bile (Burhol et al., 1980) HCl, fat, or ethanol (Schaffalitzky de Muckadell et al., 1977b), and on vagal stimulation (Schaffalitzky de Muckadell et al., 1977a). In the codfish, plasma concentrations of VIP were found to be depressed by bombesin (Holstein and Humphrey, 1980). Release of motilin by duodenal acidification in man has been described by Bloom et al. (1978). Mitznegg et al. (1977) showed that plasma motilin levels in man decreased after administration of secretin. The effect was attributed to alkalinization of the duodenal mucosa.

Release of immunoreactive GIP in man has been found to take place after the infusion into the duodenum of cattle bile (Burhol et al., 1980) and of relatively large quantities of HCl (LeRoith et al., 1980). It also followed on oral administration of glucose (Cataland et al., 1974). In dogs, glucose, but still more efficiently fat, resulted in increases of plasma immunoreactive GIP (Pederson et al., 1975). Some effects of gastrointestinal hormones on the release of nongastrointestinal hormones will be briefly mentioned in the following section.

E. EXTRAGASTROINTESTINAL ACTIONS

It has long been suggested that various gastrointestinal hormones might, in addition to their actions on organs involved in digestion, also have other actions. Today it is known that many of them can indeed be shown pharmacologically to have various such actions. It is much less clear which of these actions are physiologically important, and, if they are, to what degree their exclusion can or cannot be easily compensated for by other mechanisms.

Ross (1970) found that, on rapid intravenous injection in anesthetized cats, secretin increased cardiac output and, on close intraarterial injections into mesenteric and femoral arteries, increased blood flow in these vessels and reduced the resistance of their vascular beds. Goodhead et al. (1970) found that secretin increased cardiac output in anesthetized dogs. Kitani et al. (1978) found that, in rats, secretin significantly increased the cardiac output distribution to the stomach, small intestine, and pancreas, whereas glucagon increased cardiac output distribution to the heart, lungs, and kidneys. Chou et al. (1977) found that secretin, in anesthetized dogs, caused vasodilation in all vascular beds investigated including those of the skin and muscles of the forelimb. On perivascular injection into rats, VIP has been found to dilate pial arterioles on the convexity of the cerebral cortex (McCulloch and Edvinsson, 1980). Activation of cardiac adenylate cyclase by VIP and by secretin has been described by Chatelain et al. (1980).

The effects, or lack of effects, of secretin on renal function have long been discussed. Owen and Ivy (1931) found a partially purified preparation of secretin to have a slight, but distinct, diuretic effect in anesthetized dogs. Dragstedt and Owen (1931) considered this effect to be an indirect one, dependent on the stimulation of pancreatic bicarbonate secretion. Ågren (1934) found no diuretic effect of secretin in anesthetized cats. Baron et al. (1958) found that secretin had a distinct diuretic effect in man, but, like Dragstedt and Owen (1931), considered this to be dependent on the "alkaline tide" following the stimulation of pancreatic bicarbonate secretion. Barbezat et al. (1972) found that on intravenous injection both secretin, in large doses, and glucagon were diuretic in dogs. Marchand et al. (1972), however, found that secretin injection directly into the renal artery of anesthetized dogs did produce an increase in renal blood flow but, in contrast to glucagon, no diuresis. Levy (1975) found that although secretin did not have any effect of its own on diuresis in the anesthetized dog it inhibited, partially, the natriuretic effect of glucagon. Waldum et al. (1980a,b), in analyzing the effects of moderately large doses of secretin on diuresis in man, concluded that secretin is diuretic in man but only when administered in large doses, and that its effect is probably due to impairment of sodium reabsorption in the renal tubules caused by an increase in renal blood flow, secondary to a direct vasodilation of the renal arterioles.

Secretin has been found to stimulate lipolysis in rat adipose tissue *in vitro* (Lazarus *et al.,* 1968; Rudman and Del Rio, 1969a; Butcher and Carlson, 1970) and in free fat cells of the mouse (Rudman and Del Rio, 1969a). Other workers, however, have found no effect of secretin on cAMP levels in mouse adipose tissue (Dehaye *et al.,* 1975). VIP, like secretin, has been found to have a lipolytic effect on rat adipose tissue (Frandsen and Moody, 1973).

There is considerable interest in possible effects of gastrointestinal peptides on intake of food. MacLagan (1937) found that insulin administered, in small doses together with glucose, slightly diminished food intake in rabbits. Similar effects were observed with a preparation of posterior pituitary hormones and with a crude preparation of "enterogastrone." The effects of the latter were definite but transient. Schally *et al.* (1967) found another type of "enterogastrone" preparation to diminish food intake in mice. Stunkard *et al.* (1955) found that glucagon inhibited gastric hunger contractions and the sensation of hunger in man. Glick *et al.* (1971) found that secretin, administered intraperitoneally or intraarterially, had no effect on food intake in rats. CCK appeared to have a slight depressant effect, but this was not statistically significant. Gibbs *et al.* (1973), however, with a somewhat different experimental technique and larger doses of the hormones, confirmed that secretin was without effect on food intake in rats but that CCK definitely decreased the intake of food without influencing water intake. A satiety effect of CCK has been repeatedly confirmed by different workers in both normal and genetically obese rats (McLaughlin and Baile, 1980), in genetically obese mice (Parrot and Batt, 190), in domestic fowls (Savory and Gentle, 1980), and in rhesus monkeys (Falasco *et al.* 1979). In man, one study showed no effect of CCK on satiety (Goetz and Sturdevant, 1975), but another showed a depressant effect on appetite (Stacher *et al.,* 1979).

There is consequently no doubt that CCK has been shown to induce satiety in several vetebrate species under experimental conditions. This is obviously not a nonspecific effect caused by any gastrointestinal hormone. Neither secretin, gastrin, nor GIP had, in contrast to CCK, any significant effect on feeding behavior in sham-fed rats (Lorenz *et al.,* 1979). The mechanism of this action of CCK, on the other hand, is yet unclear. Because of its cholecystokinetic and pancreozyminic action, CCK will expel bile and pancreatic secretory proteins into the small intestine. It also strongly stimulates intestinal peristalsis. The possible effects on satiety of this does not seem to have been compensated for in the experiments hitherto described. With the exception of the work of Stacher *et al.* (1979), the doses of CCK found necessary to elicit satiety have been large. An interesting possibility is that CCK in its effects on satiety may be acting by the release of some other hormone. Anika *et al.* (1980) found that small doses of insulin decreased food intake in pigs and pointed out that insulin is known to be released by intestinal hormones like CCK and GIP. It is also known that besides insulin, CCK releases calcitonin (see below). An interesting observation (Maddison, 1977) is that, in rats, CCK elicits satiety also on intracranial injection, but that in contrast to intraperitoneal injection there is a latency period of about half an hour. It may be mentioned that an anorexogenic peptide with the sequence Glp-His-Gly has been isolated from the urine of patients with anorexia nervosa (Reichelt *et al.*, 1978).

One report described a sustained increase in plasma calcium in man following intravenous infusion of secretin (Isenberg *et al.*, 1973), but others could not confirm this finding (Thompson *et al.*, 1972; Bradley *et al.*, 1975). Interestingly, however, secretin, although at fairly high concentrations, was found to release immunoreactive parathyrin from dispersed, isolated bovine parathyroid cells (Windeck *et al.*, 1978).

In contrast to secretin, glucagon, in the dog, was found to induce hypocalcemia, presumably by release of calcitonin (Avioli *et al.*, 1969). In sheep, secretin failed to influence plasma calcitonin levels, but an extract of porcine small intestine, containing both secretin and CCK and also other peptides, stimulated calcitonin release (Care, 1970). A partially purified preparation of porcine CCK, 8-CCK, cerulein, and "pentagastrin" all stimulated calcitonin release from perfused pig thyroid glands, whereas the N-terminal hexapeptide of 33-CCK was inactive (Care *et al.*, 1971). Stimulation of calcitonin release in the pig by "pentagastrin" was demonstrated independently of the work of Care and associates by Cooper *et al.* (1971); subsequently, Cooper *et al.* (1972b) showed that also G/CCK-4 stimulated calcitonin release in the pig. The possible importance of gastrointestinal hormones for the physiological release of calcitonin has been discussed by Cooper *et al.*, 1972a).

Vasoactive intestinal polypeptide has been shown pharmacologically to cause hyperglycemia in dogs and to stimulate glycogenolysis in slices of rabbit liver *in vitro* (Kerins and Said, 1973). It has also been shown to stimulate the release of rat prolactin, both *in vivo* (Kato *et al.*, 1978) and from anterior pituitary tissue *in vitro* (Kato *et al.*, 1978;

Enjalbert *et al.*, 1980). It has been shown to stimulate thyroid hormone secretion from thyroid tissue of several species *in vitro* (Ahrén *et al.*, 1980). Somatostatin secretion from rat hypothalamus was found to be inhibited by VIP (Epelbaum *et al.*, 1979), and VIP was also found to inhibit the inhibiting action of somatostatin on somatotropin secretion from rat pituitaries *in vitro* (Tapia-Arancibia *et al.*, 1980).

The effects of various gastrointestinal hormonal peptides on the release of immunoreactive somatostatin from the perfused dog pancreas have been investigated by Ipp *et al.* (1977) and from the perfused rat stomach by Chiba *et al.* (1980).

Plasma concentrations of immunoreactive somatostatin in man have been found to be elevated by cerulein (Adrian *et al.*, 1977) and by secretin (Glaser *et al.*, 1980).

Soon after the discovery of secretin, Moore *et al.* (1906) suggested that not only the exocrine, but also the endocrine, secretion of the pancreas might be stimulated by "a hormone or secretin" of the duodenal mucous membrane. They claimed that, in a few cases of diabetes mellitus, crude extracts of porcine upper intestinal mucosa administered orally had resulted in decreased sugar excretion in the urine. Secretin was found not to have any effect on blood sugar, at any rate in cats (Mellanby, 1928; Ågren, 1934) or dogs (Ågren, 1934). La Barre (1932), however, described attempts at the purification of an antidiabetic hormone, which he named incretin, from the duodenal mucosa of pigs. Attempts to isolate or unequivocally prove the existence of incretin were, however, unsuccessful, possibly with the exception of some observations by Laughton and Macallum (1932) suggesting that the duodenal mucosa of several animal species indeed contained some substance that on intravenous injection decreased blood sugar concentrations in intact rabbits and dogs but failed to do so in depancreatized animals. Loew *et al.* (1940), however, found no evidence supporting the theory that the duodenum exerts a control over carbohydrate metabolism, and work on the isolation of incretin stopped. Interest in incretin awakened again through a different series of observations, and incretin, like enterogastrone and enterocrinin, became a concept instead of a name for a particular substance.

Staub (1921) had found that if two consecutive equal doses of glucose were administered in man, the second dose as soon as the hyperglycemia following the first had subsided, then the hyperglycemic effect due to the second dose was less pronounced and of shorter duration than that due to the first dose. Traugott (1922) made similar observations. Somersalo (1950) confirmed the existence of the "Staub effect" but found that it was seen clearly only on oral administration of glucose.

On intravenous administration, the two hyperglycemic effects were usually of equal magnitude. Scow and Cornfield (1954) found that the overall removal rate for orally administered glucose in rats was approximately three times as high as for intravenously administered glucose. With a bioassay for plasma insulin-like activity, Arnould *et al.* (1963) found that the increases in plasma insulin concentrations in dogs after oral administration of glucose, were unexpectedly high compared with what was known about the relation of insulin to blood glucose concentrations. They suggested that the oral glucose might have triggered an insulinogenic mechanism from the duodenum or the liver.

When the radioimmunoassay for insulin became available (Yalow and Berson, 1960), it was clearly demonstrated that intravenously and orally or intraduodenally administered glucose affected plasma insulin levels differently. Elrick *et al.* (1964) found that plasma insulin concentrations increased more in man if a dose of glucose was administered orally than if it was administered intravenously and suggested that some factor stimulating insulin secretion was released by the glucose from the stomach or the intestine, or by the high concentration of glucose from the liver.

McIntyre *et al.* (1965) demonstrated very clearly that, on intrajejunal administration of a certain dose of glucose, the plasma glucose concentration, in man, was lower and the plasma insulin concentration much higher than when the same dose of glucose was administered intravenously. The liver could be excluded from the discussion of this phenomenon, since the phenomenon occurred also in patients with portacaval shunts.

An important observation was made by Dupré (1964), who showed that if two consecutive equal doses of glucose were administered intravenously in man, the second dose together with a partially purified preparation of secretin, the hyperglycemic effect following on the second dose, instead of being equal to the first, was much weaker. This suggested that the secretin preparation used, contained as a contaminant a previously unidentified intestinal hormone. Unexpectedly, however, essentially pure secretin was found on intravenous administration to increase plasma concentrations of immunoreactive insulin in man, without however, affecting blood glucose concentrations (Dupré *et al.*, 1966). Stimulation by secretin of insulin release from rabbit and dog pancreas slices *in vitro* was demonstrated by Pfeiffer *et al.* (1965). An intensive period of investigation of the effects of secretin and other gastrointestinal peptides on the endocrine pancreas started in many laboratories and still continues. It was soon shown that secretin was not the only gastrointestinal hormone that could stimulate insulin release. In anesthetized dogs, stimulation of insulin secretion could be observed following endoportal injection of either secretin or partially purified preparations of CCK and of gastrin. The CCK preparation, in contrast to secretin or gastrin, also stimulated glucagon secretion. The concept of an "enteroinsular axis" came into being (Unger *et al.*, 1967). Glucagon, like secretin, was shown to stimulate insulin secretion in man (Jarett and Cohen, 1967). CCK seemed to be a particularly efficient releaser of insulin in dogs (Meade *et al.*, 1967; Buchanan *et al.*, 1968) and also from isolated rat pancreatic islets where secretin, under the experimental conditions used, had no effect (Hinz *et al.*, 1971).

Turner, however, found that under certain conditions of glucose concentration, etc., in the incubation medium, secretin did not release insulin from rabbit pancreatic tissue *in vitro*, pancreozymin had only a weak release effect, but glucagon and an extract of porcine duodenojejunal mucosa had a strong release effect. Since the extract had negligible secretin and pancreozymin activity and no glucagon-like immunoreactivity, Turner (1969) suggested that it might contain a hitherto unidentified hormone for which the old designation incretin might be used.

When it was discovered that GIP had strong insulin-releasing activity (Rabinovitch and Dupré, 1974; Dupré *et al.*, 1973), Turner *et al.* (1974) compared the insulin-releasing properties of GIP and partially purified IRP in rats and found that they were qualitatively indistinguishable, suggesting that IRP and GIP are probably very similar although not necessarily identical. Since then the insulin-releasing activity of certain partially purified CCK-preparations was found to be due in part to the GIP present in these preparations (Rabinovitch and Dupré, 1974). The obvious question is whether the observations on the insulin-releasing properties of CCK, made by the use of only partially purified preparations of it, can be attributed entirely to their GIP content. In other words, does CCK itself have insulin-releasing activity? Hedner *et al.* (1975) found no effect of 8-CCK or highly purified porcine CCK on plasma insulin concentrations in man. Rehfeld (1971), however, found that the *N*-benzyloxycarbonyl derivate of G/CCK-4 was insulinotropic in man, more so than a preparation of hog gastrin. Kaneto *et al.* (1970) had found in dogs that this derivative of G/CCK-4 released both insulin and glucagon. Frame *et al.* (1975) found that, in dogs, 8-CCK released both insulin and glucagon. Release of insulin in response to neurotensin has been described by Ishida (1977).

With the isolated perfused porcine pancreas, Jensen *et al.* (1978b) found that insulin release by secretin occurred at only high concentrations of secretin in the perfusate. In the same system, the effects of VIP were shown to be dependent on glucose concentration: At high glucose concentration, VIP released insulin but not glucagon; at low glucose concentration, glucagon was released but not insulin (Jensen *et al.*, 1978a). The physiological importance of the effects of gastrointestinal hormones on insulin and glucagon secretion is far from clear. Perley and Kipnis (1967) estimated that about half of the insulin released in response to oral glucose was released by the action of intestinal factors. As to which intestinal peptides are mainly involved in this, it was early shown that acidification of the duodenum, known to release secretin and CCK, had no influence on plasma insulin concentrations (Boyns *et al.*, 1966; Mahler and Weisberg, 1968; O'Connor *et al.*, 1976). Likewise, intraduodenal glucose, known to increase plasma insulin concentrations, had no effect on either pancreatic secretion (Sum and Preshaw, 1967) or plasma secretin concentrations (Boden *et al.*, 1974). This shows that secretin is not the insulin-releasing factor released from the intestinal wall in response to oral glucose. This does not mean that secretin cannot have an insulin-releasing effect when it is released into the blood stream in connection with a meal. In view of the fact that GIP is released in response to oral glucose (Cataland *et al.*, 1974) and has a strong insulin-releasing capacity, which is dependent on glucose concentration, it is almost certain that GIP is physiologically insulinotropic. It has been suggested that since this action of GIP may be more important physiologically then its inhibitory action on gastric secretion, GIP could be renamed "*g*lucose-dependent *i*nsulinotropic *p*olypeptide" (Brown and Pederson, 1976). The probable physiological importance of GIP is also suggested by the finding that in insulin-dependent juvenile-type diabetics there is a correlation between the concentrations of plasma insulin and of GIP, intravenous insulin leading to a decrease in GIP concentrations (Talaulicar *et al.*, 1981). Creutzfeldt (1979) considered GIP to be an important incretin, but not the only incretin, since administration of antisera to GIP only partially abolished the incretin effect in rats. This view is supported by recent work of Lauritsen *et al.* (1980).

Bourdeaux *et al.* (1980) found that lipoprotein lipase activity was stimulated in adipose tissue of fasted rats by gastrin and CCK, but not by secretin or VIP.

VIII. Structure–Activity Relationships

When oxytocin had been synthesized by Du Vigneaud and co-workers (1953b) the question was asked whether the synthetic peptide exhibited oxytocin action exclusively or if it also had some vasopressin-like action, as had been found for highly purified preparations of natural oxytocin. Bioassays provided the answer (Gyermek and Fekete, 1955; van Dyke *et al.*, 1955). Synthetic oxytocin exhibited in a low degree, but distinctly, vasopressin-like activity in addition to its strong oxytocin activity. This observation was of considerable theoretical importance and seemed to indicate that peptide hormones may differ from enzymes by being much less specific in their actions. There was also insulin, known to have all kinds of actions (Jensen, 1948), but somehow insulin had been held to be different. Oxytocin and vasopressin resemble each other chemically, and it was not too difficult to accept that they could, to some extent, exhibit each other's actions. The problem of selectivity in action again appeared when gastrin was isolated. Would gastrin clearly stimulate the secretion of gastric acid and nothing else, or would it also do a number of other things that partially purified preparations had been found to do (Blair *et al.*, 1963)? Again the answer was given by bioassays and was unequivocal: porcine gastrin stimulated, on subcutaneous injection in dogs, the secretion of gastric acid, although it inhibited it instead when given intravenously in large doses (Gregory and Tracy, 1964). It also stimulated pepsin secretion, pancreatic volume flow and enzyme secretion, gastric motility and, to a slight extent, hepatic bile flow and gallbladder contractility. On the jejunum, it had a diphasic effect, contraction being followed by decreased tone and motility. Later, as to some extent seen from the above review of the physiological effects of the gastrointestinal hormones, gastrin has been found to have still other activities.

As in the case of oxytocin, the finding that gastrin had multiple effects was of considerable theoretical importance. Especially its stimulation of pancreatic secretion of fluid seemed sensational since this, in contrast to stimulation of enzyme secretion, was at that time held to be a prerogative of secretin—and, although only little was then known about the amino acid sequence of secretin, it was known that the amino acid composition of secretin was very different from that of gastrin.

If gastrin had been found to stimulate only the secretion of gastric acid it would have fitted in well with the hypothesis of Hofmann (1960). According to this, the receptor for a peptide hormone in the plasma membrane of the target cell is a specific protein inactive by itself but forming an active enzyme when it noncovalently binds the hormone, as the inactive S-protein forms an active ribonuclease when it binds the inactive S-peptide (Richards, 1958). Because gastrin has so many different actions it seemed less probable that it was acting by the formation of some hypothetical active enzyme, selectively and directly engaged in the production of HCl by the parietal cells. Instead, it seemed more likely that it acted by some allosteric mechanism for hormone action (Monod et al., 1963). These authors found it "difficult to imagine any biochemical mechanism other than allosteric which could allow a single chemical signal to be understood and interpreted simultaneously in different ways by entirely different systems." There was, however, no direct evidence to suggest whether gastrin acted according to one or the other of these two mechanisms, or by quite some other mechanism. It could also be acting by different mechanisms on different cells. The active enzyme formation and the allosteric mechanisms were, moreover, not mutually completely exclusive in view of the hypothesis for hormone action propounded by Sutherland and his colleagues, according to which the attachment of a hormone, the first messenger, to its receptor in the plasma membrane of its target cell results in the activation of an enzyme that catalyzes the formation of an intracellular "second messenger" (Sutherland et al., 1965). However—as exemplified by the activation of cell plasma membrane adenylate cyclase with the resultant increase in intracellular concentrations of adenosine-3',5'-cyclic monophosphate (cAMP)—such activation could in the same type of cell take place by a variety of hormones with very different chemical structures; thus it seemed most improbable that the hormones participated directly in the formation of the active center of the enzyme, according to the Hofmann hypothesis. What was true of gastrin was true of the other gastrointestinal hormones—not only was, but still is. For the action of gastrin, on specifically the parietal cells, there is now some evidence *against* the enzyme activation type of mechanism although the strength of this evidence is debatable.

For all peptide hormones, consequently also the gastrointestinal, it is now generally believed that, whatever the hormone–receptor interaction is, it does not entail the formation of covalent bonds. This has by no means always been the prevalent opinion. On the contrary, at least in the case of oxytocin and vasopressin, several investigations once seemed to suggest that the formation of disulfide bridges between receptor and hormone was a prerequisite for hormone action. It was only when Rudinger and Jošt (1964) showed that an analog of oxytocin, in which the possibility of disulfide formation had been abolished by the replacement of a sulfur atom by a —CH_2— group, still showed strong oxytocin activity that the concept of covalent receptor binding fell into disrepute for oxytocin. This influenced thinking about other hormone–receptor interactions. The degree of uncertainty that, nevertheless, persists in this area may be illustrated by the finding of

Linsley *et al.* (1979) of a substantial degree of evidently covalent binding of epidermal growth factor to its cellular receptors and similar findings of Baker *et al.* (1979) concerning both epidermal growth factor and thrombin. Not even the concept that peptide hormones act exclusively on cell plasma membrane receptors has gone free of doubt in view of the finding of internalization of some peptide hormones or hormone–receptor complexes (Kolata, 1978). Experiments suggesting nuclear uptake of angiotensin were indeed described more than 10 years ago (Robertson and Khairallah, 1971). At the time when the amino acid sequence of gastrin was elucidated, an intense collaboration was in progress between organic chemists, who were synthesizing all kinds of derivatives, analogs, fragments, and elongated chain forms of peptide hormones like oxytocin, vasopressin, angiotensin, bradykinin, corticotropin, and physiologists, who compared the effects of such modified peptides with the natural ones so as to obtain information on the importance of the various structural elements in the hormones for function (Schwyzer, 1963). This type of work was with great intensity brought to bear on gastrin and later, other gastrointestinal hormones.

An important and obvious question concerning gastrin was whether all its various activities were exerted by the same part of the molecule or by different parts. Tracy and Gregory reported (1964) that, in dogs, the entire range of physiological activities displayed by natural pG-17 ns was displayed also by its C-terminal tetrapeptide amide Trp-Met-Asp-Phe-NH_2, but not any longer by the tripeptide or dipeptide amides. A possible difference was that G-4 showed, more regularly than G-17, an inhibitory action on gastric tone and motility after stimulation. Quantitatively, however, there was a considerable increase in activity on lengthening of the peptide chain toward the N terminus of G-17. Such an accumulation of all the actions of a peptide hormone to the same part of the peptide chain does not seem always to be found in peptide hormones, as discussed for somatotropin by Paladini *et al.* (1979). The concentration of the activities of gastrin to the relatively small structure of a tetrapeptide amide greatly facilitated investigations of the structural requirements for gastrin action.

It was found that blocking of the N-terminal amino group of G-4 by a benzyloxycarbonyl residue did not influence activity, but that replacement of the C-terminal amide by the methyl ester group resulted in a peptide that no longer stimulated acid secretion or intestinal motility. Interestingly, the methyl ester of G-4 did stimulate the secretion of pepsin and the pancreatic secretion of enzymes and fluid and also augmented histamine-stimulated secretion of acid. In view of this it is somewhat surprising that the N-terminal and middle peptide fragments of G-17 were investigated as to their acid secretion-stimulatory properties in the form of their C-terminal methyl esters, instead of amides. It is often stated that for gastrin activity, G-4 must be C-terminal in any gastrin and that N-terminal fragments of gastrin are inactive. From the paper of Tracy and Gregory (1964) it is seen, however, that the methyl ester of the N-terminal hexapeptide of pG-17 stimulated the secretion of pepsin and augmented histamine-stimulated acid secretion, but did not by itself stimulate acid secretion. In this it resembled the C-terminal methyl ester of G-4 itself, and it would indeed have been interesting to see what effect a replacement of the ester group by the amide group might have had for its action.

Morley *et al.* (1965) described the synthesis of 33 analogs and derivatives of G-4 and the assay of these peptides on several different functions in dogs. In general, the ability of a particular peptide to stimulate gastric acid secretion was found to be associated with the other types of activities, but there were for some peptides definite indications of partial dissociation of activities. For instance, substitution of the methionine residue by norleucine decreased activity on pancreatic enzyme secretion while retaining it on acid secretion. It may be mentioned that Beswick *et al.* (1968) found in anesthetized cats that the N-benzyloxycarbonyl derivative of G-4, in which the methionine had been substituted by leucine, stimulated the secretion of gastric acid but not of pancreatic enzymes. This interesting observation does not seem to have been followed up. Oxidation of the methionine sulfur to either the sulfoxide or sulfone abolished most, but not all, types of activity, and there seemed to be some interesting differences between the sulfoxide and the sulfone. Replacement of the N-terminal amino group of the tryptophan residue by hydrogen did not influence activity, and various modifications also in the indole ring were compatible with activity. Several modifications in the phenylalanine residue were also permissible, but the importance of the intact amide structure was confirmed. Very clearly changes in the aspartyl position, even seemingly minor modifications such as replacement of aspartyl by glutamyl, resulted in inactivation. Morley *et al.* (1965) considered their findings to suggest that in G-4, and probably also in G-17, the tryptophan, methionine, and phenylalanine residues of the tetrapeptide are binding rather than functional active sites and that the most important feature of the gastrin molecule is the relationship between the aspartic acid residue and the C-terminal amide group.

In further studies, a total of about 500 analogs of derivatives of G-4 were synthesized by Morley and his colleagues, and the results appeared to justify the conclusion that the aspartyl residue, in contradistinction to the other residues, was "functional." Especially suggestive was the finding (Morley, 1968a,b) that a tetrazolyl residue with its spatial and acidic properties, similar to those of aspartyl, could replace the latter in G-4. It indeed seemed that gastrin was, at any rate when stimulating acid secretion, acting according to the Hofmann hypothesis. However, other work suggests that this is not so. Trout and Grossman (1971) showed that the peptide Asp-Tyr(SO$_3$H)-Met-Gly-Trp-Met-Ala-Phe-NH$_2$, *i.e.*, an N-acyl derivative of G-4 in which the critical aspartic acid residue has been substituted by an alanine residue, stimulated gastric acid secretion in cats although the dose necessary for this was some 100 times larger than for G-4. This difference in dose makes it, perhaps, uncertain whether or not the two peptides stimulate acid secretion by the same mechanism, but, if they do, then a "functional" role for the aspartyl residue of G-4 can hardly be tenable (Morley, 1977). It may be mentioned, however, that substituting alanine for aspartic acid in G-4, as such, led to a peptide that did not stimulate acid secretion (Trout and Grossman, 1971) as had earlier been shown by Morley (1968b) in the rat.

Lin *et al.* (1977) found, on the other hand, that the N-1-methyl-cyclobutyl-oxycarbonyl derivative of the tripeptide Met-Asn-Phe exhibited, although at very high dose levels, acid secretion-stimulating activity in dogs. This would mean that neither the aspartyl residue nor the C-terminal amide group are necessary for this activity in G-4, although they greatly contribute to a high activity of the peptide. These findings also confirm earlier findings by Lin and coworkers that G-4 is not, strictly, the minimal active fragment of gastrin. It is evident that the synthesis of different analogs and derivatives of gastrin has done much to define the structures necessary for gastrin activity, at least strong activity.

In another of its major aspirations in this field, the construction of gastrin-related peptides with inhibitory effects on acid secretion, synthetic chemistry has been less successful, although not unsuccessful. As discussed by Morley (1968b) and by Kenner (1972) such work has followed two main lines, both borrowed from enzymology. One has been the synthesis of analogs of gastrin with low or no activity in the hope of obtaining competitive inhibitors of the hormone; the other, inspired by the synthesis of irreversible enzyme inhibitors, is the synthesis of gastrin analogs carrying groups known to react by the formation of covalent linkages to proteins, in the hope that if the receptors to gastrin are proteins they would be irreversibly modified and inactivated. Despite the large number of substances synthesized, neither approach led to the desired goal (Kenner, 1972). For example, Agarwal *et al.* (1968a) synthesized the 16-asparaginyl analog of hG-17 s, and several other analogs of hG-17 s in which the various modifications had been made in its G-4 moiety. None of the substances showed any inhibitory properties on acid secretion, and other gastrin analogs carrying reactive groups like halomethyl or maleimide were no more efficient. Despite this, there is reason to believe that further work along both these lines may be worthwhile. "Antigastrin" (2-phenyl)-2-(2 pyridyl) thioacetamide, a remote analog of the C-terminal phenylalanine amide of gastrin, synthesized by H. W. Sause, did show some inhibitory action on gastric secretion in dogs (Bedi *et al.,* 1967), although not in cats (Sewing *et al.,* 1968). More encouraging (Kaess, 1980) was the finding (Soumarmon *et al.,* 1977) that a derivative of hG-17 ns, with weak gastric acid secretion stimulatory properties in rats, in which the tryptophan residue in the G-4 moiety had been converted to an *o*-nitrophenyl-sulfonyl derivative, competed with gastrin for binding to plasma membranes from rat gastric mucosa. The binding kinetics seemed to suggest that the tryptophan residue was involved not primarily in receptor binding, but in the stimulation of acid secretion.

Bertaccini *et al.* (1974a) have described two cerulein-related peptides that seem to act as competitive inhibitors of pentagastrin-stimulated acid secretion in Heidenhain pouch dogs. Galardy and Jamieson (1975) described experiments in which photolysis of 2-nitro-5-azidobenzoyl pentagastrin (evidently the C-terminal pentapeptide of gastrin, not the "pentagastrin" of commerce) in the presence of guinea pig pancreatic lobules causes irreversible stimulation of enzyme secretion, presumably by irreversible coupling of the pentagastrin moiety to the CCK receptors. More recently, Galardy *et al.* (1980) have described similar experiments with 2-nitro-5-azidobenzoylglycyl 8-CCK.

It may be remembered that more than 700 derivatives of the relatively simple histamine molecule had to be fashioned before the clinically useful H_2 histamine receptor antagonists were discovered (Black *et al.,* 1972). The latter receptor antagonists have drawn attention away not only from selective gastrin antagonists, but also from enterogastrone.

An interesting structural problem not yet solved is the observation by Davidson *et al.* (1969b) that porcine gastrin was some 200 times more potent than human G-17 ns in stimulating acid secretion from bullfrog gastric mucose *in vitro,* despite the fact that hG-17 and pG-17 differ only in a single amino acid residue, far removed from their G-4 moieties. Unfortunately, the comparison was carried out using a mixture of pG-17 s and pG-17 ns on the one hand, and hG-17 ns on the other. The effect of sulfation of the tyrosine residue for the potency with which a gastrin peptide stimulates acid secretion seems to vary between species. In dogs, Stening and Grossman (1969a) found that pG-17 s and pG-17 ns were equipotent in this action, but on the isolated gastric mucosa of the bullfrog, G-17 s was 10 times stronger than G-17 ns (Way and Durbin, 1969). Also on secretion of enzymes from the isolated per-fused porcine pancreas, the sulfated forms of gastrin were found to be much stronger than the nonsulfated forms (Jensen et al., 1980). Gas-trins from different mammalian species differ somewhat in their po-tency to stimulate acid secretion in dogs, but these differences are quite small (Cooke, 1967; Grossman, 1970b).

Mazur et al. (1969) showed that the methyl ester of the C-terminal dispeptide of gastrin was some 100–200 times sweeter than sucrose. This ester seems to be finding use as a nutritive sweetener. A report by Potts et al. (1980) states that at 550 times higher doses than the dose expected for normal human intake it impaired learning behavior of male, but not of female, rats. The structural basis for the sweet taste is unknown.

Synthetic organic chemistry has played an important role in the elucidation of the structural requirements for the two best known ac-tions of CCK, the cholecystokinetic and the pancreozyminic. This has entailed much work on the part of physiologists without whose careful comparisons of the various synthetic analogs and derivatives of the C-terminal part of the CCK chain, of the related cerulein, and C-terminal sequences of gastrin, the synthetic work would not have been informative about function. In view of the striking structural similarity between the C-terminal octapeptide sequence of the de-capeptide amide cerulein, Glp-Gln-*Asp*-*Tyr*(SO_3H)-Thr-*Gly*-*Trp*-*Met*-*Asp*-*Phe*-*NH*$_2$, and the C-terminal octapeptide amide of CCK, *Asp*-*Tyr*(SO_3H)-Met-*Gly*-*Trp*-*Met*-*Asp*-*Phe*-*NH*$_2$, it was inevitable that investigators working with these two peptides in part doubled their work. This has in many cases, however, also led to a welcome confir-mation of results.

Very many details concerning the pharmacological effects of various modifications in the cerulein and CCK sequences have been published and will not be discussed in detail here. Such discussion may be found in articles by Ondetti et al. (1970b), Anastasi et al. (1968b), Bernardi et al. (1972), and elsewhere. The result of this work may be summarized in the recognition that, although as mentioned above, sulfation of the tyrosine residue is of little importance for the activity of gastrin, it is very important for the action of CCK, although not absolutely essen-tial. Its importance appears, however, to be much greater for cholecys-tokinetic than for pancreozyminic activity (Johnson et al., 1970). For the salmon, as for the mammalian, gallbladder sulfation of the tyrosine residue of CCK is important for strong cholecystokinetic activity. The salmon gallbladder, however, in contrast to the mammalian (Vagne and Grossman, 1968; Johnson *et al.*, 1970), does not distinguish between the two strong stimulants of the mammalian gallbladder, cerulein and CCK, in which the tyrosine-*O*-sulfate residue is separated from the C-terminal pentapeptide amide by an intervening amino acid residue and gastrin-s in which this residue is directly attached to the pentapeptide (Vigna and Gorbman, 1977). Sulfation has been shown to be important also for other actions of CCK besides the cholecystokinetic and pancreozyminic, such as the stimulation of the secretion of hepatic bile in the dog (Kaminski *et al.*, 1977) and contraction of the longitudinal muscle of the guinea pig ileum *in vitro* (Vizi *et al.*, 1974). For the latter activity, sulfation greatly increased the potency of gastrin-type peptides also.

Fara and Erde (1978) reported that the differences in cholecystokinetic potencies between cerulein and desulfated cerulein were greater if assayed *in vitro* than *in vivo*, suggesting that some modification of one or the other or both of the peptides was taking place.

It was first shown (Mutt and Jorpes, 1968) that the C-terminal octapeptide obtained on treatment of CCK with trypsin exhibited a high degree of cholecystokinetic and pancreozyminic activity. This, however, is not the minimal fragment of CCK showing strong activity, since the C-terminal heptapeptide, 7-CCK, is roughly as active as the 8-CCK (Ondetti *et al.*, 1970b). This has made the heptapeptide an object for the preparation of synthetic analogs. Bodanszky *et al.* (1980) showed that the deamino derivative of 7-CCK was roughly as active as 7-CCK in stimulating protein secretion from the pancreas of the anesthetized cat and in contraction of guinea pig gallbladder *in situ*. It also stimulated amylase release from dispersed guinea pig pancreatic acini, but in this it was distinctly weaker than 7-CCK. An analog of 7-CCK in which the N-terminal residue of tyrosine-*O*-sulfate was replaced by seryl-*O*-sulfate showed only very weak cholecystokinetic and pancreozyminic activity (Bodanszky *et al.*, 1977). Further work suggested that this decreased activity was not primarily due to the omission of the aromatic ring but rather to the changed distance of the sulfate ester group from the peptide backbone, since replacement of the seryl ester by ε-hydroxynorleucine-*O*-sulfate resulted in a 7-CCK analog with strong activities (Bodanszky *et al.*, 1978b), although not quite as strong as for 7-CCK itself.

In discussing the structural requirements for CCK activity, an unexpected complication arose by the finding that bombesin not only released gastrin (Bertaccini *et al.*, 1974b) and CCK (Fender *et al.*, 1976) in experimental animals, but also, like CCK, stimulated the release of amylase from rat pancreatic fragments *in vitro* and caused calcium efflux from isolated acinar cells (Deschodt-Lanckman *et al.,* 1976). It is evident from later work (Peikin *et al.,* 1979; Philpott and Petersen, 1979) that bombesin and CCK act on different receptors so the problem of structural differences need not be too obstructive. Nevertheless, one may ask why there should be receptors for two structurally very different peptides but with the same function on the acinar cell. When GRP, which is presumably the mammalian counterpart of bombesin, was isolated it was found to be very similar to bombesin, and consequently very dissimilar to CCK, in its active C-terminal sequence. Unexpectedly, however, the N-terminal sequences of CCK and GRP showed some, admittedly not very impressive, similarities. Perhaps CCK and GRP have evolved from a common ancestral peptide and their receptors with them. One group of investigators (Rajh *et al.,* 1980) described experiments suggesting that the tryptophan residue in the G/CCK-4 moiety of CCK may be more important for activity than previously recognized. This is interesting, but it is not very probable, however, that the requirement for the indole ring will be found to be absolute, in view of the substitutions that are known to be compatible with gastrin-like activity in G-4 (Morley, 1968b). It is interesting to note that bombesin, too, has a tryptophan residue in its active C-terminal part. A promising factor for future work is the discovery (Peikin *et al.,* 1979) that dibutyryl cGMP acts as a competitive inhibitor of CCK activity on the pancreatic acinar cell. Vigna and Gorbman (1979) found that mammalian CCK does not stimulate the contraction of the hagfish gallbladder, but does stimulate lipase secretion from such scattered cells in hagfish intestine as are considered to be homologous to the pancreatic acinar cells of higher vertebrates. The secretion of intestinal alkaline phosphatase is not stimulated.

In contrast to CCK and gastrin, no smaller fragment of the heptacosapeptide sequence of secretin with a high degree of biological activity has been found, either regarding stimulation of pancreatic secretion or, in the few cases investigated, its other activities. This could mean that the heptacosapeptide amide is in itself the minimal (substantially) active fragment, but that larger forms, not yet isolated, exist naturally. During the stepwise synthesis of secretin by Bodanszky and co-workers (1966) starting from the C-terminal valine amide, we tested the peptides of various chain lengths, which were given to us by these workers, and found that the hexacosapeptide amide Ser_2-Val_{27}-NH_2 reproducibly exhibited secretin-like activity but that the activity increased a hundredfold on addition of the His_1 residue (Mutt and Jorpes, 1967b). Solomon *et al.* (1977) carried out a comparison of the activities of secretin and de-histidyl$_1$ secretin on pancreatic secretion of bicarbonate and fluid in dogs. The de-histidyl secretin appeared to be a full agonist of secretin but had only about 1% of the activity of the latter. This is again an example of a structural moiety in a peptide hormone being important for the action of the hormone, but not indispensable. In keeping with this is the finding by Makhlouf *et al.* (1978) that the 5-27 fragment of secretin and some analogs of it show some degree of pancreatic stimulation in the rat and in the guinea pig. A similar situation regarding the N-terminal histidine residue has been found for glucagon (Lin *et al.,* 1975).

During the above-mentioned synthesis of secretin, Bodanszky and co-workers also synthesized the Asn-3 analog of secretin, and we found it to exhibit only very weak secretin-like activity (Mutt and Jorpes, 1967b). When the sequence of VIP was determined, we pointed out that not only the similarities between the three peptides glucagon, secretin, and VIP were interesting but perhaps even more so the differences, which could shed light on the reasons for hormone specificity. In particular we drew attention to those positions in which the amino acid residues were identical in secretin and VIP on the one hand, and in glucagon and VIP on the other (Mutt and Said, 1974). Such residues might have something to do with the secretin-like activity of VIP and secretin, on the one hand, and the glucagon-like activity of glucagon and VIP on the other. For secretin-like activity, Asp-3 is such a residue, and since then several studies with synthetic analogs of secretin have demonstrated the importance of this residue for secretin-like activity (Wünsch *et al.,* 1977b; Adler *et al.,* 1980). However, the very weak secretin-like activity of PHI on the mammalian pancreas (Dimaline and Dockray, 1980) shows that neither His-1 nor Asp-3 by themselves nor their correct spatial relationship in a heptacosapeptide amide are enough for strong stimulation of pancreatic secretion in mammals. In birds, however, PHI is a strong stimulant of pancreatic secretion (Dimaline and Dockray, 1980). Asp-3 is also involved, by formation of a succinimide ring with the acylated amino group of Gly-4 in one inactivation mechanism for secretin Jaeger *et al.,* 1978).

Wright and Rodbell (1979a,b) have found that Gln-3 is one of the determinants for the ability of glucagon to interact with its receptors and to activate adenylate cyclase in rat liver cell plasma membranes, since the N-terminal hexapeptide of glucagon exhibits such an activity whereas the N-terminal hexapeptide of secretin, which differs from it only by the replacement of Gln-3 by Asp-3, is inactive. The N-terminal hexapeptide of VIP is also inactive in this respect. It had been shown earlier that whereas secretin and VIP interact on receptors in the rat liver, glucagon reacts only with its own receptors (Bataille *et al.*, 1974). VIP and secretin both act, although with different affinities, on two types of receptors on guinea pig pancreatic acinar cells (Gardner *et al.*, 1976; Christophe *et al.*, 1976a) and on receptors in rat (Laburthe *et al.*, 1979) and guinea pig (Binder *et al.*, 1980) intestinal epithelial cells. An interesting observation (Adler *et al.*, 1980) is that Val_5 secretin is equipotent to porcine secretin in stimulating the flow of pancreatic juice, but that the juice secreted in response to Val_5 secretin has a lower concentration of potassium than that secreted in response to secretin.

Deschodt-Lanckman *et al.* (1975) found that in rats somatostatin-14 stimulated the secretion of pancreatic amylase and lipase, but only weakly compared to secretin and CCK. In rat pancreatic fragments *in vitro,* somatostatin by itself weakly stimulated cAMP formation but inhibited the stimulatory action of secretin on formation of cAMP. These authors considered somatostatin to be a competitive inhibitor of secretin and drew attention to the identical -Thr-Phe-Thr-Ser- sequence of amino acid residues 5–8 in secretin and 10–13 in soma- tostatin-14. Vatn *et al.* (1980) found that, in man too, somatosta- tin inhibited secretin-stimulated pancreatic secretion by an apparently competitive mechanism. In dogs, Johnson and Grossman (1969) found that secretin inhibits gastrin-stimulated acid secretion apparently noncompetitively, whereas CCK inhibits it competitively (1970); this fits in well with what would be expected from the structures of the hormones. However, the finding (Berstad and Peterson, 1970) that pentagastrin-stimulated acid secretion in man seems to be inhibited competitively by secretin may act as a warning against the drawing of too far-reaching conclusions.

Although strikingly similar in structure, glucagon and secretin dif- fer in many of their physiological or pharmacological actions. Unfor- tunately, the degree of difference is difficult to estimate from reports in the literature. Taking pancreatic secretion as an example, Necheles (1957) found that administration of glucagon transiently increased secretin-stimulated pancreatic secretion in dogs and then inhibited it. Dreiling *et al.* (1958) found no effect of glucagon- on secretin- stimulated pancreatic secretion in man. Dyck *et al.* (1970) found inhibi- tion of pancreatic secretion stimulated by secretin together with pan- creozymin, and Iwatsuki *et al.* (1976) found, with the perfused dog pancreas, that glucagon elicited a dose-dependent, weak increase in pancreatic secretion.

Despite similarities in structure, GIP and secretin differ in their actions on the pancreatic secretion that is not stimulated by GIP (Brown *et al.*, 1970), in their effects on gastric secretion where acid secretion induced by various stimuli is inhibited in different proportions by GIP and secretin, and on pepsin secretion, which is stimulated by secretin but inhibited by GIP (Pederson and Brown, 1972). In a short communication, Brown and Pederson (1970b) reported that the C-terminal fragment obtained on cleaving GIP with CNBr inhibited pentagastrin-stimulated acid secretion in vagally and sympathetically denervated fundic pouches of dogs.

Rudman and Del Rio (1969b) analyzed various fragments of porcine secretin for lipolytic activity on rat adipose tissue and found that the His_1-Arg_{14} fragment showed about 0.5%, on a molar basis, of the activity of secretin itself. Fragment Thr_5-Val_{27}-NH_2 was inactive. The authors concluded that the lipolytic activity of secretin was exerted by structures in the N-terminal half of the molecule and that the His_1-Gly_4 sequence was essential for this activity, which was enhanced by structures C-terminal to this pentapeptide sequence.

It is evident that, different from the situation in enzymology, the intense search for more than 15 years for functional groups and active centers in gastrointestinal peptide hormones has in no case led to the identification of any structure that is indispensable for activity; important, yes, but indispensable, no. One possible reason for this may be that such structures do not exist. There is no reason, apart from speculation, to assume that peptide hormones act by the formation of centers of hypothetical enzymes, or by some other catalytic mechanism. Equally probable (Monod et al., 1963) is that they act by allosterically modifying structures in plasma membranes leading to changes in transmembrane potentials and ion translocations, as has been shown for the reaction of acetylcholine with its nicotinic receptor (Heidmann and Changeux, 1978).

Such allosteric changes may result in the activation of nucleotide cyclases. In the case of adenylate cyclase it has been suggested that hormones may act by mediating the binding of purine nucleotides to a regulatory site (Ross and Gilman, 1980). The consecutive changes in intracellular concentrations of cyclic nucleotides may be involved with what is recognized as the physiological cellular response to the hormone, although as far as is known at present they may also, for some hormones, be parallel, unrelated phenomena. Peptide hormone chemistry is still at a disadvantage with respect to enzymology. In the study of enzyme action the reactants—the enzyme and its substrate—are in many cases known. For peptide hormones the counterpart of the substrates, the hormones themselves, are often known, but their receptors, the counterparts of the enzymes, are not yet known in a single case. Little is known about the similarities and differences of receptors for the same hormone in different types of cells, and of interspecies differences. It has been shown that the cholecystokinin receptor is not identical in brain and in pancreas (Innis and Snyder, 1980) and that in the sphincter of Oddi there seem to be two different receptors for CCK, one excitatory and the other inhibitory (Behar and Biancani, 1980). Already earlier it had been shown that receptors for opioid peptides were of different types (Lord *et al.*, 1977).

It is probable that when the structures of the receptors are elucidated, much more will be understood about how peptide hormones act. The possibility, however, also exists that the receptor may be there only for binding of the hormone to its target cell and that the real action of the hormone is outside of the receptor–hormone complex. That this may be so may possibly be inferred from the work of Blundell *et al.* (1976) on glucagon. Glucagon is known to have a random structure in dilute aqueous solution but to be largely helical in crystals (Edelhoch and Lippoldt, 1969). From the analysis of crystallographic data, Blundell *et al.* (1976) suggested that glucagon might take up a similar conformation on receptor binding as it has in its crystals. This would imply that the 6–27 sequence would be helical, resulting in two hydrophobic patches for interaction with presumably corresponding hydrophobic patches on the receptor. The N-terminal histidylpentapeptide, known to be important for the biological action of glucagon, would remain flexible. The authors pointed out that with few exceptions secretin, VIP, and GIP have hydrophobic amino acid residues in the same positions as glucagon, even if these hydrophobic acids are, in most of these positions, not of the same type as in glucagon. Consequently, it would appear likely that glucagon, secretin, VIP, and GIP might bind to their receptors with roughly the same regions of their peptide chains. In each case this would leave the N-terminal pentapeptides free, which may be of importance for the biological actions of VIP and secretin, presumably less so for GIP.

Bedell *et al.* (1977) have pointed out that a certain symmetry due to the presence of two hydrophobic patches may be seen not only in the glucagon group of hormones but also in several other peptide hormones. They speculated on the possibility that binding of such hormones to their receptors involves interaction between these hydrophobic areas with corresponding symmetrically situated hydrophobic areas on the receptors. This would be a mechanism for increased security for receptor recognition by the hormone. Burgen *et al.* (1975) have discussed two models for the interaction of flexible peptide hormones with their receptors. According to one, the "lock and key" model, only that fraction of the many conformational forms of the hormone in solution that happens to have the correct conformation for interaction with the receptor will react with it. According to the other, the "zipper" model, only a short segment of the hormone needs to react with the receptor for linking to occur by conformational adaptation of the hormone, or both hormone and receptor.

IX. Some Mediators of Activity

Many years before cAMP or the inhibitory effect of methyl xanthines on the phosphodiesterase catalyzing its hydrolysis to 5′-adenosine monophosphate had been discovered (Sutherland *et al.*, 1965), Roth and Ivy (1944) described experiments showing that caffeine stimulated gastric acid secretion in man and in the cat, although not in dogs.

Methyl xanthines, theophylline mainly, have been one class of tools used in the experiments carried out in many laboratories attempting to define the role, if any, of cyclic nucleotides in the actions of different gastrointestinal hormones. Often the effects of a hormone on tissue concentrations of a cyclic nucleotide have been measured. It is obvious that the interpretation of such findings has been difficult. Not only are the cells producing the various gastrointestinal hormones dispersed among other cells, so are also the target cells for their action. If a hormone effects a change in the concentration of a cyclic nucleotide in, for instance, pancreatic tissue, it will not immediately be evident whether this change is due to changes in concentration of this nucleotide in the acinar cells, duct cells, cells of the blood vessels, or, as pointed out by Haig (1974), perhaps in cells of the endocrine pancreas. It could perhaps also be possible for the nucleotide concentration to increase in one type of cell and decrease in another, so that estimating the tissue content of the nucleotide would suggest that the hormone had not at all influenced the nucleotide concentration. This problem of cellular heterogeneity in the target organs for the hormones has been recognized for a long time (Levine, 1973). It is only more recently that serious attempts have been made to obtain homogeneous cell populations for the study of specific hormonal effects. Obviously the use of such cells will lead to other kinds of difficulties in the interpretation of the effects of hormones (Dormer *et al.*, 1981), especially of their effects *in vivo,* where their target cells may be exposed to important paracrine actions of other hormones coming from neighboring cells. Many attempts have been made to determine whether cAMP is involved as a second messenger in the action of gastrin. It was shown that, in the frog gastric mucosa *in vitro,* cAMP in all probability mediates the stimulating effects of theophylline and caffeine on acid secretion (Harris *et al.,* 1969). However, it was soon found by many workers that different stimulants of acid secretion seemed to act by different mechanisms.

Nakajima *et al.* (1970) found that, for the stimulation of acid secretion in *Necturus* mucosa by aminophylline, cAMP was a necessary intermediate but that pentagastrin stimulated secretion by a different mechanism. Perrier and Laster (1970) found that in several mammalian species histamine consistently stimulated parietal mucosal adenylate cyclase four- to fivefold, but that neither choline esters nor gastrin had any such effect. Certain prostaglandins that inhibit gastric acid secretion, however, also strongly stimulated the mucosal adenylate cyclase. Karppanen *et al.* (1974), with gastric mucosa and minced gastric tissue from guinea pigs, also found that cAMP might be the intracellular mediator of histamine-induced acid secretion, but nothing indicated that it was in any way involved in the stimulation of acid secretion by "pentagastrin."

The extensive work on the role of cAMP in gastric secretion has been discussed by Soll and Grossman (1978) and will not be discussed again here. Soll and Grossman concluded that it is plausible that the action of histamine on the parietal cell may be mediated by generation of cAMP, but that the mediators for gastrin and cholinergic stimulation remained unknown. Thompson *et al.* (1981), with an isolated highly enriched population of rat parietal cells, have come to a similar conclusion. Perhaps gastrin and cholinergic agonists do not need mediators? It seems as though the long-debated role of histamine in the stimulation of gastric acid secretion is at last supported by some factual information. The strong stimulating effect of histamine on gastric secretion was discovered by Popielski (1920), and it seemed possible that histamine might be "the gastric hormone" (Sacks *et al.,* 1932) until Komarov (1942) clearly showed gastrin to be an entity distinct from histamine. When Gregory and Tracy (1964) isolated gastrin, and gastrin was found on a molar basis to be 500 times stronger than histamine in stimulating gastric secretion (Makhlouf *et al.,* 1964), the importance of histamine seemed much less. However, when it was shown (Kahlson *et al.,* 1964) that gastrin stimulated the activity of histidine decarboxylase, and thereby the production of histamine in the fundic mucosa of the rat, the possibility that histamine functioned as "the final common mediator" for all forms of stimulation of gastric acid secretion (MacIntosh, 1938; Code, 1956) appeared reasonable. However, the rat was found to be a special case, and even in the rat it was

possible to inhibit acid secretion stimulated by gastrin without influencing the activity of gastrin on histidine decarboxylase (Caren *et
al.*, 1969).

At this stage it appeared possible that histamine might physiologically not have anything to do with regulation of acid secretion
(Johnson, 1971). The discovery of the histamine H_2 receptor antagonists (Black *et al.*, 1972) abruptly changed the picture, and when it
was found that not only acid secretion stimulated by histamine, but
also by gastrin and cholinergic agents, was inhibited by the antagonists, the common mediator role for histamine once again seemed
reasonable. Konturek *et al.* (1974), however, pointed to two additional
possible explanations: the H_2 receptor antagonists might be nonselective inhibitors of parietal cell receptors, or else there could be receptors
for acetylcholine, histamine, and gastrin on the parietal cell and blocking of the histamine receptors decreased the affinity of the other two
receptors for their agonists. It would now seem that it is the last-
mentioned possibility that comes closest to the actual situation. Soll
(1978) has shown with isolated rat parietal cells that these cells do
have specific receptors for histamine, gastrin, and cholinergic agonists
and that interactions between the different secretogogues in their ability to stimulate oxygen uptake could be demonstrated. Specific blocking of histamine-stimulated cAMP production by the prostaglandins E_2
and I_2 in isolated dog parietal cells has been described by Soll (1980).

Sanyal and Waton (1976) made observations in cats suggesting that
"pentagastrin" might release 5-hydroxytryptamine.

Jung and Greengard (1933) found that the contraction-stimulating
action of CCK on the guinea pig gallbladder was not inhibited by
atropine. They also stated cursorily that the ileum behaved in this
respect like the gallbladder. Later workers have come to the same
conclusion as Jung and Greengard concerning the action of CCK on the
gallbladder (Yau *et al.*, 1973), but only in part concerning its action on
the ileum. Naito *et al.* (1963) found that, in several mammalian
species, the stimulating effect of CCK on the motor activity of the small
intestine was inhibited by atropine.

Gregory and Tracy (1964) found that atropine, in conscious dogs,
inhibited the stimulating action of gastrin on gastric tone and motility
and practically abolished its action on intestinal tone and motility.
Hedner *et al.* (1967) confirmed that atropine inhibited the effect of CCK
on the guinea pig ileum *in vitro* and on the peristaltic movements of the
cat duodenum *in vivo*.

Bennett (1965) studied the effect of pG-17 s on various types of
smooth muscle *in vitro*. Gastrin had no effect on rat uterus. Guinea pig

ileum contracted, and this effect was not abolished by hexamethonium. It was, however, abolished by atropine, suggesting a stimulation by gastrin of postganglionic parasympathetic nerves to release acetylcholine. Vizi *et al.* (1972, 1973) directly measured the concentration of acetylcholine in the organ bath in which the contraction of strips of guinea pig ileum was stimulated by pG-17 ns, 8-CCK, "pentagastrin," and cerulein. All these peptides led to release of acetylcholine, and 8-CCK was the strongest in this respect. The authors concluded that the peptides stimulated the ganglionic cells of the myenteric plexus, which then released acetylcholine from the nerve terminals. Del Tacca *et al.* (1970) also had demonstrated the release of acetylcholine from guinea pig ileum and colon under the influence of cerulein. Much of the important work carried out in many laboratories to elucidate the physiological effects of various gastrointestinal peptides on gastrointestinal smooth muscle cannot be reviewed here. It may, nevertheless, be mentioned that Hutchison and Dockray (1981) confirmed that atropine abolished the contraction stimulation effect of acetylcholine and of low doses of 8-CCK on guinea pig ileum longitudinal muscle *in vitro*. However, they also found that the effects of large doses of 8-CCK, in contrast to those of acetylcholine, were only partly inhibited by atropine. Incubation of the muscle with high concentrations of substance P, however, not only desensitized it to substance P, but also abolished the atropine-resistant action of CCK on the muscle. This and other observations suggested that CCK might be acting by releasing both acetylcholine and substance P from the myenteric plexus.

Stewart and Burks (1980) have found that the stimulation by "pentagastrin" of isolated dog intestine seems to result from an action of the peptide on nonnicotinic cholinergic receptors on postganglionic cholinergic nerves. These authors also refer to other work, not discussed here, indicating that besides its action via liberation of acetylcholine, gastrin-like peptides may have other direct, inhibitory actions on smooth muscle cells.

Hutchison and Dockray (1980) have reported the interesting observation that dibutyryl-3',5'-cyclic guanosine monophosphate is a competitive antagonist also for the action of 8-CCK on the myenteric plexus, as it earlier had been shown to be for its actions on the acinar cells of the pancreas (Peikin *et al.*, 1979).

Several workers have investigated the effects of the gastrin-CCK type of peptides on the concentrations of cyclic nucleotides in smooth muscle. Andersson *et al.* (1976a) described work showing that in the gallbladder the concentrations of cAMP decrease during stimulation of contraction by CCK, whereas they increase in the sphincter of Oddi

during CCK-stimulated relaxation. In both tissues, the phosphodiesterase hydrolyzing cAMP was found to have been stimulated by CCK,
but in the sphincter there apparently occurred a parallel stimulation of
adenylate cyclase that effectively antagonized the action of the phosphodiesterase.

Amer and McKinney (1972) described experiments in which they
obtained stimulation of cAMP hydrolyzing phosphodiesterase, partially purified from rabbit gallbladder tissue, by CCK and gastrin at
low hormone concentrations. At high concentrations, enzyme inhibition was observed instead. They also found that G/CCK-4, at all concentrations, induced inhibition. Amer (1974) reported that CCK stimulated guanylate cyclase activity in rabbit gallbladder and also raised
tissue concentrations of cGMP.

Case et al. (1969) showed that dibutyryl cAMP, especially in combination with theophyllin, elicited a secretin-like, but not a
pancreozymin-like, effect on a saline-perfused preparation of the cat
pancreas. This suggested that cAMP might be the intracellular
mediator for the effects of secretin, but not of pancreozymin, on the
pancreas. Much subsequent work, in many laboratories, has supported
this hypothesis. For instance, Domschke et al. (1976) showed that the
amount of cAMP and of bicarbonate secreted by the human pancreas in
response to different doses of secretin varied remarkably similarly. This
type of evidence, although important, is nevertheless circumstantial,
since secretin might be stimulating cAMP production in other cells in
the pancreas than those involved in bicarbonate secretion. However,
Fölsch et al. (1980) found that secretin stimulated the accumulation of
cAMP in isolated pancreatic duct fragments from the rat; VIP also
stimulated cAMP accumulation, although much more weakly than
secretin, but CCK had no effect. Thus there is scarcely any doubt left
that secretin does stimulate cAMP in its target cells for stimulation of
bicarbonate secretion, it is not known how the increase in cellular
cAMP content is related to bicarbonate secretion, or, indeed, if it is
related.

Dopamine is known to stimulate pancreatic secretion. A possible
relation between the mechanism by which it does this and the known
secretin mechanism has been discussed by Vaysse et al. (1978).

A finding that secretin activates guanylate cyclase in various tissues
(Thompson et al., 1974) does not seem to have been followed up. It has
been clearly demonstrated that VIP stimulates adenylate cyclase activity in various tissues (Amiranoff et al., 1980). Whether this and the
ensuing increases in tissue cAMP concentrations are obligatory intermediate steps for the stimulating action of VIP on intestinal secretion

is not known. Some work suggests that they may not be so (Mailman, 1978; Lee and Coupar, 1980; Camilleri *et al.*, 1981).

It has been suggested that the action of VIP on cerebral arterioles may be mediated by prostaglandins (Wei *et al.*, 1980) and that its action on prolactin release is regulated by steroids (Rotsztejn *et al.*, 1980). Hokin and Hokin (1956) showed that pancreozymin, like acetylcholine, stimulated incorporation of ^{32}P into phospholipids in pigeon pancreas slices *in vitro*.

Bauduin and Cantraine (1972) found that this "phospholipid effect," in the rat pancreas *in vitro*, is not seen at low levels of stimulation of enzyme secretion, showing that it is not a necessary component of the secretory process as such. It seems, however, always to appear over a certain level of stimulation. It has generally been assumed to be due to turnover of already existing phospholipids, but some workers have found evidence that it also involves de novo synthesis of phospholipids (Patapanian *et al.*, 1981).

Kulka and Sternlicht (1968) found that a preparation of pancreozymin stimulated enzyme secretion from mouse pancreas *in vitro* and that this was accompanied by an increase of the pancreatic content of cAMP. Since then a vast amount of work has been carried out to analyze the effects of various peptide hormones on pancreatic enzyme secretion.

In parallel with this there has been an intense interest in the role of calcium in hormone-stimulated pancreatic enzyme secretion. Calcium in the incubation medium was found to be essential for the stimulation of steroid synthesis in adrenal rat glands *in vitro* by corticotropin (Birmingham *et al.*, 1953) and for the stimulation of amylase secretion from pigeon pancreas slices *in vitro* by acetylcholine (Hokin, 1966). The importance of calcium for intercellular communication was evident early (Douglas, 1968; Rasmussen, 1970). Attention was often paid to the effects on various secretory and contractile processes of calcium in the extracellular medium and to the uptake of calcium by cells. Friedmann and Park (1968) found that catecholamines and glucagon caused an efflux of Ca^{2+} from the perfused rat liver and that the efflux was apparently mediated by cAMP. Zimmerman *et al.* (1967) showed that the concentration of pancreatic juice calcium in dogs fell during stimulation of secretion with secretin. When, during continued secretin stimulation, enzyme secretion was induced by CCK the concentration of calcium in the juice increased markedly. Similar observations concerning pancreatic secretion of calcium were made in man by Goebell *et al.* (1970).

Case and Clausen (1973) suggested that the primary action of both

CCK and acetylcholine on the isolated uncinate pancreas of rats might be to increase influx of Na^+ into the acinar cells. This would result in release of Ca^{2+} from intracellular stores and enzyme secretion, provided that the cell membrane had not been depleted of calcium. In calcium-free media, CCK still stimulated release of calcium but no longer of enzymes. Atropine abolished the stimulatory effect of acetylcholine on release of both calcium and enzymes, but did not influence the effect of CCK.

Matthews et al. (1973) found that acetylcholine induced membrane depolarization, Ca^{2+} efflux, and amylase release, each with a similar dose-dependence, in segments of mouse pancreas in vitro. The effect of acetylcholine on Ca^{2+} efflux was inhibited by atropine, whereas the similar effect of pancreozymin was not affected. The authors considered the evidence to indicate the existence of two distinct membrane receptors, one responsive to pancreozymin and the other to acetylcholine. Activation of the receptors would result in membrane depolarization because of increased cation permeability, Ca^{2+} efflux, and amylase secretion.

Bauduin et al. (1971) found that although exogenous cAMP or dibutyryl cAMP did induce enzyme secretion in rat pancreas in vitro, the maximal effect was low compared to that achieved by pancreozymin or cholinergic stimulation. This made it doubtful that cAMP could function as an important mediator of the effects of the physiological stimulants. Furthermore, certain metabolic effects in the pancreas that followed on cholinergic stimulation or stimulation with pancreozymin did not take place on stimulation with the nucleotide.

Marois et al. (1972) showed that both secretin and CCK stimulated adenylate cyclase activity in homogenates of rat pancreas. Rutten et al. (1972) made the same observation, but found that a hundred times higher concentration of CCK than of secretin was necessary to obtain the same effect on the cyclase. Neither glucagon nor gastrin activated the cyclase.

Case (1973) considered the evidence implicating cAMP in the regulation of pancreatic enzyme secretion to be somewhat equivocal. He also pointed to a difference, in relation to calcium, of the release of certain hormones where the release is dependent on extracellular calcium concentrations and hormone-stimulated release of pancreatic enzymes where calcium is released from an intracellular pool instead.

A new element was brought into the discussion by the finding (Deschodt-Lanckman et al., 1974) that CCK could influence intracellular concentrations of cGMP. They found that the concentrations of rat pancreatic cAMP were elevated both in vivo and in vitro by secretin and by VIP, but not by pancreozymin, cerulein, or carbamylcholine. The levels of cGMP, however, were elevated by pancreozymin. The authors suggested that cAMP mediates the effects of the hormones that stimulate the secretion of water and inorganic electrolytes by the pancreas and that cGMP may be involved in the action of those hormones that stimulate the secretion of enzymes. For investigations in this field, the divalent cation ionophore A23187 (Reed and Lardy, 1972) has been very useful. Eimerl *et al.* (1974) found that A23187 stimulated enzyme secretion from rat pancreas *in vitro* and that the effect was not inhibited by atropine. The effect was, however, dependent on the presence of calcium in the incubation medium. Like carbamylcholine, the ionophore selectively stimulated the secretion of digestive enzymes. The secretion of lactic dehydrogenase was not influenced. The authors suggested that elevation of intracellular cGMP might be a function of the activation of the muscarinic cholinergic receptor and that calcium might be acting as a messenger from the receptor to the guanylate cyclase.

Williams and Lee (1974) found that stimulation of amylase secretion from mouse pancreas fragments *in vitro* was dependent on the presence of Ca^{2+} in the incubation medium but pointed out that this did not imply that calcium influx was necessary for stimulation of enzyme secretion by physiological stimulants.

Schreurs *et al.* (1976), with the isolated rabbit pancreas and pancreatic fragments, found that the stimulating effect of carbachol on enzyme secretion was only partly dependent on the presence of Ca^{2+} in the perfusate or incubation medium. Carbachol caused an efflux of Ca^{2+} from the pancreatic tissue. A23187, on the other hand, stimulated enzyme secretion only in the presence of extracellular calcium. The authors concluded that stimulation of enzyme secretion was in both cases dependent on an increase of cytoplasmic Ca^{2+} concentrations, the ionophore acting by increasing the permeability of the plasma membrane to Ca^{2+}, and carbachol acting by releasing Ca^{2+} from intracellular stores. As to the nature of these intracellular stores, Clemente and Meldolesi (1975) found that in guinea pig pancreatic tissue lobules very little calcium occurred free in the cytoplasm, most of it being distributed among the various particulate fractions with substantial variations in concentrations from one fraction to another.

An extensive investigation of the effects of CCK and other hormonal peptides on dispersed guinea pig pancreatic acinar cells has been carried out by Gardner and colleagues.

Christophe *et al.* (1976b) found that 8-CCK, as well as carbamylcholine, stimulated calcium efflux, amylase secretion, and increase of cellular cGMP content in such cells. The action of carbamylcholine, but not of 8-CCK, was inhibited by atropine. These effects still took place in a calcium-free incubation medium. Secretin did not influence cellular cGMP or calcium concentrations. A23187, like 8-CCK and carbamylcholine, also increased cellular cGMP concentrations and in this action it was not dependent on extracellular calcium, calcium outflux, and amylase secretion. However, it differed from the other two stimulants by increasing initial calcium influx also. The findings were interpreted to indicate that in pancreatic acinar cells the initial steps in the mechanism of action of 8-CCK and carbamylcholine were mobilization of cellular calcium followed by increases in cGMP concentrations.

Long and Gardner (1977) found that although 8-CCK did not activate adenylate cyclase in dispersed pancreatic cells, in high doses it could inhibit the stimulation of the cyclase by secretin. In homogenates of these cells, 8-CCK did activate adenylate cyclase.

It is impossible here to review all of the many important investigations that have been carried out on the role of cyclic nucleotides and of calcium in hormone-stimulated secretion of pancreatic enzymes, but see reviews by Case (1978), Christophe et al. (1980), and Gardner (1979). Relevant problems in electrophysiology have been discussed by Petersen (1976). Gardner (1979) has suggested, as a working hypothesis, that the pancreatic acinar cell carries specific receptors for cholinergic agents and for certain classes of peptides. The receptor class to which the CCK receptor belongs contains receptors also to gastrin and other gastrin-CCK related peptides. Likewise, the secretin receptor class has receptors for VIP and secretin. At least in some species, high doses of VIP or secretin may stimulate enzyme secretion concomitant with increases in intracellular cAMP. CCK, on reaction with its receptor, induces release of cellular calcium from storage pool(s), increases cellular cGMP concentrations, enzyme secretion, and depolarization of the cell plasma membrane, and causes electrical uncoupling of the cell when in situ in its tissue. Calcium efflux on stimulation with betanechol could also be demonstrated in isolated pancreatic acini (Dormer et al., 1981), where the electrical coupling of the cells (Iwatsuki and Petersen, 1978) presumably is intact. There is no general agreement on all details of this picture. Although most workers have found that CCK and cholinergic agents stimulate only efflux of Ca^{2+} from pancreatic acinar cells, others have found that influx of Ca^{2+} is stimulated also (Kondo and Schulz, 1976). Likewise, although most workers have found that the acinar cell membrane becomes depolarized under the impact of CCK, others have observed hyperpolarization instead (Kanno, 1972).

An obviously important question is how the calcium efflux and in-crease in intracellular cGMP are related to the actual process of en-zyme secretion. Some observations suggest that the rise in cGMP is not at all related to enzyme secretion but is a parallel, unrelated phenome-non (Gunther and Jamieson, 1979; Gardner and Rottman, 1980). Characterization of nucleotide-dependent pancreatic protein kinases (Mangeat *et al.*, 1978; Jensen and Gardner, 1978) and of the proteins that have been found to be phosphorylated in connection with secretagogue-stimulated secretion of pancreatic enzymes (Lambert *et al.*, 1975) may perhaps shed more light on this question.

X. (SUBGROUP 3b) HYPOTHETICAL HORMONES

This term does not refer here to the "candidate hormones" (Grossman, 1975), known endogenous substances that show hormone-like activities pharmacologically but whose hormonal status in phys-iology is yet unclear. It refers instead to the hypothetical substances of subgroup 3b (p. 238). One does not have to read long in gastrointestinal physiology before encountering phenomena that *might* be explained by the actions of substances of hormonal nature, although other explana-tions may seem reasonable also. Some examples, chosen from among many, more or less at random, follow. Annis and Hallenbeck (1951) found that exclusion of the pancreatic juice from the duodenum in fed dogs led to an increase in the secretion of pancreatic juice and that this could be prevented by replacement of the juice by a corresponding amount of bicarbonate solution. However, Hong *et al.* (1967) found that replacement of the excluded juice by normal pancreatic juice resulted in a much more pronounced inhibitory effect on pancreatic secretion and that this difference disappeared if the juice had been boiled. Does pan-creatic juice contain an inhibitory hormone for pancreatic secretion, or some substance releasing one? It has been shown, in rats and in chick-ens, that the feeding of trypsin inhibitors leads to an increase in the secretion of pancreatic enzymes (Lyman and Lepkovsky, 1957; Geratz and Hurt, 1970). Green and Lyman (1972) suggested that the effect of the inhibitors was indirect: trypsin, somehow, inhibited enzyme secre-tion, and this inhibition was removed by the trypsin inhibitors. Green and Lyman further suggested, on the basis of their own observations and with reference to the findings of others, that trypsin might act by preventing release of CCK. This is a plausible hypothesis, although the mechanism by which it could do so is not clear. Other explanations, including the involvement of hormonal factors other than CCK in trypsin-induced inhibition of pancreatic secretion, have not yet been ruled out.

Schulak and Kaplan (1975) found that, in addition to its known effect in thyroid-intact rats, gastrin also induced hypocalcemia in thyroparathyroidectomized rats. Consequently, there was some mechanism other than release of calcitonin involved in this case. The effect was abolished by gastrectomy. This might mean that gastrin is releasing a yet unknown hypocalcemic factor from the gastric tissue. Andersson and Uvnäs (1961) found that acidification of isolated duodenal pouches in dogs with fundic Pavlov pouches resulted in a pronounced inhibition of postprandial acid secretion in the pouches. Subsequently, Andersson et al. (1965) showed that acidification of the isolated duodenal bulb inhibited acid secretion in both Pavlov- and Heidenhain-type pouches, provided that this secretion had been evoked by gastrin. Secretion, in response to histamine, was not significantly inhibited. Acidification of short segments of the distal duodenum did not inhibit the effect of "pentagastrin." The name of bulbogastrone has been given to the substance(s) present in the duodenal bulb responsible for the inhibition of gastrin-stimulated acid secretion (Andersson et al., 1973). The nature of bulbogastrone is not yet known.

Stadil and Rehfeld (1974) found that in vagotomized duodenal ulcer patients, aspiration of the stomach contents markedly lowered plasma gastrin concentrations and hypothesized that some intraluminal gastrin-releasing factor was removed by the aspiration. Since the effect was seen only after vagotomy, this hypothetical factor might normally be suppressed by vagal branches to the gastric body or be dependent on intragastric pH. Is this hypothetical factor a hypothetical hormone?

Kelly et al. (1964) had found that in antrectomized Heidenhain pouch dogs the output of acid increased after total abdominal vagal denervation as compared to the output when vagal innervation was intact.

Stening and Grossman (1970) found that extragastric vagotomy in dogs increased the acid response to pentagastrin in previously vagally denervated pouches but not in the innervated stomach. They postulated that the extragastric vagatomy removed the effect of an inhibitor of unknown source and nature that was released by the vagal tone.

Lebedinskaja (1933) found that construction of a portacaval shunt in dogs strongly increased the secretion of gastric acid in the animals. Following this lead, an "intestinal phase hormone" of gastric secretion has been extensively purified by Orloff and co-workers (1979).

Skvortsova et al. (1972) found that removal of the duodenum in cats was followed by pronounced disturbances in the microstructure of the thyroid gland. This suggests that the duodenum may normally be exerting some kind of hormonal trophic influence on the thyroid gland.

Felber *et al.* (1974) described experiments in rats showing that extracts prepared from duodeni exposed to glucose stimulated pancreatic amylase, but not trypsin secretion, whereas extracts of duodeni exposed to a protein hydrolyzate stimulated secretion of trypsin, but not of amylase.

Some investigations suggest that the "gastrozymin" described by Blair *et al.* (1953) may indeed exist as a separate entity (Vagne and Mutt, 1977; Braganza *et al.,* 1976). A peptide fraction that induces the absorption of water and sodium in the rat duodenum has been obtained from porcine upper small intestine, and the active substance in it has been named sorbin (Pansu *et al.,* 1981). Inhibition of pancreatic secretion and gallbladder contraction by the assumably specific hormone(s) pancreotone (Harper *et al.,* 1979) or by the anticholecystokinetic hormone (Sarles *et al.,* 1979) has been described.

Comparing the incretin effect and plasma GIP concentrations in patients with small bowel resection, Lauritsen *et al.* (1980) concluded that as yet unknown intestinal hormonal factors act as incretins in concert with GIP.

An incretin released from the intestine, not only by glucose but also by inorganic electrolytes, has been described by Levin *et al.* (1979). Partial purification of villikinin (Kokas and Ludány, 1930, 1934) has been described (Kokas and Johnston, 1965; Kokas *et al.,* 1971), but final characterization remains.

XI. Conclusions

The field of gastrointestinal hormones is rapidly expanding, and the combined number of publications describing the cellular origins of these substances, their biosynthesis, isolation, structures, evolutionary relationships, organic chemical synthesis, physiological and pharmacological actions, involvement in pathological states, clinical applications, and so on is now running into tens of thousands. Despite the vast amount of information available, it is as yet possible only to tell *what* these hormones do (stimulate the secretion of pancreatic bicarbonate, activate adenylate cyclase, etc.), not *how* they do it.

There are still many observations in physiology suggesting the involvement of hormonal factors where the presumptive hormone has not yet been identified, either as being one of the already known hormones, possibly acting in concert with some other hormone or modifying neural activity, or as a previously unknown hormone.

With the continuing development of even more efficient methods for the isolation of peptides and for the determination of peptide structures, it may be expected that an increasing number of naturally occurring peptides will be isolated. This will place a heavy responsibility on physiologists and pharmacologists not to overlook the properties of such peptides as may be useful for physiological and pharmacological experimentation or for use in medicine.

REFERENCES

Abel, J. J. (1926). Crystalline insulin. *Proc. Natl. Acad. Sci. U.S.A.* **12**, 132–136.

Adelson, J. W., and Rothman, S. S. (1974). Selective pancreatic enzyme secretion due to a new peptide called chymodenin. *Science* **183**, 1087–1089.

Adelson, J. W., Nelbach, M. E., Chang, R., Glaser, C. B., and Yates, G. B. (1980). Chymodenin: Between "factor" and "hormone." *In* "Gastrointestinal Hormones" (G. B. J. Glass, ed.), pp. 387–396. Raven, New York.

Adkins, R. B., Ende, N., and Gobbel, W., Jr. (1967). A correlation of parietal cell activity with ultrastructural alterations. *Surgery* **62**, 1059–1069.

Adler, M., Mestdagh, M., De Neef, Ph., König, W., Christophe, J., and Robberecht, P. (1980). In vivo effects of five secretin analogs on fluid and potassium secretions from the rat pancreas. *Life Sci.* **26**, 1175–1181.

Adrian, T. E., Bloom, S. R., Besteman, H. S., Barnes, A. J., Cooke, T. J. C., Russell, R. C. G., and Faber, R. G. (1977). Mechanism of pancreatic polypeptide release in man. *Lancet* **I**, 161–164.

Agarwal, K. L., Kenner, G. W., and Sheppard, R. C. (1968a). Peptides. Part XXVII. Synthesis of five heptadecapeptides related to human gastrin. *J. Chem. Soc. (C)* 1384–1391.

Agarwal, K. L., Beacham, J., Bentley, P. H., Gregory, R. A., Kenner, G. W., Sheppard, R. C., and Tracy, H. J. (1968b). Isolation, structure and synthesis of ovine and bovine gastrins. *Nature (London)* **219**, 614–615.

Agarwal, K. L., Kenner, G. W., and Sheppard, R. C. (1969a). Structure and synthesis of canine gastrin. *Experientia* **25**, 346–348.

Agarwal, K. L., Kenner, G. W., and Sheppard, R. C. (1969b). Feline gastrin. An example of peptide sequence analysis by mass spectrometry. *J. Am. Chem. Soc.* **91**, 3096–3097.

Agarwal, K. L., Grudzinski, S., Kenner, G. W., Rogers, N. H., Sheppard, R. C., and McGuigan, J. E. (1971). Immunochemical differentiation between gastrin and related peptide hormones through a novel conjugation of peptides to proteins. *Experientia* **27**, 514–515.

Ågren, G. (1934). Über die pharmakodynamischen Wirkungen und chemischen Eigenschaften des Sekretins. *Scand. Arch. Physiol.* **70**, 10–87.

Ahrén, B., Alumets, J., Ericsson, M., Fahrenkrug, J., Fahrenkrug, L., Håkanson, R., Hedner, P., Lorén, I., Melander, A., Rerup, C., and Sundler, F. (1980). VIP occurs in intrathyroidal nerves and stimulates thyroid hormone secretion. *Nature (London)* **287**, 343–345.

Albinus, M., Blair, E. L., Grund, E. R., Reed, J. D., Sanders, D. J., Gomez-Pan, A., Schally, A. V., and Besser, G. M. (1975). The mechanism whereby growth hormone-release inhibiting hormone (somatostatin) inhibits food stimulated gastric acid secretion in the cat. *Agents Actions* **5**, 306–309.

Alumets, J., Håkanson, R., Sundler, F., and Chang, K. J. (1978). Leu-enkephalin-like material in nerves and enterochromaffin cells in the gut. *Histochemistry* **56**, 187–196.

Alumets, J., Schaffalitzky de Muckadell, O., Fahrenkrug, J., Sundler, F., Håkanson, R., and Uddman, R. (1979). A rich VIP nerve supply is characteristic of sphincters. *Nature (London)* **280**, 155–156.

Amer, M. S. (1974). Cyclic guanosine 3′,5′-monophosphate and gall bladder contraction. *Gastroenterology* **67**, 333–337.

Amer, M. S., and McKinney, G. R. (1972). Studies with cholecystokinin in vitro. IV. Effects of cholecystokinin and related peptides on phosphodiesterase. *J. Pharmacol. Exp. Ther.* **183**, 535–548.

Amiranoff, B., Laburthe, M., and Rosselin, G. (1980). Potentiation by guanine nucleotides of the VIP-induced adenylate cyclase stimulation in intestinal epithelial cell membranes. *Life Sci.* **26**, 1905–1911.

Anastasi, A., Erspamer, V., and Cei, J. M. (1964). Isolation and amino acid sequence of physalaemin, the main active polypeptide of the skin of *Physalaemus fuscumaculatus*. *Arch. Biochem. Biophys.* **108**, 341–348.

Anastasi, A., Erspamer, V., and Endean, R. (1967). Isolation and structure of caerulein, an active decapeptide from the skin of *Hyla caerulea*. *Experientia* **23**, 699–700.

Anastasi, A., Erspamer, V., and Endean, R. (1968a). Isolation and amino acid sequence of caerulein, the active decapeptide of the skin of *Hyla caerulea*. *Arch. Biochem. Biophys.* **125**, 57–68.

Anastasi, A., Bernardi, L., Bertaccini, G., Bosisio, G., de Castiglione, R., Erspamer, V., Goffredo, O., and Impicciatore, M. (1968b). Synthetic peptides related to caerulein. Note 1. *Experientia* **24**, 771–773.

Anastasi, A., Erspamer, V., and Bucci, M. (1971). Isolation and structure of bombesin and alytesin, two analogous active peptides from the skin of the European amphibians Bombina and Alytes. *Experientia* **27**, 166–167.

Anderson, J. C., Barton, M. A., Gregory, R. A., Hardy, P. M., Kenner, G. W., MacLeod, J. K., Preston, J., Sheppard, R. C., and Morley, J. S. (1964). Synthesis of gastrin. *Nature (London)* **204**, 933–934.

Andersson, K.-E., Andersson, R. G. G., Hedner, P., and Persson, C. G. A. (1976a). Effect of cholecystokinin on the adenylate cyclase activity in cat sphincter of Oddi. *Acta Physiol. Scand.* **98**, 269–271.

Andersson, S. (1973). *Proc. Nobel Symp., 16th, Stockholm, 1970*.

Andersson, S., and Nilsson, G. (1974). Appearance of gastrin in perfusates from the isolated gastric antrum of dogs. *Scand. J. Gastroenterol.* **9**, 619–621.

Andersson, S., and Uvnäs, B. (1961). Inhibition of postprandial gastric secretion in Pavlov pouches by instillation of hydrochloric acid into the duodenal bulb. *Gastroenterology* **41**, 486–490.

Andersson, S., Elwin, C.-E., and Uvnäs, B. (1958). The effect of exclusion of the antrum and duodenum, and subsequent resection of the antrum, on the acid secretion in Pavlov pouch dogs. *Gastroenterology* **34**, 636–658.

Andersson, S., Nilsson, G., and Uvnäs, B. (1965). Inhibition of gastric secretion by acid in proximal and distal duodenal pouches. *Acta Physiol. Scand.* **65**, 191–192.

Andersson, S., Nilsson, G., Sjödin, L., and Uvnäs, B. (1973). Mechanism of duodenal inhibition of gastric acid secretion. *Proc. Nobel Symp., 16th, Stockholm 1970* pp. 223–238.

Andersson, S., Chang, D., Folkers, K., and Rossell, S. (1976). Inhibition of gastric acid secretion in dogs by neurotensin. *Life Sci.* **19**, 367–370.

André, C., Lambert, R., and Vagne, M. (1972). Effect of secretin on gastric mucus secretions in humans. *Acta Hepato-Gastroenterol.* **19**, 12.

Anika, S. M., Houpt, T. R., and Houpt, K. A. (1980). Insulin as a satiety hormone. *Physiol. Behav.* **25**, 21–23.

Annis, D., and Hallenbeck, G. A. (1951). Effect of excluding pancreatic juice from duodenum on secretory response of pancreas to a meal. *Proc. Soc. Exp. Biol. Med.* **77**, 383–388.

Arimura, A., Sato, H., Dupont, A., Nishi, N., and Schally, A. V. (1975). Somatostatin: abundance of immunoreactive hormone in rat stomach and pacnreas. *Science* **189**, 1007–1009.

Arnould, Y., Bellens, R., Franckson, J. R. M., and Conrad, V. (1963). Insulin response and glucose-C^{14} disappearance rate during the glucose tolerance test in the unanesthetized dog. *Metabolism* **12**, 1122–1131.

Assan, R., and Slusher, N. (1972). Structure/function and structure/immunoreactivity relationships of the glucagon molecule and related synthetic peptides. *Diabetes* **21**, 843–855.

Assan, R., Rosselin, G., and Dolais, J. (1967). Effets sur la glucagonémie des perfusions et ingestions d'acides aminés. *J. Annu. Diabetol. Hotel Dieu* **7**, 25–41.

Austen, B. M. (1979). Predicted secondary structures of amino-terminal extension sequences of secreted proteins. *FEBS Lett.* **103**, 308–313.

Avioli, L. V., Birge, S. J., Scott, S., and Shieber, W. (1969). Role of the thyroid gland during glucagon-induced hypocalcemia in the dog. *Am. J. Physiol.* **216**, 939–945.

Aviv, P., and Leder, P. (1972). Purification of biologically active globin messenger RNA by chromatography on oligothymidylic acid-cellulose. *Proc. Natl. Acad. Sci. U.S.A.* **69**, 1408–1412.

Babkin, B. P. (1950). "Secretory Mechanism of the Digestive Glands." Harper (Hoeber), New York.

Baker, J. B., Simmer, R. L., Glenn, K. C., and Cunningham, D. D. (1979). Thrombin and epidermal growth factor become linked to cell surface receptors during mitogenic stimulation. *Nature (London)* **278**, 743–745.

Banting, F. G., Best, C. H., Collip, J. B., and McLeod, J. J. R. (1922). The preparation of pancreatic extracts containing insulin. *Trans. R. Soc. Can.* **16**, 27–29.

Barbezat, G. O., and Grossman, M. I. (1971). Intestinal secretion: stimulation by peptides. *Science* **174**, 422–423.

Barbezat, G. O., and Grossman, M. I. (1975). Release of cholecystokinin by acid. *Proc. Soc. Exp. Biol. Med.* **148**, 463–467.

Barbezat, G. O., Isenberg, J. I., and Grossman, M. I. (1972). Diuretic action of secretin in dog. *Proc. Soc. Exp. Biol. Med.* **139**, 211–215.

Barlet, J. P. (1974). The influence of porcine calcitonin given intragastrally on restraint-induced gastric ulcers in pigs. *Horm. Metab. Res.* **6**, 517–521.

Barnes, A. J., and Bloom, S. R. (1976). Pancreatectomised man: a model for diabetes without glucagon. *Lancet* **I**, 219–221.

Baron, D. N., Newman, F., and Warrick, A. (1958). The effects of secretin on urinary volume and electrolytes in normal subjects and patients with chronic pancreatic disease. *Experientia* **14**, 30–32.

Barreras, R. F. (1973). Calcium and gastric secretion. *Gastroenterology* **64**, 1168–1184.

Barrowman, J. A., and Mayston, P. D. (1971). The influence of chronic administration of pentagastrin upon the pancreas of hypophysectomized rats. *J. Physiol. (London)* **219**, 26p–28p.

Barrowman, J. A., and Mayston, P. D. (1974). The trophic influence of cholecystokinin on the rat pancreas. *J. Physiol. (London)* **238**, 73p–75p.

Basso, N., Lezoche, E., Speranza, V., and Walsh, J. H. (1981). *Int. Symp. Brain-Gut Axis, New Frontier Abstr.*

Bataille, D., Freychet, P., and Rosselin, G. (1974). Interactions of glucagon, gut glucagon, vasoactive intestinal polypeptide and secretin with liver and fat cell plasma membranes: Binding to specific sites and stimulation of adenylate cyclase. *Endocrinology* **95**, 713–721.

Bataille, D., Gespach, C., Tatemoto, K., Marie, J. C., Coudray, A. M., Rosselin, G., and Mutt, V. (1981). Bioactive enteroglucagon (oxyntomodulin): Present knowledge on its chemical structure and its biological activities. *Peptides* **2** (Suppl. 2), 41–44.

Bauduin, H., and Cantraine, F. (1972). "Phospholipid effect" and secretion in the rat pancreas. *Biochim. Biophys. Acta* **270**, 248–253.

Bauduin, H., Rochus, L., Vincent, D., and Dumont, J. E. (1971). Role of cyclic 3′,5′-AMP in the action of physiological secretagogues on the metabolism of rat pancreas in vitro. *Biochim. Biophys. Acta* **252**, 171–183.

Bayliss, W. M. (1920). "Principles of General Physiology," 3rd Ed. Longman Green, London.

Bayliss, W. M., and Starling, E. H. (1902a). On the causation of the so-called "peripheral reflex secretion" of the pancreas. *Proc. R. Soc.* **69**, 352–353.

Bayliss, W. M., and Starling, E. H. (1902b). The mechanism of pancreatic secretion. *J. Physiol. (London)* **28**, 325–353.

Bayliss, W. M., and Starling, E. H. (1904). The chemical regulation of the secretory process. *Proc. R. Soc.* **73**, 310–322.

Beacham, J., Bentley, P. H., Gregory, R. A., Kenner, G. W., MacLeod, J. N., and Sheppard, R. C. (1966). Synthesis of human gastrin I. *Nature (London)* **209**, 585–586.

Becker, H. D., Reeder, D. D., and Thompson, J. C. (1973). Effect of glucagon on circulating gastrin. *Gastroenterology* **65**, 28–35.

Becker, N. M. (1893). Contributions à la physiologie et à la pharmacologie de la glande pancreatique. *Arch. Sci. Biol. St. Petersburg* **II**, 433–461.

Beddell, C. R., Sheppey, G. C., Blundell, T. L., Sasaki, K., Dockerill, S., and Goodford, P. J. (1977). Symmetrical features in polypeptide hormone–receptor interactions. *Int. J. Pept. Protein Res.* **9**, 161–165.

Bedi, B. S., Gillespie, G., and Gillespie, I. E. (1967). Effects of a specific gastrin antagonist on gastric acid secretion in pouch dogs. *Lancet* **I**, 1240–1243.

Behar, J., and Biancani, P. (1977). Effect of cholecystokinin-octapeptide on lower esophageal sphincter. *Gastroneterology* **73**, 57–61.

Behar, J., and Biancani, P. (1980). Effect of cholecystokinin and the octapeptide of cholecystokinin on the feline sphincter of Oddi and gall bladder. *J. Clin. Invest.* **66**, 1231–1239.

Beijer, H. J. M., Hulstaert, P. F., Brouwer, F. A. S., and Charbon, G. A. (1979). The effect of secretin on peripheral arterial blood flow. *Arch. Int. Pharmacodyn.* **240**, 269–277.

Bennett, A. (1965). Effect of gastrin on isolated smooth muscle preparations. *Nature (London)* **208**, 170–173.

Benoit, R., Böhlen, P., Brazeau, P., Ling, N., and Guillemin, R. (1980). Isolation and characterization of rat pancreatic somatostatin. *Endocrinology* **107**, 2127–2129.

Bentley, P. H., Kenner, G. W., and Sheppard, R. C. (1966). Structures of human gastrins I and II. *Nature (London)* **209**, 583–585.

Bernardi, L., Bertaccini, G., Bosisio, G., Bucci, R., de Castiglione, R., Erspamer, V., Goffredo, O., and Impicciatore, M. (1972). Synthetic peptides related to caerulein. Note 2. *Experientia* **28**, 7–9.

Berson, S. A., and Yalow, R. S. (1958). Isotopic tracers in the study of diabetes. *Adv. Biol. Med. Phys.* **6**, 349–421.

Berson, S. A., and Yalow, R. S. (1959). Quantitative aspects of the reaction between insulin and insulin-binding antibody. *J. Clin. Invest.* **38**, 1996–2016.

Berson, S. A., and Yalow, R. S. (1971). Nature of immunoreactive gastrin extracted from tissues of gastrointestinal tract. *Gastroenterology* **60**, 215–222.

Berson, S. A., and Yalow, R. S. (1973). "Methods in Investigative and Diagnostic Endocrinology," Vol. 2B, Part 3. North-Holland Publ., Amsterdam.

Berstad, A. (1969). Stimulation of gastric secretion of pepsin by secretin in man. *Scand. J. Gastroenterol.* **4**, 617–622.

Berstad, A., and Petersen, H. (1970). Dose–response relationship of the effect of secretin on acid and pepsin secretion in man. *Scand. J. Gastroenterol.* **5**, 647–654.

Bertaccini, G., and Dobrilla, G. (1980). Histamine H_2-receptor antagonists: old and new generation. Pharmacology and clinical use. *Ital. J. Gastroenterol.* **12**, 309–314.

Bertaccini, G., de Castiglione, R., and Impicciatore, M. (1974a). Preliminary data on the inhibition of pentagastrin stimulated gastric secretion induced by some natural and synthetic peptides. *Br. J. Pharmacol.* **52**, 463p.

Bertaccini, G., Erspamer, V., Melchiorri, P., and Sopranzi, N. (1974b). Gastrin release by bombesin in the dog. *Br. J. Pharmacol.* **52**, 219–225.

Beswick, F. B., Howat, H. T., and Morris, A. I. (1968). The effects of gastrin and peptide analogues related to gastrin on cats. *J. Physiol. (London)* **197**, 71p–72p.

Beubler, E., and Lembeck, F. (1979). Inhibition of stimulated fluid secretion in the rat small and large intestine by opiate agonists. *Naunyn-Schmiedebergs Arch. Pharmacol.* **306**, 113–118.

Binder, H. J., Lemp, G. F., and Gardner, J. D. (1980). Receptors of vasoactive intestinal peptide and secretion on small intestinal epithelial cells. *Am. J. Physiol.* **238**, G190–G196.

Birmingham, M. K., Elliot, F. H., and Valère, P. H.-L. (1953). The need for the presence of calcium for the stimulation in vitro of rat adrenal glands by adrenocorticotrophic hormone. *Endocrinology* **53**, 687–689.

Black, J. W., Duncan, W. A. M., Durant, C. J., Ganellin, C. R., and Parsons, E. M. (1972). Definition and antagonism of histamine H_2-receptors. *Nature (London)* **236**, 385–390.

Blair, E. L., Harper, A. A., and Lake, H. J. (1953). The pepsin-stimulating effects of gastric and intestinal extracts in cats. *J. Physiol. (London)* **121**, 20p–21p.

Blair, E. L., Harper, A. A., Lake, H. J., Reed, J. D., and Scratcherd, T. (1961). A simple method of preparing gastrin. *J. Physiol. (London)* **156**, 11p–13p.

Blair, E. L., Harper, A. A., Lake, H. J., and Reed, J. D. (1963). Characteristics of responses to "gastrin" extracts. *J. Physiol. (London)* **165**, 81p–82p.

Blair, E. L., Brown, J. C., Harper, A. A., and Scratcherd, T. (1966). A gastric phase of pancreatic secretion. *J. Physiol. (London)* **184**, 812–824.

Blanchard, M. H., and King, M. V. (1966). Evidence of association of glucagon from optical rotatory dispersion and concentration-difference spectra. *Biochem. Biophys. Res. Commun.* **25**, 298–303.

Bleich, H. E., Cutnell, J. D., and Glasel, J. A. (1976). Intramolecular microdynamical and conformational parameters of peptides from ^1H and ^{13}C NMR spin-lattice relaxation. Tetragastrin. *Biochemistry* **15**, 2455–2466.

Blobel, G., and Dobberstein, B. (1975). Transfer of proteins across membranes. I. Presence of proteolytically processed and unprocessed nascent immunoglobulin light chains on membrane-bound ribosomes of murine myeloma. *J. Cell. Biol.* **67**, 835–851.

Blobel, G., and Sabatini, D. D. (1971). Ribosome-membrane interaction in eukaryotic cells. *In* "Biomembranes" (L. A. Manson, ed.), Vol. 2, pp. 193–195. Plenum, New York.

Bloom, S. R. (1977). Hormones of the gastrointestinal tract. *Rec. Adv. Med.* **17**, 357–386.

Bloom, S. R., ed. (1978). "Gut Hormones." Churchill, London.

Bloom, S. R., and Edwards, A. V. (1979). The relationship between release of vasoactive intestinal peptide in the salivary gland of the cat in response to parasympathetic stimulation and the atropine resistant vasodilatation. *J. Physiol. (London)* **295**, 35p–36p.

Bloom, S. R., and Polak, J. M. (1978). Gut hormone overview. *In* "Gut Hormones" (S. R. Bloom, ed.), pp. 3–18. Churchill, London.

Bloom, S. R., and Polak, J. M. (1980a). *Int. Symp. Gut Horm., 3rd, Cambridge, Sept. 14–18* (Abstr.).

Bloom, S. R., and Pollak, J. M. (1980b). Gut hormones. *Adv. Clin. Chem.* **21**, 177–244.

Bloom, S. R., and Polak, J. M. (1981). "Gut Hormones," 2nd Ed. Churchill, London.

Bloom, S. R., Mitchell, S. J., Greenberg, G. R., Christofides, N., Domschke, W., Domschke, S., Mitznegg, P., and Demling, L. (1978). Release of VIP, secretin and motilin after duodenal acidification in man. *Acta Hepato-Gastroenterol.* **25**, 365–368.

Bloom, S. R., Bryant, M. G., Polak, J. M., van Noorden, S., and Wharton, J. (1979). Vasoactive intestinal peptide-like immunoreactivity in salivary glands of the rat. *J. Physiol. (London)* **289**, 23 p.

Blundell, T. L., Cutfield, J. F., Cutfield, S. M., Dodson, E. J. Dodson, G. G., Hodgkin, D. C., Mercola, D. A., and Vijayan, M. (1971). Atomic postitions in rhombohedral 2-zinc insulin crystals. *Nature (London)* **231**, 506–511.

Blundell, T. L., Dockerill, S., Sasaki, K., Tickle, I. J., and Wood, S. P. (1976). The relation of structure to storage and receptor binding of glucagon. *Metabolism* **25** (Suppl. 1), 1331–1339.

Bodanszky, A., Ondetti, M. A., Mutt, V., and Bodanszky, M. (1969). Synthesis of secretin. IV. Secondary structure in a miniature protein. *J. Am. Chem. Soc.* **91**, 944–949.

Bodanszky, A., Bodanszky, M., Jorpes, E. J., Mutt, V., and Ondetti, M. A. (1970). Molecular architecture of peptide hormones optical rotatory dispersion of cholecystokinin-pancreozymin, bradykinin and 6-glycine bradykinin. *Experientia* **26**, 948–950.

Bodanszky, M., and Fink, M. L. (1976). Studies on the conformation of secretin. The position of the helical stretch. *Bioorg. Chem.* **5**, 275–282.

Bodanszky, M., Ondetti, M. A., Levine, S. D., Narayanan, V. L., von Saltza, M., Sheehan, J. T., Williams, N. J., and Sabo, E. F. (1966). Synthesis of a heptacosapeptide amide with the hormonal activity of secretin. *Chem. Ind. (London)* 1757–1758.

Bodanszky, M., Ondetti, M. A., Levine, S. D., and Williams, N. J. (1967). Synthesis of secretin. II. The stepwise approach. *J. Am. Chem. Soc.* **89**, 6753–6757.

Bodanszky, M., Chaturvedi, N., Hudson, D., and Itoh, M. (1972). Cholecystokinin-pancreozymin. I. The synthesis of peptides corresponding to the N-terminal sequence. *J. Org. Chem.* **37**, 2303–2307.

Bodanszky, M., Bodanszky, A., Klausner, Y. S., and Said, S. I. (1974a). A preferred conformation in the vasoactive intestinal peptide (VIP). Molecular architecture of gastrointestinal hormones. *Bioorg. Chem.* **3**, 133–140.

Bodanszky, M., Klausner, Y. S., Lin, C. Y., Mutt, V., and Said, S. I. (1974b). Synthesis of the vasoactive intestinal peptide (VIP). *J. Am. Chem. Soc.* **96**, 4973–4978.

Bodanszky, M., Fink, M. L., Funk, K. W., and Said, S. I. (1976). A re-examination of the conformation of secretin in water. *Clin. Endocrinol.* **5** (Suppl.), 195s–200s.

Bodanszky, M., Natarajan, S., Hahne, W., and Gardner, J. D. (1977). Cholecystokinin (pancreozymin). 3. Synthesis and properties of an analogue of the C-terminal heptapeptide with serine sulfate replacing tyrosine sulfate. *J. Med. Chem.* **20,** 1047–1050.

Bodanszky, M., Bodanszky, A., and Said, S. I. (1978a). Synthesis of the avian vasoactive intestinal peptide (VIP). *Fed. Proc. Fed. Am. Soc. Exp. Biol.* **37,** 1829/3071.

Bodanszky, M., Martinez, J., Priestley, G. P., Gardner, J. D., and Mutt, V. (1978b). Cholecystokinin (pancreozymin). 4. Synthesis and properties of a biologically active analogue of the C-terminal heptapeptide with ε-hydroxynorleucine sulfate replacing the tyrosine sulfate. *J. Med. Chem.* **21,** 1030–1035.

Bodanszky, M., Martinez, J., Walker, M., Gardner, J. D., and Mutt, V. (1980). Cholecystokinin (pancreozymin). 5. Hormonally active desamino derivative of Tyr(SO₃H)-Met-Gly-Trp-Met-Asp-Phe-NH₂. *J. Med. Chem.* **23,** 82–85.

Boden, G., Essa, N., Owen, O. E., and Reichle, F. A. (1974). Effects of intraduodenal administration of HCl and glucose on circulating immunoreactive secretin and insulin concentrations. *J. Clin. Invest.* **53,** 1185–1193.

Boden, G., Essa, N., and Owen, O. E. (1975). Effects of intraduodenal amino acids, fatty acids, and sugars on secretin concentrations. *Gastroenterology* **68,** 722–727.

Böhlen, P., Brazeau, P., Benoit, R., Ling, N., Esch, F., and Guillemin, R. (1980). Isolation and amino acid composition of two somatostatin-like peptides from ovine hypothalamus: somatostatin-28 and somatostatin-25. *Biochem. Biophys. Res. Commun.* **96,** 725–734.

Boissonnas, R. A., Guttmann, St., and Jaquenoud, P.-A. (1960). Synthèse de la l-arginyl-l-propyl -1-propyl-glycyl-1- phénylalanyl-l- séryl-1-propyl-1-phénylalanyl -1-arginine, un nonapeptide présentant les propriétés de la bradykinine. *Helv. Chim. Acta* **43,** 1349–1358.

Boissonnas, R. A., Franz, J., and Stürmer, E. (1963). On the chemical characterization of substance P. *Ann. N.Y. Acad. Sci.* **104,** 376–377.

Bolton, J. E., Munday, K. A., Parsons, B. J., and Poat, J. A. (1974). Effects of angiotensin on fluid transport by rat jejunum in vivo. *J. Physiol. (London)* **241,** 33p–34p.

Bonfils, S., Fromageot, P., and Rosselin, G. (1977). "Hormonal Receptors in Digestive Tract Physiology." North-Holland Publ., Amsterdam.

Bornet, H., and Edelhoch, H. (1971). Polypeptide hormone interaction. I. Glucagon detergent interaction. *J. Biol. Chem.* **246,** 1785–1792.

Bourdaux, A.-M., Giudicelli, Y., Rebourcet, M.-C., Nordmann, J., and Nordmann, R. (1980). Influence of some gastrointestinal hormones on adipose tissue lipoprotein lipase activity in vitro: evidence of a stimulatory effect of pancreozymin and gastrin. *Biochem. Biophys. Res. Commun.* **95,** 212–219.

Boyns, D. R., Jarrett, R. J., and Keen, H. (1966). Intestinal hormones and plasma-insulin. *Lancet* **I,** 409–410.

Bradley, E. L., III, Wenger, J., Smith, R. B., III, and Galambos, J. T. (1975). Serum calcium responses to exogenous secretin. *Arch. Surg.* **110,** 1221–1223.

Braganza, J. M., Howat, H. T., and Kay, G. H. (1976). A comparison of the pepsin stimulating effects of secretin preparations. *J. Physiol. (London)* **258,** 63–72.

Brawerman, G., Mendecki, J., and Lee, S. Y. (1972). A procedure for the isolation of mammalian messenger ribonucleic acid. *Biochemistry* **11,** 637–641.

Brazeau, P., Vale, W., Burgus, R., Ling, N., Butcher, M., Rivier, J., and Guillemin, R. (1973). Hypothalamic polypeptide that inhibits the secretion of immunoreactive pituitary growth hormone. *Science* **179,** 77–79.

Brewer, H. B., Jr., Keutmann, H. T., Potts, J. T., Jr., Reisfeld, R. A., Schlueter, R., and Munson, P. L. (1968). Isolation and chemical properties of porcine thyrocalcitonin. *J. Biol. Chem.* **243,** 5739–5747.

Bromer, W. W., Sinn, L. G., Staub, A., and Behrens, O. K. (1956). The amino acid sequence of glucagon. *J. Am. Chem. Soc.* **78**, 3858–3860.

Bromer, W. W., Sinn, L. G., and Behrens, O. K. (1957). The amino acid sequence of glucagon. V. Location of amide groups, acid degradation studies and summary of sequential evidence. *J. Am. Chem. Soc.* **79**, 2807–2810.

Bromer, W. W., Boucher, M. E., and Koffenberger, J. E., Jr. (1971). Amino acid sequence of bovine glucagon. *J. Biol. Chem.* **246**, 2822–2827.

Broomé, A., and Olbe, L. (1969). Studies on the mechanism of the antrectomy-induced suppression of the maximal acid response to histamine in duodenal ulcer patients. *Scand. J. Gastroenterol.* **4**, 281–289.

Brown, J. C. (1967). Presence of a gastric motor-stimulating property in duodenal extracts. *Gastroenterology* **52**, 225–229.

Brown, J. C. (1974). "Enterogastrone" and other new gut peptides. *Med. Clin. North Am.* **58**, 1347–1358.

Brown, J. C., and Dryburgh, J. R. (1971). A gastric inhibitory polypeptide II: The complete amino acid sequence. *Can. J. Biochem.* **49**, 867–872.

Brown, J. C., and Parkes, C. O. (1967). Effect on fundic pouch motor activity of stimulatory and inhibitory fractions separated from pancreozymin. *Gastroenterology* **53**, 731–736.

Brown, J. C., and Pederson, R. A. (1970a). A multiparameter study on the action of preparations containing cholecystokinin-pancreozymin. *Scand. J. Gastroenterol.* **5**, 537–541.

Brown, J. C., and Pederson, R. A. (1970b). Cleavage of a gastric inhibitory polypeptide with cyanogen bromide and the physiological action of the C-terminal fragment. *J. Physiol. (London)* **210**, 52p–53p.

Brown, J. C., and Pederson, R. A. (1976). Gi hormones and insulin secretion. *Proc. Int. Congr. Endocrinol., 5th* **2**, 568–570.

Brown, J. C., Johnson, L. P., and Magee, D. F. (1966). Effect of duodenal alkalinization on gastric motility. *Gastroenterology* **50**, 333–339.

Brown, J. C., Harper, A. A., and Scratcherd, T. (1967). Potentiation of secretin stimulation of the pancreas. *J. Physiol. (London)* **190**, 519–530.

Brown, J. C., Pederson, R. A., Jorpes, E., and Mutt, V. (1969). Preparation of highly active enterogastrone. *Can. J. Physiol. Pharmacol.* **47**, 113–114.

Brown, J. C., Mutt, V., and Pederson, R. A. (1970). Further purification of a polypeptide demonstrating enterogastrone activity. *J. Physiol. (London)* **209**, 57–64.

Brown, J. C., Mutt, V., and Dryburgh, J. R. (1971). The further purification of motilin, a gastric motor activity stimulating polypeptide from the mucosa of the small intestine of hogs. *Can. J. Physiol. Pharmacol.* **49**, 399–405.

Brown, J. C., Cook, M. A., and Dryburgh, J. R. (1972). Motilin, a gastric motor activity-stimulating polypeptide: final purification, amino acid composition and C-terminal residues. *Gastroenterology* **62**, 401–404.

Brown, J. C., Cook, M. A., and Dryburgh, J. R. (1973). Motilin, a gastric motor activity stimulating polypeptide: the complete amino acid sequence. *Can. J. Biochem.* **51**, 533–537.

Brown, J. C., Frost, J. L., Kwauk, S., Otte, S. C., and McIntosh, C. H. S. (1980). Gastric inhibitory polypeptide (GIP): isolation, structure and basic functions. *In* "Gastrointestinal Hormones" (G. B. J. Glass, ed.), pp. 223–232. Raven, New York.

Brownstein, M., Arimura, A., Sato, M., Schally, A. V., and Kizer, J. S. (1975). The regional distribution of somatostatin in the rat brain. *Endocrinology* **96**, 1456–1461.

Buchanan, K. D., Vance, J. E., Aokir, T., and Williams, R. H. (1967). Rise in serum immunoractive glucagon after intrajejunal glucose in pancreatectomized dogs. *Proc. Soc. Exp. Biol. Med.* **126,** 813–815.

Buchanan, K. D., Vance, J. E., Morgan, A., and Williams, R. H. (1968). Effect of pancreozymin on insulin and glucagon levels in blood and bile. *Am. J. Physiol.* **215,** 1293–1298.

Buchanan, K. D., Flanagan, R. W. J., Murphy, R. F., O'Connor, F. A., and Shahidullah, M. (1974). Immunological characterization of glucagon-like immunoreactivity. *Eur. J. Clin. Invest.* **4,** 326–327.

Bünzli, H. F., Glatthaar, B., Kunz, P., Mülhaupt, E., and Humbel, R. E. (1972). Amino acid sequence of the two insulins from mouse (*Mus musculus*). *Hoppe-Seylers Z. Physiol. Chem.* **353,** 451–458.

Burgen, A. S. V., Roberts, G. C. K., and Feeney, J. (1975). Binding of flexible ligands to macromolecules. *Nature (London)* **253,** 753–755.

Burhol, P. G. (1974). Gastric stimulation by intravenous injection of cholecystokinin and secretin in fistula chickens. *Scand. J. Gastroenterol.* **9,** 49–53.

Burhol, P. G., Lygren, I., Waldum, H. L., and Jorde, R. (1980). The effect of duodenal infusion of bile on plasma VIP, GIP, and secretin and on duodenal bicarbonate secretion. *Scand. J. Gastroenterol.* **15,** 1007–1011.

Burr, H., and Lingrel, J. B. (1971). Poly A sequences at the 3′ termini of rabbit globin mRNAs. *Nature (London) New Biol.* **233,** 41–43.

Butcher, R. W., and Carlson, L. A. (1970). Effects of secretin on fat mobilizing lipolysis and cyclic AMP levels in rat adipose tissue. *Acta Physiol. Scand.* **79,** 559–563.

Camilleri, M., Cooper, B. T., Adrian, T. E., Bloom, S. R., and Chadwick, V. S. (1981). Effects of vasoactive intestinal peptide and pancreatic polypeptide in rabbit intestine. *Gut* **22,** 14–18.

Caple, I., and Heath, T. (1972). Regulation of output of electrolytes in bile and pancreatic juice in sheep. *Aust. J. Biol. Sci.* **25,** 155–165.

Care, A. D. (1970). The effects of pancreozymin and secretin on calcitonin release. *Fed. Proc. Fed. Am. Soc. Exp. Biol.* **29,** 253/38.

Care, A. D., Bruce, J. B., Boelkins, J., Kenny, A. D., Conaway, H., and Anast, C. S. (1971). Role of pancreozymin-cholecystokinin and structurally related compounds as calcitonin secretagogues. *Endocrinology* **89,** 262–271.

Caren, J. F., Aures, D., and Johnson, L. R. (1969). Effect of secretin and cholecystokinin on histidine decarboxylase activity in the rat stomach. *Proc. Soc. Exp. Biol. Med.* **131,** 1194–1197.

Carlquist, M., Mutt, V., and Jörnvall, H. (1979). Isolation and characterization of bovine vasoactive intestinal peptide (VIP). *FEBS Lett.* **108,** 457–460.

Carlquist, M., Jörnvall, H., and Mutt, V. (1981). Isolation and amino acid sequence of bovine secretin. *FEBS Lett.* **127,** 71–74.

Carlquist, M., McDonald, T. J., Go, V. L. W., Bataille, D., Johansson, C., and Mutt, V. (1982). Isolation and amino acid composition of human vasoactive intestinal peptide. *Horm. Metab. Res.* **14,** 28–29.

Carpenter, G. (1978). The regulation of cell proliferation: Advances in the biology and mechanism of action of epidermal growth factor. *J. Invest. Dermatol.* **71,** 283–287.

Carraway, R., and Leeman, S. E. (1971). The isolation of a new hypotensive peptide from bovine hypothalami. *Fed. Proc. Fed. Am. Soc. Exp. Biol.* **30,** 215/117.

Carraway, R., and Leeman, S. E. (1973). The isolation of a new hypotensive peptide, neurotensin, from bovine hypothalami. *J. Biol. Chem.* **248,** 6854–6861.

Carraway, R., and Leeman, S. E. (1975a). The amino acid sequence of a hypothalamic peptide, neurotensin. *J. Biol. Chem.* **250,** 1907–1911.

Carraway, R., and Leeman, S. E. (1975b). The synthesis of neurotensin. *J. Biol. Chem.* **250**, 1912–1918.

Carraway, R., and Leeman, S. E. (1976). Characterization of radioimmunoassayable neurotensin in the rat. Its differential distribution in the central nervous system, small intestine and stomach. *J. Biol. Chem.* **251**, 7045–7052.

Carraway, R., and Leeman, S. E. (1979). The amino acid sequence of bovine hypothalamic substance P. Identity to substance P from colliculi and small intestine. *J. Biol. Chem.* **254**, 2944–2945.

Carraway, R., Kitabgi, P., and Leeman, S. E. (1978). The amino acid sequence of radioimmunoassayable neurotensin from bovine intestine. Identity to neurotensin from hypothalamus. *J. Biol. Chem.* **253**, 7996–7998.

Carrea, G., Pasta, P., Castellato, M. M., Manera, E., and Lugaro, G. (1976). Purification and properties of a porcine duodenal glycoprotein with gastric antisecretory activity. *Int. J. Biochem.* **7**, 209–214.

Carter, D. C., Taylor, I. L., Elashoff, J., and Grossman, M. I. (1979). Reappraisal of the secretory potency and disappearance rate of pure human minigastrin. *Gut* **20**, 705–708.

Case, R. M. (1973). Calcium and gastrointestinal secretion. *Digestion* **8**, 269–288.

Case, R. M. (1978). Synthesis, intracellular transport and discharge of exportable proteins in the pancreatic acinar cell and other cells. *Biol. Rev.* **53**, 211–354.

Case, R. M., and Clausen, T. (1973). The relationship between calcium exchange and enzyme secretion in the isolated rat pancreas. *J. Physiol. (London)* **235**, 75–102.

Case, R. M., and Goebell, H. (1976). *Proc. Int. Conf., 1975, Titisee, Germany.*

Case, R. M., Laundy, T. J., and Scratcherd, T. (1969). Adenosine 3′,5′-monophosphate (cyclic AMP) as the intracellular mediator of the action of secretin on the exocrine pancreas. *J. Physiol. (London)* **204**, 45P–47P.

Castell, D. O., and Harris, L. D. (1970). Hormonal control of gastroesophageal-sphincter strength. *N. Engl. J. Med.* **282**, 886–889.

Cataland, S., Crockett, S. E., Brown, J. C., and Mazzaferri, E. L. (1974). Gastric inhibitory polypeptide (GIP) stimulation by oral glucose in man. *J. Clin. Endocrinol. Metab.* **39**, 223–228.

Celestine, L. R. (1967). Gastrin-like effects of cholecystokinin-pancreozymin. *Nature (London)* **215**, 763–764.

Chan, S. J., Keim, P., and Steiner, D. F. (1976). Cell-free synthesis of rat preproinsulins: Characterization and partial amino acid sequence determination. *Proc. Natl. Acad. Scu. U.S.A.* **73**, 1964–1968.

Chance, R. E., Ellis, R. M., and Bromer, W. W. (1968). Porcine proinsulin: Characterization of amino acid sequence. *Science* **161**, 165–167.

Chang, J. Y., Brauer, D., and Wittmann-Liebold, B. (1978). Micro-sequence analysis of peptides and proteins using 4-*NN*-dimethyl aminoazobenzene, 4′-isothiocyanate/phenylisothiocyanate double coupling method. *FEBS Lett.* **93**, 205–214.

Chang, M. M., and Leeman, S. E. (1970a). Isolation of a sialogogic peptide from bovine hypothalami; its identification as substance P. *Fed. Proc. Fed. Am. Soc. Exp. Biol.* **29**, 282/202.

Chang, M. M., and Leeman, S. E. (1970b). Isolation of a sialogogic peptide from bovine hypothalamic tissue and its characterization as substance P. *J. Biol. Chem.* **245**, 4784–4790.

Chang, M. M., Leeman, S. E., and Niall, H. D. (1971). Amino acid sequence of substance P. *Nature (London) New Biol.* **232**, 86–87.

Chang, R. C. C., Huang, W-Y., Redding, T. W., Arimura, A., Coy, D. H., and Schally, A. V.

(1980). Isolation and structure of several peptides from porcine hypothalami. *Biochim. Biophys. Acta* **625**, 266–273.

Chariot, J., Lehy, T., Nasca, S., and Dubrasquet, M. (1974). Effets de l' hypergastrinie prolongée sur la pancréas de rat. *Biol. Gastroenterol.* **7**, 221–236.

Chatelain, P., Robberecht, P., De Neef, P., Camus, J.-C., Heuse, D., and Cristophe, J. (1980). Secretin and VIP-stimulated adenylate cyclase from rat heart. *Pflügers Arch.* **389**, 29–35.

Cherrrington, A. D., Kawamori, R., Pek, S., and Vranic, M. (1974). Arginine infusion in dogs. Model for the roles of insulin and glucagon in regulating glucose turnover and free fatty acid levels. *Diabetes* **23**, 805–815.

Chey, W. Y., and Brooks, F. P. (1974). "Endocrinology of the Gut." Slack, Thorofare, New Jersey.

Chey, W. Y., and Gutierrez, J. G. (1978). The endocrine control of gastrointestinal function. *Adv. Int. Med.* **23**, 61–84.

Chey, W. Y., Hitanant, S., Hendricks, J., and Lorber, S. H. (1970). Effect of secretin and cholecystokinin on gastric emptying and gastric secretion in man. *Gastroenterology* **58**, 820–827.

Chey, W. Y., Oliai, A., and Boehm, M. (1974). Radioimmunoassay (RIA) of secretin II. Studies on correlation between RIA secretin levels and biological investigations. *In* "Endocrinology of the Gut" (W. Y. Chey and F. P. Brooks eds.), pp. 320–326. Slack, Thorofare, New Jersey.

Chiba, T., Taminato, T., Kadowaki, S., Inoue, Y., Mori, K., Seino, Y., Abe, H., Chihara, K., Matsukura, S., Fujita, T., and Goto, Y. (1980). Effects of various gastrointestinal pepetides on gastric somatostain release. *Endocrinology* **106**, 145–149.

Chijikwa, J. B., and Davison, J. S. (1974). The action of gastrin-like polypeptides on the peristaltic reflex in the guinea-pig intestine. *J. Physiol. (London)* **238**, 68p–70p.

Chou, C. C., Hsieh, C. P., and Dabney, J. M. (1977). Comparison of vascular effects of gastrointestinal hormones on various organs. *Am. J. Physiol.* **232**, H103–H109.

Chou, P. Y., and Fasman, G. D. (1975). The conformation of glucagon: Predictions and consequences. *Biochemistry* **14**, 2536–2541.

Choudhury, A. M., Kenner, G. W., Moore, S., Ramage, R., Richards, P. M., Thorpe, W. D., Moroder, L., Wendlberger, G., and Wünsch, E. (1979). Synthesis of human big gastrin-I. *Proc. Eur. Peptide Symp., 14th, 1976* pp. 257–261.

Choudhury, A. M., Chu, K. Y., Kenner, G. W., Moore, S., Ramachandran, K. L., and Ramage, R. (1979). N-terminal sequence of porcine big gastrin: Sequence, synthesis, and immunochemical studies. *Biorg. Chem.* **8**, 471–483.

Choudhury, A. M., Kenner, G. W., Moore, S., Ramachandran, K. L., Thorpe, W. D., Ramage, R., Dockray, G. J., Gregory, R. A., Hood, L., and Hunkapiller, M. (1980). N-terminal sequence of human big gastrin: Sequence, synthetic and immunochemical studies. *Hoppe-Seylers Z. Physiol. Chem.* **361**, 1719–1733.

Chrétien, M., and Li, C. H. (1967). Isolation, purification, and characterization of γ-lipotropic hormone from sheep pituitary glands. *Can. J. Biochem.* **45**, 1163–1174.

Christensen, J. (1975). Pharmacology of the esophageal motor function. *Annu. Rev. Pharmacol.* **15**, 243–258.

Christiansen, J., and Borgeskov, S. (1974). The effect of glucagon and the combined effect of glucagon and secretin on lower esophageal sphincter pressure in man. *Scand. J. Gastroenterol.* **9**, 615–618.

Christiansen, J., Bech, A., Fahrenkrug, J., Holst, J. J., Lauritsen, K., Moody, A. J., and Schaffalitzky de Muckadell, O. (1979). Fat-induced jejunal inhibition of gastric acid secretion and release of pancreatic glucagon, enteroglucagon, gastric inhibitory polypeptide, and vasoactive intestinal polypeptide in man. *Scand. J. Gastroenterol.* **14,** 161–166.

Christophe, J. P., Conlon, T. P., and Gardner, J. D. (1976a). Interaction of porcine vasoactive intestinal peptide with dispersed pancreatic acinar cells from the guinea pig. Binding of radioiodinated peptide. *J. Biol. Chem.* **251,** 4629–4634.

Christophe, J. P., Frandsen, E. K., Conlon, T. P., Krishna, G., and Gardner, J. D. (1976b). Action of cholecystokinin, cholinergic agents, and A-23187 on accumulation of guanosine $3':5'$-monophosphate in dispersed guinea pig pancreatic acinar cells. *J. Biol. Chem.* **251,** 4640–4645.

Christophe, J., Svoboda, M., Calderon-Attas, P., Lambert, M., Vandermeers-Pirte, M. C., Vandermeers, A., Deschodt-Lanckman, M., and Robberecht, P. (1980). Gastrointestinal hormone–receptor interactions in the pancreas. *In* "Gastrointestinal Hormones" (G. B. J. Glass, ed.), pp. 451–476. Raven, New York.

Clemente, F., and Meldolesi, J. (1975). Calcium and pancreatic secretion-dynamics of subcellular calcium pools in resting and stimulated acinar cells. *Br. J. Pharmacol.* **55,** 369–379.

Clendinnen, B. G., Reeder, D. D., Davidson, W. D., and Thompson, J. C. (1970). Effect of gastrointestinal hormones on salivation in the dog. *Arch. Surg.* **101,** 596–598.

Code, C. F. (1956). Histamine and gastric secretion. *CIBA Found. Symp. Histamine* pp. 189–219.

Cohen, M. L., and Landry, A. S. (1980). Vasoactive intestinal polypeptide: increased tone, enhancement of acetylcholine release, and stimulation of adenylate cyclase in intestinal smooth muscle. *Life Sci.* **26,** 811–822.

Cohen, N., Mazure, P., Dreiling, D. A., and Janowitz, H. D. (1959). Effect of glucagon on histamine-stimulated gastric secretion in man. *Fed. Proc. Fed. Am. Soc. Exp. Biol.* **18,** 28/108.

Cohen, S. (1962). Isolation of a mouse submaxillary gland protein accelerating incisor eruption and eyelid opening in the new-born animal. *J. Biol. Chem.* **237,** 1555–1562.

Cohen, S. (1972). The hormonal regulation of lower esophageal sphincter competence. *Digestion* **6,** 231–240.

Cohen, S., and Carpenter, G. (1975). Human epidermal growth factor: Isolation and chemical and biological properties. *Proc. Natl. Acad. Sci. U.S.A.* **72,** 1317–1321.

Cohen, S., and Harris, L. D. (1972). The lower esophageal sphincter. *Gastroenterology* **63,** 1066–1073.

Cohen, S., and Lipshultz, W. (1971). Hormonal regulation of human lower esophageal sphincter competence: Interaction of gastrin and secretin. *J. Clin. Invest.* **50,** 449–454.

Colvin, J. R., Smith, D. B., and Cook, W. H. (1954). The microheterogeneity of proteins. *Chem. Rev.* **54,** 687–711.

Conlon, J. M. (1980). The glucagon-like polypeptides—order out of chaos? *Diabetologia* **18,** 85–88.

Conlon, J. M. Murphy, R. F., and Buchanan, K. D. (1979). Physicochemical and biological properties of glucagon-like polypeptides from porcine colon. *Biochim. Biophys. Acta* **577,** 229–240.

Contaxis, C. C., and Epand, R. M. (1974). A study of the conformational properties of glucagon in the presence of glycols. *Can. J. Biochem.* **52,** 456–468.

Cooke, A. R. (1967). Comparison of acid and pepsin outputs from gastric fistula dogs in response to histamine, gastrin and related peptides. *Gastroenterology* **53,** 579–583.

Coons, A. H., Leduc, E. H., and Connolly, J. M. (1955). Studies on antibody production;

method for histochemical demonstration of specific antibody and its application to study of hyperimmune rabbit. *J. Exp. Med.* **102**, 49–60.

Cooper, C. W., Schwesinger, W. H., Mahgoub, A. M., and Ontjes, D. A. (1971). Thyrocalcitonin: Stimulation of secretion by pentagastrin. *Science* **172**, 1238–1240.

Cooper, C. W., Schwesinger, W. H., Mahgoub, A. M., Ontjes, D. A., Gray, T. K., and Munson, P. L. (1972a). Regulation of secretion of thyrocalcitonin. *In* "Calcium, Parathyroid Hormone and the Calcitonins" (R. V. Talmage and P. L. Munson, eds.), pp. 128–139. Excerpta Medica, Amsterdam.

Cooper, C. W., Schwesinger, W. H., Ontjes, D. A., Mahgoub, A. M., and Munson, P. L. (1972b). Stimulation of secretion of pig thyrocalcitonin by gastrin and related hormonal peptides. *Endocrinology* **91**, 1079–1089.

Craig, L. C. (1962). Countercurrent distribution. *Comp. Biochem.* **4**, 1–31.

Crean, G. P., Rumsey, R. D. E., Hogg, D. F., and Marshall, M. W. (1968). Experimental hyperplasia of the gastric mucosa. *In* "The Physiology of Gastric Secretion" (L. S. Semb and J. Myren, eds.), pp. 82–85. Universitetsforlaget, Oslo.

Crean, G. P., Hogg, D. F., and Rumsey, R. D. E. (1969a). Hyperplasia of the gastric mucosa produced by duodenal obstruction *Gastroenterology* **56**, 193–199.

Crean, G. P., Marshall, M. W., and Rumsey, R. D. E. (1969b). Parietal cell hyperplasia induced by the administration of pentagastrin (ICI 50,123) to rats. *Gastroenterology* **57**, 147–155.

Creuzfeldt, W. (1979). The incretin concept today. *Diabetologia* **16**, 75–85.

Creuzfeldt, W., Arnold, R., Creutzfeldt, C., Feurle, G., and Ketterer, H. (1971). Gastrin and G-cells in the antral mucosa of patients with pernicious anaemia, acromegaly and hyperparathyroidism and in a Zollinger–Ellison tumour of the pancreas. *Eur. J. Clin. Invest.* **1**, 461–479.

Creutzfeldt, W., Creutzfeldt, C., and Arnold, R. (1974). Gastrin-producing cells. *In* "Endocrinology of the Gut" (W. Y. Chey and F. P. Brooks, eds.), pp. 35–62. Slack, Thorndale, New Jersey.

Creutzfeldt, W., Arnold, R., Creutzfeldt, C., and Track, N. S. (1975). Pathomorphologic, biochemical, and diagnostic aspects of gastrinomas (Zollinger–Ellison syndrome). *Hum. Pathol.* **6**, 47–76.

Crick, J., Harper, A. A., and Raper, H. S. (1950). On the preparation of secretin and pancreozymin. *J. Physiol. (London)* **110**, 367–376.

Csendes, A., and Grossman, M. I. (1972). d- and l-isomers of serine and alanine equally effective as releasers of gastrin. *Experientia* **28**, 1306–1307.

Dahlgren, Sven (1966). Cholecystokinin: Pharmacology and clinical use. *Acta Chir. Scand. Suppl.* **357**, 256–260.

Daly, M. M., Allfrey, V. G., and Mirsky, A. E. (1952). Uptake of glycine-N^{15} by components of cell nuclei. *J. Gen. Physiol.* **36**, 173–179.

Darnell, J. E., Wall, R., and Tushinski, R. J. (1971). An adenylic acid-rich sequence in messenger RNA of HeLa cells and its possible relationship to reiterated sites in DNA. *Proc. Natl. Acad. Sci. U.S.A.* **68**, 1321–1325.

Davidson, W. D., Lemmi, C. A. E., and Thompson, J. C. (1966). Action of gastrin on the isolated gastric mucosa of the blullfrog. *Proc. Soc. Exp. Biol. Med.* **121**, 545–547.

Davidson, W. D., Urushibara, O., and Thompson, J. C. (1969a). Action of pancreozymincholecystokinin on the isolated gastric mucosa of the bullfrog. *Proc. Soc. Exp. Biol. Med.* **129**, 711–713.

Davidson, W. D., Urushibara, O., and Thompson, J. C. (1969b). Comparison of the effects of human and porcine gastrin on isolated gastric mucosa of the bullfrog. *Proc. Soc. Exp. Biol. Med.* **130**, 204–206.

Dayhoff, M. O. (1972). "Atlas of Protein Sequence and Structure," Vol 5. Natl. Biomed. Res. Found., Washington, D.C.

Dean, P. M., and Matthews, E. K. (1972). Pancreatic acinar cells: Measurement of membrane potential and miniature depolarization potentials. *J. Physiol. (London)* **255**, 1–13.

Debas, H. T. (1979). Clinical implications of the gastointestinal hormones. *Can. J. Surg.* **22**, 10–16.

Debas, H. T., and Grossman, M. I. (1973). Pure cholecystokinin: Pancreatic protein and bicarbonate response. *Digestion* **9**, 469–481.

Debas, H. T., Walsh, J. H., and Grossman, M. I. (1974a). Pure human minigastrin: Secretory potency and disappearance rate. *Gut* **15**, 686–689.

Debas, H. T., Csendes, A., Walsh, J. H., and Grossman, M. I. (1974b). Release of antral gastrin. *In* "Endocrinology of the Gut" (W. Y. Chey and F. P. Brooks, eds.), pp. 222–232. Slack, Thorndale, New Jersey.

Debas, H. T., Farooq, O., and Grossman, M. I. (197). Inhibition of gastric emptying is a physiological action of cholecystokinin. *Gastroenterology* **68**, 1211–1217.

Dehaye, J., Winand, J., Robberecht, P., and Christophe, J. (1975). Variations in cyclic AMP levels in the epididymal adipose tissue of normal and congenitally obese mice. *Arch. Int. Physiol. Biochim.* **83**, 177–178.

Dembinski, A. B., and Johnson, L. R. (1979). Growth of pancreas and gastrointestinal mucosa in antrectomized and gastrin-treated rats. *Endocrinology* **105**, 769–773.

Dembinski, A. B., and Johnson, L. R. (1980). Stimulation of pancreatic growth by secretin, caerulein, and pentagastrin. *Endocrinology* **106**, 323–328.

Demling, L. (1972). "Gastrointestinal Hormones." Thieme, Stuttgart.

Demol, P., Laugier, R., Dagorn, J. C., and Sarles, H. (1979). Inhibition of rat pancreatic secretion by neurotensin: Mechanism of action. *Arch. Int. Pharmacodyn.* **242**, 139–148.

Denniss, A. R., and Young, J. A. (1978). Modification of salivary duct electrolyte transport in rat and rabbit by physalaemin, VIP, GIP and other enterohormones. *Pflügers Arch.* **376**, 73–80.

Dent, J., Dodds, W. J. Hogan, W. J., Arndorfer, R. C., and Teeter, B. C. (1980). Effect of cholecystokinin-octapeptide on opossum lower esophageal sphincter. *Am. J. Physiol.* **239**, G230–G235.

Deranleau, D. A., Ross, J. B. A., Rousslang, K. W., and Kwiram, A. L. (1978). Conformations of polypeptide hormones by optically detected magnetic resonance and a Zimm–Bragg analysis of helical folding in glucagon. *J. Am. Chem. Soc.* **100**, 1913–1917.

Deschodt-Lanckman, M., Robberecht, P., De Neef, Ph., and Christophe, J. (1974). Teneur en AMP-cyclique et GMP-cyclique du pancréas de rat stimulé in vivo et in vitro par des hormones gastro-intestinales. *Arch. Int. Physiol. Biochim.* **82**, 180.

Deschodt-Lanckman, M., Robberecht, P., Pector, J. C., and Christophe, J. (1975). Effects of somatostatin on pancreatic exocrine function. Interaction with secretin. *Arch. Int. Physiol. Biochim.* **83**, 960–961.

Deschodt-Lanckman, M., Robberecht, P., de Neef, Ph., Lammens, M., and Christophe, J. (1976). In vitro action of bombesin and bombesin-like peptides on amylase secretion, calcium efflux, and adenylate cyclase activity in the rat pancreas. *J. Clin. Invest.* **58**, 891–898.

Devillers -Thiery, A., Kindt, T., Scheele, G., and Blobel, G. (1975). Homology in amino-terminal sequence of precursors to pancreatic secretory proteins. *Proc. Natl. Acad. Sci. U.S.A.* **72**, 5016–5020.

Diamond, J. S., Siegel, S. A., Gall, M. B., and Karlen, S. (1939). The use of secretin as a clinical test of pancreatic function. *Am. J. Dig. Dis.* **6** 366–372.

DiMagno, E. P., Hendricks, J. C., Dozois, R. R., and Go, V. L. W. (1981). Effect of secretin on pancreatic duct pressure, resistance to pancreatic flow, and duodenal motor activity in the dog. *Dig. Dis. Sci.* **26**, 1–6.

Dimaline, R., and Dockray, G. J. (1978). Multiple immunoreactive forms of vasoactive intestinal peptide in human colonic mucosa. *Gastroenterology* **75**, 387–392.

Dimaline, R., and Dockray, G. J. (1980). Actions of a new peptide from porcine intestine (PHI) on pancreatic secretion in the rat and turkey. *Life Sci.* **27**, 1947–1951.

Dinoso, V. P., Jr., Meshkinpour, H., Lorber, S. H., Gutierrez, J. G., and Chey, W. Y. (1973). Motor responses of the sigmoid colon and rectum to exogenous cholecystokinin and secretin. *Gastroenterology* **65**, 438–444.

Dockray, G. J. (1973). Vasoactive intestinal peptide: Secretin-like action on the avian pancreas. *Experientia* **29**, 1510–1511.

Dockray, G. J. (1976). Immunochemical evidence of cholecystokinin-like peptides in brain. *Nature (London)* **264**, 568–570.

Dockray, G. J. (1977). Immunoreactive component resembling cholecystokinin octapeptide in intestine. *Nature (London)* **270**, 359–361.

Dockray, G. J. (1979a). Comparative physiology and biochemistry of gut hormones. *Annu. Rev. Physiol.* **41**, 83–96.

Dockray, G. J. (1979b). Evolutionary relationships of the gut hormones. *Fed. Proc. Fed. Am. Soc. Exp. Biol.* **38**, 2295–2301.

Dockray, G. J., and Gregory, R. A. (1980). Does the C-terminal tetrapeptide of gastrin and CCK exist as an entity? *Nature)London)* **286**, 742.

Dockray, G. J., and Walsh, J. H. (1975). Amino terminal gastrin fragment in serum of Zollinger–Ellison syndrome patients. *Gastroenterology* **68**, 222–230.

Dockray, G. J., Gregory, R. A., Hutchison, J. B., Harris, J. I., and Runswick, M. J. (1978a). Isolation, structure and biological activity of two cholecystokinin octapeptides from sheep brain. *Nature (London)* **274**, 711–713.

Dockray, G. J., Gregory, R. A., and Kenner, G. W. (1978b). Immunochemical differences between natural and synthetic big gastrins. *Gastroenterology* **75**, 556.

Dockray, G. J., Gregory, R. A., Hood, L., and Hunkapiller, M. (1979a). NH_2-terminal dodecapeptide of porcine big gastrin: Revised sequence and confirmation of structure by immunochemical analysis. *Bioorg. Chem.* **8**, 465–470.

Dockray, G., Rehfeld, J. F., and Walsh, J. H. (1979b). Naming gastrin and cholecystokinin peptides. *In* "Gastrins and the Vagus" (J. F. Rehfeld and E. Amdrup, eds.), pp. 95–97. Academic press, New York.

Dodds, W. J., Dent, J., Hogan, W. J., Patel, G. K., Toouli, J., and Arndorfer, R. C. (1981). Paradoxial lower esophageal sphincter contraction induced by cholecystokinin-octapeptide in patients with achalasia. *Gastroenterology* **80**, 327–333.

Doi, K., Prentki, M., Yip, C., Muller, W. A., Jeanrenaud, B., and Vranic, M. (1979). Identical biological effects of pancreatic glucagon and a purified moiety of canine gastric immunoreactive glucagon. *J. Clin. Invest.* **63**, 525–531.

Dolinsky, I. L. (1894). Influence of acids on the secretion of the pancreatic gland. *Arch. Sci. Biol. St. Petersburg* **3**, 399–427.

Domschke, S., Domschke, W., Rösch, W., Konturek, S. J., Wünsch, E., and Demling, L. (1976). Bicarbonate and cyclic AMP content of pure human pancreatic juice in response to graded doses of synthetic secretin. *Gastroenterology* **70**, 533–536.

Domschke, S., Domschke, W., Rösch, W., Konturek, S. J., Sprügel, W., Mitznegg, P., Wünsch, E., and Demling, L. (1977). Vasoactive intestinal peptide: A secretin-like partial agonist for pancreatic secretion in man. *Gastroenterology* **73**, 478–480.

Doolittle, R. F. (1972). Terminal pyrrolidonecarboxylic acid: Cleavage with enzymes. *Methods Enzymol.* **25 B**, 231–244.

Dormer, R. L., Poulsen, J. H., Licko, V., and Williams, J. A. (1981). Calcium fluxes in isolated pancreatic acini: Effects of secretagogues. *Am. J. Physiol.* **240**, G38–G49.

Douglas, W. W. (1968). Stimulus-secretion coupling: the concept and clues from chromaffin and other cells. *Br. J. Pharmacol.* **34**, 451–474.

Douglas, M., and Duthie, H. L. (1971). Pancreozymin and secretin in the control of pancreatic exocrine secretion. *Gut.* **12**, 862.

Dragstedt, C. A., and Owen, S. E. (1931). The mechanism of the diuretic action of secretin preparations. *Am. J. Physiol.* **27**, 286–290.

Dreiling, D. A., and Janowitz, H. D. (1962). The measurement of pancreatic secretory function. *In* "The Exocrine Pancreas" (A. V. S de Reuck and M. P. Cameron, eds.), pp. 225–258. Churchill, London.

Dreiling, D. A., Janowitz, H. D., Haemmerli, U. P., and Marshall, D. (1958). The effect of glucagon on the exocrine pancreatic secretion of man. *J. M. Sinai Hosp. N.Y.* **25**, 240–243.

Du Pont, C., Gespach, C., Chenut, B., and Rosselin, G. (1980). Regulation by vasoactive intestinal peptide of cyclic AMP accumulation in gastric epithelial glands. *FEBS Lett.* **113**, 25–28.

Dupré, J. (1964). An intestinal hormone affecting glucose: Disposal in man. *Lancet* **II**, 672–673.

Dupré, J., Rojas, L., White, J. J., Unger, R. H., and Beck, J. C. (1966). Effects of secretin on insulin and glucagon in portal and peripheral blood in man. *Lancet* **II**, 26–27.

Dupré, J., Ross, S. A., Watson, D., and Brown, J. C. (1973). Stimulation of insulin secretion by gastric inhibitory polypeptide in man. *J. Clin. Endocrinol. Metab.* **37**, 826–828.

Du Vigneaud, V., Ressler, C., and Trippett, S. (1953a). The sequence of amino acids in oxytocin, with a proposal for the structure of oxytocin. *J. Biol. Chem.* **205**, 949–957.

Du Vigneaud, V., Ressler, C., Swan, J. M., Roberts, C. W. Katsoyannis, P. G., and Gordon, S. (1953b). The synthesis of an octapeptide amide with the hormonal activity of oxytocin. *J. Am. Chem. Soc.* **75**, 4879–4880.

Dyck, W. P., Texter, E. C., Jr., Lasater, J. M., and Hightower, N. C., Jr. (1970). Influence of glucagon on pancreatic exocrine secretion in man. *Gastroenterology* **58**, 532–539.

Dyck, W. P., Bonnet, D., Lasater, J., Stinson, C., and Hall, F. F. (1974). Hormonal stimulation of intestinal disaccharidase release in the dog. *Gastroenterology* **66**, 533–538.

Dyke, H. B., van, Adamsons, K., Jr., and Engel, S. L. (1955). Aspects of the biochemistry and physiology of the neurohypophyseal hormones. *Recent Prog. Horm. Res.* **11**, 1–41.

Ebeid, A. M., Soeters, P. B., Murray, P., and Fischer, J. E. (1977a). Release of vasoactive intestinal peptide (VIP) by intraluminal osmotic stimuli. *J. Surg. Res.* **23**, 25–30.

Ebeid, A. M., Murray, P., Soeters, P. B., and Fischer, J. E. (1977b). Release of VIP by calcium stimulation. *Am. J. Surg.* **133**, 140–144.

Edelhoch, H., and Lippoldt, R. E. (1969). Structural studies on polypeptide hormones. I. Fluorescence. *J. Biol. Chem.* **244**, 3876–3883.

Edin, R., Lundberg, J. M., Ahlman, H., Dahlström, A., Fahrenkrug, J., Hökfelt, T., and Kewenter, J. (1979). On the VIP-ergic innervation of the feline pylorus. *Acta Physiol. Scand.* **107**, 185–187.

Edkins, J. S. (1905). On the chemical mechanism of gastric secretion. *Proc. R. Soc. London Ser. B* **76**, 376.

Edkins, J. S. (1906). The chemical mechanism of gastric secretion. *J. Physiol. (London)* **34**, 133–144.

Edman, P. (1950). Method for determination of the amino acid sequence in peptides. *Acta Chem. Scand.* **4**, 283–293.

Edman, P., and Begg, G. (1967). A protein sequenator. *Eur. J. Biochem.* **1**, 80–91.

Edmonds, M., Vaughan, M. H., Jr. and Nakazato, H. (1971). Polyadenylic acid sequences in the heterogeneous nuclear RNA and rapidly-labeled polyribosomal RNA of HeLa cells: Possible evidence for a precursor relationship. *Proc. Natl. Acad. Sci. U.S.A.* **68**, 1336–1340.

Eimerl, S., Savion, N., Heichal, O., and Selinger, Z. (1974). Introduction of enzyme secretion in rat pancreatic slices using the ionophore A-23187 and calcium. *J. Biol. Chem.* **249**, 3991–3993.

Eisentraut, A., Ohneda, A., Parada, E., and Unger, R. H. (1968). Immunologic discrimination between pancreatic glucagon and eneteric glucagon-like immunoreactivity (GLI) in tissues and plasma. *Diabetes* **17** (Suppl.), 321–322.

Eklund, S., Jodal, M., Lundgren, O., and Sjöqvist, A. (1979). Effects of vasoactive intestinal polypeptide on blood flow, motility and fluid transport in the gastrointestinal tract of the cat. *Acta Physiol. Scand.* **105**, 461–468.

Elde, R., Hökfelt, T., Johansson, O., and Terenius, L. (1976). Immunohistochemical studies using antibodies to leucine-enkephalin: initial observations on the nervous system of the rat. *Neuroscience* **1**, 349–351.

Elder, J. B., Ganguli, P. C., Gillespie, I. E., Gerring, E. L., and Gregory, H. (1975). Effect of urogastrone on gastric secretion and plasma gastrin levels in normal subjects. *Gut* **16**, 887–893.

Elder, J. B., Williams, G., Lacey, E., and Gregory, H. (1978). Cellular localisation of human urogastrone/epidermal growth factor. *Nature (London)* **271**, 466–467.

Elliott, D. F., Lewis, G. P., and Horton, E. W. (1960). The structure of bradykinin—a plasma kinin from ox blood. *Biochem. Biophys. Res. Commun.* **3**, 87–91.

Eloy, R., Vaultier, J. P., Raul, F., Mirhom, R., Clendinnen, G., and Grenier, J. F. (1978). Hormonal stimulation of intestinal brush border enzymes release. *Res. Exp. Med.* **172**, 109–121.

Elrick, H., Stimmler, L., Hlad, C. J., Jr., and Arai, Y. (1964). Plasma insluin response to oral and intravenous glucose administration. *J. Clin. Endocrinol. Metab.* **24**, 1076–1082.

Elwin, C.-E. (1974). Gastric acid responses to antral application of some amino acids, peptides, and isolated fractions of a protein hydrolysate. *Scand. J. Gastroenterol.* **9**, 239–247.

Enjalbert, A., Arancibia, S., Ruberg, M., Priam, M., Bluet-Pajot, M. T., Rotsztejn, W. H., and Kordon, C. (1980). Stimulation of in vitro prolactin release by vasoactive intestinal peptide. *Neuroendocrinology* **31**, 200–204.

Enochs, M. R., and Johnson, L. R. (1974). Pentagastrin stimulates tissue growth in stomach and duodenal tissues by stimulating protein and nucleic acid synthesis. *Fed. Proc. Fed. Am. Soc. Exp. Biol.* **33**, 309/594.

Enochs, M. R., and Johnson, L. R. (1977). Trophic effects of gastrointestinal hormones: Physiological implications. *Fed. Proc. Fed. Am. Soc. Exp. Biol.* **36**, 1942–1947.

Enriques, E., and Hallion, L. (1903). Réflexe acide de Pavloff et sécrétine : méchanisme humoral commun. *C. R. Soc. Biol. Paris* **55**, 233–234.

Epand, R. M., and Grey, V. (1973). Conformational and biological properties of partial squences of glucagon. *Can. J. Physiol. Pharmacol* **51**, 243–248.

Epand, R. M., and Scheraga, H. A. (1968). The influence of long-range interactions on the structure of myoglobin. *Biochemistry* **7**, 2864–2872.

Epelbaum, J., Tapia-Arancibia, L., Besson, J., Rotsztejn, W. H., and Kordon, C. (1979). Vasoactive intestinal peptide inhibits release of somatostatin from hypothalamus in vitro. *Eur. J. Pharmacol.* **58**, 493–495.

Erspamer, V. (1971). Biogenic amines and active polypeptides of the amphibian skin. *Annu. Rev. Pharmacol.* **11**, 327–350.

Erspamer, V., and Melchiorri, P. (1975). Actions of bombesin on secretions and motility of the gastrointestinal tract. *In* "Gastrointestinal Hormones" (J. C. Thompson, ed.), pp. 575–589. Univ. of Texas Press, Austin.

Erspamer, V., Melchiorri, P., Falconieri-Erspamer, C., and Negri, L. (1978). Polypeptides of the amphibian skin active on the gut and their mammalian counterparts. *Adv. Exp. Med. Biol.* **106**, 51–64.

Esteller, A., Lopez, M. A., and Murillo, A. (1977). The effect of secretin and cholecystokinin-pancreozymin on the secretion of bile in the anaesthetized rabbit. *Q. J. Exp. Physiol.* **62**, 353–359.

Estivariz, F. E., Hope, J., McLean, C., and Lowry, P. J. (1980). Purification and characterization of a γ-melanotropin precursor from frozen human pituitary glands. *Biochem. J.* **191**, 125–132.

v. Euler, U. S. (1936). *Naunyn-Schmiedebergs Arch. Exp. Pathol. Pharmacol. Untersuchungen* über Substanz P, die atropinfeste, darmerregende und gefässerweiternde Substanz aus Darum und Hirn. **181**, 181–197.

v. Euler, U. S. (1942). Herstellung und Eigenschaften von Substanz P. *Acta Physiol. Scand.* **4**, 373–735.

v. Euler, U. S., and Gaddum, J. H. (1931). An unidentified depressor substance in certain tissue extracts. *J. Physiol. (London)* **72**, 74–87.

Evans, D. C., and Lin, T.-M. (1971). Actions of pentagastrin (PG) on the incorporation of 1-histine (H) and 1-phenylalanin (P) into the proteins of the rat stomach. *Fed. Proc. Fed. Am. Soc. Exp. Biol.* **30**, 478/1583.

Fahrenkrug, J., Schaffalitzky de Muckadell, O. B., Holst, J. J., and Jensen, S. L. (1979). Vasoactive intestinal polypeptide in vagally mediated pancreatic secretion of fluid and HCO_3. *Am. J. Physiol.* **237**, E535–E540.

Falasco, J. D., Smith, G. P., and Gibbs, J. (1979). Cholecystokinin suppresses sham feeding in the Rhesus monkey. *Physiol. Behav.* **23**, 887–890.

Fara, J. W., and Erde, S. M. (1978). Comparison of in vivo and in vitro responses to sulfated and nonsulfated ceruletide. *Eur. J. Pharmacol.* **47**, 359–363.

Fara, J. W., and Madden, K. S. (1975). Effect of secretin and cholecystokinin on small intestinal blood flow distribution. *Am. J. Physiol.* **229**, 1365–1370.

Fasth, S., and Hultén, L. (1971). The effect of glucagon on intestinal motility and blood flow. *Acta Physiol. Scand.* **83**, 169–173.

Feeney, J., Robert, G. C. K., Brown, J. P., Burgen, A. S. V., and Gregory, H. (1972). Conformational study of some component peptides of pentagastrin. *J. Chem. Soc. Perkin Trans.* **II**, 601–604.

Felber, J. P., Zermatten, A., and Dick, J. (1974). Modulation, by food, of hormonal system regulating rat pancreatic secretion. *Lancet* **II**, 185–188.

Feldman, E. J., and Grossman, M. I. (1980). Liver extract and its free amino acids equally stimulate gastric acid secretion. *Am. J. Physiol.* **239**, G493–G496.

Fender, H. R., Curtis, P. J., Rayford, P. L., and Thompson, J. C. (1976). Effect of bombesin on serum gastrin and cholecystokinin in dogs. *Surg. Forum* **26**, 414–416.

Feurle, G. E., Weber, U., and Helmstaedter, V. (1980). Corticotropin-like substances in human gastric antrum and pancreas. *Biochem. Biophys. Res. Commun.* **95**, 1656–1662.

Feyrter, F. (1952). Über die These von den peripheren endokrinen (parakrinen) Drüsen. *Acta Neuroveg.* **4**, 409–424.

Fischer, E. (1906). Untersuchungen über Aminosäuren, Polypeptide und Proteine. *Ber. Dtsch. Chem. Ges.* **39**, 551–610.

Fisher, R. S., Lipshutz, W., and Cohen, S. (1973). The hormonal regulation of pyloric sphincter function. *J. Clin. Invest.* **52**, 1289–1296.

Fisher, R. S., DiMarino, A. J., and Cohen, S. (1975). Mechanism of cholecystokinin inhibition of lower esophageal sphincter pressure. *Am. J. Physiol.* **228**, 1469–1473.

Fitch, W. M. (1976). The deduction of messenger RNA sequences from amino acid sequences is, to date, a total failure. *J. Theor. Biol.* **59**, 251–252.

Folkers, K., Chang, D., Humphries, J., Carraway, R., Leeman, S. E., and Bowers, C. Y. (1976). Synthesis and activities of neurotensin, and its acid and amide analogs: Possible natural occurrence of (Gln⁴)-neurotensin. *Proc. Natl. Acad. Sci. U.S.A.* **73**, 3833–3837.

Fölsch, U. R., Winckler, K., and Wormsley, K. G. (1978). Influence of repeated administration of cholecystokinin and secretin on the pancreas of the rat. *Scand. J. Gastroenterol.* **13**, 663–671.

Fölsch, U. R., Fischer, H., Söling, H.-D., and Creuzfeldt, W. (1980). Effects of gastrointestinal hormones and carbamylcholine on cAMP accumulation in isolated pancreatic duct fragments from the rat. *Digestion* **20**, 277–292.

Forrell, M. M. (1973). Bile salts as stimulants of pancreatic secretion. *Proc. Nobel Symp., 16th, Stockholm* pp. 277–282.

Forell, M. M., Stahlheber, H., and Scholz, F. (1965). Galle als Reiz der Enzymsekretion des Pankreas. *Dtsch. Med. Wochenschr.* **90**, 1128–1132.

Frame, C. M. (1976). The contribution of the distal gastrointestinal tract to glucagon-like immunoreactivity secretion in the rat. *Proc. Soc. Exp. Biol. Med.* **152**, 667–670.

Frame, C. M. (1977). Regional release of glucagon-like immunoreactivity from the intestine of the cat. *Horm. Metab. Res.* **9**, 117–120.

Frame, C. M., Davidson, M. B., and Sturdevant, R. A. L. (1975). Effects of the octapeptide of cholecystokinin on insulin and glucagon secretion in the dog. *Endocrinology* **97**, 549–553.

Frandsen, E. K., and Moody, A. J. (1973). Lipolytic action of a newly isolated vasoactive intestinal polypeptide. *Horm. Metab. Res.* **5**, 196–199.

Friedman, M. H. F., Recknagel, R. O., Sandweiss, D. J., and Patterson, T. L. (1939). Inhibitory effect of urine extracts on gastric secretion. *Proc. Soc. Exp. Biol. Med.* **41**, 509–511.

Friedmann, N., and Park, C. R. (1968). Early effects of 3',5'-adenosine monophosphate on the fluxes of calcium and potassium in the perfused liver of normal and adrenalectomized rats. *Proc. Natl. Acad. Sci. U.S.A.* **61**, 504–508.

Friesen, S. R. (1968). A gastric factor in the pathogenesis of the Zollinger–Ellison syndrome. *Ann. Surg.* **168**, 483–501.

Frigo, G. M., Lecchini, S., Falaschi, C., Del Taca, M., and Crema, A. (1971). On the ability of caerulein to increase propulsive activity in the isolated small and large intestine. *Naunyn-Schmiedebergs Arch. Pharmakol. Exp. Pathol.* **268**, 44–58.

Galardy, R. E., and Jamieson, J. D. (1975). Photoaffinity labeling of secretagogue receptors in the pancreatic exocrine cell. *In* "Gastrointestinal Hormones" (J. C. Thompson, ed.), pp. 345–365. Univ. of Texas Press, Austin.

Galardy, R. E., Hull, B. E., and Jamieson, J. D. (1980). Irreversible photoactivation of a pancreatic secretagogue receptor with cholecystokinin COOH-terminal octapeptides. *J. Biol. Chem.* **255**, 3148–3155.

Gardner, J. D. (1979). Regulation of pancreatic exocrine function in vitro: Initial steps in the actions of secretagogues. *Annu. Rev. Physiol.* **41,** 55–66.

Gardner, J. D., and Rottman, A. J. (1980). Evidence against cyclic GMP as a mediator of the actions of secretagogues on amylase release from guinea pig pancreas. *Biochim. Biophys. Acta* **627,** 230–243.

Gardner, J. D., Peskin, G. W., Cerda, J. J., and Brooks, F. P. (1967). Alterations of in vitro fluid and electrolyte absorption by gsatrointestinal hormones. *Am. J. Surg.* **113,** 57–64.

Gardner, J. D., Conlon, T. P., Fink, M. L., and Bodanszky, M. (1976). Interaction of peptides related to secretin with hormone receptors on pancreatic acinar cells. *Gastroenterology* **71,** 965–970.

Gayet, R., and Guillaumie, M. (1930). La relations quantitatives réciproques de la sécrétion du suc pancréatique et du débit sanguin. *C. R. Soc. Biol.* **103,** 1216–1219.

Geratz, J. D., and Hurt, J. P. (1970). Regulation of pancreatic enzyme levels by trypsin inhibitors. *Am. J. Physiol.* **219,** 705–711.

Gibbs, J., Young, R. C., and Smith, G. P. (1973). Cholecystokinin decreases food intake in rats. *J. Comp. Physiol. Psychol.* **84,** 488–495.

Giles, G. R., Mason, M. C., Humphries, C., and Clark, C. G. (1969). Action of gastrin on the lower oesophageal sphincter in man. *Gut* **10,** 730–734.

Gilham, P. T. (1964). The synthesis of polynucleotide-celluloses and their use in the fractionation of polynucleotides. *J. Am. Chem. Soc.* **86,** 4982–4989.

Gillespie, I. E., and Grossman, M. I. (1962). Effect of acid in pyloric pouch on response of fundic pouch to injected gastrin. *Am. J. Physiol.* **203,** 557–559.

Gillespie, I. E., and Grossman, M. I. (1963). Inhibition of gastric secretion by extracts containing gastrin. *Gastroenterology* **44,** 301–310.

Gillespie, I. E., and Grossman, M. I. (1964a). Potentiation between urecholine and gastrin extract and between urecholine and histamine in the stimulations of Heidenhain pouches. *Gut* **5,** 71–76.

Gillespie, I. E., and Grossman, M. I. (1964b). Inhibitory effect of secretin and cholecystokinin on Heidenhain pouch responses to gastrin extract and histamine. *Gut* **5,** 342–345.

Gillespie, I. E., Clark, D. H., Kay, A. W., and Tankel, H. I. (1960). Effect of antrectomy, vagotomy with gastrojejunostomy, and antrectomy with vagotomy on the spontaneous and maximal gastric acid output in man. *Gastroenterology* **38,** 361–367.

Glaser, B., Vinik, A. I., Sive, A. A., and Floyd, J. C., Jr. (1980). Plasma human pancreatic polypeptide responses to administrated secretin: Effects of surgical vagotomy, cholinergic blockade, and chronic pancreatitis. *J. Clin. Endocrinol. Metab.* **50,** 1094–1099.

Glass, G. B. J. (1980). "Gastrointestinal Hormones." Raven, New York.

Glazer, G., SIlverman, S., and Steer, M. (1976). Parallel secretion of amylase, trypsinogen and chymotrypsinogen from the in vitro rabbit pancreas. *J. Physiol. (London)* **258,** 88p–90p.

Glick, Z., Thomas, D. W., and Mayer, J. (1971). Absence of effect of injections of the intestinal hormones secretin and cholecystokinin-pancreozymin upon feeding behavior. *Physiol. Behav.* **6,** 5–8.

Goebell, H., Bode, Ch., and Horn, H. D. (1970). Einfluss von Sekretin und Pankreozymin auf die Calciumsekretion im menschlichen Duodenalsaft bei normaler und gestörter Pankreasfunktion. *Klin. Wochenschr.* **48,** 330–1339.

Goetz, H., and Sturdevant, R. (1975). Effect of cholecystokinin on food intake in man. *Clin. Res.* **23,** 98A.

Goldman, R. B., Kim, Y. S., Jones, R. S., and Sleisenger, M. H. (1971). The effect of glucagon on enterokinase secretion from Bruner's gland pouches in dogs. *Proc. Soc. Exp. Biol. Med.* **138**, 562–565.

Goodhead, B., Himal, H. S., and Zanbilowicz, J. (1970). Relationship between pancreatic secretion and pancreatic blood flow. *Gut* **11**, 62–68.

Goodman, I., and Hiatt, R. B. (1972). Coherin: a new peptide of the bovine neurohypophysis with activity on gastrointestinal motility. *Science* **178**, 419–421.

Goodman, R. H., Jacobs, J. W., Chin, W. W., Lund, P. K., Dee, P. C., and Habener, J. F. (1980a). Nucleotide sequence of a cloned structural gene coding for a precursor of pancreatic somatostatin. *Proc. Natl. Acad. Sci. U.S.A.* **77**, 5869–5873.

Goodman, R. H., Lund, P. K., Jacobs, J. W., and Habener, J. F. (1980b). Pre-prosomatostatins. Products of cell-free translations of messenger RNAs from anglerfisch islets. *J. Biol. Chem.* **255**, 6549–6552.

Götze, H. Adelson, J. W., Hadorn, H. B., Portmann, R., and Troesch, V. (1972). Hormone-elicited enzyme release by the small intestinal wall. *Gut* **13**, 471–476.

Goyal, R. K., and McGuigan, J. E. (1976). Is gastrin a major determinant of basal lower esophageal sphincter pressure? *J. Clin. Invest.* **57**, 291–300.

Gratzer, W. B., and Beaven, G. H. (1969). Relation between conformation and association state. A study of the association equilibrium of glucagon. *J. Biol. Chem.* **224**, 6675–6679.

Gratzer, W. B., Beaven, G. H., Rattle, H. W. E., and Bradbury, E. M. (1968). A conformational study of glucagon. *Eur. J. Biochem.* **3**, 276–283.

Gratzer, W. B., Greth, K. M., and Beaven, G. H. (1972). Presence of trimers in glucagon solution. *Eur. J. Biochem.* **31**, 505–509.

Gray, J. S., Bradley, WM. B., and Ivy, A. C. (1937). On the preparation and biological assay of enterogastrone. *Am. J. Physiol.* **118**, 463–476.

Gray, J. S., Wieczorowski, E., and Ivy, A. C. (1939). Inhibition of gastric secretion by extracts of normal male urine. *Science* **89**, 489–490.

Gray, J. S., Culmer, C. U., Wieczorowski, E., and Adkison, J. L. (1940). Preparation of pyrogene-free urogastrone. *Proc. Soc. Exp. Biol. Med.* **43**, 225–228.

Gray, T. K., Brannan, P., Juan, D., Morawski, S. G., and Fordtran, J. S. (1976). Ion transport changes during calcitonin-induced intestinal secretion in man. *Gastroenterology* **71**, 392–398.

Gray, W. R., and Hartley, B. S. (1963). The structure of a chymotryptic peptide from *Pseudomonas* cytochrome c-551. *Biochem. J.* **89**, 379–380.

Green, G. M., and Lyman, R. L. (1972). Feedback regulation of pancreatic enzyme secretion as a mechanism for trypsin inhibitor-induced hypersecretion in rats. *Proc. Soc. Exp. Biol. Med.* **140**, 6–12.

Greengard, H. (1948). Hormones of the gastrointestinal tract. *In* "The Hormones" (G. Pincus and K. V. Thimann, eds.), Vol. I, pp. 201–254. Academic Press, New York.

Greengard, H., and Ivy, A. C. (1938). The isolation of secretin. *Am. J. Physiol.* **124**, 427–434.

Greenlee, H. B., Longhi, E. H., Guerrero, J. D., Nelsen, T. S., El-Bedri, A. L., and Dragstedt, L. R. (1957). Inhibitory effect of pancreatic secretin on gastric secretion. *Am. J. Physiol.* **190**, 396–402.

Greenwell, J. R. (1975). The effects of cholecystokinin-pancreozymin, acetylcholine and secretin on the membrane potentials of mouse pancreatic cells in vitro. *Pflügers Arch.* **353**, 159–170.

Gregory, H. (1975). Isolation and structure of urogastrone and its relationship to epidermal growth factor. *Nature (London)* **257**, 325–327.

Gregory, H., and Preston, B. M. (1977). The primary structure of human urogastrone. *Int. J. Pept. Protein Res.* **9**, 107–118.

Gregory, H., Hardy, P. M., Jones, D. S., Kenner, G. W., and Sheppard, R. C. (1964). The antral hormone gastrin. Structure of gastrin. *Nature (London)* **204**, 931–933.

Gregory, R. A. (1955). New method for preparation of urogastrone. *J. Physiol. (London)* **129**, 528–546.

Gregory, R. A. (1962a). Gastric secretion: A review of its chief nervous and hormonal mechanisms. *In* "Surgical Physiology of the Gastro-Intestinal Tract, Symposium" (A. N. Smith, ed.), pp. 57–70. Edinburgh Royal Coll., Edinburgh.

Gregory, R. A. (1962b). "Secretory Mechanisms of the Gastrointestinal Tract." Monograph of the Physiological Society. Arnold, London. Book.

Gregory, R. A. (1967). Enterogastrone—a reappraisal of the problem. *In* "Gastric Secretion. Mechanisms and Control" (T. K. Shnitka *et al.*, eds.), pp. 469–477. Oxford Univ. Press, London and New York.

Gregory, R. A. (1968). Recent advances in the physiology of gastrin. *Proc. R. Soc. Ser. B* **170**, 81–88.

Gregory, R. A. (1974). The gastrointestinal hormones: A review of recent advances. *J. Physiol. (London)* **241**, 1–32.

Gregory, R. A. (1979a). A review of some recent developments in the chemistry of the gastrins. *Bioorg. Chem.* **8**, 497–511.

Gregory, R. A. (1979b). Some aspects of the structure of gastrin and gastrin-like forms and fragments in gut and brain. *In* "Gastrins and the Vagus" (J. F. Rehfeld and E. Amdrup, eds.), pp. 47–55. Academic Press, New York.

Gregory, R. A., and Tracy, H. J. (1963). Constitution and properties of two gastrins extracted from hog antral mucosa. *J. Physiol. (London)* **169**, 18p–19p.

Gregory, R. A., and Tracy, H. J. (1964). The constitution and properties of two gastrins extracted from hog antral mucosa. *Gut* **5**, 103–114.

Gregory, R. A., and Tracy, H. J. (1972). Isolation of two "big gastrins" from Zollinger–Ellison tumour tissue. *Lancet* **II**, 797–799.

Gregory, R. A., and Tracy, H. J. (1973). Big gastrin. *J. Med. M. Sinai N.Y.* **40**, 359–364.

Gregory, R. A., and Tracy, H. J. (1974). Isolation of two minigastrins from Zollinger–Ellison tumour tissue. *Gut* **15**, 683–685.

Gregory, R. A., and Tracy, H. J. (1975). The chemistry of the gastrins: Some recent advances. *In* "Gastrointestinal Hormones" (J. C. Thompson, ed.), pp. 13–24. Univ. of Texas Press, Austin.

Gregory, R. A., Tracy, H. J., and Grossman, M. I. (1966). Isolation of two gastrins from human antral mucosa. *Nature (London)* **209**, 583.

Gregory, R. A., Tracy, H. J., Grossman, M. I., de Valois, D., and Lichter, R. (1969a). Isolation of canine gastrin. *Experientia* **25**, 345–346.

Gregory, R. A., Tracy, H. J., Agarwal, K. L., and Grossman, M. I. (1969b). Amino acid constitution of two gastrins isolated from Zollinger–Ellison tumour tissue. *Gut* **10**, 603–608.

Gregory, R. A., Tracy, H. J., Harris, J. I., Runswick, M. J., Moore, S., Kenner, G. W., and Ramage, R. (1979). Minigastrin: Corrected structure and synthesis. *Hoppe-Seylers Z. Physiol. Chem.* **360**, 73–80.

Gross, E. (1972). Structural relationships in and between peptides with α,β-unsaturated amino acids. *In* "Chemistry and Biology of Peptides" (J. Meienhofer, ed.), pp. 671–678. Ann Arbor Science Publ., Ann Arbor, Michigan.

Grossman, M. I. (1950). Gastrointestinal hormones. *Phys. Rev.* **30**, 33–90.

Grossman, M. I. (1966). "Gastrin." UCLA Forum in Medical Sciences No. 5. Univ. of California Press, Los Angeles.

Grossman, M. I. (1970a). Proposal: Use the term cholecystokinin in place of cholecystokinin-pancreozymin. *Gastroenterology* **58**, 128.

Grossman, M. I. (1970b). Gastrin and its activities. *Nature (London)* **228**, 1147–1150.

Grossman, M. I. (1974). Candidate hormones of the gut. I. Introduction. *Gastroenterology* **67**, 730–731.

Grossman, M. I. (1975). Additional candidate hormones of the gut. *Gastroenterology* **69**, 570–571.

Grossman, M. I. (1979a). Chemical messengers: a view from the gut. *Fed. Proc. Fed. Am. Soc. Exp. Biol.* **38**, 2341–2343.

Grossman, M. I. (1979b). Neural and hormonal regulation of gastrointestinal function: an overview. *Annu. Rev. Physiol.* **41**, 27–33.

Grossman, M. I., and Ivy, A. C. (1946). Effect of alloxan upon external secretion of the pancreas. *Proc. Soc. Exp. Biol. Med.* **63**, 62–63.

Grossman, M. I., and Konturek, S. J. (1974). Gastric acid does drive pancreatic bicarbonate secretion. *Scand. J. Gastroenterol.* **9**, 299–302.

Grossman, M. I., Roberston, C. R., and Ivy, A. C. (1948). Proof of a hormonal mechanism for gastric secretion—the humoral transmission of the distension stimulus. *Am. J. Physiol.* **153**, 1–9.

Grossman, M. I., Speranza, V., Basso, N., and Lezoche, E. (1978)."Gastrointestinal Hormones and Pathology of the Digestive System." Plenum, New York.

Grube, D., and Forssmann, W. G. (1979). Morphology and function of the enteroendocrine cells. *Horm. Metab. Res.* **11**, 589–606.

Gunther, G. R., and Jamieson, J. D. (1979). Increased intracellular cyclic GMP does not correlate with protein discharge from pancreatic acinar cells. *Nature (London)* **280**, 318–320.

Gustavsson, S., Johansson, H., Lundqvist, G., and Nilsson, F. (1977). Effects of vasoactive intestinal peptide and pancreatic polypeptide on small bowel propulsion in the rat. *Scand. J. Gastroenterol.* **12**, 993–997.

Gutiérrez, J. G., Chey, W. Y., and Dinoso, V. P. (1974). Actions of cholecystokinin and secretin on the motor activity of the small intestine in man. *Gastroenterology* **67**, 35–41.

Gutman, R. A., Fink, G., Voyles, N., Selawry, H., Penhos, J. C., Lepp, A., and Recant, L. (1973). Specific biologic effects of intestinal glucagon-like materials. *J. Clin. Invest.* **52**, 1165–1175.

Gyermek, L., and Fekete, G. (1955). On the vasopressor and antidiuretic activities of synthetic oxytocin. *Experientia* **11**, 238.

Habener, J. F., Potts, J. T., Jr., and Rich, A. (1976). Pre-proparathyroid hormone. *J. Biol. Chem.* **251**, 3893–3899.

Habener, J. F., Kemper, B. W., Rich, A., and Potts, J. T., Jr. (1977). Biosynthesis of parathyroid hormone. *Recent Progr. Horm. Res.* **33**, 249–308.

Habener, J. F., Rosenblatt, M., Kemper, B., Kronenberg, H. M., Rich, A., and Potts, J. T., Jr. (1978). Pre-proparathyroid hormone: Amino acid sequence, chemical synthesis, and some biological studies of the precursor region. *Proc. Natl. Acad. Sci. U.S.A.* **75**, 2616–2620.

Häcki, W. H., Greenberg, G. R., and Bloom, S. R. (1978). Role of secretin in man. *In* "Gut Hormones" (S. R. Bloom, ed.), pp. 182–192. Churchill, London.

Haig, T. H. B. (1974). Regulation of pancreatic acinar function: Effects of cyclic AMP, dibutyryl cyclic AMP, and theophylline in vitro. *Can. J. Physiol. Pharmacol.* **52**, 780–785.

Håkanson, R., Ekman, R., Sundler, F., and Nilsson, R. (1980). A novel fragment of the corticotropin-β- lipotropin precursor. The missing amino-terminal portion. *Nature (London)* **283**, 789–792.

Hallenga, K., van Binst, G., Knappenberg, M., Brison, J., Michel, A., and Dirkx, J. (1979). The conformational properties of some fragments of the peptide hormone somatostatin. *Biochim. Biophys. Acta* **577**, 82–101.

Hamilton, J. W., Niall, H. D., Jacobs, J. W., Keutman, H. T., Potts, J. T., Jr., and Cohn, D. V. (1974). The N-terminal amino acid sequence of bovine proparathyroid hormone. *Proc. Natl. Acad. Sci. U.S.A.* **71**, 653–656.

Hammarsten, E., Ågren, G., Hammarsten, H., and Wilander, O. (1933). Versuche zur Reinigung von Sekretin. V. *Biochem. Z.* **264**, 275–284.

Hammer, R. A., Carraway, R., Williams, R. H., and Leeman, S. E. (1979). Isolation of human intestinal neurotensin (NT). *Gastroenterology* **76**, 1150.

Hansky, J., Soveny, C., and Korman, M. G. (1971). Effect of secretin on serum gastrin as measured by immunoassay. *Gastroenterology* **61**, 62–68.

Hansky, J., Soveny, C., and Korman, M. G. (1973a). The effect of glucagon on serum gastrin. I. Studies in normal subjects. *Gut* **14**, 457–461.

Hansky, J., Royle, J. P., Soveny, C., and Korman, M. G. (1973b). Relationship of immunoreactivity to biological activity of gastrin. *Gastroenterology* **64**, A-56/739.

Harper, A. A. (1972). The control of pancreatic secretion. *Gut* **13**, 308–317.

Harper, A. A., and Raper, H. S. (1943). Pancreozymin, a stimulant of the secretion of pancreatic enzymes in extracts of the small intestine. *J. Physiol. (London)* **102**, 115–125.

Harper, A. A., Hood, A. J. C., Mushens, J., and Smy, J. R. (1979). Pancreotone, an inhibitor of pancreatic secretion in extracts of ileal and colonic mucosa. *J. Physiol. (London)* **292**, 455–467.

Harris, J. B., Nigon, K., and Alonso, D. (1969). Adenosine 3',5'-monophosphate: Intracellular mediator for methyl xanthine stimulation of gastric secretion. *Gastroenterology* **57**, 377–384.

Harvey, R. F., Dowsett, L., and Read, A. E. (1974). Studies on the nature of cholecystokinin-pancreozymin in small-intestinal mucosal extracts. *Gut* **15**, 838–839.

Hayes, J. R., Ardill, J., Kennedy, T. L. Shanks, R. G., and Buchanan, K. D. (1972). Stimulation of gastrin release by catecholamines. *Lancet* **I**, 819–821.

Heding, L. G. (1969). The production of glucagon antibodies in rabbits. *Horm. Metab. Res.* **1**, 87–88.

Heding, L. G. (1971). Radioimmunological determination of pancreatic and gut glucagon in plasma. *Diabetologia* **7**, 10–19.

Hedner, P., Persson, H., and Rorsman, G. (1967). Effect of cholecystokinin on small intestine. *Acta Physiol. Scand.* **70**, 250–254.

Hedner, P., Persson, G., and Ursing, D. (1975). Insulin release in fasting man induced by impure but not by pure preparations of cholecystokinin. *Acta Med. Scand.* **197**, 109–112.

Heidmann, T., and Changeux, J.-P. (1978). Structural and functional properties of the acetylcholine receptor protein in its purified and membrane-bound states. *Annu. Rev. Biochem.* **47**, 317–357.

Heitz, P., Kasper, M., van Noorden, S., Polak, J. M., Gregory, H., and Pearse, A. G. E. (1978). Urogastrone is produced by Brunner glands. *J. Endocrinol.* **77**.

Hellerström, C., Howell, S. L., Edwards, J. C., and Andersson, A. (1972). An investigation of glucagon biosynthesis in isolated pancreatic islets of guinea pigs. *FEBS Lett.* **27**, 97–101.

Hemmasi, B., and Bayer, E. (1977). The solid phase synthesis of porcine secretin with full biological activity. *Int. J. Pept. Protein Res.* **9**, 63–70.

Henriksen, F. W. (1969). Effect of vagotomy or atropine on the canine pancreatic response to secretin and pancreozymin. *Scand. J. Gastroenterol.* **4**, 137–144.

Henriksen, F. W., and Möller, S. (1971). Effect of secretin on the pancreatic secretion of protein. *Scand. J. Gastroenterol. Suppl.* **9**, 181–187.

Henriksen, F. W., and Worning, H. (1967). The interaction of secretin and pancreozymin on the external pancreatic secretion in dogs. *Acta Physiol. Scand.* **70**, 241–249.

Herbert, E., Budarf, M., Phillips, M., Rosa, P., Policastro, P., Oates, E., Roberts, J. L., Seidah, N. G., and Chrétien, M. (1980). Presence of a presequence (signal sequence) in the common precursor to ACTH and endorphin and the role of glycosylation in processing of the precursor and secretion of ACTH and endorphin. *Ann. N.Y. Acad. Sci.* **343**, 79–93.

Hickson, J. C. D. (1970). The secretory and vascular response to nervous and hormonal stimulation in the pancreas of the pig. *J. Physiol. (London)* **206**, 299–322.

Hinz, M., Katsilambros, N., Schweitzer, B., Raptis, S., and Pfeiffer, E. F. (1971). The role of the exocrine pancreas in the stimulation of insulin secretion by intestinal hormones. *Diabetologia* **7**, 1–5.

Hobart, P., Crawford, R., Shen, L.-P., Pictet, R., and Rutter, W. J. (1980). Cloning and sequence analysis of cDNAs encoding two distinct somatostatin precursors found in the endocrine pancreas of anglerfish. *Nature (London)* **288**, 137–141.

Hofmann, K. (1960). Preliminary observations relating structure and function in some pituitary hormones. *Brookhaven Symp. Biol.* **13**, 184–202.

Hogan, W. J., Dodds, W. J., Hoke, S. E., Reed, D. P., Kalkhoff, R. K., and Arndorfer, R. C. (1975). Effect of glucagon on esophageal motor function. *Gastroenterology* **69**, 160–165.

Hoke, S. E., Reid, D. P., Hogan, W. J., Dodds, W. J., Kalkhoff, R. K., and Arndorfer, R. C. (1972). The effect of glucagon on esophageal motor function. *Clin. Res.* **20**, 732A.

Hokin, L. E. (1966). Effect of calcium omission on acetylcholine-stimulated amylase secretion and phospholipid synthesis in pigeon pancreas slices. *Biochim. Biophys. Acta* **115**, 219–221.

Hokin, L. E., and Hokin, M. R. (1956). The actions of pancreozymin in pancreas slices and the role of phospholipids in enzyme secretion. *J. Physiol. (London)* **132**, 442–453.

Holladay, L. A., and Puett, D. (1976). Somatostatin conformation: Evidence for a stable intramolecular structure from circular dichroism, diffusion and sedimentation equilibrium. *Proc. Natl. Acad. Sci. U.S.A.* **73**, 1199–1202.

Hollenberg, M. D. (1979). Epidermal growth factor-urogastrone, a polypeptide acquiring hormonal status. *Vitamins Horm.* **37**, 69–110.

Hollenberg, M. D., and Gregory, H. (1980). Epidermal growth factor-urogastrone: Biological activity and receptor binding of derivatives. *Mol. Pharmacol.* **17**, 314–320.

Holst, J. J. (1977). Extraction, gel filtration pattern, and receptor binding of porcine gastrointestinal glucagon-like immunoreactivity. *Diabetologia* **13**, 159–169.

Holst, J. J. (1978). Extrapancreatic glucagons. *Digestion* **17**, 168–190.

Holstein, B., and Humphrey, C. S. (1980). Stimulation of gastric acid secretion and supression of VIP-like immunoreactivity by bobesin in the Atlantic codfish, *Gadus morhua. Acta Physiol. Scand.* **109**, 217–223.

Holtermüller, K. H. (1976). Cholecystokinetic action of magnesium and calcium: A speculative proposal. *Acta Hepato-Gastroenterol.* **23**, 305–307.

Holtermüller, K. H., Malagelada, J.-R., McCall, J. T., and Go, V. L. W. (1976). Pancreatic, gallbladder, and gastric responses to intraduodenal calcium perfusion in man. *Gastroenterology* **70**, 693–696.

Holton, P. (1973). "Pharmacology of Gastrointestinal Motility and Secretion" Vol. I and II. Pergamon, Oxford.

Hong, S. S., Nakamura, M., and Magee, D. F. (1967). Relationship between duodenal pH and pancreatic secretion in dogs and pigs. *Ann. Surg.* **166**, 778–782.

Hotz, J., Goebell, H., Hirche, H., Minne, H., and Ziegler, R. (1980). Inhibition of human gastric secretion by intragastrically administrated calcitonin. *Digestion* **20**, 180–189.

Howell, W. H. (1898). The physiological effects of extracts of the hypophysis cerebri and infundibular body. *J. Exp. Med.* **3**, 245–258.

Hughes, J., Smith, T. W., Kosterlitz, H. W., Fothergill, L. A., Morgan, B. A., and Morris, H. R. (1975). Identification of two related pentapeptides from the brain with potent opiate agonist activity. *Nature (London)* **258**, 577–579.

Hunkapiller, M. W., and Hood, L. E. (1978). Direct microsequence analysis of polypeptides using an improved sequenator, a nonprotein carrier (polybrene), and high pressure liquid chromatography. *Biochemistry* **17**, 2124–2133.

Hunt, J. N., and Ramsbottom, N. (1967). Effect of gastrin II on gastric emptying and secretion during a test meal. *Br. Med. J.* **4**, 386–390.

Hunt, T. E. (1957). Mitotic activity in the gastric mucosa of the rat after fasting and refeeding. *Anat. Rec.* **127**, 539–550.

Hutchison, J. B., and Dockray, G. J. (1980). Inhibition of the action of cholecystokinin octapeptide on the guinea pig ileum myenteric plexus by dibutyryl cyclic guanosine monophosphate. *Brain Res.* **202**, 501–505.

Hutchison, J. B., and Dockray, G. J. (1981). Evidence that the action of cholecystokinin octapeptide on the guinea pig ileum longitudinal muscle is mediated in part by substance P release from the myenteric plexus. *Eur. J. Pharmacol.* **69**, 87–93.

Ihse, I., Arnesjö, B., and Lundquist, I. (1976). Effects on exocrine and endocrine rat pancreas of long-term administration of CCK-PZ (cholecystokinin-paancreozymin) or synthetic octapeptide—CCK-PZ. *Scand. J. Gastroenterol.* **11**, 529–535.

Impicciatore, M., Debas, H., Walsh, J. H., Grossman, M. I., and Bertaccini, G. (1974). Release of gastrin and stimulation of acid secretion by bombesin in dog. *Rend. Gastro-Enterol.* **6**, 99–101.

Impicciatore, M., Hansen, D. G., Rachmilewitz, D., Maitra, S. K., Lugaro, G., and Grossman, M. I. (1980). Comparison of human urine gastric inhibitory (HUGI) and bacterial endotoxin as inhibitors of acid secretion. *Eur. J. Pharmacol.* **65**, 365–368.

Innis, R. B., and Snyder, S. H. (1980). Distinct cholecystokinin receptors in brain and pancreas. *Proc. Natl. Acad. Sci. U.S.A.* **77**, 6917–6921.

Ipp, E., Dobbs, R. E., Arimura, A., Vale, W., Harris, V., and Unger, R. H. (1977). Release of immunoreactive somatostatin from the pancreas in response to glucose, amino acids, pancreozymin-cholecystokinin and tolbutamide. *J. Clin. Invest.* **60**, 760–765.

Ippoliti, A. F., Isenberg, J. I., and Hagie, L. (1981). Effect of oral and intravenous 16,16-dimethyl prostaglandin E₂ in duodenal ulcer and Zollinger–Ellison syndrome patients. *Gastroenterology* **80**, 55–59.

Isenberg, J. I., Walsh, J. H., Passaro, E., Jr., Moore, E. W., and Grossman, M. I. (1972). Unusual effect of secretin on serum gsatrin, serum calcium and gastric secretion in a patient with suspected Zollinger–Ellison syndrome. *Gastroenterology* **62**, 626–631.

Isenberg, J. I., Brickman, A. S., and Moore, E. W. (1973). The effect of secretin on serum calcium in man. *J. Clin. Endocrinol. Metab.* **37**, 30–33.

Ishida, T. (1977). Stimulatory effect of neurotensin on insulin and gastrin secretion in dogs. *Endocrinol. Jpn.* **24**, 335–342.

Itakura, K., Hirose, T., Crea, R., Riggs, A. D., Heyneker, H. L., Bolivar, F., and Boyer,

H. W. (1977). Expression in *Escherichia coli* of a chemically synthesized gene for the hormone somatostatin. *Science* **198**, 1056–1063.

Ito, S., Takai, K., Shibata, A., Matsubara, Y., and Yanaihara, N. (1979). Met-enkephalin-immunoreactive and gastrin-immunoreactive cells in the human and canine pyloric antrum. *Gen. Comp. Endocrinol.* **38**, 238–245.

Itoh, Z., Honda, R., Hiwatashi, K., Takeuchi, S., Aizawa, I., Takayanagi, R., and Couch, E. F. (1976). Motilin-induced mechanical activity in the canine alimentary tract. *Scand. J. Gastroenterol.* **11** (Suppl.) 39 93–110.

IUPAC–IUB Commission on Biochemical Nomenclature (CBN). (1968). A one letter notation for amino acid sequences. *Eur. J. Bochem.* **5**, 151–153.

IUPAC–IUB Commission on Biochemical Nomenclature (CBN). (1977). Nomenclature of multiple forms of enzymes. Recommendations (1976). *J. Biol. Chem.* **252**, 5939–5941.

Ivy, A. C. (1930). The role of hormones in digestion. *Physiol. Rev.* **10**, 282–335.

Ivy, A. C., and Oldberg, E. (1928). A hormone mechanism of gall-bladder contraction and evacuation. *Am. J. Physiol.* **86**, 599–613.

Ivy, A. C., Kloster, G., Lueth, H. C., and Drewyer, G. E. (1929a). On the preparation of "cholecystokinin." *Am. J. Physiol.* **91**, 336–344.

Ivy, A. C., Lueth, H. C., and Kloster, G. (1929b). Vasodepressor phenomenon caused by some cholecystokinin preparations. *Proc. Soc. Exp. Biol. Med.* **26**, 309–311.

Iwatsuki, K., Ono, H., and Hashimoto, K. (1976). Effects of glucagon on pancreatic secretion in the dog. *Clin. Exp. Pharmacol. Physiol.* **3**, 59–65.

Iwatsuki, N., and Petersen, O. H. (1978). Electrical coupling and uncoupling of exocrine acinar cells. *J. Cell. Biol.* **79**, 533–545.

Izeboud, E., and Beyerman, H. C. (1980). Synthesis of porcine motilin via its sulfoxides. *J. R. Neth. Chem. Soc.* **99**, 124–130.

Jackson, B. M., Reeder, D. D., and Thompson, J. C. (1972). Dynamic characteristics of gastrin release. *Ann. J. Surg.* **123**, 137–142.

Jacobsen, H., Demand, A., Moody, A. J., and Sundby, F. (1977). Sequence analysis of porcine gut GLI-1. *Biochim. Biophys. Acta* **493**, 452–459.

Jacobson, E. D., Swan, K. G., and Grossman, M. I. (1967). Blood flow and secretion in the stomach. *Gastroenterology* **52**, 414–420.

Jaeger, E., Knof, S., Scharf, R., Lehnert, P., Schulz, I., and Wünsch, E. (1978). Chemical evidence for the mechanism of inactivation of secretin. *Scand. J. Gastroenterol.* **13** (Suppl.), 49 (Abstr. 93).

Jaeger, E., Filippi, B., Knof, S., Lehnert, P., Moroder, L., and Wünsch, E. (1979). Circular dichroism studies on secretin and some analogues with different biological activities. *In* "Hormone Receptors in Digestion and Nutrition" (G. Rosselin *et al.* eds.), pp. 25–32. Elsevier, Masterdam.

Jaffe, B. M. (1979). Hormones of the gastrointestinal tract. *In* "Endocrinology" (L. J. de Groot *et al.*, eds.), Vol. 3, pp. 1669–1698. Grune & Stratton, New York.

Jansson, R., Steen, G., and Svanvik, J. (1978). Effects of intravenous vasoactive intestinal peptide (VIP) on gallbladder function in the cat. *Gastroenterology* **75**, 47–50.

Jarrett, R. J., and Cohen, N. M. (1967). Intestinal hormones and plasma-insulin. *Lancet* **II**, 861–863.

Jauregui-Adell, J., and Marti, J. (1975). Acidic cleavage of the aspartyl-proline bond and the limitations of the reaction. *Anal. Biochem.* **69**, 468–473.

Jensen, H. (1948). The internal secretion of the pancreas. *In* "The Hormones" (G. Pincus and K. V. Thimann, eds.), Vol. I, pp. 301–332. Academic Press, New York.

Jensen, R. T., and Gardner, J. D. (1978). Cyclic nucleotide-dependent protein kinase activity in acinar cells from guinea pig pancreas. *Gastroenterology* **75**, 806–817.

Jensen, R. T., Moody, T., Pert, C., Rivier, J. E., and Gardner, J. D. (1978). Interaction of bombesin and litorin with specific membrane receptors on pancreatic acinar cells. *Proc. Natl. Acad. Sci. U.S.A.* **75**, 6139–6143.

Jensen, S. L., Fahrenkrug, J., Holst, J. J., Kühl, C., Nielsen, O. V., and Schaffalitzky de Muckadell, O. B. (1978a). Secretory effects of secretin on isolated perfused porcine pancreas. *Am. J. Physiol.* **235**, E381–E386.

Jensen, S. L., Fahrenkrug, J., Holst, J. J., Nielsen, O. V., and Schaffalitzky de Muckadell, O. B. (1978b). Secretory effects of VIP on isolated perfused canine pancreas. *Am. J. Physiol.* **235**, E387–E391.

Jensen, S. L., Rehfeld, J. F., Holst, J. J., Fahrenkrug, J., Nielsen, O. V., and Schaffalitzky de Muckadell, O. B. (1980). Secretory effects of gastrins on isolated perfused porcine pancreas. *Am. J. Physiol.* **238**, E186–E192.

John, M. J., Borjesson, B. W., Walsh, J. R., and Niall, H. D. (1981). Limited sequence homology between porcine and rat relaxins; Implications for physiological studies. *Endocrinology* **108**, 726–729.

Johnson, L. R. (1971). Control of gastric secretion: no room for histamine? *Gastroenterology* **61**, 106–118.

Johnson, L. R. (1976). The trophic action of gastrointestinal hormones. *Gastroenterology* **70**, 278–288.

Johnson, L. R. (1977). New aspects of the trophic action of the gastrointestinal hormones. *Gastroenterology* **72**, 788–792.

Johnson, L. R., and Chandler, A. M. (1973). RNA and DNA of gastric and duodenal mucosa in antrectomized and gastrin-treated rats. *Am. J. Physiol.* **224**, 937–940.

Johnson, L. R., and Grossman, M. I. (1969). Characteristics of inhibition of gastric secretion by secretin *Am. J. Physiol.* **217**, 1401–1404.

Johnson, L. R., and Grossman, M. I. (1970). Analysis of inhibition of acid secretion by cholecystokinin in dogs. *Am. J. Physiol.* **218**, 550–554.

Johnson, L. R., and Grossman, M. I. (1971). Intestinal hormones as inhibitors of gastric secretion. *Gastroenterology* **60**, 120–144.

Johnson, L. R., and Guthrie, P. D. (1974a). Mucosal DNA synthesis: a short term index of the trophic action of gastrin. *Gastroenterology* **67**, 453–459.

Johnson, L. R., and Guthrie, P. D. (1974b). Secretin inhibition of gastrin-stimulated deoxyribonucleic acid synthesis. *Gastroenterology* **67**, 601–606.

Johnson, L. R., and Guthrie, P. (1976). Effect of cholecystokinin and 16,16-dimethyl prostaglandin E_2 on RNA and DNA of gastric and duodenal mucosa. *Gastroenterology* **70**, 59–65.

Johnson, L. R., and Guthrie, P. D. (1978). Effect of secretin on colonic DNA synthesis. *Proc. Soc. Exp. Biol. Med.* **158**, 521–523.

Johnson, L. R., Aures, D., and Yuen, L. (1969a). Pentagastrin-induced stimulation of protein synthesis in the gastrointestinal tract. *Am. J. Physiol.* **217**, 251–254.

Johnson, L. R., Aures, D., and Håkanson, R. (1969b). Effect of gastrin on the in vitro incorporation of ^{14}C-leucine into protein of the digestive tract. *Proc. Soc. Exp. Biol. Med.* **132**, 996–998.

Johnson, L. R., Stening, G. F., and Grossman, M. I. (1970). Effect of sulfation on the gastrointestinal actions of caerulein. *Gastroenterology* **58**, 208–216.

Johnson, L. R., Copeland, E. M., Dudrick, S. J., Lichtenberger, L. M., and Castro, G. A. (1975a). Structural and hormonal alterations in the gastrointestinal tract of parenterally fed rats. *Gastroenterology* **68**, 1177–1183.

Johnson, L. R., Lichtenberger, L. M., Copeland, E. M., Dudrick, S. J., and Castro, G. A. (1975b). Action of gastrin on gastrointestinal structure and function. *Gastroenterology* **68**, 1184–1192.

Johnson, R. E., Hruby, V. J., and Rupley, J. A. (1979). Thermodynamics of glucagon aggregation. *Biochemistry* **18**, 1176–1179.

Jones, R. S., and Grossman, M. I. (1970). Choleretic effects of cholecystokinin, gastrin II, and caerulein in the dog. *Am. J. Physiol.* **219**, 1014–1018.

Jones, R. S., and Hall, A. D. (1969). The effects of glucagon on Brunner's gland secretion in dogs. *Proc. Soc. Exp. Biol. Med.* **132**, 1159–1161.

Jones, R. S., and Meyers, W. C. (1979). Regulation of hepatic biliary secretion. *Annu. Rev. Physiol.* **41**, 67–82.

Jordan, P. H., and Peterson, N. D. (1962). Effects of secretin upon gastric secretion. *Ann. Surg.* **156**, 914–923.

Jordan, P. H., and Yip, B. S. S. C. (1972). The canine secretory response to gastrin extracted from gastric juice of man. *Surgery* **72**, 624–629.

Jörnvall, H., Carlquist, M., Kwauk, S., Otte, S. C., McIntosh, C. H. S., Brown, J. C., and Mutt, V. (1981a). Amino acid sequence and heterogeneity of gastric inhibitory polypeptide (GIP). *FEBS Lett.* **123**, 205–210.

Jörnvall, H., Carlström, A., Pettersson, T., Jacobsson, B., Persson, M., and Mutt, V. (1981b). Structural homologies between prealbumin, gastrointestinal prohormones and other proteins. *Nature (London)* **291**, 261–263.

Jörnvall, H., Mutt, V., and Persson, M. (1982). Structural similarities among gastrointestinal hormones and related active peptides. *Hoppe-Seylers Z. Physiol. Chem.* **363**, 475–483.

Jorpes, J. E. (1968). The isolation and chemistry of secretin and cholecystokinin. *Gastroenterology* **55**, 157–164.

Jorpes, J. E., and Mutt, V. (1961a). On the biological activity and amino acid composition of secretin. *Acta Chem. Scand.* **15**, 1790–1791.

Jorpes, J. E., and Mutt, V. (1961b). The gastrointestinal hormones, secretin and cholecystokinin-pancreozymin. *Ann. Int. Med.* **55**, 394–405.

Jorpes, J. E., and Mutt, V. (1961c). Process for the production of gastrointestinal hormones and hormone concentrate. USA Pat. No. 3.013.944.

Jorpes, J. E., and Mutt, V. (1964). Gastrointestinal hormones. *In* "The Hormones" (G. Pincus, K. V. Thimann, and E. B. Astwood, eds.), Vol. IV, pp. 365–385. Academic Press, New York.

Jorpes, J. E., and Mutt, V. (1966). Cholecystokinin and pancreozymin, one single hormone? *Acta Physiol. Scand.* **66**, 196–202.

Jorpes, J. E., and Mutt, V. (1973). Secretin and cholecystokinin (CCK). *In* "Handbook of Experimental Pharmacology" (O. Eichler *et al.*, eds.), pp. 1–179. Springer Verlag, Berlin and New York.

Jorpes, J. E., Mutt, V., Magnusson, S., and Steele, B. B. (1962). Amino acid composition and N-terminal amino acid sequence of porcine secretin. *Biochem. Biophys. Res. Commun.* **9**, 275–279.

Jorpes, E., Mutt, V., and Toczko, K. (1964). Further purification of cholecystokinin and pancreozymin. *Acta Chem. Scand.* **18**, 2408–2410.

Jorpes, J. E., Mutt, V., Jonson, G., Thulin, L., and Sundman, L. (1965). Influence of secretin and cholecystokinin on bile flow. *In* "The Biliary System" (W. Taylor, ed.), pp. 293–301. Blackwell, Oxford.

Jung, F. T., and Greengard, H. (1933). Response of the isolated gall bladder to cholecystokinin. *Am. J. Physiol.* **103**, 275–278.

Kachelhoffer, J., Eloy, M. R., Pousse, A., Hohmatter, D., and Grenier, J. F. (1974). Mesenteric vasomotor effects of vasoactive intestinal polypeptide. Study on perfused isolated intestinal canine jejunal loops. *Pflügers Arch.* **352**, 37–46.

Kachelhoffer, J., Mendel, C., Dauchel, J., Hohmatter, D., and Grenier, J. F. (1976). The effects of VIP on intestinal motility: Study on ex vivo perfused isolated canine jejunal loops. *Am. J. Dig. Dis.* **21**, 957–962.

Kacian, D. L., Spiegelman, S., Bank, A., Terada, M., Metafora, S., Down, L., and Marks, P. A. (1972). In vitro synthesis of DNA components of human genes for globins. *Nature (London) New Biol.* **235**, 167–169.

Kaess, H. (1980). Le dérivé ortho-nitrophényl- sulfényl de la pentagastrine: un antagoniste des récepteurs a gastrine? Une voie de recherche prometteuse. *Gastroenterol. Clin. Biol.* **4**, 751–753.

Kahlson, G., Rosengren, E., Svahn, D., and Thunberg, R. (1964). Mobilization and formation of histamine in the gastric mucosa as related to acid secretion. *J. Physiol. (London)* **174**, 400–416.

Kaminiski, D. L., and Deshpande, Y. G. (1979). Effect of gastrin I and gastrin II on canine bile flow. *Am. J. Physiol.* **236**, E584–E588.

Kaminski, D. L., and Nahrwold, D. L. (1979). Neurohormonal control of biliary secretion and gallbladder function. *World J. Surg.* **3**, 449–456.

Kaminski, D. L., Ruwart, M. J., and Jellinek, M. (1977). Structure–function relationships of peptide fragments of gastrin and cholecystokinin. *Am. J. Physiol.* **233**, E286–E292.

Kamionkowski, M., Grossman, S., and Fleshler, B. (1964). The inhibitory effect of secretin on broth-stimulated gastric secretion in human subjects. *Gut* **5**, 237–240.

Kanda, T., Goodman, deWitt, S., Canfield, R. E., and Morgan, F. J. (1974). The amino acid sequence of human plasma prealbumin. *J. Biol. Chem.* **249**, 6796–6805.

Kaneko, T., Cheng, P. Y., Toda, G., Oka, H., Oda, T., Yanaihara, N., Yanaihara, C., Mihara, S., Nishida, T., Kaise, N., Shin, S., and Imagawa, K. (1979). Biological binding activities of synthetic possible C-terminal fragments of glicentin in rat liver plasma membranes. *In* "Gut Peptides" (A. Miyoshi and M. I. Grossman, eds.), pp. 157–161. Elsevier, Amsterdam.

Kaneto, A., Mizuno, Y., Tasaka, Y., and Kosaka, K. (1970). Stimulation of glucagon secretion by tetragastrin. *Endocrinology* **86**, 1175–1180.

Kanno, T. (1972). Calcium-dependent amylase release and electrophysiological measurements in cells of the pancreas. *J. Physiol. (London)* **226**, 353–371.

Karppanen, H. O., Neuvonen, P. J., Bieck, P. R., and Westermann, E. (1974). Effect of histamine, pentagastrin and theophylline on the production of cyclic AMP in isolated gastric tissue of the guinea pig. *Naunyn-Schmiederbergs Arch. Pharmacol.* **284**, 15–23.

Kato, Y., Iwasaki, Y., Iwasaki, J., Abe, H., Yanaihara, N., and Imura, H. (1978). Prolactin release by vasoactive intestinal polypeptide in rats. *Endocrinology* **103**, 554–558.

Kaura, R., Allen, A., and Hirst, B. H. (1980). Mucus in the gastric juice of cats during pentagastrin and secretin infusions: The viscosity in relation to glycoprotein structure and concentration. *Biochem. Soc. Trans.* **8**, 52–53.

Kelly, K. A., Nyhus, L. M., and Harkins, H. N. (1964). The vagal nerve and intestinal phase of gastric secretion. *Gastroenterology* **46**, 163–166.

Kemper, B., Habener, J. F., Mulligan, R. C., Potts, J. T., Jr., and Rich, A. (1974). Preparathyroid hormone: A direct translation product of parathyroid messenger RNA. *Proc. Natl. Acad. Sci. U.S.A.* **71**, 3731–3735.

Kenner, G. W. (1972). The chemistry of gastrin, a peptide hormone. *Chem. Ind.* 791–794.

Kenny, A. J., and Say, R. R. (1962). Glucagon-like activity extractable from the gastrointestinal tract of man and other animals. *J. Endocrinol.* **25**, 1–7.

Kerins, C., and Said, S. I. (1973). Hyperglycemic and glycogenolytic effects of vasoactive intestinal polypeptide. *Proc. Soc. Exp. Biol. Med.* **142**, 1014–1017.

Kimmel, J. R., Pollock, H. G., and Hazelwood, R. L. (1968). Isolation and characterization of chicken insulin. *Endocrinology* **83**, 1323–1330.

Kimmel, J. R., Hayden, L. J., and Pollock, H. G. (1975). Isolation and characterization of a new pancreatic polypeptide hormone. *J. Biol. Chem.* **250**, 9369–9376.

King, M. V. (1959). The unit cell and space group of cubic glucagon. *J. Mol. Biol.* **1**, 375–378.

Kita, T., Inoue, A., Nakanishi, S., and Numa, S. (1979). Purification and characterization of the messenger RNA coding for bovine corticotropin/β-lipotropin precursor. *Eur. J. Biochem.* **93**, 213–220.

Kitabgi, P., and Freychet, P. (1978). Effects of neurotensin on isolated intestinal smooth muscles. *Eur. J. Pharmacol.* **50**, 349–357.

Kitabgi, P., Carraway, R., and Leeman, S. E. (1976). Isolation of a tridecapeptide from bovine intestinal tissue its partial characterization as neurotensin. *J. Biol. Chem.* **251**, 7053–7058.

Kitani, K., Suzuki, Y., and Miura, R. (1978). Differences in the effects of secretin and glucagon on the blood circulation in unanesthetized rats. *Acta Hepato-Gastroenterol.* **25**, 470–473.

Klaff, L. J., Hudson, A., Sheppard, M., and Tyler, M. (1981). In vitro release of cholecystokinin octapeptide-like immunoreactivity from rat brain synaptosomes. *S. Afr. Med. Tydskr.* 158–160.

Klapdor, R. (1979). Gastrointestinale Hormone: Gegenwärtiger Stand. *Med. Lab.* **32**, 71–88.

Klausner, Y. S., and Bodanszky, M. (1977). Cholecystokinin-pancreozymin. 2. Synthese of a protected heptapeptide hydrazide corresponding to sequence 17–23. *J. Org. Chem.* **42**, 147–149.

Klein, M. S., and Winawer, S. J. (1974). Intermittent basal gastric hypersecretion following small bowel resection. *Am. J. Gastroenterol.* **61**, 470–475.

Koelz, H. R., Drack, G. Th., and Blum, A. L. (1976). Calcitonin und Speicheldrüsen-Amylase- sekretion in vivo und in vitro. *Schweiz. Med. Wochenschr.* **106**, 298–299.

Kokas, E., and Johnston, C. L., Jr. (1965). Influence of refined villikinin on motility of intestinal villi. *Am. J. Physiol.* **208**, 1196–1202.

Kokas, E., and Ludány, G. (1930). Weitere Untersuchungen über die Bewegung der Darmzottern. *Pflügers Arch. Physiol.* **225**, 421–428.

Kokas, E., and Ludány, G. (1934). Die hormonale Regelung der Darmzottenbewegung. II. Das Villikinin. *Pflügers Arch. Physiol.* **234**, 182–186.

Kokas, E., Davis, J. L., III., and Brunson, W. D. (1971). Separation of villikinin-like substance from intestinal mucosal extract. *Arch. Int. Pharmacodyn. Ther.* **191**, 310–317.

Kolata, G. B. (1978). Polypeptide hormones:What are they doing in cells? *Science* **201**, 895–897.

Komarov, S. A. (1942). Studies on gastrin. I. Methods of isolation of a specific gastric secretagogue from the pyloric mucus membrane and its chemical properties. *Rev. Can. Biol.* **1**, 191–205.

Kondo, S., and Schulz, I. (1976). Calcium ion uptake in isolated pancreas cells induced by secretagogues. *Biochim. Biophys. Acta* **419**, 76–92.

Konturek, S. J., Tasler, J., and Obtulowicz, W. (1972). Effect of atropine on pancreatic responses to endogenous and exogenous cholecystokinin. *Am. J. Dig. Dis.* **17**, 911–917.

Konturek, S. J., Demitrescu, T., and Radecki, T. (1974). The role of histamine receptors in the stimulation of gastric acid secretion. *Am. J. Dig. Dis.* **19,** 999–1006.

Konturek, S. J., Thor, P., Dembinski, A., and Krol, R. (1975). Comparison of secretin and vasoactive intestinal peptide on pancreatic secretion in dogs. *Gastroenterology* **68,** 1527–1535.

Konturek, S. J., Tasler, J., Ortukowicz, W., and Cieszkowski, M. (1976a). Comparison of amino acids bathing the oxyntic gland area in the stimulation of gastric secretion. *Gastroenterology* **70,** 66–69.

Konturek, S. J., Dembiński, A., Thor, P., and Król, R. (1976b). Comparison of vasoactive intestinal peptide (VIP) and secretin in gastric secretion and mucosal blood flow. *Pflügers Arch.* **361,** 175–181.

Kosaka, T., and Lim, R. K. S. (1930). Demonstration of the humoral agent in fat inhibition of gastric secretion. *Proc. Soc. Exp. Biol. Med.* **27,** 890–891.

Kowalewski, K., Pachkowski, T., and Kolodej, A. (1978). Effect of secretin on mucinous secretion by the isolated canine stomach perfused extracorporeally. *Pharmacology* **16,** 78–82.

Kraut, H., Frey, E. K., and Werle, E. (1930). The circulatory hormone. IV. Demonstration of a circulatory hormone in the pancreas. *Z. Physiol. Chem.* **189,** 97–106.

Kreil, G., Haiml, L., and Suchanek, G. (1980). Stepwise cleavage of the two part of promellitin by dipeptidyl-peptidase IV. Evidence for a new type of precursor—product conversion. *Eur. J. Biochem.* **11,** 49–58.

Krejs, G. J., Fordtran, J. S., Bloom, S. R., Fahrenkrug, J., Schaffalitzky De Muckadell, O. B., Fischer, J. E. Humphrey, C. S., O'Dorisio, T. M., Said, S. I., Walsh, J. H., and Shulkes, A. A. (1980). Effect of VIP infusion on water and ion transport in the human jejunum. *Gastroenterology* **78,** 722–727.

Kronenberg, H. M., Roberts, B. E., Habener, J. F., Potts, J. T., Jr., and Rich, A. (1977). DNA complementary to parathyroid mRNA directs synthesis of preproparathyroin hormone in a linked transcription–translation system. *Nature (London)* **267,** 804–807.

Kronenberg, H. M., McDevitt, B. E., Majzoub, J. A., Nathans, J., Sharp, P. A., Potts, J. T., Jr., and Rich A. (1979). Cloning and nucleotide sequence of DNA coding for bovine preproparathyroid hormone. *Proc. Natl. Acad. Sci. U.S.A.* **76,** 4981–4985.

Krutzsch, H. C. (1980). Determination of polypeptide amino acid sequences from the carboxyl terminus using angiotensin I converting enzyme. *Biochemistry* **19,** 5290–5296.

Kudrewetzky, B. B. (1894). Materiale zur Physiologie der Bauchspeicheldrüse. *Arch. Physiol. (Lipzig)* 83–116.

Kulka, R. G., and Sternlicht, E. (1968). Enzyme secretion in mouse pancreas mediated by adenosine-3'5'- cyclic phosphate and inhibited by adenosine-3'-phosphate. *Proc. Natl. Acad. Sci. U.S.A.* **61,** 1123–1128.

La Barre, M. J. (1932). Sur le possibilités d' un traitment du diabète par l'incrétine. *Bull. Acad. Med. Belg.* **12,** 620–634.

Laburthe, M., Prieto, J. C., Amiranoff, B., Dupont, C., Hui Bon Hoa, D., and Rosselin, G. (1979). Interaction of vasoactive intestinal peptide with isolated intestinal epithelial cells from rat. *Eur. J. Biochem.* **96,** 239–248.

Lagerlöf, H. O. (1942). Pancreatic function and pancreatic disease studied by means of secretin. *Acta Med. Scand. Suppl.* **128.**

Lambert, M., Camus, J., and Christophe, J. (1975). Phosphorylation in vitro of proteins in the pancreas and parotids of rats: effects of hormonal secretagogues and cyclic nucleotides. *Biochem. Pharmacol.* **24,** 1755–1758.

Lamers, C. B. (1978). Clinical aspects of gastrointestinal hormones. *Neth. J. Med.* **21,** 77–82.

Lanciault, G., Merritt, A., Rosato, E. Bonoma, C., and Brooks, F. P. (1972). Comparative relationship between serum gastrin concentration and gastric acid output. *Am. J. Dig. Dis.* **17,** 523–526.

Lanciault, G., Bonoma, C., and Brooks, F. P. (1973). Vagal stimulation, gastrin release, and acid secretion in anesthetized dogs. *Am. J. Physiol.* **225,** 546–552.

Larsson, L. I. (1977). Corticotropin-like peptides in central nervous and in endocrine cells of gut and pancreas. *Lancet* **II,** 1321–1323.

Larsson, L. I. (1978). Gastrin and ACTH-like immunoreactivity occurs in two ultrastructurally distinct cell types of rat antropyloric mucosa. *Histochemistry* **58,** 33–48.

Lauber, M., Camier, M., and Cohen, P. (1979). Higher molecular weight forms of immunoreactive somatostatin in mouse hypothalamic extracts: Evidence of processing in vtro. *Proc. Natl. Acad. Sci. U.S.A.* **76,** 6004–6008.

Laughton, N. B., and Macallum, A. B. (1932). The relation of the duodenal mucosa to the internal secretion of the pancreas. *Proc. R. Soc. Ser. B* **111,** 37–46.

Lauritsen, K. B., Moody, A. J., Christensen, K. C., and Jensen, S. L. (1980). Gastric inhibitory polypeptide (GIP) and insulin release after small-bowel resection in man. *Scand. J. Gastroenterol.* **15,** 833–840.

Lawrence, A. M. (1966). Radioimmunoassayable glucagon levels in man: effects of starvation, hypoglycemia, and glucose administration. *Proc. Natl. Acad. Sci. U.S.A.* **55,** 316–320.

Laycock, D. G., and Hunt, J. A. (1969). Synthesis of rabbit globin by a bacterial cell free system. *Nature (London)* **221,** 1118–1122.

Lazarus, L. H., Linnoila, R. I., Hernandes, O., and DiAugustine, R. P. (1980). A neuropeptide in mammalian tissues with physalaemin-like immunoreactivity. *Nature (London)* **287,** 555–558.

Lazarus, N. R., Voyles, N. R., Devrim, S., Tanese, T., and Recant, L. (1968). Extragastrointestinal effects of secretin, gastrin, and pancreozymin. *Lancet* **II,** 248–250.

Lebedinskaja, S. I. (1933). Uber die Magensekretion bei Eckschen Fistelhunden. *Z. Ges. Exp. Med.* **88,** 264–270.

Lee, M. K., and Coupar, I. M. (1980). Inhibition of intestinal secretion without reduction of cyclic AMP levels. *Eur. J. Pharmacol.* **68,** 501–503.

Lee, S. Y., Mendecki, J., and Brawerman, G. (1971). A polynucleotide segment rich in adenylic acid in the rapidly-labeled polyribosomal RNA component of mouse sarcoma 180 ascites cells. *Proc. Natl. Acad. Sci. U.S.A.* **68,** 1331–1335.

Leeman, S. E., and Carraway, R. E. (1977). Discovery of a sialogogic peptide in bovine hypothalamic extracts: Its isolation, characterization as substance P, structure and synthesis. *In* "Substance P" (U.S. von Euler and B. Pernow, eds.), pp. 5–13. Raven, New York.

Leeman, S. E., and Hammerschlag, R. (1967). Stimulation of salivary secretion by a factor extracted from hypothamic tissue. *Endocrinology* **81,** 803–810.

Lehy, T., Voillemot, N., Dubrasquet, M., and Dufougeray, F. (1975). Gastrin cell hyperplasia in rats with chronic antral stimulation. *Gastroenterology* **68,** 71–82.

Lembeck, F., and Starke, K. (1968). Substanz P und Speichersekretion. *Naunyn-Schmiedebergs Arch. Pharmacol. Pathol.* **259,** 375–385.

Leppäluoto, J., Koivusalo, F., and Kraama, R. (1977). Existence of TRF-like immunoreactivity in neuroectodermal tissues. *Proc. Int. Union Physiol. Sci.* **13,** 440.

Leppäluoto, J., Koivusalo, F., and Kraama, R. (1978). Thyrotropin-releasing factor: Distribution in neural and gastrointestinal tissues. *Acta Physiol. Scand.* **104,** 175–179.

Lernmark, A., Chan, S. J., Choy, R., Nathans, A., Carroll, R., Tager, H. S., Rubenstein, A. H., Swift, H. H., and Steiner, D. F. (1976). Biosynthesis of insulin and glucagon: a view of the current state of the art. In "The Peptide Hormones, Molecular and Cellular Aspects" (R. Porter and D. Fitzsimons, eds.), pp. 7–30. Elsevier, Amsterdam.

LeRoith, D., Spitz, I. M., Ebert, R., Liel, Y., Odes, S., and Creuzfeldt, W. (1980). Acid-induced gastric inhibitory polypeptide secretion in man. J. Clin. Endocrinol. Metab. 51, 1385–1389.

Leroy, J., Morisset, J. A., and Webster, P. D. (1971). Dose-related response of pancreatic synthesis and secretion to cholecystokinin-pancreozymin. J. Lab. Clin. Med. 78, 149–157.

Leuret, F., and Lassaigne, J. L. (1825). "Recherches Physiologiques et Chimiques pour Servir a l'Histoire de la Digestion." Huzard, Paris.

Levant, J., Walsh, J. H., and Isenberg, J. I. (1973). Stimulation of gastric secretion and gastrin release by single oral doses of calcium carbonate in man. New Engl. J. Med. 289, 555–558.

Levin, S. R., Pehlevanian, M. Z., Lavee, A. E., and Adachi, R. I. (1979). Secretion of a insulinotropic factor from isolated, perfused rat intestine. Am. J. Physiol. 236, E710–E720.

Levine, R. A. (1973). Cyclic AMP in digestive physiology. Am. J. Clin. Nutr. 26, 876–881.

Levine, S. D., and Bodanszky, M. (1966). Secretin. The synthesis of a "wrong" hexapeptide amide, sequence 22–27. Biochemistry 5, 3441–3443.

Levy, M. (1975). Further observations on the response of the glomerular filtration rate to glucagon: comparison with secretin. Can. J. Physiol. Pharmacol. 53, 81–85.

Li, C. H. (1952). Recent studies on the problems involved in the preparation, properties and bioassay of adrenocorticotrophic hormone. Acta Endocrinol. 10, 255–296.

Li, C. H. (1968). β-lipotropin, a new pituitary hormone. Arch. Biol. Med. Exp. 5, 55–61.

Li, C. H., Chung, D., Yamashiro, D., and Lee, C. Y. (1978). Isolation, characterization, and synthesis of a corticotropin-inhibiting peptide from human pituitary glands. Proc. Natl. Acad. Sci. U.S.A. 75, 4306–4309.

Lichtenberger, L., and Johnson, L. R. (1974). Gastrin in the ontogenic development of the small intestine. Am. J. Physiol. 227, 390–395.

Lichtenberger, L., Miller, L. R., Erwin, D. N., and Johnson, L. R. (1973). Effect of pentagastrin on adult rat duodenal cells in culture. Gastroenterology 65, 242–251.

Lichtenberger, L., Welsh, J. D., and Johnson, L. R. (1976). Relationship between the changes in gastrin levels and intestinal properties in the starved rat. Am. J. Dig. Dis. 21, 33–38.

Lim, L., and Canellakis, E. S. (1970). Adenine-rich polymer associated with rabbit reticulocyte messenger RNA. Nature (London) 227, 710–712.

Lin, M. C., Wright, D. E., Hruby, V. J., and Rodbell, M. (1975). Structure–function relationships in glucagon; properties of highly purified des-His¹-, monoiodo-, and (des-Asn²⁸,Thr²⁹)(homoserine lactone²⁷)-glucagon. Biochemistry 14, 1559–1563.

Lin, T.-M., and Chance, R. E. (1974). Candidate hormones of the gut. VI. Bovine pancreatic polypeptide (BPP) and avian pancreatic polypeptide (APP). Gastroenterology 67, 737–738.

Lin, T.-M., Spray, G. F., and Southard, G. L. (1977). Dispensability of both the amide of phenylalanine and the carboxyl group of aspartic acid for the stimulation of gastric acid secretion by gastrin peptides in dogs. Gastroenterology 72, 566–568.

Ling, N., Esch, F., Davis, D., Mercado, M., Regno, M., Bohlen, P., Brazeau, P., and Guillemin, R. (1980). Solid phase synthesis of somatostatin-28. *Biochem. Biophys. Res. Commun.* **95,** 945–951.

Linsley, P. S., Blifeld, C., Wrann, M., and Fox, C. F. (1979). Direct linkage of epidermal growth factor to its receptor. *Nature (London)* **278,** 745–748.

Livermore, A. H., and du Vigneaud, V. (1949). Preparation of high potency oxytocic material by the use of countercurrent distribution. *J. Biol. Chem.* **180,** 365–373.

Lockard, R. E., and Lingrel, J. B. (1969). The synthesis of mouse hemoglobin β-chains in a rabbit reticulocyte cell-free system programmed with mouse reticulocyte 9s RNA. *Biochem. Biophys. Res. Commun.* **37,** 204–212.

Loew, E. R., Gray, J. S., and Ivy, A. C. (1940). Is a duodenal hormone involved in carbohydrate metabolism? *Am. J. Physiol.* **129,** 659–663.

Lomedico, P. T. (1975). Cell-free translation of pancreatic mRNA: Synthesis of immunoreactive insuline. *Diabetes* **24** (Suppl. 2), 405 (Abstr. 52).

Lomedico, P. T., Chan, S. J., Stiner, D. F., and Saunders, G. F. (1977). Immunological and chemical characterization of bovine preproinsulin. *J. Biol. Chem.* **252,** 7971–7978.

Long, B. W., and Gardner, J. D. (1977). Effects of cholecystokinin and adenylate cyclase activity in dispersed pancreatic acinar cells. *Gastroenterology* **73,** 1008–1014.

Long, M. M., Urry, D. W., and Stoekenius, W. (1977). Circular dichroism of biological membranes: purple membrane of *Halobacterium halobium. Biochem. Biophys. Res. Commun.* **75,** 725–731.

Lord, J. A. H., Waterfield, A. A., Hughes, J., and Kosterlitz, H. W. (1977). Endogenous opioid peptides: multiple agonists and receptors. *Nature (London)* **267,** 495–499.

Lorenz, D. N., Kreielsheimer, G., and Smith, G. P. (1979). Effect of cholecystokinin, gastrin, secretin, and GIP on sham feeding in the rat. *Physiol. Behav.* **23,** 1065–1072.

Love, J. W., Walder, A. I., and Bingham, C. (1968). Effect of pure natural and synthetic secretin on Brunner's gland secretion in dogs. *Nature (London)* **219,** 731–732.

Lowe, B. W., Lovell, F. M., and Rudko, A. D. (1971). Reply to "Prediction of α-helices in glucagon" by Schiffer and Edmundson. *Biophys. J.* **11,** 235.

Lowry, P. J., Hope, J., and Silman, R. E. (1976). The evolution of corticotrophin, melanothrophin and lipotrophin. *Proc. Int. Congr. Endocrinol., 5th, Hamburg* **2,** 71–76.

Luft, R., Efendic, S., Hökfelt, T., Johansson, O., and Arimura, A. (1974). Immunohistochemical evidence for the localization of somatostatin-like immunoreactivity in a cell population of the pancreatic islets. *Med. Biol.* **52,** 428–430.

Lugaro, G., Pasta, P., Casellato, M. M., Mazzola, G., and Carrea, G. (1976). Chemical and physical properties of the human urinary glycoprotein with gastric antisecretory activity. *Biochem. J.* **153,** 641–646.

Lund, P. K., Sanders, D. J., and Zahedi-Asl, S. (1979). Gastric juice gastrin. *J. Physiol. (London)* **296,** 35P.

Lund, P. K., Goodman, R. H., Jacobs, J. W., and Habener, J. F. (1980). Glucagon precursors identified by immunoprecipitation of products of cell-free translation of messenger RNA. *Diabetes* **29,** 583–586.

Lundberg, J. M., Hökfelt, T., Schultzenberg, M., Uvnäs-Wallensten, K., Köhler, C., and Said, S. I. (1979). Occurrence of vasoactive intestinal polypeptide (VIP)-like immunoreactivity in certain cholinergic neurons of the cat: evidence from combined immunohistochemistry and acetylcholinesterase staining. *Neuroscience* **4,** 1539–1559.

Lundberg, J. M., Änggård, A., Fahrenkrug, J., Hökfelt, T., and Mutt, V. (1980a). Vasoactive intestinal polypeptide in cholinergic neurons of exocrine glands: Functional significance of coexisting transmitters for vasodilation and secretion. *Proc. Natl. Acad. Sci. U.S.A.* **77,** 1651–1655.

Lundberg, J. M., Änggård, A., Hökfelt, T., and Kimmel, J. (1980b). Avian pancreatic polypeptide (APP) inhibits atropine resistant vasodilation in cat submandibular salivary gland and nasal mucosa: Possible interaction with VIP. *Acta Physiol. Scand.* **10,** 199–201.

Luyckx, A. S., and Lefebvre, P. J. (1969). Release of glucagon or a glucagon-like immunoreactive material by rat jejunum incubated in vitro. *In* "Protein and Polypeptide Hormones" (M. Margoulis, ed.), pp. 884–886. Excerpta Medica, Amsterdam.

Lyman, R. L., and Lepkovsky, S. (1957). The effect of raw soybean meal and trypsin inhibitor diets on pancreatic enzyme secretion in the rat. *J. Nutr.* **62,** 269–284.

Lyons, W. R. (1937). Preparation and assay of mammotropic hormone. *Proc. Soc. Exp. Biol. Med.* **35,** 645–648.

McBride-Warren, P. A., and Epand, R. M. (1972). Evidence for the compact conformation of monomeric glucagon. Hydrogen–tritium exchange studies. *Biochemistry* **11,** 3571–3575.

McCulloch, J., and Edvinsson, L. (1980). Cerebral circulatory and metabolic effects of vasoactive intestinal polypeptide. *Am. J. Physiol.* **238,** H449–H456.

McDonald, J. K., Callahan, P. X., Zeitman, B. B., and Ellis, S. (1969). Inactivation and degradation of glucagon by dipeptidyl aminopeptidase I (Cathepsin C) of rat liver. Including a comparative study of secretin degradation. *J. Biol. Chem.* **244,** 6199–6208.

McDonald, T. J., Nilsson, G., Vagne, M., Ghatei, M., Bloom, S. R., and Mutt, V. (1978). A gastrin releasing peptide from the porcine nonantral gastric tissue. *Gut* **19,** 767–774.

McDonald, T. J., Jörnvall, H., Nilsson, G., Vagne, M., Ghatei, M., Bloom, S. R., and Mutt, V. (1979). Characterization of a gastrin releasing peptide from porcine nonantral gastric tissue. *Biochem. Biophys. Res. Commun.* **90,** 227–233.

McDonald, T. J., Jörnvall, H., Ghatei, M., Bloom, S. R., and Mutt, V. (1980). Characterization of an avian gastric (proventricular) peptide having sequence homology with the porcine gastrin-releasing peptide and the amphibian peptides bombesin and alytesin. *FEBS Lett.* **122,** 45–58.

McGuigan, J. E. (1974). Gastrin. *Vitamins Horm.* **32,** 47–88.

McGuigan, J. E. (1978). Gastrointestinal hormones. *Annu. Rev. Med.* **29,** 307–318.

MacIntosh, F. C. (1938). Histamine as a normal stimulant of gastric secretion. *Q. J. Exp. Physiol.* **28,** 87–98.

McIntosh, C., Arnold, R., Botte, E., Becker, H., Kobberling, J., and Creutzfeldt, W. (1978). Gastrointestinal somatostatin in man and dog. *Metabolism* **27** (Suppl. 1), 1317–1320.

McIntyre, N., Holdsworth, C. D., and Turner, D. S. (1965). Intestinal factors in the control of insulin secretion. *J. Clin. Endocrinol.* **25,** 1317–1324.

Maclagan, N. F. (1937). The role of appetite in the control of body weight. *J. Physiol. (London)* **90,** 385–394.

McLaughlin, C. L., and Baile, C. A. (1980). Decreased sensitivity of Zucker obese rats to the putative satiety agent cholecystokinin. *Physiol. Behav.* **25,** 543–548.

Maddison, S. (1977). Intraperitoneal and intracranial cholecystokinin depress operant responding for food. *Physiol. Behav.* **19,** 819–824.

Magee, D. F., and Nakamura, M. (1966). Action of pancreozymin preparations on gastric secretion. *Nature (London)* **212,** 1487–1488.

Magee, D. F., and Nakajima, S. (1968a). Stimulatory action of secretin on gastric pepsin secretion. *Experientia* **24**, 689–690.

Magee, D. F., and Nakajima, S. (1968b). The effects of antral acidification on the gastric secretion stimulated by endogenous and exogenous gastrin. *J. Physiol. (London)* **196**, 713–721.

Mahler, R. J., and Weisberg, H. (1968). Failure of endogenous stimulation of secretin and pancreozymin release to influence serum-insulin. *Lancet* **I**, 448–451.

Mailman, D. (1978). Effects of vasoactive intestinal polypeptide on intestinal absorption and blood flow. *J. Physiol. (London)* **279**, 121–132.

Mains, R. E., and Eipper, B. A. (1980). Biosynthetic studies on ACTH, β-endorphin, and α-melanotropin in the rat. *Ann. N.Y. Acad. Sci.* **343**, 94–110.

Mains, R. E., Eipper, B. A., and Ling, N. (1977). Common precursor to corticotropins and endorphins. *Proc. Natl. Acad. Sci. U.S.A.* **74**, 3014–3018.

Mainz, D. L., Black, O., and Webster, P. D. (1973). Hormonal control of pancreatic growth. *J. Clin. Invest.* **52**, 2300–2304.

Majumdar, A. P. N. (1979). Effects of fasting and pentagastrin on protein synthesis by different classes of polyribosomes of gastric mucosa of rabbits. *Biochem. Med.* **22**, 288–298.

Makhlouf, G. M., McManus, J. P. A., and Card, W. I. (1964). The action of gastrin II on gastric-acid secretion in man. Comparison of the "maximal" secretory response to gastrin II and histamine. *Lancet* **II**, 485–489.

Maklouf, G. M., Bodanszky, M., Fink, M. L., and Schebalin, M. (1978). Pancreatic secretory activity of secretin$_{5-27}$ and substituted analogues. *Gastroenterology* **75**, 244–248.

Makman, M. H., and Sutherland, E. W., Jr. (1964). Use of liver adenyl cyclase for assay of glucagon in human gastrointestinal tract and pancreas. *Endocrinology* **75**, 127–134.

Malagelada, J., Go, V. L. W., Dimagno, E. P., and Summerskill, W. H. J. (1972). Bile acids inhibit cholecystokinin (CCK) release in man. *J. Clin. Invest.* **51**, 59a–60a.

Malagelada, J., Go, V. L. W., and Summerskill, W. H. J. (1973). Differing sensitivities of gallbladder and pancreas to cholecystokinin-pancreozymin (CCK-PZ) in man. *Gastroenterology* **64**, 950–954.

Malfertheiner, P., Fussgänger, R., Minne, H., and Ditschuneit, H. (1980). Influence of gastrointestinal hormones on human salivary secretion. *Horm. Metab. Res.* **12**, 485.

Mangeat, P. H., Chahinian, H., and Marchis-Mouren, G. J. (1978). Characterization of the cyclic AMP-dependent protein kinase from rat pancreas, further purification of the catalytic subunit, substrate specificity, effect of the pancreatic heat stable inhibitor. *Biochimie* **60**, 777–785.

Marchand, G. R., Hubel, K. A., and Williamson, H. E. (1972). Effects of secretin on renal hemodynamics and excretion. *Proc. Soc. Exp. Biol. Med.* **139**, 1356–1358.

Markussen, J. (1971). Mouse insulins—separation and structures. *Int. J. Pept. Protein Res.* **3**, 149–155.

Markussen, J., and Sundby, F. (1973). Separation and characterization of glucagon-like immunoreactive components from gut extracts by electrofocusing. *In* "Protides of the Biological Fluids" (H. Peeters, ed.), Vol. 17, pp. 471–474. Pergaman, Oxford.

Markussen, J., Frandsen, E., Heding, L. G., and Sundby, F. (1972). Turkey glucagon: Crystallization, amino acid composition and immunology. *Horm. Metab. Res.* **4**, 360–363.

Marois, C., Morisset, J., and Dunnigan, J. (1972). Presence and stimulation of adenyl cyclase in pancreas homogenate. *Rev. Can. Biol.* **31**, 253–257.

Martin, F., MacLeod, I. B., and Sircus, W. (1970). Effects of antrectomy on the fundic mucosa of the rat. *Gastroenterology* **59**, 437–444.

Mashiter, K., Harding, P. E., Chou, M., Mashiter, G. D., Stout, J., Diamond, D., and

Field, J. B. (1975). Persistent pancreatic glucagon but not insulin response to arginine in pancreatectomized dogs. *Endocrinology* **96**, 678–693.

Mason, J. C., Murphy, R. F., Henry, R. W., and Buchanan, K. D. (1979). Starvation-induced changes in secretin-like immunoreactivity of human plasma. *Biochim. Biophys. Acta* **582**, 322–331.

Matsuyama, T., and Foà, P. P. (1974). Plasma glucose, insulin, pancreatic, and enteroglucagon levels in normal and depancreatized dogs. *Proc. Soc. Exp. Biol. Med.* **147**, 97–102.

Matthews, E. K., Petersen, O. H., and Williams, J. A. (1973). Pancreatic acinar cells: acetylcholine-induced membrane depolarization, calcium efflux and amylase release. *J. Physiol. (London)* **234**, 689–701.

Matuchansky, C., Huet, P. M., Mary, J. Y., Rambaud, J. C., and Bernier, J. J. (1972). Effects of cholecystokinin and metoclopramide on jejunal movements of water and electrolytes and on transit time of luminal fluid in man. *Eur. J. Clin. Invest.* **2**, 169–175.

Maxam, A. M., and Gilbert, W. (1977). A new method for sequencing DNA. *Proc. Natl. Acad. Sci. U.S.A.* **74**, 560–564.

Maxwell, V., Shulkes, A., Brown, J. C., Solomon, T. E., Walsh, J. H., and Grossman, M. I. (1980). Effect of gastric inhibitory polypeptide on pentagastrin-stimulated acid secretion in man. *Dig. Dis. Sci.* **25**, 113–116.

del Mazo, J. (1977). Measurement of immunoreactive CCK-PZ in the GI tract and in the central nervous system of several animal species. *Gastroenterology* **72**, A-24/1047.

Mazur, R. H., Schlatter, J. M., and Goldkamp, A. H. (1969). Structure–tastte relationships of some dipeptides. *J. Am. Chem. Soc.* **91**, 2684–2691.

Meade, R. C., Kneubuhler, H. A., Schulte, W. J., and Barboriak, J. J. (1967). Stimulation of insulin secretion by pancreozymin. *Diabetes* **16**, 141–144.

Mehlis, B., Böhm, S., Becker, M., and Bienert, M. (1975). Circular dichroism and infrared studies of substance P and C-terminal analogues. *Biochem. Biophys. Res. Commun.* **66**, 1447–1453.

Melchiorri, P. (1980). Bombesin-like peptides in the gastrointestinal tract of mammals and birds. *In* "Gastrointestinal Hormones" (G. B. J. Glass, ed.), pp. 717–725. Raven, New York.

Mellanby, J. (1925). The mechanism of pancreatic digestion—the function of secretin. *J. Physiol (London)* **60**, 85–91.

Mellanby, J. (1926). The secretion of pancreatic juice. *J. Physiol. (London)* **61**, 419–435.

Mellanby, J. (1928). The isolation of secretin—its chemical and physiological properties. *J. Physiol. (London)* **66**, 1–17.

Mevarech, M., Noyes, B. E., and Agarwal, K. L. (1979). Detection of gastrin-specific mRNA using oligodeoxynucleotide probes of defined sequence. *J. Biol. Chem.* **254**, 7472–7475.

Meves, M., Beger, H. G., Haubold, U., and Hüthwohl, B. (1975). The slowing of gastric emptying by intestinal hormones. *Br. J. Surg.* **62**, 154.

Meyer, J. H., and Grossman, M. I. (1972a). Comparison of D- and L-phenylalanine as pancreatic stimulants. *Am. J. Physiol.* **222**, 1058–1063.

Meyer, J. H., and Grossman, M. I. (1972b). Release of secretin and cholecystokinin. *In* "Gastrointestinal Hormones" (L. Demling, ed.), pp. 43–55. Thieme, Stuttgart.

Meyer, J. H., Spingola, L. J., and Grossman, M. I. (1971). Endogenous cholecystoinin potentiates exogenous secretin on pancreas of dog. *Am. J. Physiol.* **221**, 742–747.

Miller, L. R., Jacobson, E. D., and Johnson, L. R. (1973). Effect of pentagastrin on gstric mucosal cells grown in tissue culture. *Gastroenterology* **64**, 254–267.

Miller, T. A., Tepperman, F. S., Fang, W.-F., and Jacobson, E. D. (1979). Effect of somatostatin on pancreatic protein secretion induced by cholecystokinin. *J. Surg. Res.* **26,** 488–493.

Milstein, C., Brownlee, C. G., Harrison, T. M., and Mathews, M. B. (1972). A possible precursor of immunoglobulin light chain. *Nature (London) New Biol.* **239,** 117–120.

Mitznegg, P., Domschke, W., Domschke, S., Belohlavek, D., Sprügel, W., Struntz, U., Wünsch, E., Jaeger, E., and Demling, L. (1975). Protein synthesis in human gastric mucosa: effects of pentagastrin, secretin and 13-Nle-motilin. *Acta Hepato-Gastroenterol.* **22,** 333–335.

Mitznegg, P., Bloom, S. R., Domschke, W., Haecki, W. H., Domschke, S., Belohlayek, D., Wünsch, E., and Demling, L. (1977). Effect of secretin on plasma motilin in man. *Gut* **18,** 468–471.

Miyoshi, A. (1979). "Gut Peptides." Elsevier, Amsterdam.

Monod, J., Changeaux, J.-P., and Jacob, F. (1963). Allosteric proteins and cellular control system. *J. Mol. Biol.* **6,** 306–329.

Monod, M. E. (1964). Action entérokinétique de la Cecekine. *Arch. Mal. Appar. Dig.* **53,** 607–608.

Moody, A. J., Jacobsen, H., and Sundby, F. (1978). Gastric glucagon and gut glucagon-like immunoreactants. *In* "Gut Hormones" (S. R. Bloom, ed.), pp. 369–378. Churchill, London.

Moore, B., Edie, E. S., and Abram, J. H. (1906). On the treatment of diabetes mellitus by acid extract of duodenal mucous membrane. *Biochem. J.* **1,** 28–39.

Moossa, A. R., Hall, A. W., Skinner, D. B., and Winans, C. S. (1976). Effect of fifty percent small bowel resection on gastric secretory function in rhesus monkeys. *Surgery* **80,** 208–213.

Moran, E. C., Chou, P. Y., and Fasman, G. D. (1977). Conformational transitions of glucagon in solution: the $\alpha-\beta$ transition. *Biochem. Biophys. Res. Commun.* **77,** 1300–1306.

Morin, G., Besancon, F., Grall, A., Debray, C., and Garat, J.-P. (1966). La cholécys-tokinine appliquée au radiodiagnostic usuel de l'intestin gréle: nouvelle technique de radiocinématographie complète en quelques minutes, avec 62 observations. *Radiologie* **9,** 247–250.

Morisset, J., and Dunnigan, J. (1967). Exocrine pancreas adaptation to diet in vag-otomized rats. *Rev. Can. Biol.* **26,** 11–16.

Morita, S., Doi, K., Yip, C. C., and Vranic, M. (1976). Measurement and partial charac-terization of immunoreactive glucagon in gastrointestinal tissues of dogs. *Diabetes* **25,** 1018–1025.

Moritz, M., Finkelstein, G., Meshkinpour, H., Fingerut, J., and Lorber, S. H. (1973). Effect of secretin and cholecystokinin on the transport of electrolyte and water in human jejunum. *Gastroenterology* **64,** 76–80.

Morley, J. E. (1979). Extrahypothalamic thyrotropin-releasing hormone (TRH)—its dis-tribution and its function. *Life Sci.* **25,** 1539–1550.

Morley, J. E., Garvin, T. J., Pekary, A. E., and Hershman, J. M. (1977). Thyrotropin-releasing hormone in the gastrointestinal tract. *Biochem. Biophys. Res. Commun.* **79,** 314–318.

Morley, J. S. (1968a). Structure–function relationships in gastrin-like peptides. *Proc. Soc. Ser. B* **170,** 97–111.

Morley, J. S. (1968b). Structure–activity relationships. *Fed. Proc. Fed. Am. Soc. Exp. Biol.* **27,** 1314–1317.

Morley, J. S. (1977). Information about peptide hormone receptors from structure–activity studies. *In* "Hormonal Receptors in Digestive Tract Physiology" (S. Bonfils *et al.,* eds.), pp. 3–18. Elsevier, Amsterdam.

Morley, J. S., Tracy, H. J., and Gregory, R. A. (1965). Structure–function relationships in the active C-terminal tetrapeptide sequence of gastrin. *Nature (London)* **207,** 1356–1359.

Moroder, L., Wilschowitz, L. Jaeger, E., Knof, S., Thamm, P., and Wünsch, E. (1979). Synthese von Tyrosin-*O*-sulfat-haltigen Peptiden. *Hoppe-Seylers Z. Physiol. Chem.* **360,** 787–790.

Mroz, E. A., and Leeman, S. E. (1977). Substance P. *Vitamins Horm.* **35,** 209–281.

Mukhopadhyay, A. K. (1978). Effect of substance P on the lower esophageal sphincter of the opossum. *Gastroenterology* **75,** 278–282.

Mulcahy, H., Fitzgerald, O., and McGeeney, K. F. (1972). Secretin and pancreozymin effect on salivary amylase concentration in man. *Gut* **13,** 850.

Muller, J. E., Straus, E., and Yalow, R. S. (1977). Cholécystokinin and its COOH-terminal octapeptide in the pig brain. *Proc. Natl. Acad. Sci. U.S.A.* **74,** 3035–3037.

Muller, W. A., Brennan, M. F., Tan, M. H., and Aoki, T. T. (1974). Studies on glucagon secretion in pancreatectomized patients. *Diabetes* **23,** 512–516.

Multicenter Pilot Study (1967). Pentagastrin as a stimulant of maximal gastric acid response in man. *Lancet* **I,** 291–295.

Murat, J. E., and White, T. T. (1966). Stimulation of gastric secretion by commercial cholecystokinin extracts. *Proc. Soc. Exp. Biol. Med.* **123,** 593–594.

Murphy, R. F. (1979). The chemical characterization of gastrointestinal hormones. *Clin. Endocrinol. Metab.* **8,** 281–298.

Murphy, R. F., Elmore, D. T., and Buchanan, K. D. (1971). Isolation of glucagon-like immunoreactivity of gut by affinity chromatography. *Biochem. J.* **125,** 61p–62p.

Murphy, R. F., Buchanan, K. D., and Elmore, D. T. (1973). Isolation of glucagon-like immunoreactivity of gut by affinity chromatography on anti-glucagon antibodies coupled to sepharose 4B. *Biochim. Biophys. Acta* **303,** 118–127.

Mutt, V. (1972). Some recent developments in the field of the intestinal hormones. *In* "Endocrinology 1971" (S. Taylor, ed.), pp. 250–256.

Mutt, V. (1974). The intestinal hormones in 1973. *In* "Endocrinology 1973" (S. Taylor, ed.), pp. 100–116. Heineman, London.

Mutt, V. (1976). Further investigations on intestinal hormonal polypeptides. *Clin. Endocrinol.* **5** (Suppl.), 175s–183s.

Mutt, V. (1978). Progress in intestinal hormone research. *In* "Gastrointestinal Hormones and Pathology of the Digestive System" (M. Grossman *et al.,* eds.), pp. 133–146. Plenum, New York.

Mutt, V., and Jorpes, J. E. (1966). Secretin: Isolation and determination of structure. *IUPAC Int. Congr. Chem. Natural Products, Stockholm* Sect. 2 C-1, p. 119.

Mutt, V., and Jorpes, J. E. (1967a). Isolation of aspartyl-phenylalanine amide from cholecystokinin-pancreozymin. *Biochem. Biophys. Res. Commun.* **26,** 392–397.

Mutt, V., and Jorpes, J. E. (1967b). Contemporary developments in the biochemistry of the gastrointestinal hormones. *Recent Prog. Horm. Res.* **23,** 483–503.

Mutt, V., and Jorpes, J. E. (1968). Structure of porcine cholecystokinin-pancreozymin. 1. Cleavage with thrombin and with trypsin. *Eur. J. Biochem.* **6,** 156–162.

Mutt, V., and Jorpes, J. E. (1971). Hormonal polypeptides of the upper intestine. *Biochem. J.* **125,** 57p–58p.

Mutt, V., and Said, S. I. (1974). Structure of the porcine vasoactive intestinal octacosapeptide. The amino-acid sequence. Use of kallikrein in its determination. *Eur. J. Biochem.* **42,** 581–589.

Mutt, V., and Söderberg, U. (1959). On the assay of secretin. *Ark. Kem.* **15,** 63–68.

Mutt, V., Jorpes, J. E., and Magnusson, S. (1970). Structure of porcine secretin. The amino acid sequence. *Eur. J. Biochem.* **15,** 513–519.

Mutter, M., Mutter, H., Uhmann, R., and Bayer, E. (1976). Konformationsuntersuchungen an Oligoalanin, Substanz P und der Myoglobinsequenz (66-73). Der Zirkulardichroismus von polyäthylenglykolgebundenen Peptiden. *Biopolymers* **15**, 917–927.

Myren, J., Schrumpf, E., Hansen, L. E., and Vatn, M. (1978). *Scand. J. Gastroenterol.* **13**, (Suppl.), 49.

Naito, S., Iwata, R., and Saito, T. (1963). Etudes sur la cholecystokinin, son mode d'action sur la contraction de la vésicule biliaire. *Presse Med.* **71**, 2688–2689.

Nakajima, S., and Magee, D. F. (1968). Effect of gastrin pentapeptide on pepsin secretion. *Gastroenterology* **54**, 134–135.

Nakajima, S., and Magee, D. F. (1970a). Inhibitory action of cholecystokinin-pancreozymin on gastric pepsin secretion. *Experientia* **26**, 159.

Nakajima, S., and Magee, D. F. (1970b). Influences of duodenal acidification on acid and pepsin secretion of the stomach in dogs. *Am. J. Physiol.* **218**, 545–549.

Nakajima, S., Shoemaker, R. L., Hirschowitz, B. I., and Sachs, G. (1970). Comparison of actions of aminophylline and pentagastrin on Necturus gastric mucosa. *Am. J. Physiol.* **219**, 1259–1262.

Nakanishi, S., Inoue, A., Kita, T., Nakamura, M., Chang, A. C. Y., Cohen, S. N., and Numa, S. (1979). Nucleotide sequence of cloned cDNA for bovine corticotropin-β-lipotropin precursor. *Nature (London)* **278**, 423–427.

Nakazato, H., and Edmonds, M. (1972). The isolation and purification of rapidly labeled polysome-bound ribonucleic acid on polythymidylate cellulose. *J. Biol. Chem.* **247**, 3365–3367.

Nasset, E. S. (1938). Enterocrinin, a hormone, which excites the glands of the small intestine. *Am. J. Physiol.* **121**, 481–487.

Nasset, E. S. (1972). Succus entericus secretion stimulated by cholecystokinin and its C-terminal octapeptide. *Fed. Proc. Fed. Am. Soc. Exp. Biol.* **31**, 354/779.

Necheles, H. (1957). Effects of glucagon on external secretion of the pancreas. *Am. J. Physiol.* **191**, 595–597.

Niada, R., Prino, G., Lugaro, G., Carrea, G., Pasta, P., and Casellato, M. M. (1979). Inhibition of gastric acid secretion by a glycoprotein isolated from human urine (human urinary gastric inhibitor). *Eur. J. Pharmacol.* **56**, 217–223.

Niall, H. D., Hogan, M. L., Saer, R., Rosenblum, I. Y., and Greenwood, F. C. (1971). Sequences of pituitary and placental lactogenic and growth hormones: Evolution from a primordial peptide by gene reduplication. *Proc. Natl. Acad. Sci. U.S.A.* **68**, 866–869.

Nilsson, A. (1975). Structure of the vasoactive intestinal octacosapeptide from chicken intestine. The amino acid sequence. *FEBS Lett.* **60**, 322–325.

Nilsson, A., Carlquist, M., Jörnvall, H., and Mutt, V. (1980). Isolation and characterization of chicken secretin. *Eur. J. Biochem.* **112**, 383–388.

Noe, B. D., and Bauer, E. G. (1971). Evidence for glucagon biosynthesis involving a protein intermediate in islets of the anglerfish (*Lophius americanus*). *Endocrinology* **89**, 642–651.

Noe, B. D., Spiess, J., Rivier, J. E., and Vale, W. (1979). Isolation and characterization of somatostatin from anglerfish pancreatic islet. *Endocrinology* **105**, 1410–1415.

Nolan, C., Margoliash, E., Peterson, J. D., and Steiner, D. F. (1971). The structure of bovine proinsulin. *J. Biol. Chem.* **246**, 2780–2795.

Nordström, C. (1972). Release of enteropeptidase and other brush-border enzymes from the small intestinal wall in the rat. *Biochim. Biophys. Acta* **289**, 367–377.

Noyes, B. E., Mevarech, M., Stein, R., and Agarwal, K. L. (1979). Detection and partial sequence analysis of gastrin mRNA by using an oligodeoxynucleotide probe. *Proc. Natl. Acad. Sci. U.S.A.* **76**, 1770–1774.

O'Connor, F. A., Buchanan, K. D., Connon, J. J., and Shahidullah, M. (1976). Secretin and insulin: response to intraduodenal acid. *Diabetologia* **12**, 145–148.

O'Connor, F. A., Conlon, J. M., Buchanan, K. D., and Murphy, R. F. (1979). The use of perfused rat intestine to characterise the gluagon-like immunoreactivity released into serosal secretions following stimulation by glucose. *Horm. Metab. Res.* **11**, 19–23.

O'Connor, K. J., Gay, A., and Lazarus, N. R. (1973). The biosynthesis of glucagon in perfused rat pancreas. *Biochem. J.* **134**, 473–480.

Ohneda, A., Horigome, K., Kai, Y., Itabashi, H., Ishii, S., and Yamagata, S. (1976). Purification of canine gut glucagon-like immunoreactivity (GLI) and its insulin releasing activity *Horm. Metab. Res.* **8**, 170–174.

Olbe, L. (1966). Vagal release of gastrin. *In* "Gastrin" (M. I. Grossman, ed.), pp. 83–107. Univ. of California Press, Los Angeles.

Oliver, G., and Schäfer, E. A. (1894). On the physiological action of extract of the suprarenal capsules. *J. Physiol. (London)* **16**, i–iv.

Oliver, G., and Schäfer, E. A. (1895a). The physiological effects of extracts of the suprarenal capsules. *J. Physiol. (London)* **18**, 230–276.

Oliver, G., and Schäfer, E. A. (1895b). On the physiological actions of extracts of pituitary body and certain other glandular organs. *J. Physiol. (London)* **18**, 277–279.

Ondetti, M. A., Plusec, J., Sabo, E. F., Sheehan, J. T., and Williams, N. (1970a). Synthesis of cholecystokinin-pancreozymin. I. The C-terminal dodecapeptide. *J. Am. Chem. Soc.* **92**, 195–199.

Ondetti, M. A., Rubin, B., Engel, S. L., Plusec, J., and Sheehan, J. T. (1970b). Cholecystokinin-pancreozymin: Recent developments. *Am. J. Dig. Dis.* **15**, 149–156.

Orci, L., Baetens, O., Rufener, C., Brown, M., Vale, W., and Guillemin, R. (1976). Evidence for immunoreactive neurotensin in dog intestinal mucosa. *Life Sci.* **19**, 559–562.

Orloff, M. J., Hyde, P. V. B., Kosta, L. D., Guillemin, R. C. L., and Bell, R. H., Jr. (1979). The intestinal phase hormone. *World J. Surg.* **3**, 523–538.

Ormsbee, H. S., III, Koehler, S. L. Jr. and Telford, G. L. (1978). Somatostatin inhibits motilin-induced interdigestive contractile activity in the dog. *Am. J. Dig. Dis.* **23**, 781–788.

Orth, D. N., and Nicholson, W. E. (1977). Different molecular forms of ACTH. *Ann. N.Y. Acad. Sci.* **297**, 27–48.

Osnes, M., Hanssen, L. E., Lehnert, P., Flaten, O., Larsen, S., Londong, W., and Otte, M. (1980). Exocrine pancreatic secretion and immunoreactive secretin release after repeated intraduodenal infusions of bile in man. *Scand. J. Gastroenterol.* **15**, 1033–1039.

Owen, S. E., and Ivy, A. C. (1931). The diuretic action of secretin preparations. *Am. J. Physiol.* **97**, 276–281.

Oyama, H., Bradshaw, R. A., Bates, O. J., and Permutt, A. (1980). Amino acid sequence of catfish pancreatic somatostatin I. *J. Biol. Chem.* **255**, 2251–2254.

Palacios, R., Sullivan, D., Summer, N. M., Kiely, M. L., and Schimke, R. T. (1973). Purification of ovalbumin ribonucleic acid by specific immunoadsorption of ovalbumin-synthesizing polysomes and millipore partition of ribonucleic acid. *J. Biol. Chem.* **248**, 540–548.

Paladini, A. C., Peña, C., and Retegui, L. A. (1979). The intriguing nature of the multiple actions of growth hormone. *Trends Biochem. Sci.* **4**, 256–260.

Paléus, S., and Nielands, J. B. (1950). Preparation of cytochrome c with the aid of ion exchange resin. *Acta Chem. Scand.* **4**, 1024–1030.

Panijpan, B., and Gratzer, W. B. (1974). Conformational nature of monomeric glucagon. *Eur. J. Biochem.* **45**, 547–553.

Pansu, D., Berard, A., Dechelette, M. A., and Lambert, R. (1974). Influence of secretin and pentagastrin on the circadian rhythm of cell proliferation in the intestinal mucosa in rats. *Digestion* **11**, 266–274.

Pansu, D., Vagne, M., Bosshard, A., and Mutt. V. (1981). Sorbin, a peptide contained in porcine upper small intestine which induces the absorption of water and sodium in the rat duodenum. *Scand. J. Gastrenterol.* **16**, 193–199.

Parker, J. G., and Beneventano, T. C. (1970). Acceleration of small bowel contrast study by cholecystokinin. *Gastroenterology* **58**, 679–684.

Parrott, R. F., and Batt, R. A. L. (1980). The feeding response of obese mice (genotype, ob ob) and their wild-type littermates to cholecystokinin (pancreozymin). *Physiol. Behav.* **24**, 751–753.

Passaro, E. P., Jr., Gillespie, I. E., and Grossman, M. I. (1963). Potentiation between gastrin and histamine in stimulation of gastric secretion. *Proc. Soc. Exp. Biol. Med.* **114**, 50–52.

Patapanian, H., Pirola, R. C., and Somer, J. B. (1981). Increased de novo phospholipid biosynthesis in the stimulated rat exocrine pancreas. *Biochem. Biophys. Res. Commun.* **99**, 319–323.

Patel, D. J., Bodanszky, M., and Ondetti, M. A. (1970). Proton nuclear magnetic resonance study of secretin. *Macromolecules* **3**, 694–698.

Patzelt, C., Tager, H. S., Carroll, R. J., and Steiner, D. F. (1979). Identification and processing of proglucagon in pancreatic islets. *Nature (London)* **282**, 260–266.

Paul, F. (1974). Quantitative Untersuchungen der Wirkung von Pankreas-Glukagon und Sekretin auf die Magen-Darm-Motorik mittels elektromanometrischer Simultanregisteierungen beim Menschen. *Klin. Wochenschr.* **52**, 983–939.

Pavlov, J. P. (1900). Ein Vortrag. "Das Experiment als zeitgemässe und einheitliche Methode medizinischer Forschung," pp. 1–48. Bergmann, Wiesbaden.

Pearl, J. M., Ritchie, W. P., Jr., Gilsdorf, R. B., Delaney, J. P., and Leonard, A. S. (1966). Hypothalamic stimulation and feline gastric mucosal cellular populations. Factors in the etiology of the stress ulcer. *J. Am. Med. Assoc.* **195**, 281–284.

Pearse, A. G. E. (1968). Common cytochemical and ultrastructural characteristics of cells producing polypeptide hormones (the APUD series) and their relevance to thyroid and ultimobrnachial C cells and calcitonin. *Proc. R. Soc. Ser. B* **170**, 71–80.

Pearson, D., Shively, J. E., Clark, B. R., Geschwind, I. I., Barkley, M., Nishioka, R. S., and Bern, H. A. (1980). Urotensin II: A somatostatin-like peptide in the caudal neurosecretory system of fishes. *Proc. Natl. Acad. Scu. U.S.A.* **77**, 5021–5024.

Pederson, R. A., and Brown, J. C. (1972). Inhibition of histamine-, pentagastrin-, and insulin-stimulated canine gastric secretion by pure "gastric inhibitory polypeptide." *Gastroenterology* **62**, 393–400.

Pederson, R. A., Schubert, H. E., and Brown, J. C. (1975). Gastric inhibitory polypeptide. Its physiologic release and insulinotropic action in the dog. *Diabetes* **24**, 1050–1056.

Peikin, S. R., Costenbader, C. L., and Gardner, J. D. (1979). Actions of derivatives of cyclic nucleotides on dispersed acini from guinea pig pancreas. Discovery of a competitive antagonist of the action of cholecystokinin. *J. Biol. Chem.* **254**, 5321–5327.

Perley, M. J., and Kipnis, D. M. (1967). Plasma insulin responses to oral and intravenous glucose: studies in normal and diabetic subjects. *J. Clin. Invest.* **46**, 1954–1962.

Permutt, M. A., and Boime, I. (1975). Isolation of biologically active fish islets messenger

RNA by oligo-dT cellulose affinity chromatography. *Diabetes* **24** (Suppl. 2), 405 (Abstr. 51).

Pernow, B. (1953). Studies on substance P. Purification, occurrence and biological actions. *Acta Physiol. Scand.* **29** (Suppl. 105), 1–90.

Perrier, C. V., and Laster, L. (1970). Adenyl cyclase activity of guinea pig gastric mucosa: stimulation by histamine and prostaglandins. *J. Clin. Invest.* **49**, 73a.

Petersen, H., Berstad, A., and Myren, J. (1973). Bicarbonate response to graded doses of secretin in patients with different gastric acid secretory capacity. *Acta Hepato-Gastroenterol.* **20**, 421–427.

Petersen, H., Solomon, T., and Grossman, M. I. (1978). Effect of chronic pentagastrin, cholecystokinin, and secretin on pancreas of rats. *Am. J. Physiol.* **234**, E286–E293.

Petersen, H., Solomon, T. E., and Grossman, M. I. (1979). Pancreatic secretion in rats after chronic treatment with secretin plus caerulein. *Gastroenterology* **76**, 790–794.

Petersen, O. H. (1976). Electrophysiology of mammalian gland cells. *Physiol. Rev.* **56**, 535–577.

Petersen, O. H., and Ueda, N. (1975). Pancreatic acinar cells: effect of acetylcholine, pancreozymin, gastrin and secretin on membrane potential and resistance in vivo and in vitro. *J. Physiol. (London)* **247**, 461–471.

Pe Thein, M., and Schofield, B. (1959). Release of gastrin from the pyloric antrum following vagal stimulation by sham feeding in dogs. *J. Physiol (London)* **148**, 291–305.

Petrin, A. (1974). Wirkung von Calcitonin auf die Magen- und Pankreas-Sekretion. *Dtsch. Med. Wochenschr.* **99**, 2368–2371.

Pfeiffer, E. F., Telib, M., Ammon, J., Melani, F., and Ditschuneit, H. (1965). Direkte Stimulierung der Insulin-Sekretion in Vitro durch Sekretin. *Dtsch. Med. Wochenschr.* **90**, 1663–1669.

Pham Van Chuong, P., Penke, B., de Castiglione, R., and Fromageot, P. (1979). Conformational study of gastrin and C-terminal peptides by circular dichroism. *In* "Hormone Receptors in Digestion and Nutrition" (G. Rosselin *et al.*, eds.), pp. 33–44. Elsevier, Amsterdam.

Philpott, H. G., and Petersen, O. H. (1979). Separate activation sites for cholecystokinin and bombesin on pancreatic acini. An electrophysiological study employing a competitive antagonist for the action of CCK. *Pflügers Arch.* **382**, 263–267.

Piszkiewicz, D. (1974). pH-dependent conformational change of gastrin. *Nature (London)* **248**, 341–342.

Piszkiewicz, D., Landon, M., and Smith, E. L. (1970). Anomalous cleavage of aspartyl-proline peptide bonds during amino acid sequence determinations. *Biochem. Biophys. Res. Commun.* **40**, 1173–1178.

Pitts, J. E., Blundell, T. L., Tickle, I. J., and Wood, S. P. (1979). X-Ray analysis and the conformation of pancreatic polypeptide, PP. *In* "Peptides: Structure and Biological Function" (E. Gross and J. Meienhofer, eds.), pp. 1011–1016. Pierce Chemical Company, Rockford, Illinois.

Polacek, M. A., and Ellison, E. H. (1963). A comparative study of parietal cell mass and distribution in normal stomachs, in stomachs with duodenal ulcer and in stomachs of patients with pancreatic adenoma. *Surg. Forum* **14**, 343–345.

Polak, J. M., Pearse, A. G. E., Grimelius, L., Bloom, S. R., and Arimura, A. (1975). Growth-hormone release-inhibiting hormone in gastrointestinal and pancreatic D cells. *Lancet* **I**, 1220–1222.

Polak, J. M., Bloom, S. R., Hobbs, S., Solcia, E., and Pearse, A. G. E. (1976). Distribution of bombesin-like peptide in human gastrointestinal tract. *Lancet* **I**, 1109–1110.

Polak, J. M., Sullivan, S. N., Bloom, S. R., Buchan, A. M. J., Facer, P., Brown, M. R., and

Pearse, A. G. E. (1977a). Specific localisation of neurotensin to the N-cell in human intestine by radioimmunoassay and immunocytochemistry. *Nature (London)* **270**, 183–184.

Polak, J. M., Sullivan, S. N., Bloom, S. R., Facer, P., and Pearse, A. G. E. (1977b). Enkephalin-like immunoreactivity in the human gastrointestinal tract. *Lancet* **I**, 972–974.

Pollok, H. G., and Kimmel, J. R. (1975). Chicken glucagon. Isolation and amino acid sequence studies. *J. Biol. Chem.* **250**, 9377–9380.

Popielski, L. (1901). Ueber das periphertsche reflectorische Nervencentrum des Pankreas. *Pflügers Arch. Physiol.* **86**, 215–246.

Popielski, L. (1909). Über die physiologische Wirkung von Extrakten aus sämtlichen Teilen des Verdauungskanales (Magen, Dick- und Dünndarm), sowie des Gehirns, Pankreas und Blutes und über die chemischen Eigenschaften des darin wirkenden Körpers. *Pflügers Arch. Physiol.* **128**, 191–221.

Popielski, L. (1920). β-Imidazolyläthylamin und die Organextrakte. *Pflügers Arch. Physiol.* **178**, 237–259.

Porath, J., and Flodin, P. (1959). Gel filtration: a method for desalting and group separation. *Nature (London)* **123**, 1657–1659.

Potts, J. T., Jr. (1970). Recent advances in thyrocalcitonin research. *Fed. Proc. Fed. Am. Soc. Exp. Biol.* **29**, 1200–1205.

Potts, J. T., Jr., Niall, H. D., Keutman, H. T., Brewer, H.B., Jr., and Deftos, L. J. (1968). The amino acid sequence of porcine thyrocalcitonin. *Proc. Natl. Acad. Sci. U.S.A.* **59**, 1321–1328.

Potts, W. J., Bloss, J. L., and Nutting, E. F. (1980). Biological properties of aspartame. I. Evaluation of central nervous system effects. *J. Environ. Pathol. Toxicol.* **3**, 341–353.

Pradayrol, L., Jörnvall, H., Mutt, V., and Ribet, A. (1980). N-terminally extended somatostatin: the primary structure of somatostatin-28. *FEBS Lett.* **109**, 55–58.

del Prato, S., Riva, F., Devidé, A., Nosadini, R., Fedele, D., and Tiengo, A. (1980). Glucagon levels and ketogenesis in human diabetes following total or partial pancreatectomy and severe chronic pancreatitis. *Acta Diabetol. Lat.* **17**, 111–118.

Pratt, C. L. G. (1940). The influence of secretin on gastric secretion. *J. Physiol. (London)* **98**, 1p–2p.

Preshaw, R. M., and Grossman, M. I. (1965). Stimulation of pancreatic secretion by extracts of the pyloric gland area of the stomach. *Gastroenterology* **48**, 36–44.

Putz, P., Bazira, L., and Willems, G. (1980). The effect of caerulein on epithelial growth in the mouse gall bladder. *Experientia* **36**, 429–430.

Rabinovitch, A., and Dupré, J. (1974). Effects of the gastric inhibitory polypeptide present in impure pancreozymin-cholecystokinin on plasma insulin and glucagon in the rat. *Endocrinology* **94**, 1139–1144.

Racusen, L. C., and Binder, H. J. (1977). Alteration of large intestinal electrolyte transport by vasoactive intestinal polypeptide in the rat. *Gastroenterology* **73**, 790–796.

Rajh, H. M., Smyth, M. J., Renckens, B. A. M., Jansen, J. W. C. M., De Pont, J. J. H. H. M., Bonting, S. L., Tesser, G. I., and Nivard, R. J. F. (1980). Role of the tryptophan residue in the interaction of pancreozymin with its receptor. *Biochim. Biophys. Acta* **632**, 386–398.

Rasmussen, H. (1970). Cell communication, calcium ion, and cyclic adenosine monophosphate. *Science* **170**, 404–412.

Rattan, S., Said, S. I., and Goyal, R. K. (1977). Effect of vasoactive intestinal polypeptide (VIP) on the lower esophageal sphincter pressure (LESP). *Proc. Soc. Exp. Biol. Med.* **155**, 40–43.

Rayford, P. L., Miller, T. A., and Thompson, J. C. (1976a). Secretin, cholecystokinin and newer gastrointestinal hormones. (First of two parts). *New Engl. J. Med.* **249,** 1093–1101.

Rayford, P. L., Miller, T. A., and Thompson, J. C. (1976b). Secretin, cholecystokinin and newer gastrointestinal hormones. (Second of two parts). *New Engl. J. Med.* **249,** 1157–1164.

Redman, C. M., Siekevitz, P., and Palade, G. E. (1966). Synthesis and transfer of amylase in pigeon pancreatic microsomes. *J. Biol. Chem.* **241,** 1150–1158.

Reed, P. W., and Lardy, H. A. (1972). A23187: A divalent cation inonophore. *J. Biol. Chem.* **247,** 6970–6977.

Reeder, D. D., Conlee, J. L., and Thompson, J.C. (1971). Calcium carbonate antacid and serum gastrin concentration in duodenal ulcer. *Surg. Forum* **22,** 308–310.

Rehfeld, J. F. (1971). Effect of gastrin and its C-terminal tetrapeptide on insulin secretion in man. *Acta Endocrinol.* **66,** 169–176.

Rehfeld, J. F. (1972). Three components of gastrin in human serum. Gel filtration studies on the molecular size of immunoreactive serum gastrin. *Biochim. Biophys. Acta* **285,** 364–372.

Rehfeld, J. F. (1973). Gastrins in serum. A review of gastrin radioimmunoanalysis and the discovery of gastrin heterogeneity in serum. *Scand. J. Gastroenterol.* **8,** 577–583.

Rehfeld, J. F. (1977). Cholecystokinins and gastrins in brain and gut. *Acta Pharmacol. Toxicol.* **41** (Suppl. IV), 24.

Rehfeld, J. F. (1978a). Immunochemical studies on cholecystokinin. I. Development of sequence-specific radioimmunoassays for porcine triacontatriapeptide cholecystokinin. *J. Biol. Chem.* **253,** 4016–4021.

Rehfeld, J. F. (1978b). Immunochemical studies on cholecystokinin. II. Distribution and molecular heterogeneity in the central nervous system and small intestine in man and hog. *J. Biol. Chem.* **253,** 4022–4030.

Rehfeld, J. F. (1979). Heterogeneity of gastrointestinal hormones. *World J. Surg.* **3,** 415–422.

Rehfeld, J. F. (1980). COOH-terminal extended endogenous gastrin. *Biochem. Biophys. Res. Commun.* **92,** 811–818.

Rehfeld, J. F., and Amdrup, E. (1979). "Gastrin and the Vagus." Academic Press, New York.

Rehfeld, J. F., and Larsson, L.-I. (1979). The predominating antral gastrin and intestinal cholecystokinin is the common COOH-terminal tetrapeptide amide. *In* "Gastrin and the Vagus" (J. F. Rehfeld and E. Amdrup, eds.), pp. 85–94. Academic Press, New York.

Rehfeld, J. F., Stadil, F., and Vikelsøe, J. (1974). Immunoreactive gastrin components in human serum. *Gut* **15,** 102–111.

Rehfeld, J. F., Stadil, F., Malmström, J., and Miyata, M. (1975). Gastrin heterogeneity in serum and tissue. *In* "Gastrointestinal Hormones" (J. C. Thompson, ed.), pp. 43–58. Univ. of Texas Press, Austin.

Rehfeld, J. F., Larsson, L.-I., Golterman, N. R., Schwartz, T. W., Holst, J. J., Jensen, S. L., and Morley, J. S. (1980). Reply: Does the C-terminal tetrapeptide of gastrin and CCK exist as an entity? *Nature (London)* **286,** 742.

Reichelt, K. L., Foss, I., Trygstad, O., Edminson, P. D., Johansen, J. H., and Bøler, J. B. (1978). Humoral control of apetite—II. Purification and characterization of an anorexogenic peptide from human urine. *Neuroscience* **3,** 1207–1211.

Resin, H., Stern, D. H., Sturdevant, R. A. L., and Isenberg, J. I. (1973). Effect of the C-terminal octapeptide of cholecystokinin on lower esophageal sphincter pressure in man. *Gastroenterology* **64,** 946–949.

Rhodes, R., Tai, H. H., and Chey, W. Y. (1974). Observations on plasma secretin responses to a meat meal and intraduodenal infusion of HCl solution in man. *Clin. Res.* **22,** 695A.

Riccardi, R. P., Miller, J. S., and Roberts, B. E. (1979). Purification and mapping of specific mRNAs by hybridization-selection and cell-free translation. *Proc. Natl. Acad. Sci. U.S.A.* **76,** 4927–4931.

Richards, F. M. (1958). On the enzymic activity of subtilisin-modified ribonuclease. *Proc. Natl. Acad. Sci. U.S.A.* **44,** 162–166.

Richardson, P. D. I., and Withrington, P. G. (1977). The effects of glucagon, secretin, pancreozymin and pentagastrin on the hepatic arterial vascular bed of the dog. *Br. J. Pharmacol.* **59,** 147–156.

Rigopoulou, D., Valverde, I., Marco, J., Faloona, G., and Unger, R. H. (1970). Large glucagon immunoreactivity in extracts of pancreas. *J. Biol. Chem.* **245,** 496–501.

Robberecht, P., Deschodt-Lanckman, M., and Vanderhaegen, J. J. (1978). Demonstration of biological activity of brain gastrin-like peptidic material in the human: Its relationship with the COOH-terminal octapeptide of cholecystokinin. *Proc. Natl. Acad. Sci. U.S.A.* **75,** 524–528.

Roberts, J. L., and Herbert, E. (1977a). Characterization of a common precursor to corticotropin and β-lipotropin: Cell-free synthesis of the precursor and identification of corticotropin peptides in the molecule. *Proc. Natl. Acad. Sci. U.S.A.* **74,** 4826–4830.

Roberts, J. L., and Herbert, E. (1977b). Characterization of common precursor to corticotropin and β-lipotropin: Identification of β-lipotropin peptides and their arrangement relative to corticotropin in the precursor synthetized in a cell-free system. *Proc. Natl. Acad. Sci. U.S.A.* **74,** 5300–5304.

Robertson, A. L., Jr., and Khairallah, P. A. (1971). Angiotensin II: Rapid localization in nuclei of smooth and cardiac muscle. *Science* **172,** 1138–1139.

Robertson, C. R., Langlois, K., Martin, C. G., Slezak, G., and Grossman, M. I. (1950). Release of gastrin in reponse to bathing the pyloric mucosa with acetylcholine. *Am. J. Physiol.* **163,** 27–33.

Robinson, R. M., Harris, K., Hlad, C. J., and Eiseman, B. (1957). Effect of glucagon on gastric secretion. *Proc. Soc. Exp. Biol. Med.* **96,** 518–520.

Rocha e Silva, M., Beraldo, W. T., and Rosenfeld, G. (1949). Bradykinin, a hypotensive and smooth muscle stimulating factor released from plasma globulin by snake venoms and by trypsin. *Am. J. Physiol.* **156,** 261–273.

Rommel, K., and Böhmer, R. (1974). Influence of secretin and cholecystokinin on maltase, sucrase and lactase in the jejunum of the rat. *Digestion* **11,** 194–198.

Rorstad, O. P., Epelbaum, J., Brazeau, P., and Martin, J. B. (1979). Chromatographic and biological properties of immunoreactive somatostatin in hypothalamic and extrahypothalamic brain regions of the rat. *Endocrinology* **105,** 1083–1092.

Rösch, W. (1974). Die hormonelle und pharmakologische Beeinflussbarkeit des unteren Ösophagussphinkters. *Fortschr. Med.* **92,** 1261–1263.

Rosell, S., Thor, K. Rökaeus, Å., Nyquist, O., Lewenhaupt, A., Kager, L., and Folkers, K. (1980). Plasma concentration of neurotensin-like immunoreactivity (NTLI) and lower esophageal sphincter (LES) pressure in man following infusion of (Gln⁴)-neurotensin. *Acta Physiol. Scand.* **109,** 369–375.

Ross, E. M., and Gilman, A. G. (1980). Biochemical properties of hormone-sensitive adenylate cyclase. *Annu. Rev. Biochem.* **49,** 533–564.

Ross, G. (1970). Cardiovascular effects of secretin. *Am. J. Physiol.* **218,** 1166–1170.

Ross, J., Aviv, H., Scolnick, E., and Leder, P. (1972). In vitro synthesis of DNA complementary to purified rabbit globin mRNA. *Proc. Natl. Acad. Sci. U.S.A.* **69,** 264–268.

Ross, J. B. A., Rousslang, K. W., Deranleau, D. A., and Kwiram, A. L. (1977). Glucagon conformation: Use of optically detected magnetic resonance and phosphorescence of tryptophan to evaluate critical requirements for folding of the polypeptide chain. *Biochemistry* **16**, 5398–5402.

Rosselin, G., Fromageot, P., and Bonfils, S. (1979). "Hormone Receptors in Digestion and Nutrition." Elsevier, Amsterdam.

Roth, J. A., and Ivy, A. C. (1944). The effect of caffein upon gastric secretion in the dog, cat and man. *Am. J. Physiol.* **141**, 454–461.

Rothman, S. S. (1977). The digestive enzymes of the pancreas: A mixture of inconstant proportions. *Annu. Rev. Physiol.* **39**, 373–389.

Rothman, S. S., and Wells, H. (1967). Enhancement of pancreatic enzyme synthesis by pancreozymin. *Am. J. Physiol.* **213**, 215–218.

Rotsztejn, W., Benoist, L., Besson, J., and Duval, J. (1980). Régulation par la dexaméthasone de la libération de prolactine induite par le peptide vasoactif intestinal (VIP). *C. R. Acad. Sci. Paris D* **290**, 791–793.

Rozé, C. (1980). Control of esophageal and gastric motility. Recent physiological and pharmacological aspects (Part I: Esophagus). *Gastroenterol. Clin. Biol.* **4**, 486–496.

Rudinger, J., and Jošt, K. (1964). A biologically active analogue of oxytocin not containing a disulfide group. *Experientia* **20**, 570–571.

Rudman, D., and Del Rio, A. E. (1969a). Lipolytic activity of synthetic porcine secretin. *Endocrinology* **85**, 214–217.

Rudman, D., and Del Rio, A. E. (1969b). Lipolytic activity of a peptide fragment of porcine secretin. *Endocrinology* **85**, 610–611.

Rudo, N. D., Rosenberg, I. H., and Wissler, R. W. (1976). The effect of partial starvation and glucagon treatment on intestinal villus morphology and cell migration. *Proc. Soc. Exp. Biol. Med.* **152**, 277–280.

Rufener, C., Dubois, M. P., Malaisse-Lagae, F., and Orci, L. (1975). Immuno-fluorescent reactivity to anti-somatostatin in the gastrointestinal mucosa of the dog. *Diabetologia* **11**, 321–324.

Ruppin, H., Domschke, S., Domschke, W., Wünsch, E., Jaeger, E., and Demling, L. (1975). Effects of 13-Nle-motilin in man—Inhibition of gastric evacuation and stimulation of pepsin secretion. *Scand. J. Gastroenterol.* **10**, 199–202.

Russel, J. H., and Geller, D. M. (1975). The structure of rat proalbumin. *J. Biol. Chem.* **250**, 3409–3413.

Russell, T. R., Searle, G. L., and Scott Jones, R. (1975). The choleretic mechanisms of sodium, taurocholate, secretin, and glucagon. *Surgery* **77**, 498–504.

Rutten, W. J., De Pont, J. J. H. M., and Bonting, S. L. (1972). Adenylate cyclase in the rat pancreas. Properties and stimulation by hormones. *Biochim. Biophys. Acta* **271**, 201–213.

Ryan, J., and Cohen, S. (1977). Effect of vasoactive intestinal polypeptide on basal and cholecystokinin-induced gallbladder pressure. *Gastroenterology* **73**, 870–872.

Ryder, S. W., Eng, J., Straus, E., and Yalow, R. S. (1981). Extraction and immunochemical characterization of cholecystokinin-like peptides from pig and rat brain. *Proc. Natl. Acad. Sci. U.S.A.* **78**, 3892–3896.

Ryle, A. P., Sanger, F., Smith, L. F., and Kitai, R. (1955). The disulphide bonds of insulin. *Biochem. J.* **60**, 541–556.

Sabatini, D. D., Tashiro, Y., and Palade, G. E. (1966). On the attachment of ribosomes to microsomal membranes. *J. Mol. Biol.* **19**, 503–524.

Sacks, J., Ivy, A. C., Burgess, J. P., and Vandolah, J. E. (1932). Histamine as hormone for gastric secretion *Am. J. Physiol.* **101**, 331–338.

Said, S. I., and Mutt, V. (1970a). Polypeptide with broad biological activity: Isolation from small intestine. *Science* **169**, 1217–1218.

Said, S. I., and Mutt, V. (1970b). Potent periferal and splanchnic vasodilator peptide from normal gut. *Nature (London)* **225**, 863–864.

Said, S. I., and Mutt, V. (1972). Isolation from porcine-intestinal wall of a vasoactive octacosapeptide related to secretin and to glucagon. *Eur. J. Biochem.* **28**, 199–204.

Salganik, R. I., Argutinskaya, S. V., and Bersimbaev, R. I. (1971). Induction of transcription in the stimulating action of a gastrin pentapeptide on gastric acid secretion. *Experientia* **27**, 53–54.

Samols, E., and Marks, V. (1967). Nouvelles conceptions sur la signification fonctionnelle du glucagon (pancréatique et extrapancréatique.) *J. Annu. Diabetol. Hotel Dieu* **7**, 43–66.

Samols, E., Marri, G., and Marks, V. (1965a). Promotion of insulin secretion by glucagon. *Lancet* **II**, 415–416.

Samols, E., Tyler, J., Marri, G., and Marks, V. (1965b). Stimulation of glucagon secretion by oral glucose. *Lancet* **II**, 1257–1259.

Samols, E., Tyler, J., Megyesi, C., and Marks, V. (1966). Immunochemical glucagon in human pancreas, gut, and plasma. *Lancet* **II**, 727–729.

Sandblom, P., Voegtlin, W. L., and Ivy, A. C. (1935). The effect of cholecystokinin on the choledocho-duodenal mechanism (Sphincter of Oddi). *Am. J. Physiol.* **113**, 175–180.

Sandweiss, D. J. (1943). The immunizing effect of the anti-ulcer factor in normal human urine (Anthelone) against the experimental gastrojejunal (peptic) ulcer in dogs. *Gastroenterology* **1**, 965–969.

Sanger, F. (1945). The free amino groups of insulin. *Biochem. J.* **39**, 507–515.

Sanger, F. (1949). Species differences in insulins. *Nature (London)* **164**, 529.

Sanger, F., Air, G. M., Barrell, B. G., Brown, N. L., Coulson, A. R., Fiddes, J. C., Hutchison, C. A., III, Slocombe, P. M., and Smith, M. (1977). Nucleotide sequence of bacteriophage ΦX174 DNA. *Nature (London)* **265**, 687–695.

Sanyal, A. K., and Waton, N. G. (1976). The possible mechanism for the "fade" in acid gastric secretion during continuous infusions of pentagastrin. *J. Physiol. (London)* **261**, 445–451.

Sarles, H., Hage, G., Laugier, R., Demol, P., and Bataille, D. (1979). Present status of the anticholecystokinin hormone. *Digestion* **19**, 73–76.

Sasaki, H., Rubaclava, B., Baetens, D., Blazquez, E., Srikant, C. B., Orci, L., and Unger, R. H. (1975a). Identification of glucagon in the gastrointestinal tract. *J. Clin. Invest.* **56**, 135–145.

Sasaki, K., Docerill, S., Adamiak, D. A., Tickle, I. J., and Blundell, T. (1975b). X-ray analysis of glucagon and its relationship to receptor binding. *Nature (London)* **257**, 751–757.

Savage, C. R., Jr., Inagami, T., and Cohen, S. (1972). The primary structure of epidermal growth factor. *J. Biol. Chem.* **247**, 7612–7621.

Savory, C. J., and Gentle, M. J. (1980). Intravenous injections of cholecystokinin and caerulein suppress food intake in domestic fowls. *Experientia* **36**, 1191–1192.

Schachter, M. (1969). Kallikreins and kinins. *Physiol. Rev.* **49**, 509–547.

Schaffalitzky de Muckadell, O. B., Fahrenkrug, J., and Holst, J. J. (1977a). Release of vasoactive intestinal polypeptide (VIP) by electric stimulation of the vagal nerves. *Gastroenterology* **72**, 373–375.

Schaffalitzky de Muckadell, O. B., Fahrenkrug, J., Holst, J. J., and Lauritsen, K. B. (1977b). Release of vasoactive intestinal polypeptide (VIP) by intraduodenal stimuli. *Scand. J. Gastroenterol.* **12**, 793–799.

Schally, A. V., Redding, T. W., Lucien, H. W., and Meyer, J. (1967). Enterogastrone inhibits eating by fasted mice. *Science* **157**, 210–211.

Schally, A. V., Dupont, A., Arimura, A., Redding, T. W., and Linthicum, G. L. (1975). Isolation of porcine GH-release inhibiting hormone (GH-RIH): The existence of 3 forms of GH-RIH. *Fed. Proc. Fed. Soc. Exp. Biol.* **34**, 584/2065.

Schally, A. V., Dupont, A., Arimura, A., Redding, T. W., Nishi, N., Linthicum, G. L., and Schlesinger, D. H. (1976). Isolation and structure of somatostatin from porcine hypothalami. *Biochemistry* **15**, 509–514.

Schally, A. V., Huang, W.-Y., Chang, R. C. C., Arimura, A., Redding, T. W., Millar, R. P., Hunkapiller, M. W., and Hood, L. E. (1980). Isolation and structure of prosomatostatin: A putative somatostatin precursor from pig hypothalamus. *Proc. Natl. Acad. Sci. U.S.A.*, **77**, 4489–4493.

Schapiro, H. (1975). Inhibitory action of antidiuretic hormone on canine pancreatic exocrine flow. *Am. J. Dig. Dis.* **20**, 853–857.

Schapiro, H., and Woodward, E. R. (1965). Inhibition of the secretin mechanism by local anesthetics. *Am. Surg.* **31**, 139–141.

Schechter, I. (1973). Biologically and chemically pure mRNA coding for a mouse immunoglobulin L-chain prepared with the aid of antibodies and immobilized oligothymine. *Proc. Natl. Acad. Sci. U.S.A.* **70**, 2256–2260.

Schiffer, M., and Edmundson, A. B. (1970). Prediction of α-helices in glucagon. *Biophys. J.* **10**, 293–295.

Schiller, P. W., Natarajan, S., and Bodanszky, M. (1978). Determination of the intramolecular tyrosine–tryptophan distance in a 7-peptide releated to the C-terminal sequence of cholecystokinin. *Int. J. Pept. Protein Res.* **12**, 139–142.

Schreurs, V. V. A. M., Swarts, H. G. P., De Pont, J. J. H. H. M., and Bonting, S. L. (1976). Role of calcium in exocrine pancreatic secretion. II. Comparison of the effects of carbachol and the ionophore A-23187 on enzyme secretion and calcium movements in rabbit pancreas. *Biochim. Biophys. Acta* **419**, 320–330.

Schubert, H., and Brown, J. C. (1974). Correction to the amino acid sequence of porcine motilin. *Can. J. Biochem.* **52**, 7–8.

Schulak, J. A., and Kaplan, E. L. (1975). The importance of the stomach in gastrin-induced hypocalcemia in the rat. *Endocrinology* **96**, 1217–1220.

Schulz, G. E., and Schirmer, R. H. (1979). "Principles of Protein Structure." Springer-Verlag, Berlin and New York.

Schulz, I., Yamagata, A., and Weske, M. (1969). Micropuncture studies on the pancreas of the rabbit. *Pflügers Arch.* **308**, 277–290.

Schwyzer, R. (1960). The chemistry and pharmacology of angiotensin. *Vitamins Horm.* **18**, 237–288.

Schwyzer, R. (1963). Chemical structure and biological activity in the field of polypeptide hormones. *Pure Appl. Chem.* **6**, 265–295.

Scow, R. O., and Cornfield, J. (1954). Quantitative relations between the oral and intravenous glucose tolerance curves. *Am. J. Physiol.* **179**, 435–438.

Scratcherd, T. (1965). Electrolyte composition and control of biliary secretion in the cat and rabbit. *In* "The Biliary System" (W. Taylor, ed.), pp. 515–529. Blackwell, Oxford.

Seeburg, P. H., Shine, J., Martial, J. A., Ullrich, A., Baxter, J. D., and Goddman, H. M. (1977a). Nucleotide sequence of part of the gene for human chorionic somatomammotropin: Purification of DNA complementary to predominant mRNA species. *Cell* **12**, 157–165.

Seeburg, P. H., Shine, J., Martial, J. A., Baxter, J. D., and Goodman, H. M. (1977b).

Nucleotide sequence and amplification in bacteria of structural gene for rat growth hormone. *Nature (London)* **270**, 486–494.

Seidah, N. G., Benjannet, S., Routhier, R., De Serres, G., Rochemont, J., Lis, M., and Chrétien, M. (1980). Purification and characterization of the N-terminal fragment of pro-opiomelanocortin from human pituitaries: Homology to the bovine sequence. *Biochem. Biophys. Res. Commun.* **95**, 1417–1424.

Seino, S., Seino, Y., Taminato, T., Mori, K., Matsukura, S., Yawata, M., and Imura, H. (1980). Effect of adrenergic blocking agents on plasma gastrin and secretin levels in man. *Am. J. Gastroenterol.* **73**, 137–140.

Senyk, G., Nitecki, D. E., Spitler, L., and Goodman, J. W. (1972). The immune response to glucagon in conjugate form. *Immunochemistry* **9**, 97–110.

Seppälä, M., and Wahlström, T. (1980). Identification of lutenizing hormone-releasing factor and alpha-subunit of glycoprotein hormones in human pancreatic islets. *Life Sci.* **27**, 395–397.

Sewing, K.-Fr., Gorinsky, P. D., and Lembeck, F. (1968). Failure of "antigastrin" (SC-15 396) to inhibit gastric acid and pepsin secretion in anesthetized gastric fistula cats. *Naunyn-Schmiedebergs Arch. Pharmakol. Exp. Pathol.* **261**, 89–92.

Shaw, R. A., and Jones, R. S. (1978). The choleretic action of cholecystokinin and cholecystokinin octapeptide in dogs. *Surgery* **84**, 622–625.

Shields, D. (1980). In vitro biosynthesis of fish islet preprosomatostatin: Evidence of processing and segregation of a high molecular weight precursor. *Proc. Natl. Acad. Sci. U.S.A.* **77**, 4074–4078.

Shields, D., and Blobel, G. (1977). Cell-free synthesis of fish preproinsulin, and processing by heterologous mammalian microsomal membranes. *Proc. Natl. Acad. Sci. U.S.A.* **74**, 2059–2063.

Shine, J., Seeburg, P. H., Martial, J. A., Baxter, J. D., and Goodman, H. M. (1977). Construction and analysis of recombinant DNA for human chorionic somatomammotropin. *Nature (London)* **270**, 494–499.

Siewert, R., Weiser, F., Jennewein, H. M., and Waldeck, F. (1974a). Clinical and manometric investigations of the lower esophageal sphincter and its reactivity to pentagastrin in patients with Hiatus hernia. *Digestion* **10**, 287–297.

Siewert, R., Waldeck, F., and Peiper, H.-J. (1974b). Gastrointestinale Hormone und unterer Oesophagussphincter. *Chirurg* **45**, 28–33.

Simon, B., and Kather, H. (1980). Human colonic adenylate cyclase. Stimulation of enzyme activity by vasoactive intestinal peptide and various prostaglandins via distinct receptor sites. *Digestion* **20**, 62–67.

Sinar, D. R., O'Doriso, T. M., Mazzaferri, E. L., Mekhjian, H. S., Caldwell, J. H., and Thomas, F. B. (1978). Effect of gastric inhibitory polypeptide on lower esophageal sphincter pressure in cats. *Gastroenterology* **75**, 263–267.

Sjödin, L. (1972). Influence of secretin and cholecystokinin on canine gastric secretion elicited by food and by exogenous gastrin. *Acta Physiol. Scand.* **85**, 110–117.

Sjödin, L., and Miura, S. (1974). Secretin-induced inhibition of acid secretion before and after vagal denervation of canine gastric pouches. *Scand. J. Gastroenterol.* **9**, 185–190.

Skvortsova, N. B., Lyalin, E. A., and Ugolev, A. M. (1972). Influence of the removal and isolation of the duodenum on the thyroid gland in cats. Possibility of the existence of a thyroid-stimulating hormone of the duodenum. *Dokl. Akad. Nauk SSSR* **207**, 501–503.

Slayback, J. B., Swena, E. M., Thomas, J. E., and Smith, L. L. (1967). The pancreatic secretory response to topical anesthetic block of the small bowel. *Surgery* **61**, 591–595.

Smith, A. N., and Hogg, D. (1966). Effect of gastrin II on the motility of the gastrointestinal tract. *Lancet* **I** 403–404.

Smith, C. L., Kewenter, J., Connell, A. M., Ardill, J., Hayes, R., and Buchanan, K. (1975). Control factors in the release of gastrin by direct electrical stimulation of the vagus. *Am. J. Dig. Dis.* **20,** 13–22.

Smith, C. W., and Walter, R. (1978). Vasopressin analog with extraordinary high antidiuretic potency: A study of conformation and activity. *Science* **199,** 297–299.

Smith, L. F. (1966). Species variation in the amino acid sequence of insulin. *Am. J. Med.* **40,** 662–666.

Smyth, D. G. (1975). The peptide hormones; molecular and cellular aspects. *Nature (London)* **257,** 89–90.

Snape, W. J., Jr., and Cohen, S. (1976). Hormonal control of esophageal function. *Arch. Intern. Med.* **136,** 538–542.

Snyder, S. H. (1980). Brain peptides as neurotransmitters. *Science* **209,** 976–983.

Sober, H. A., and Peterson, E. A. (1954). Chromatography of proteins on cellulose ion-exchangers. *J. Am. Chem. Soc.* **76,** 1711–1712.

Solcia, E., Polak, J. M., Pearse, A. G. E., Forssmann, W. G., Larsson, L.-I., Sundler, F., Lechago, J., Grimelius, L. Fujita, T., Creutzfeldt, W., Getps, W., Falkmer, S., Lefranc, G., Hietz, P., Hage, E., Buchan, A. M. J., Bloom, S. R., and Grossman, M. I. (1978). Lausanne 1977 classification of gastroenteropancreatic endocrine cells. *In* "Gut Hormones" (S. R. Bloom, ed.), pp. 40–48. Churchill, London.

Soll, A. H. (1978). The interaction of histamine with gastrin and carbamylcholine on oxygen uptake by isolated mammalian parietal cells. *J. Clin. Invest.* **61,** 381–389.

Soll, A. H. (1980). Specific inhibition by prostaglandins E_2 and I_2 of histamine-stimulated (^{14}C)aminopyrine accumulation and cyclic adenosine monophosphate generation by isolated canine parietal cells. *J. Clin. Invest.* **65,** 1222–1229.

Soll, A. H., and Grossman, M. I. (1978). Cellular mechanisms in acid secretion. *Annu. Rev. Med.* **29,** 495–507.

Solomon, T. E., and Grossman, M. I. (1979). Effect of atropine and vagotomy on response of transplanted pancreas. *Am. J. Physiol.* **236,** E186–E190.

Solomon, T. E., Beyerman, H. C., and Grossman, M. I. (1977). Potency of des-histidyl[1]-secretin for pancreatic secretion in dogs. *Clin. Res.* **25,** A 547.

Somersalo, O. (1950). Staub effect in children. Studies of the blood sugar regulation by means of double and triple glucose tolerance tests. *Acta Paediat. Suppl.* **78.**

Soumarmon, A., Lewin, M., Dubrasquet, M., Bonfils, S., Girma, J. P., Morgat, J. L., and Fromageot, P. (1977). TM-gastrin as a gastrin receptor antagonist in gastric mucosa. *In* "Hormonal Receptors in Digestive Tract Physiology" (S. Bonfils *et al.,* eds.), p. 404. Elsevier, Amsterdam.

Spiess, J., and Vale, W. (1980). Multiple forms of somatostatin-like activity in rat hypothalamus. *Biochemistry* **19,** 2861–2866.

Spiess, J., Rivier, J. E., Rodkey, J. A., Bennett, C. D., and Vale, W. (1979). Isolation and characterization of somatostatin from pigeon pancreas. *Proc. Natl. Acad. Sci. U.S.A.* **76,** 2974–2978.

Srikant, C. B., McCorkle, K., and Unger, R. H. (1977). Properties of immunoreactive glucagon fractions of canine stomach and pancreas. *J. Biol. Chem.* **252,** 1847–1851.

Stacher, G., Bauer, H., and Steinringer, H. (1979). Cholecystokinin decreases appetite and activation evoked by stimuli arising from the preparation of a meal in man. *Physiol. Behav.* **23,** 325–331.

Stadil, F., and Rehfeld, J. F. (1974). Gastrin response to insulin after selective, highly selective and truncal vagotomy. *Gastroenterology* **66,** 7–15.

Stanley, M. D., Coalson, R. E., Grossman, M. I., and Johnson, L. R. (1972). Influence of secretin and pentagastrin on acid secretion and parietal cell number in rats. *Gastroenterology* **63,** 264–269.

Starling, E. H. (1905). The chemical correlation of the functions of the body. *Lancet* **II,** 339–341.

Stasiewicz, J., and Wormsley, K. G. (1974). Functional control of the biliary tract. *Acta Hepato-Gastroenterol.* **21,** 450–468.

Staub, A., Sinn, L., and Behrens, O. K. (1953). Purification and crystallization of hyperglycemic glycogenolytic factor (HGF). *Science* **117,** 628–629.

Staub, A., Sinn, L., and Behrens, O. K. (1955). Purification and crystallization of glucagon. *J. Biol. Chem.* **214,** 619–632.

Staub, H. (1921). Untersuchungen über den Zuckerstoffwechsel des Menschen. *Z. Klin. Med.* **91,** 44–60.

Steiner, D. F., and Oyer, P. E. (1967). The biosynthesis of insulin and a probable precursor of insulin by a human islet cell adenoma. *Proc. Natl. Acad. Sci. U.S.A.* **57,** 473–480.

Steiner, D. F., Clark, J. L., Nolan, C., Rubenstein, A. H., Margoliash, E., Aten, B., and Oyer, P. E. (1969). Proinsulin and the biosynthesis of insulin. *Recent Prog. Horm. Res.* **25,** 207–282.

Stening, G. F., and Grossman, M. I. (1969a). Gastrin-related peptides as stimulants of pancreatic and gastric secretion. *Am. J. Physiol.* **217,** 262–266.

Stening, G. F., and Grossman, M. I. (1969b). Hormonal control of Brunner's glands. *Gastroenterology* **56,** 1047–1052.

Stening, G. F., and Grossman, M. I. (1970). Gastric acid response to pentagastrin and histamine after extragastric vagotomy in dogs. *Gastroenterology* **59,** 364–371.

Stening, G. F., Johnson, L. R., and Grossman, M. I. (1969a). Effect of secretin on acid and pepsin secretion in cat and dog. *Gastroenterology* **56,** 468–475.

Stening, G. F., Johnson, L. R., and Grossman, M. I. (1969b). Effect of cholecystokinin and caerulein on gastrin- and histamine-evoked gastric secretion. *Gastroenterology* **57,** 44–50.

Stewart, J. J., and Burks, T. F. (1980). Actions of pentagastrin on smooth muscle of isolated dog intestine. *Am. J. Physiol.* **239,** G295–G299.

Straaten, Th. (1933). Die Bedeutung der Pylorusdrüsenzone für die Magensaftsekretion. *Arch. Klin. Chir.* **176,** 236–251.

Straus, E. (1978). The explosion of gastrointestinal hormones. Their clinical significance. *Med. Clin. North Am.* **62,** 21–37.

Straus, E., and Yalow, R. S. (1978). Species specificity of cholecystokinin in gut and brain of several mammalian species. *Proc. Natl. Acad. Sci. U.S.A.* **75,** 486–489.

Strosser, M. T., Cohen, L., Harvey, S., and Mialhe, P. (1980). Somatostatin stimulates glucagon secretion in ducks. *Diabetologia* **18,** 319–322.

Studer, R. O., Trzeciak, H., and Lergier, W. (1973). Isolierung und Aminosäuresquenz von Substanz P aus Pferdedarm. *Helv. Chim. Acta* **56,** 860–866.

Stunkard, A. J., Van Itallie, T. B., and Resis, B. B. (1955). The mechanism of satiety: Effect of glucagon on gastric hunger contractions in man. *Proc. Soc. Exp. Biol. Med.* **89,** 258–261.

Suchanek, G., and Kreil, G. (1977). Translation of melittin messenger RNA in vitro yields a product terminating with glutaminylglycin rather than with glutaminamide. *Proc. Natl. Acad. Sci. U.S.A.* **74,** 975–978.

Sum, P. T., and Preshaw, R. M. (1967). Intraduodenal glucose infusion and pancreatic secretion in man. *Lancet* **II,** 340–341.

Sundby, F., Frandsen, E., Thomsen, J., Kristiansen, K., and Brunfeldt, K. (1972). Crystallization and amino acid sequence of duck glucagon. *FEBS Lett.* **26,** 289–293.

Sundby, F., Markussen J., and Danho, W. (1974). Camel glucagon: Isolation, crystallization and amino acid composition. *Horm. Metab. Res.* **6**, 425.

Sundby, F., Jacobsen, H., and Moody, A. J. (1976). Purification and characterization of a protein from porcine gut with glucagon-like immunoreactivity. *Horm. Metab. Res.* **8**, 366–371.

Sutherland, E. W., and de Duve, C. (1948). Origin and distribution of the hyperglycemic-glycogenolytic factor of the pancreas. *J. Biol. Chem.* **175**, 663–674.

Sutherland, E. W., Øye, I., and Butcher, R. W. (1965). The action of epinephrine and the role of the adenyl cyclase system in hormone action. *Recent Prog. Horm. Res.* **21**, 623–646.

Sutton, D., and Donaldson, R. M. (1974). In vitro biosynthesis and secretion of pepsinogen by rabbit gastric mucosa. *Gastroenterology* **66**, A-132/786.

Swann, J. C., and Hammes, G. G. (1969). Self-association of glucagon. Equilibrium studies. *Biochemistry* **8**, 1–7.

Szokolow, A. (1904). Zur Analyse der Abscheidungsarbeit des Magens bei Hunden. *Jahrb. Fortschr. Tierchem.* **34**, 469–470.

del Tacca, M., Soldani, G., and Crema, A. (1970). Experiments of the mechanism of action of caerulein at the level of the guinea-pig ileum and colon. *Agents Actions* **1**, 176–182.

Tager, H. S., and Markese, J. (1979). Intestinal and pancreatic glucagon-like peptides. Evidence for identity of higher molecular weight forms. *J. Biol. Chem.* **254**, 2229–2233.

Tager, H. S., and Steiner, D. F. (1973). Isolation of a glucagon-containing peptide: Primary structure of a possible fragment of proglucagon. *Proc. Natl. Acad. Sci. U.S.A.* **70**, 2321–2325.

Tager, H. S., Patzelt, C., Assoian, R. K., Chan, S. J., Duguid, J. R., and Steiner, D. F. (1980a). Biosynthesis of islet cell hormones. *Ann. N.Y. Acad. Sci.* **343**, 133–147.

Tager, H., Thomas, N., Assoian, R., Rubenstein, A., Saekow, M., Olefsky, J., and Kaiser, E. T. (1980b). Semisynthesis and biological activity of porcine (leu^{B24}) insulin and (leu^{B25}) insulin. *Proc. Natl. Acad. Sci. U.S.A.* **77**, 3181–3185.

Takabatake, Y., and Sachs, H. (1964). Vasopressin biosynthesis. III. In vitro studies. *Endocrinology* **75**, 934–942.

Talaulicar, M., Ebert, R., Willms, B., and Creuzfeldt W. (1981). Effect of exogenous insulin on fasting serum levels of gastric inhibitory polypeptide (GIP) in juvenile diabetes. *Clin. Endocrinol.* **14**, 175–180.

Tapia-Arancibia, L., Arancibia, S., Bluet-Pajot, M.-T., Enjalbert, A., Epelbaum, J., Priam, M., and Kordon, C. (1980). Effect of vasoactive intestinal peptide (VIP) on somatostatin inhibition of pituitary growth hormone secretion in vitro. *Eur. J. Pharmacol.* **63**, 235–236.

Tatemoto, K. (1980). Chemical assay for natural peptides: Application to the isolation of candidate hormones. *In* "Gastrointestinal Hormones" (G. B. J. Glass, ed.), pp. 975–977. Raven, New York.

Tatemoto, K., and Mutt, V. (1980). Isolation of two novel candidate hormones using a chemical method for finding naturally occurring polypeptides. *Nature (London)* **285**, 417–418.

Terhorst, C., Robb, R., Jones, C., and Strominger, J. L. (1977). Further structural studies of the heavy chain of HLA antigens and its similarity to immunoglobulins. *Proc. Natl. Acad. Sci. U.S.A.* **74**, 4002–4006.

Thim, L., and Moody, A. J. (1981). The primary structure of porcine glicentin (Proglucagon). *Regul. Pept.* **2**, 139–150.

Thomas, J. E. (1950). "The External Secretion of the Pancreas." Thomas, Springfield, Illinois.

Thomas, J. E., and Crider, J. O. (1940). A quantitative study of acid in the intestine as a stimulus for the pancreas. Am. J. Physiol. 131, 349–356.

Thomas, J. E., and Crider, J. O. (1941). The pancreatic secretagogue action of products of protein digestion. Am. J. Physiol. 134, 656–663.

Thompson, J. C. (1975). "Gastrointestinal Hormones." Univ. of Texas Press, Austin.

Thompson, J. C., Reeder, D. D., Bunchman, H. H., Becker, H. D., and Brandt, E. N., Jr. (1972). Effect of secretin on circulating gastrin. Ann. Surg. 176, 384–393.

Thompson, W. J., Johnson, D. G., Lavis, V. R., and Williams, R. H. (1974). Effects of secretin on guanyl cyclase of various tissues. Endocrinology 94, 276–278.

Thompson, W. J., Chang, L. K., and Rosenfeld, G. C. (1981). Histamine regulation of adenylyl cyclase of enriched rat gastric parietal cells. Am. J. Physiol. 240, G76–G84.

Thulin, L., and Samnegård, H. (1978). Circulatory effects of gastrointestinal hormones and related peptides. Acta Chir. Scand. Suppl. 482, 73–74.

Tigerstedt, R., and Bergman, P. G. (1898). Niere und Kreislauf. Skand. Arch. Physiol. 8, 223–271.

Timson, C. M., Polak, J. M., Warton, J., Ghatei, M. A., Bloom, S. R., Usellini, L., Capella, C., Solcia, E., Brown, M. R., and Pearse, A. G. E. (1979). Bombesin-like immunoreactivity in the avian gut and its localisation to a distinct cell type. Histochemistry 61, 213–221.

Toouli, J., and Watts, J. McK. (1972). Actions of cholecystokinin/pancreozymin, secretin and gastrin on extra-hepatic biliary tract motility in vitro. Ann. Surg. 175, 439–447.

Track, N. S. (1976). Evolution of the gastrointestinal hormones. In "Endocrinology of the Gut" (N. S. Track, ed.), pp. 126–139. McMaster Univ. Symp., Hamilton Canada.

Tracy, H. J., and Gregory, R. A. (1964). Physiological properties of a series of synthetic peptides structurally related to gastrin I. Nature (London) 204, 935–938.

Trakatellis, A. C., Tada, K., Yamaji, K., and Gardiki-Kouidou, P. (1975). Isolation and partial characterization of anglerfish proglucagon. Biochemistry 14, 1508–1512.

Traugott, K. (1922). Uber das Verhalten des Blutzucker-Spiegels bei wiederholter und verschiedener Art enteraler Zuckerzufuhr und dessen Bedeutung für die Leberfunktion. Klin. Wochenschr. 1, 892–894.

Tregear, G. W., Niall, H. D., Potts, J. T., Jr., Leeman, S. E., and Chang, M. M. (1971). Synthesis of substance P. Nature (London) New Biol. 232, 87–89.

Trout, H. H., and Grossman, M. I. (1971). Penultimate aspartyl unnecessary for stimulation of acid secretion by gastrin-related peptide. Nature (London) New Biol. 234, 256.

Trudeau, W. L., and McGuigan, J. E. (1969). Effects of calcium on serum gastrin levels in the Zollinger–Ellison syndrome. New Engl. J. Med. 281, 862–866.

Tumpson, D. B., and Johnson, L. R. (1969). Effect of secretin and cholecystokinin on the response of the gastric fistula rat to pentagastrin. Proc. Soc. Exp. Biol. Med. 131, 186–188.

Tung, A. K., and Zerega, F. (1971). Biosynthesis of glucagon in isolated pigeon islets. Biochem. Biophys. Res. Commun. 45, 387–395.

Tuppy, H. (1953). The amino-acid sequence of oxytocin. Biochim. Biophys. Acta 11, 449–450.

Turner, D. S. (1969). Intestinal hormones and insulin release: In vitro studies using rabbit pancreas. Horm. Metab. Res. 1, 168–174.

Turner, D. S., Etheridge, L., Marks, V., Brown, J. C., and Mutt, V. (1974). Effectiveness of the intestinal polypeptides, IRP, GIP, VIP and motilin on insulin release in the rat. *Diabetologia* **10**, 459–463.

Ugolev, A. M. (1975). Non-digestive functions of the intestinal hormones (Enterines). New data and hypotheses based on experimental duodenectomy. *Acta Hepato-Gastroenterol.* **22**, 320–326.

Ullrich, A., Shine, J., Chirgwin, J., Pictet, R., Tischer, E., Rutter, W. J., and Goodman, H. M. (1977). Rat insulin genes: Construction of plasmids containing the coding sequences. *Science* **196**, 1313–1319.

Unger, R. H. (1976). Glucagon Symposium: Foreword. Report of the nomenclature committee. *Metabolism* **25** (Suppl. 1), IX.

Unger, R. H., Eisentraut, A. M., McCall, M. S., Keller, S., Lanz, H. C., and Madison, L. L. (1959). Glucagon antibodies and their use for immunoassay for glucagon. *Proc. Soc. Exp. Biol. Med.* **102**, 621–623.

Unger, R. H., Eisentraut, A. M., McCall, M. S., and Madison, L. L. (1961a). Glucagon antibodies and an immunoassay for glucagon. *J. Clin. Invest.* **40**, 1280–1289.

Unger, R. H., Eisentraut, A., Sims, K., McCall, M. S., and Madison, L. L. (1961b). Sites of origin of glucagon in dogs and humans. *Clin. Res.* **9**, A53.

Unger, R. H., Ketterer, H., and Eisentraut, A. M. (1966). Distribution of immunoassayable glucagon in gastrointestinal tissues. *Metabolism* **15**, 865–867.

Unger, R. H., Ketterer, H., Dupré, J., and Eisentraut, A. M. (1967). The effects of secretin, pancreozymin, and gastrin on insulin and glucagon secretion in anesthetized dogs. *J. Clin. Invest.* **46**, 630–645.

Unger, R. H., Ohneda, A., Valverde, I., Eisentraut, A. M., and Exton, J. (1968). Characterization of the responses of circulating glucagon-like immunoreactivity to intraduodenal and intravenous administration of glucose. *J. Clin. Invest.* **47**, 48–65.

Urry, D. W. (1972). Protein conformation in biomembranes: optical rotation and absorption of membrane suspensions. *Biochim. Biophys. Acta* **265**, 115–168.

Uvnäs, B. (1942). The part played by the pyloric region in the cephalic phase of gastric secretion. *Acta Physiol. Scand. Suppl.* **13**.

Uvnäs-Wallensten, K. (1977). Occurrence of gastrin in gastric juice, in antral secretion, and in antral perfusates of cats. *Gastroenterology* **73**, 487–491.

Uvnäs-Wallensten, K., and Rehfeld, J. F. (1976). Molecular forms of gastrin in antral mucosa, plasma and gastric juice during vagal stimulation of anesthetized cats. *Acta Physiol. Scand.* **98**, 217–226.

Uvnäs-Wallensten, K., Rehfeld, J. F., Larsson, L.-I., and Uvnäs, B. (1977). Heptadecapeptide gastrin in the vagal nerve. *Proc. Natl. Acad. Sci. U.S.A.* **74**, 5707–5710.

Vagne, M., and Fargier, M.-C. (1973). Effect of pentagastrin and secretin on gastric mucus secretion in conscious cats. *Gastroenterology* **65**, 757–763.

Vagne, M., and Grossman, M. I. (1968). Cholecystokinetic potency of gastrointestinal hormones and related peptides. *Am. J. Physiol.* **215**, 881–884.

Vagne, M., and Mutt, V. (1977). Pepsin stimulant from intestinal mucosa. *Gastroenterology* **72**, A 16/826.

Vaillant, C., Dockray, G. J., and Walsh, J. H. (1979). The avian proventriculus is an abundant source of endocrine cells with bombesin-like immunoreactivity. *Histochemistry* **64**, 307–314.

Valenzuela, J. E. (1976). Effect of intestinal hormones and peptides on intragastric pressure in dogs. *Gastroenterology* **71**, 766–769.

Valverde, I., Rigopoulou, D., Exton, J., Ohneda, A., Eisentraut, A., and Unger, R. H. (1968). Demonstration and characterization of a second fraction of glucagon-like immunoreactivity in jejunal extracts. *Am. J. Med. Sci.* **255**, 415–420.

Valverde, I., Rigopoulou, D., Marco, J., Faloona, G. R., and Unger, R. H. (1970a). Characterization of glucagon-like immunoreactivity (GLI). *Diabetes* **19**, 614–623.

Valverde, I., Rigopoulou, D., Marco, J., Faloona, G. R., and Unger, R. H. (1970b). Molecular size of extractable glucagon and glucagon-like immunoreactivity (GLI) in plasma. *Diabetes* **19**, 624–629.

Valverde, I., Villanueva, M. L., Lozano, I., Román, D., Díaz-Fierros, M., and Marco, J. (1973). Chromatographic pattern of human intestinal glucagon-like immunoreactivity (GLI). *J. Clin. Endocrinol. Metab.* **36**, 185–187.

Varró, V. (1976). Clinical significance and perspectives of gastrointestinal peptide hormones. *Acta Physiol. Acad. Sci. Hung.* **47**, 369–378.

Vatn, M. H., Schrumpf, E., Hanssen, K. F., and Myren, J. (1980). A small dose of somatostatin inhibits the secretin stimulated secretion of bicarbonate, amylase, and chymotrypsin in man. *J. Endocrinol. Invest.* **3**, 279–282.

Vaysse, N., Martinel, C., Lacroix, A., Pascal, J. P., and Ribet, A. (1973). Effet de la cholécystokinine-pancréozymine GIH sur la vasomotricité du pancréas isolé du chien. Relations entre l'effet vaso-moteur et la résponse sécrétoire. *Biol. Gastroenterol. (Paris)* **6**, 33–40.

Vaysse, N., Esteve, J. P., Brenac, B., Moatti, J. P., and Pascal, J. P. (1978). Action of dopamine on cyclic AMP-tissue level in the rat pancreas. Interaction with secretin. *Biomedicine* **28**, 342–347.

Verma, I. M., Temple, G. F., Fan, H., and Baltimore, D. (1972). In vitro synthesis of DNA complementary to rabbit reticulocyte 10S RNA. *Nature (London) New Biol.* **235**, 163–167.

Vigna, S. R., and Gorbman, A. (1977). Effects of cholecystokinin, gastrin, and related peptides on coho salmon gallbladder contraction in vitro. *Am. J. Physiol.* **232**, E485–E491.

Vigna, S. R., and Gorbman, A. (1979). Stimulation of intestinal lipase secretion by porcine cholecystokinin in the hagfish, *Eptatretus stouti. Gen. Comp. Endocrinol.* **38**, 356–359.

Vigouroux, N., and Thomas, M. (1978). Les hormones du tube digestif. *Med. Chir. Dig.* **7**, 195–211.

Villar, H. V., Fender, H. R., Rayford, P. L., Bloom, S. R., Ramus, N. I., and Thompson, J. C. (1976). Suppression of gastrin release and gastric secretion by gastric inhibitory polypeptide (GIP) and vasoactive intestinal polypeptide (VIP). *Ann. Surg.* **184**, 97–103.

Vizi, E. S., Bertiaccini, G., Impicciatore, M., and Knoll, J. (1972). Acetylcholine-releasing effect of gastrin and related polypeptides. *Eur. J. Pharmacol.* **17**, 175–178.

Vizi, E. S., Bertaccini, G., Impicciatore, M., and Knoll, J. (1973). Evidence that acetylcholine released by gastrin and related polypeptides contributes to their effect on gastrointestinal motility. *Gastroenterology* **64**, 268–277.

Vizi, E. S., Bertaccini, G., Impicciatore, M., Mantovani, P., Zseli, J., and Knoll, J. (1974). Structure–activity relationship of some analogues of gastrin and cholecystokinin on intestinal smooth muscle of the guinea pig. *Naunyn-Schimedebergs Arch. Pharmacol.* **284**, 233–243.

Vogler, K., Haefely, W., Hurlimann, A., Studer, R. O., Lergier, W., Strassle, R., and Berneis, K. H. (1963). A new purification procedure and biological properties of substance P. *Ann. N.Y. Acad. Sci.* **104**, 378–390.

Vranic, M., Pek, S., and Kawamori, L. (1974). Increased glucagon immunoreactivity in plasma of totally depancreatized dogs. *Diabetes* **23**, 905–912.

Waldeck, F., Siewert, R., Jennewein, H.-M., and Weiser, F. (1973). Das Druckprofil im unterer Ösophagussphinkter beim Menschen und seine Beeinflussung durch Gastrin, Calcitonin und Glucagon. *Dtsch. Med. Wochenschr.* **98**, 1059–1063.

Waldum, H. L., Aanstad, U., Burhol, P. G., and Berstad, A. (1980a). The diuretic effect of secretin in man. *Scand. J. Clin. Lab. Invest.* **40**, 381–387.

Waldum, H. L., Sundsfjord, J. A., Aanstad, U., and Burhol, P. G. (1980b). The effect of secretin on renal haemodynamics in man. *Scand. J. Clin. Lab. Invest.* **40**, 475–478.

Waller, S. L., Carvalhinhos, A., Misiewicz, J. J., and Russell, R. I. (1973). Effect of cholecystokinin on colonic motility. *Lancet* **I**, 264.

Wallis, M., and Davies, R. V. (1976). Studies on the chemistry of bovine and rat growth hormones. *In* "Growth Hormone and Related Peptides" (A. Pecile and E. E. Müller, eds.), pp. 1–14. Excerpta Medica, Amsterdam.

Walsh, J. H. (1975). Circulating gastrin. *Annu. Rev. Physiol.* **37**, 81–104.

Walsh, J. H., and Grossman, M. I. (1973). Circulating gastrin in peptic ulcer disease. *Mt. Sinai J. Med.* **40**, 374–381.

Walsh, J. H., and Holmquist, A. L. (1976). Radioimmunoassay of bombesin peptides: identification of bombesin-like immunoreactivity in vertebrate gut extracts. *Gastroenterology* **70**, A90/948.

Walsh, J. H., Debas, H. T., and Grossman, M. I. (1974). Pure human big gastrin: Immunochemical properties, half life disappearance and acid-stimulating action in dogs. *J. Clin. Invest.* **54**, 477–485.

Walter, R. (1971). Conformations of oxytocin and lysine-vasopressin and their relationships to the biology of neurohypophyseal hormones. *Excerpta. Med. Int. Congr. Ser.* **241**, 181–193.

Wang, C. C., and Grossman, M. I. (1951). Physiological determination of release of secretin and pancreozymin from intestine of dogs with transplanted pancreas. *Am. J. Physiol.* **164**, 527–545.

Wang, C. C., Grossman, M. I., and Ivy, A. C. (1948). Effect of secretin and pancreozymin on amylase and alkaline phosphatase secretion by the pancreas in dogs. *Am. J. Physiol.* **154**, 358–368.

Warnes, T. W., Hine, P., and Kay, G. (1969). Alkaline phosphatase in duodenal juice following secretin and pancreozymin. *Gut* **10**, 1049.

Way, L. W. (1971). Effect of cholecystokinin and caerulein on gastric secretion in cats. *Gastroenterology* **60**, 560–565.

Way, L. W., and Durbin, R. P. (1969). Response of the bullfrog gastric mucosa to gastrin I and gastrin II. *Gastroenterology* **56**, 1266 (Abstr.).

Weber, H. E. (1975). Partial purification and translation of proinsulin messenger RNA. *Diabetes* **24** (Suppl. 2), 405 (Abstr. 50).

Webster, P. D., and Tyor, M. P. (1966). Effect of intravenous pancreozymin on amino acid incorporation in vitro by pancreas tissue. *Am. J. Physiol.* **211**, 157–160.

Wei, E. P., Kontos, H. A., and Said, S. I. (1980). Mechanism of action of vasoactive intestinal polypeptide on cerebral arterioles. *Am. J. Physiol.* **239**, H765–H768.

Wertheimer, E., and Lepage, L. (1901). Sur le fonctions réflexes des ganglions abdomineaux du sympathique dans l'innervation sécrétoire du pancréas. *J. Physiol. Pathol. Gen.* **3**, 335–348.

Wilhelmj, C. M., McCarthy, H. H., and Hill, F. C. (1937). Acid inhibition of the intestinal and intragastric chemical phases of gastric secretion. *Am. J. Physiol.* **118**, 766–774.

Willems, G., and Vansteenkiste, Y. (1974). Resistance of the antral mucosa to the trophic effect of gastrin in the dog. *Biol. Gastroenterol.* **7**, 237–240.

Willems, G., Wansteenkiste, Y., and Limbosch, J. M. (1972). Stimulating effect of gastrin on cell proliferation kinetics in canine fundic mucosa. *Gastroenterology* **62**, 583–589.

Williams, J. A., and Lee, M. (1974). Pancreatic acinar cells: use of Ca^{++} ionophore to separate enzyme release from the earlier steps in stimulus-secretion coupling. *Biochem. Biophys. Res. Commun.* **60**, 542–548.

Williamson, R. C. N., Bauer, F. L. R., Ross, J. S., and Malt, R. A. (1978). Proximal enterectomy stimulates distal hyperplasia more than bypass or pancreaticobilliary diversion. *Gastroenterology* **74**, 16–23.

Winckler, K., Hesch, R.-D., and Schmidt, H. (1973). Hemmung der Gallaenblasenkontraktion durch Calcitonin. *Dtsch. Med. Wochenschr.* **98**, 957–959.

Windeck, R., Brown, E. M., Gardner, D. G., and Aurbach, G. D. (1978). Effect of gastrointestinal hormones on isolated bovine parathyroid cells. *Endocrinology* **103**, 2020–2026.

Wingate, D. (1976). Intestinal potential difference during glucose absorption. *Lancet* **II**, 529–532.

Wingate, D. L., Ruppin, H., Thompson, H. H., Green, W. E. R., Domschke, W., Wünsch, E., Demling, L., and Ritchie, H. D. (1975). 13-norleucine motilin versus pentagastrin: Contrasting and competitive effects on gastrointestinal myoelectric activity in the conscious dog. *Acta Hepato-Gastroenterol.* **22**, 409–410.

Wittmann-Liebold, B. (1980). Current advances in sequencing as applied to the structure determination of ribosomal proteins. *In* "Polypeptide Hormones" (R. F. Beers, Jr. and E. G. Bassett, eds.), pp. 87–120. Raven, New York.

Woo, S. L. C., Rosen, J. M., Liarakos, C. D., Choi, Y. C., Busch, H., Means, A. R., and O'Malley, B. W. (1975). Physical and chemical characterization of purified ovalbumin messenger RNA. *J. Biol. Chem.* **250**, 7027–7039.

Woodward, E. R., Lyon, E. S., Landor, J., and Dragstedt, L. R. (1954). The physiology of the gastric antrum. *Gastroenterology* **27**, 766–785.

Wormsley, K. G. (1968a). The action of secretin on the secretion of enzymes by the human pancreas. *Scand. J. Gastroenterol.* **3**, 183–188.

Wormsley, K. G. (1968b). Gastric response to secretin and pancreozymin in man. *Scand. J. Gastroenterol.* **3**, 632–636.

Wormsley, K. G., and Grossman, M. I. (1964). Inhibition of gastric acid secretion by secretin and by endogenous acid in the duodenum. *Gastroenterology* **47**, 72–81.

Wright, D. E., and Rodbell, M. (1979a). Glucagon$_{1-6}$ binds to the glucagon receptor and activates hepatic adenylate cyclase. *J. Biol. Chem.* **254**, 268–269.

Wright, D. E., and Rodbell, M. (1979b). Gastrointestinal hormone–receptor recognition: Position three is a determining residue for glucagon, secretin, and VIP. *In* "Peptides, Structure and Biological Function" (E. Groos and J. Meienhofer, eds.), pp. 1029–1031. Pierce Chem., Rockford, Illinois.

Wu, Z. C., O'Dorisio, T. M., Cataland, S., Mekhjian, H. S., and Gaginella, T. S. (1979). Effects of pancreatic polypeptide and vasoactive intestinal polypeptide on rat ileal and colonic water and electrolyte transport in vivo. *Dig. Dis. Sci.* **24**, 625–630.

Wünsch, E. (1972). Zur Synthese von biologisch voll-aktivem Sekretin. *Naturwissenschaften* **59**, 239–246.

Wünsch, E., Jaeger, E., and Scharf, R. (1968). Reindarstellung des synthetischen Glucagons. *Chem. Ber.* **101**, 3664–3670.

Wünsch, E., Jaeger, E., Knopf, S., Scharf, R., and Thamm, P. (1976). Zur Synthese von Motilin. III. Reindarstellung und Charakterisierung von (13-Norleucin)motilin und (13-Leucin)motilin. *Hoppe-Seylers Z. Physiol. Chem.* **357**, 467–476.

Wünsch, E., Wendlberger, G., Hallett, A., Jaeger, E., Knopf, S., Moroder, L., Scharf, R., Schmidt, I., Thamm, P., and Wilschowitz, L. (1977a). Zur Totalsynthese des Human-Big-Gastrins I und seines 32-Leucin-Analogons. *Z. Naturforsch.* **32c**, 495–506.

Wünsch, E., Jaeger, E., and Moroder, L. (1977b). Progress in the problem of structure–activity relations of gastrointestinal hormones. *In* "Hormonal Receptors in Digestive Tract Physiology" (S. Bonfils *et al.*, eds.), pp. 19–27. Biomedic. Press, Amsterdam.

Wünsch, E., Moroder, L., Gemeiner, M., and Jaeger, E. (1980). Totalsynthese von Somatostatin-28 (Big-Somatostatin). *Z. Naturforsch.* **35b**, 911–919.

Wünsch, E., Moroder, L., WIlschowitz, L., Göhring, W., Scharf, R., and Gardner, J. D. (1981a). Zur Totalsynthese von Cholecystokinin-Pankerozymin. Darstellung des ver-knüpfungsfähigen "Schlüsselfragments" des Sequenz 24–33. *Hoppe-Seylers Z. Physiol. Chem.* **362**, 143–152.

Wünsch, E., Wendlberger, G., Mladenova-Orlinova, L., Göhring, W., Jaeger, E., and Scharf, R. (1981b). Totalsynthese des Human-Big-Gastrins. I. Revidierte Primärstruktur. *Hoppe-Seylers Z. Physiol. Chem.* **362**, 179–183.

Yajima, H., Kai, Y., and Kawatani, H. (1975a). Synthesis of the docosapeptide corre-sponding to entire amino-acid sequence of porcine motilin. *J. C. S. Chem. Commun.* 159–160.

Yajima, H., Ogawa, H., Kubota, M., Tobe, T., Fujimura, M., Hemmi, K., Torizuka, K., Adachi, H., Imura, H., and Taminato, T. (1975b). Synthesis of the tritetracontapep-tide corresponding to the entire amino acid sequence of gastric inhibitor polypeptide. *J. Am. Chem. Soc.* **97**, 5593–5594.

Yajima, H., Mori, Y., Koyama, K., Tobe, T., Setoyama, M., Adachi, H., Kanno, T., and Saito, A. (1976). Studies on peptides. LXVIII. Synthesis of the tritriacontapeptide amide corresponding to the entire amino acid sequence of the desulfated form of porcine cholecystokinin-pancreozymin (CCK-PZ). *Chem. Pharm. Bull.* **24**, 2794–2802.

Yajima, H., Takeyama, M., Koyama, K., Tobe, T., Inoue, K., Kawano, T., and Adachi, H. (1980). Synthesis of an octacosapeptide amide corresponding to the entire amino acid sequence of chicken vasoactive intestinal polypeptide (VIP). *Int. J. Pept. Protein Res.* **16**, 33–47.

Yalow, R. S., and Berson, S. A. (1960). Immunoassay of endogenous plasma insulin in man. *J. Clin. Invest.* **39**, 1157–1175.

Yalow, R. S., and Berson, S. A. (1970). Size and charge distinctions between endogenous human plasma gastrin in periferal blood and hetadecapeptide gastrins. *Gastroen-terology* **58**, 609–615.

Yalow, R. S., and Berson, S. A. (1971a). Further studies on the nature of immunoreactive gastrin in human plasma. *Gastroenterology* **60**, 203–214.

Yalow, R. S., and Berson, S. A. (1971b). Size heterogeneity of immunoreactive human ACTH in plasma and in extracts of pituitary glands and ACTH-producing thymoma. *Biochem. Biophys. Res. Commun.* **44**, 439–445.

Yalow, R. S., and Berson, S. A. (1972). And now, "big, big" gastrin. *Biochem. Biophys. Res. Commun.* **48**, 391–395.

Yalow, R. S., and Wu, N. (1973). Additional studies on the nature of big big gastrin. *Gastroenterology* **65**, 19–27.

Yamaguchi, K., Abe, K., Miyakawa, S., Ohnami, S., Sakagami, M., and Yanaihara, N. (1980). The presence of macromolecular vasoactive intestinal polypeptide (VIP) in VIP-producing tumors. *Gastroenterology* **79**, 687–694.

Yamashiro, D., Aanning, H. L., and du Vigneaud, V. (1965). Inactivation of oxytocin by acetone. *Proc. Natl. Acad. Sci. U.S.A.* **54**, 166–171.

Yau, W. M., Makhlouf, G. M., Edwards, L. E., and Farrar, J. T. (1973). Mode of action of cholecystokinin and related peptides on gallbladder muscle. *Gastroenterology* **65**, 451–456.

Yip, C. C., Hew, C.-L., and Hsu, H. (1975). Translation of messenger ribonucleic acid from isolated pancreatic islets and human insulinomas. *Proc. Natl. Acad. Sci. U.S.A.* **72**, 4777–4779.

Zandomenghi, R., and Buchanan, K. D. (1972). A method for measuring the release of gut glucagon-like immunoreactivity from rat jejunum "in vitro." *Diabetologia* **8**, 283–286.

Zelenkova, J., and Gregor, O. (1971). Development of gastrin activity. *Scand. J. Gastroenterol.* **6**, 653–656.

Zetler, G., and Baldauf, J. (1967). Chromatographische Analyse eines Substanz P-Präparates aus Gehirn. *Naunyn Schmiedebergs Arch. Pharmacol. Exp. Pathol.* **256**, 86–98.

Zimmerman, M. J., Dreiling, D. A., Rosenberg, I. R., and Janowitz, H. D. (1967). Secretion of calcium by the canine pancreas. *Gastroenterology* **52**, 865–870.

Zimmerman, M., Mumford, R. A., and Steiner, D. F. (1980). Precursor processing in the biosynthesis of proteins *Ann. N.Y. Acad. Sci.* **343**.

Zimmerman, E. G. (1979). Peptides of the brain and gut. Introductory remarks. *Fed. Proc. Fed. Am. Soc. Exp. Biol.* **38**, 2286–2287.

Zingg, H. H., and Patel, Y. C. (1979). Somatostatin precursors: Evidence for presence in and release from rat median eminence and neurohypophysis. *Biochem. Biophys. Res. Commun.* **90**, 466–472.

van Zon, A., and Beyerman, H. C. (1976). Synthesis of the gastrointestinal peptide hormone secretin by the repetitive excess mixed anhydride (REMA) method. *Helv. Chim. Acta* **59**, 1112–1126.

Zuber, H. (1963). Isolation of substance P from bovine brain. *Ann. N.Y. Acad. Sci.* **104**, 391–392.

Zyznar, E. S., Conlon, J. M., Schusdziarra, V., and Unger, R. H. (1979). Properties of somatostatin-like immunoreactive polypeptides in the canine extrahypothalamic brain and stomach. *Endocrinology* **105**, 1426–1431.

NOTE ADDED IN PROOF

The amino acid sequences of PHI and of PYY have recently been published. The sequence of PHI is (K. Tatemoto and V. Mutt, *Proc. Natl. Acad. Sci. U.S.A.* **78**, 6603–6607, 1981)

His-Ala-Asp-Gly-Val-Phe-Thr-Ser-Asp-Phe-Ser-Arg-Leu-Leu-Gly-Gln-Leu-Ser-
Ala-Lys-Lys-Tyr-Leu-Glu-Ser-Leu-Ile-NH$_2$

and that of PYY (K. Tatemoto, *Proc. Natl. Acad. Sci. U.S.A.* **79**, 2514–2518, 1982)

Tyr-Pro-Ala-Lys-Pro-Glu-Ala-Pro-Gly-Glu-Asp-Ala-Ser-Pro-Glu-Glu-Leu-Ser-Arg-
Tyr-Tyr-Ala-Ser-Leu-Arg-His-Tyr-Leu-Asn-Leu-Val-Thr-Arg-Gln-Arg-Tyr-NH$_2$

Other interesting developments have been the isolation from porcine pituitary (A. Goldstein, W. Fischli, L. I. Lowney, M. Hunkapiller, and L. Hood, *Proc. Natl. Acad. Sci. U.S.A.* **78**, 7219–7223, 1981) and from porcine duodenum (S. Tachibana, K. Araki, S. Ohya, and S. Yoshida, *Nature (London)* **295**, 339–340, 1982) of an identical opioid heptadecapeptide, dynorphin, with the amino acid sequence

Tyr-Gly-Gly-Phe-Leu-Arg-Arg-Ile-Arg-Pro-Lys-Leu-Lys-Trp-Asp-Asn-Gln

and the isolation from human brain and intestine and from *Hydra attenuata* and the sea anemone *Anthopleura elegantissima* of an identical undecapeptide with the sequence Glp-Pro-Pro-Gly-Gly-Ser-Lys-Val-Ile-Leu-Phe (H. C. Schaller and H. Bodenmüller, *Proc. Natl. Acad. Sci. U.S.A.* **78,** 7000–7004, 1981). In the hydra this peptide acts as a head-inducing morphogen. Its role in more developed organisms is not clear.

Index

A

Antithyroid drugs, mechanism of action, iodide and, 213–214

Arachidonic acid, transformation in polymorphonuclear leukocytes, 1–3

B

Bityrosine formation, effect of iodide on, 214

Blood flow, gastrointestinal hormones and, 317–319

Bombesin-related gastrin-releasing polypeptide, amino acid sequence, 252–255

C

Cholecystokinin, amino acid sequences of, 240–246

Chymodenin, partial sequence of, 261

Coupling reaction, effect of iodide on, 213–214

D

Dihydroxyeicosatetraenoic acids, epoxide intermediate in formation, 3–6

Diiodotyrosine, effects on iodination and coupling reactions, 217–220

E

Enterogastrone, 306–311

Epoxide, as intermediate in dihydroxy-eicosatetraenoic acid formation, 3–6

Esophageal sphincter pressure, gastrointestinal hormones and, 304–306

F

Factors, insulin-mimicking, 167–168

Fat, metabolism, insulin and, 161–163

G

Gas chromatography-mass spectrometry identification of steroids and, 65–82 quantitation of steroids and, 87–94

Gas chromatography-resolution mass spectrometry, quantitation of steroids and, 94–96

Gas-liquid chromatography, quantitation of steroids and, 86–87

Gastric acid, secretion, 306–311

Gastric emptying and motility, 306–311

Gastric inhibitory peptide, amino acid sequence of, 250–252

Gastrin
amino acid sequences of, 238–240
heterogeneity of, 276–286

Gastrointestinal hormones
general sequence characteristics of, 296–301
heterogeneity
of gastrin, 276–286
peptides reacting with antibodies to glucagon, 266–276
types of, 262–266
hypothetical, 363–365
isolation of 286–289
mediators of activity, 354–363
physiological aspects, 301–303
blood flow through gastrointestinal organs, 317–319
extragastrointestinal effects, 334–340
motility and secretion and, 303–317
release of hormones, 326–334
trophic effects, 319–326
structure-activity relationships, 340–356
synthesis, 299–301
work on structures, 289–296

Glicentin, amino acid sequence of, 260–261

Date Due

Science

UML 735